Contents

Preface vi

General pathological, immunopathological,
and genetic background of skeletal muscle disorders 1

Diseases associated with sarcolemmal and
extracellular matrix defects 5
Dystrophinopathies 6
Sarcoglycanopathies 24
Dysferlinopathies 29
Caveolinopathies 33
Laminin α2 (merosin) gene mutations 37
Collagen VI gene mutations. Bethlem myopathy/Limb-girdle
muscular dystrophy 41
Heparin sulfate proteoglycan (perlecan) deficiency
Schwartz-Jampel syndrome 43
Muscular dystrophy caused by α7 integrin deficiency 45

Diseases associated with myonuclear abnormalities 47
Defects of nuclear membrane related proteins (emerin, lamins A/C) 48
Abnormalities in nuclear positioning (centronuclear myopathies) 57

Myofibrillar and internal cytoskeletal proteins 61
Actinopathies 62
Core Diseases
Central core disease 65
Multi-minicore disease 68
Desmin-related myopathies 70
Nemaline myopathies 74
Plectin deficiency 78
Telethonin deficiency 81
Myotilinopathy 82
Myosin heavy chain depletion syndrome 83
Autosomal dominant myosin heavy chain IIa myopathy 85

Diseases associated with ion channel and
ion transporter defects 89
Myotonia and paramyotonia 90
Dyskalemic episodic weakness 95
Malignant hyperthermia and central core disease
associated with defects in Ca2+ channels of the
sarcotubular system 99
Brody disease associated with defects in a Ca2+ pump 103

Myopathies based on complex molecular defects 107
Repeat expansion diseases
The myotonic dystrophies 108
PABPN1 dysfunction in oculopharyngeal muscular dystrophy 115
Large telomeric deletion disease, Facioscapulohumeral dystrophy 119

Developmental disorders of skeletal muscle 123
X-linked myotubular myopathy 124
Congenital fibre type disproportion 130

8. Disorders of catabolic mechanisms 133
Lysosomal disorders
Alpha glucosidase deficiency syndromes 134
LAMP-2 deficiency 142
X-linked myopathy with excessive autophagy 145
Proteolytic disturbances
Defects of non-lysosomal proteolysis: Calpain3 deficiency 148

9. Neuromuscular transmission defects 155
Myasthenia gravis 156
The Lambert-Eaton myasthenic syndrome 166
Congenital myasthenic syndromes 170

10. Myopathies affecting fuel and energy metabolism 181
Selected disorders of carbohydrate metabolism 182
Defects of fatty acid metabolism 189
Oxidative phosphorylation defects 202
Myoadenylate deaminase deficiency 214

11. Dysimmune and infectious myopathies 217
Dysimmune myopathies. Definition of entities and
experimental models of myositis 218
Polymyositis and dermatomyositis 221
Inclusion body myositis 228
Viral myositis 231
Bacterial myositis 236
Fungal, protozoal, and other parasitic infections 238

12. Toxic and iatrogenic disorders 245

13. Effects of chronic denervation and disuse on muscle 251
Effects of denervation on muscle 252
Effects of disuse on muscle 257

14. Endocrine disorders and myotrophic molecules 259

15. Miscellaneous myopathies 265
Cancer-related muscle disease 266
Effects of ageing on skeletal muscles and
their clinical significance 270
Hereditary inclusion body myopathies 274
Marinesco-Sjögren syndrome 277
Osteomalacia myopathy 279
Vitamin E deficiency 282
Amyloid myopathy 284
Rare myopathies of childhood 287

16. Neuromuscular resources on the Internet 291

17. The principles of therapies and prevention
based on cellular and molecular mechanisms of
muscle disease 295

Contributors 305
Acknowledgments 309
Index 310

Structural and Molecular Basis of Skeletal Muscle Diseases

Volume Editor

George Karpati

Advisory Editors

Maria Molnar

Hans H. Goebel

Kiichi Arahata

Alan E. H. Emery

Eric Hoffman

Eric Shoubridge

This volume is the result of a collaboration between the World Federation of Neurology, Research Group on Neuromuscular Diseases and the International Society of Neuropathology.

To be cited as: Karpati G, *Structural and Molecular Basis of Skeletal Muscle Diseases*, ISN Neuropath Press, Basel 2002, 312 pages.

Structural and Molecular Basis of Skeletal Muscle Diseases

Volume Editor	George Karpati, Montreal, Canada
Advisory Editors	Maria Molnar, Budapest, Hungary
	Hans H. Goebel, Mainz, Germany
	Kiichi Arahata, Tokyo, Japan
	Alan E. H. Emery, Exeter, United Kingdom
	Eric Hoffman, Washington DC, United States
	Eric Shoubridge, Montreal, Canada
Production Editors	Yngve Olsson, Uppsala, Sweden
	representing International Society of Neuropathology
	P. K. Thomas, London, United Kingdom
	representing World Federation of Neurology, Research Group on Neuromuscular Diseases
Layout	Duncan MacRae, Los Angeles, United States
Editorial Assistants	Margaritka Dikova-Sorge, Munich, Germany
	Angelica Tibbling, Uppsala, Sweden
Printed by	Allen Press, Inc.
	Lawrence, KS, United States
Publisher	ISN Neuropath Press
	International Society of Neuropathology
	Institute of Pathology
	Schönbeinstrasse 40
	CH - 4003 Basel
	Switzerland

Pathology & Genetics

Pathology & Genetics is a book series published by the International Society of Neuropathology (ISN) in collaboration with other international organisations. The first volume on tumours of the nervous system, initiated by Dr. Paul Kleihues, Lyon, France was published 1997 together with WHO. A second edition of this volume published by WHO in 2000 can be purchased from IARC Press, Lyon, France (Fax: +33 4 7273 8302).

The ISN General Council elected in 2000 Dr Yngve Olsson, Uppsala, Sweden to serve as a Series Editor for additional volumes. This book on muscle diseases is volume 2 in the ISN Book Series.

The International Society of Neuropathology welcomes requests for permission to reproduce or translate this publication, in part or in full.

Requests for permission to reproduce figures or charts from this publication should be directed to the respective contributor. The authors alone of the various chapters are responsible for views expressed in this publication. The contents of the preambles represent the views of the editors.

Dr Kiichi Arahata, Japan started to serve as a very important member of the Advisory Board for this book. We deeply regret that he is no longer among us and would therefore like to dedicate this book to the memory of this eminent scientist with such a refined personality.

Preface

Over the past 10 years, the impact of modern microscopic pathology and molecular genetics on the diagnostic accuracy and understanding of the pathogenesis of muscle disease has been enormous. The resourceful and skilled application of the modern techniques of molecular genetics has been revolutionary. The initial and best example was the discovery of the gene whose mutation is the cause of Duchenne muscular dystrophy (DMD). This discovery bore fruit. It made possible the routine use of mutational analysis of patients for a precise diagnosis; in particular to distinguish Duchenne from Becker muscular dystrophies. Furthermore, it permitted a more refined and reliable method of carrier detection and prenatal diagnosis for these disorders.

The identification of the protein product of this gene allows us to use microscopic or immunoblot display of dystrophin for diagnostic purposes. Furthermore, it permitted at least 4 additional developments. Firstly, it led to the discoveries of several other molecules at the surface membrane of muscle fibers whose functional partnership is essential for the integrity of the muscle cell. Mutations of the genes encoding these molecules themselves can cause different forms of muscular dystrophies. Secondly, the discovery of dystrophin led to a better understanding of many aspects of the physiology and biochemistry of the muscle fiber surface membrane and made DMD a biologically highly informative experiment of nature. Thirdly, the molecular understanding of dystrophin deficiency and its deleterious consequences promise the development of truly effective therapy. Lastly, the example of the success of the discovery of dystrophin was heralding the molecular age of myology. It spurred feverish activities in molecular research, the fruits of which are represented by the discoveries of the molecular background of scores of other inherited muscle diseases.

Along with these momentous developments in molecular genetics, the microscopic pathology of skeletal muscle has also enjoyed a parallel surge of sophistication and practical informativeness. This is exemplified by increasing availability of highly specific and powerful antibodies for the qualitative and quantitative display of protein products of most of the genes whose mutation can cause muscle disease. Thus, the immunocytochemical profile obtained can be correlated with traditional microscopic pathological alterations at the light and electron microscopic level providing a powerful tool for a better understanding of the pathophysiology of muscle fiber damage or destruction in a given disease. It will also enable us to monitor directly the efficacy and safety of therapeutic interventions. In selected cases, microscopic techniques permit direct demonstration of genetic alterations (ie, flourescent in situ hybriodization or other forms of in situ hybridization) or even the study of the expression of specific genes by in situ reverse transcriptase polymerase chain reaction (RT-PCR).

The foregoing developments also pose challenges in designing modern educational formats, which are the most suitable to present current comprehensive knowledge of muscle disease for pathologists, clinicians and researchers. The Editors of this volume also faced that dilemma. One option was to follow the traditional categories of muscle disease and with each entity highlight the relevant state of knowledge of the molecular and microscopic features and correlate it with clinical phenotype and treatment options. Most current texts of myology have been written along these lines.

The other approach is less traditional and would take advantage of the vastly improved knowledge of the pathogenesis of muscle disease. By this approach, we would group diseases according to common basic etiological and/or pathogenic features. We recognize the fact that there are still quite a few muscle diseases in which the lack of precise pathogenic knowledge does not permit the latter approach. However, the number of these diseases is fast decreasing. Another problem with this approach is that it necessitated the creation of a "miscellaneous" category for some muscular dystrophies where the molecular defects do not have a common denominator other than being "dystrophygenic."

Furthermore, there are disorders, which on pathogenic basis, could be equally grouped in 2 categories, eg, the *congenital myasthenic syndromes*, which could be listed either under *ion channel disorders* or *neuromuscular transmission defects*. Other examples are *nemaline myopathies* and *central core disease* that could belong to either *developmental disorders* or *myofibrillar disorders*. Nevertheless, we decided to organize the categories of muscle diseases according to the "pathogenic" approach. We have not allowed the molecular and pathological facts to hang in a void, so the authors have provided a brief initial clinical correlation for each disease. Subsequently, they presented and illustrated the essential up-to-date knowledge of molecular and microscopical facts, which are indispensable for the formulation of the pathogenesis, which is the key point for each entity. In allowing this routine, we tried to remain thoroughly factual, but we did not refrain from attractive hypotheses when they were applicable.

We trust that the new system of organization of clinical myology will not confuse the readers but it will emphasise the tremendous impact of microscopic pathology and molecular science in the field.

George Karpati

General pathological, immunopathological, and genetic background of skeletal muscle disorders

George Karpati

Most diseases of skeletal muscle are caused by either genetic defects or abnormal immune regulation, or exogenous toxins and drugs (7, 8). In the premolecular era, these diseases were characterized mainly by the microscopic pathological appearance of muscle displayed by relatively simple histological staining methods, as well as by certain electrophysiological features and by the clinical phenotype. The modern era of molecular medicine has provided opportunities to determine more sophisticated features by which the scope of characterization of these diseases has become much broader (12). These features are best appreciated in genetic muscle diseases (1, 14) and are illustrated in Figure 1.

Genetically determined muscle diseases

The gene defect. Single gene defects have been identified as the primary cause of many muscle diseases (1, 14). Most of these are discussed in this volume from the pathogenetic point of view. In genetic diseases there are several characteristic features of the gene which can help to understand the pathogenesis of a disease. These features include the chromosomal location, size, exon number, promoter/enhancer profile, transcription characteristics, as well as the nature and extent of the pathogenic mutations.

The consequences of nuclear genetic defects may depend on whether one or both copies of the genes carry deleterious mutations. In recessive diseases, both alleles of the same gene carry the same or different pathogenic mutation. By contrast, in dominant diseases a pathogenic mutation is present only in one of the alleles and will still produce a pathological consequence (dominant-negative effect). Myotonic

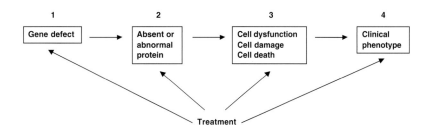

Figure 1. General paradigm of the principle events in genetic diseases.

dystrophy (chapter 6.1.1) and oculopharyngeal dystrophy (chapter 6.1.2) fall into this category (3, 9).

It is to be noted that mutation of the same gene may cause different pathological consequences and clinical phenotypes. For example, mutations at different points of the dysferlin gene may cause either 2B type of limb-girdle dystrophy or Miyoshi's distal myopathy (10). Additional factors that influence the genotype-phenotype relation is the presence of compensating or modifying alleles of genes other than the one harboring the primary pathogenic mutation. For example, overexpression of the utrophin gene can clearly mitigate the deleterious effects of dystrophin deficiency.

Many muscle diseases are caused by mutations of mitochondrial genes or nuclear genes encoding mitochondrial molecules (13). Because of many unique features of mitochondrial genes and their expression, these diseases have special characteristics that are discussed in chapter 10.3 of this volume.

The determination of pathogenic gene defects has become a powerful tool in the diagnosis and pathogenic understanding of skeletal muscle diseases.

The effect of mutation on the relevant protein. Pathogenic mutations may cause either a total or near complete absence of the corresponding protein, or at least a functional alteration that quantitatively and/or qualitatively significantly alters the relevant protein (1). That protein may be a structural molecule, an enzyme, a receptor, or an ion channel component, etc. It may be part of a cellular component (Table 1), or a functional system (Table 2). The affected protein may be either intra or extracellular, eg, matrix molecule.

Several muscle diseases are related to abnormalities of matrix proteins (11), such as the merosin-deficient congenital muscular dystrophy or a perlecan-deficient chondrodystrophic myotonic myopathy. Cells or tissues where the altered or deficient protein normally plays a significant role will suffer deleterious consequences (*vide infra*). The demonstration of a genetically determined absence or altered nature of a protein is the other powerful diagnostic tool in myology. This can take the form of microscopic histo- and cytochemistry, immunoblot analysis, or functional tests of the activity of the molecule in question, eg, enzyme assays.

The light and electron microscopic demonstration of the involved protein is usually achieved by immunocytochemistry using specific antibodies targeting a single specific epitope (monoclonal) or multiple epitopes (polyclonal) (5). Efficient demonstration of the bound antibody by various display systems (eg, fluorochromes, peroxidase) permits the generation of at least semi-quantitative results. By contrast,

• Basal lamina
• Plasma membrane, T tubule
• Mitochondria
• Sarcoplasmic reticulum
• Myofibrils
• Myonuclei

Table 1. Components of the skeletal muscle fibre that may suffer primary damage in disease.

• Ion fluxes
• Neuromuscular transmission
• Excitation-contraction coupling
• Oxidative phosphorylation
• mRNA transport

Table 2. Functional systems of the muscle fibre that can suffer primary damage in disease.

immunoblot not only confirms a deficient or altered protein, it also provides a more precise quantitative measurement. The significance of this is best illustrated in the case of Becker's dystrophy (chapter 2.1), where the amount and quality of altered dystrophin may differ so little from the normal that its detection may escape the sensitivity of microscopic immunocytochemistry and require demonstration by immuno-blot analysis.

Myopathology now greatly depends on microscopic immunocytochemistry for routine diagnosis and research. Application of immunocytochemistry to fine structural studies provides added information when the subcellular localization of the culprit molecule is in question. This point is well illustrated by the early confusion about subcellular localization of dystrophin. Initially, it was believed to be localized to the triad of the sarcoplasmic reticulum when in reality it is at the cell surface.

Deleterious consequences of the deficiency or abnormality of a protein. In tissues and cells where the culprit protein normally plays a significant

role and the normal function and/or integrity of the cell depends on it, its deficiency will cause deleterious cellular effects. These include microscopically discernable features, eg, sub-necrotic microscopic pathological alterations, necrosis, apoptosis, or functional disturbances that cannot be ascertained by presently available microscopic techniques. Examples of the latter scenario include ion channel disorders and some metabolic myopathies where the muscle fibres may appear normal with microscopic techniques, but physiologically or clinically show significantly abnormal function. In the relevant chapters of this book, appropriate myopathological alterations will be described and illustrated mainly for the better understanding of the pathogenesis of a given disease.

The question of apoptosis of skeletal muscle fibres deserves special mention at this point (5). Several publications reported "apoptosis" of skeletal muscle fibres in microscopic preparations or provide bulk tissue evidence of apoptosis (DNA "laddering"). It is important to bear in mind that in pathological muscle tissue, cells other than muscle fibres may be present in abundance in some diseases, ie, macrophages in necrotic processes or inflammatory cells in the inflammatory myopathies or myasthenia gravis. In such instances, cells that appear apoptotic by the Tunel technique may not actually represent nuclei of muscle fibres but of non-muscle cells. Furthermore, in skeletal muscle fibre, being a multinucleated cell containing usually thousands of muscle fibres with substantial overlap of the nuclear domains, cell death by apoptosis would only occur if the full apoptotic cascade would take place in at least hundreds of adjacent myonuclei of the same fibre. This is a highly unlikely event. On the other hand, apoptosis occurring in a limited number of adjacent myonuclei of the same fibre may cause segmental atrophy provided the satellite cells compensation of lost myonuclei does not occur.

The clinical phenotype

The cascade of genetic defect→absent or abnormal proteins→cell dysfunction or cell death leads to symptoms and signs of a more or less specific clinical phenotype (Figure 1) (4). In everyday practice we take advantage of the information in the above cited domains for establishing a precise diagnosis and determine the most effective and safe available treatment. However, in this volume, the focus is on the understanding of the details in these domains for the purpose of creating cohesive and logical pathogenic paradigms for the major muscle diseases. This methodical approach first identifies the full genetic background, then studies the consequent protein profile (proteomics) and correlates the protein abnormalities with cellular pathology, and ultimately, with the clinical phenotype.

While this "pathogenic approach" may appear to be too "scientific" for a clinical practitioner of myology, logical and promising therapeutic approaches are best designed using the paradigm shown in Figure 1. More concretely, for therapeutic purposes, we may try to fix the genetic defect, replace or beneficially alter the deficient or abnormal protein, or modify certain features in the biology of the affected cells by which they can compensate for the deleterious effects of the absent or abnormal proteins and the resultant clinical phenotype.

Dysimmune muscle diseases

There are entities that are caused by dysimmune mechanism(s) (6). In this volume, chapter 11 on inflammatory myopathies and chapter 9 about myasthenia gravis are devoted to these important diseases. In these chapters, the relevant immunopathology will be dissected by providing answers to several essential questions:

What is the evidence for it being a fundamentally dysimmune disease? What is the primary offending antigen? Is it extrinsic or an intrinsic molecule? Are secondary antigens operating? Which are the antigen-presenting cells?

- Muscle fibre
    General
    Specific, eg, motor endplate

- Blood vessels
    Large (artery, vein)
    Medium
    Capillaries

- Motor nerve endings

Table 3. Possible targets of immunological attack in muscle diseases.

Where is the antigen presentation taking place? What are the principal cytokines and chemokines that serve as molecules for the immune cells to signal and adhere, as well as the efficient immunoeffector molecules? What is the principal type of the dysimmune process? Is it cellular or humoral or both? What structures of the muscle are the primary targets of the immune attack (Table 3)? Is continued antigenic stimulation necessary for the disease to become chronic or is it an inductive process? Are there external or intrinsic adjuvants, ie, diet, environment, stress or predisposing genes? What are the most effective means of mitigating or neutralizing the deleterious dysimmune responses?

Unfortunately, at this time, not every question is answerable with full precision in all diseases. However, what is available is invaluable for designing treatment strategies.

Myopathies due to toxic agents

Myopathies due to exogenous toxic agents are relatively rare (2). It appears that the susceptibility of skeletal muscle fibres to damage by drugs or environmental toxins is far less than that of peripheral nerves or central nervous system cells. However, the toxicity of certain molecules of skeletal muscle fibres is clinically important, as well as informative from the biological point of view. Therefore, a special chapter has been devoted to this topic as well.

References

1. Anderson LVB (2001) The molecular basis of muscle disease. In *Disorders of Voluntary Muscle*, G Karpati, D Hilton-Jones, RC Griggs (eds). Oxford Unviersity Press: New York. pp. 60-79

2. Argov Z, Kaminski HJ, Mudallal AA, Ruff RL (2001) Toxic and iatrogenic myopathies and neuromuscular disorders. In *Disorders of Voluntary Muscle*, G Karpati, D Hilton-Jones, RC Griggs (eds). Oxford Unviersity Press: New York. pp. 676-688

3. Brais B (2001) Oculopharyngeal muscular dystrophy. In *Disorders of Voluntary Muscle*, G Karpati, D Hilton-Jones, RC Griggs (eds). Oxford Unviersity Press: New York. pp. 497-502

4. Brooke MH (1986) *A Clinician's View of Neuromuscular Disease*. Williams & Wilkins: Baltimore.

5. Carpenter S, Karpati G (2001) *Pathology of Skeletal Muscle*. Oxford University Press: New York.

6. Dalakas MC (1995) Immunopathogenesis of inflammatory myopathies. *Ann Neurol* 37: 74-86

7. Engel AG, Franzini-Armstrong C (1994) *Myology*. McGraw Hill: New York.

8. Griggs RC, Mendell RJ, Miller RG (1995) *Evaluation and Treatment of Myopathies*. F.A. Davies: Philadelphia.

9. Harper PS (2001) *Myotonic Dystrophy*. Saunders: London.

10. Ho MF, Amato A, Brown RH (2002) Dysferlinopathies. In *Structural and Molecular Basis of Skeletal Muscle Diseases*, G Karpati (ed). ISN Neuropath Press: Basel. Chapter 2. 4

11. Hoffman EP, Pegoraro E (2002) Merosinopathies and other extracellular matrix defects. In *Structural and Molecular Basis of Skeletal Muscle Diseases*, G Karpati (ed). ISN Neuropath Press: Basel. Chapter 2. 3

12. Karpati G, Hilton-Jones D, Griggs RC (2001) *Disorders of Voluntary Muscle*. Cambridge University Press: Cambridge.

13. Shoubridge E, Molnar MJ (2002) Respiratory Chain Defects. In *Structural and Molecular Basis of Skeletal Muscle Diseases*, G Karpati (ed). ISN Neuropath Press: Basel. Chapter 10.3

14. Worton RV, Molnar MJ, Brais B, Karpati G (200l) The muscular dystrophies. In *The Metabolic and Molecular Basis of Inherited Diseases*, CR Scriver *et al*.

CHAPTER 2

Diseases associated with sarcolemmal and extracellular matrix defects

2.1 Dystrophinopathies   6
2.2 Sarcoglycanopathies   24
2.4 Dysferlinopathies   29
2.5 Caveolinopathies   33
2.6 Laminin α2 (merosin) gene mutations   37
2.7 Collagen VI gene mutations (Bethlem myopathy/Limb-girdle muscular dystrophy)   41
2.8 Schwartz-Jampel syndrome:Heparin sulfate proteoglycan (perlecan) deficiency   43
2.9 α7-integrin deficiency   45

The surface membrane of muscle fibres (sarcolemma) is a critically important structure. It is made up of two distinct components: the basal lamina, and the plasma membrane or plasmalemma. The basal lamina is part of the extracellular matrix and, as such, it maintains a mechanical liaison between the muscle fibre itself and the endomysial connective tissue. It may also have a signaling role. The basal lamina survives segmental muscle fibre necrosis in disease and serves as a platform for satellite cell proliferation and fusion during regeneration.

There are several molecules of the basal lamina whose genetically determined alterations are the cause of distinct muscle diseases. These are discussed in this chapter including primary merosin deficiency in congenital muscular dystrophy, secondary merosin deficiencies in Fukuyama's disease, perlecan deficiency in chondrodystrophic myopathy (Schwartz-Jampel syndrome) and integrin VII deficiency in a limb girdle syndrome.

The other component of the sarcolemma is plasmalemma, which forms a physical and functional barrier between the extra-and intracellular space. It is of paramount importance for the health and even survival of the muscle fibre. The plasmalemma is also subjected to various mechanical stresses and strains that are incident to the contractile activity of muscle such as shortening and stretch.

The plasmalemma contains many molecules that serve numerous important functions (receptors, signaling molecules, ion channels, adhesion molecules, etc.) There are specialized regions of the plasmalemma such as caveolae, and the T tubules that are extensions of the plasmalemma. The plasmalemma is also associated with an elaborate subsarcolemmal cytoskeletal system of which β actin and dystrophin are key elements. Dissolution of the plasmalemma is the earliest event in necrosis.

Genetic deficiencies of several plasmalemmal molecules are the cause of several muscle diseases. These molecules include dystrophin, sarcoglycans, dysferlin, and caveolin, whose deficiencies or abnormalities are discussed in this chapter.

Dystrophinopathies

Louise V. B. Anderson

AAV	adeno-associated viruses
BMD	Becker muscular dystrophy
CH	calponin homology
AChR	acetylcholine esterase receptor
CK	creatine kinase
DAGs	dystrophin-associated glycoproteins
DAPs	dystrophin-associated proteins
DGC	dystrophin glycoprotein complex
DMD	Duchenne muscular dystrophy
MD	muscular dystrophy
NMJs	neuromuscular junctions
nNOS	neuronal nitric oxide synthase
NO	nitric oxide
XLDC	X-linked dilated cardiomyopathy

Definition of entities

Duchenne muscular dystrophy. Duchenne muscular dystrophy (DMD) is the best known and most severe form of myopathy caused by dystrophin deficiency. It has been estimated to affect approximately 1 in 3 500 live born males (43), and although there are other claims to the "first" clinical descriptions, the disease took the name of Duchenne following a series of articles published in 1868 (46). Before the first physical symptoms of DMD, muscle histology is abnormal and the levels of muscle enzymes like creatine kinase increase in the circulation. Occasionally, mothers may feel that an affected son is floppy compared to an unaffected sibling, but the most common early feature is a delay in walking, until 18 months or longer. Affected boys may never run properly and may appear clumsy. A waddling gait, combined with the use of Gower's manoeuvre to rise from the floor, and difficulties with climbing stairs, are typical for a boy presenting at about 4 years of age. Pseudohypertrophy of the calf muscles is present in almost all cases, and may affect other muscles in some instances. Wasting and weakness chiefly affects the proximal limb-girdle musculature, with lower limbs being more affected. Early muscle involvement is highly selective and symmetrical, but with time, the differential muscle involvement becomes less clear (45).

As the disease progresses, an affected boy may start to need a wheelchair and will lose independent ambulation by the age of 12 years. Uncommonly, more mildly affected boys, defined as becoming wheelchair bound between the ages of 12 and 16 years, may be classified as having muscular dystrophy of intermediate or D/BMD severity (patients who remain ambulant beyond 16 years are generally considered as having Becker muscular dystrophy). As muscle weakness becomes more profound, contractures develop and respiratory problems are aggravated by thoracic deformity and the weakness of the intercostal muscles. Cardiac problems may also be present, developing insidiously during the first decade, when skeletal muscle weakness is already significant (45). Intriguingly, despite the basic clinical entity being recognised for more than a century, the fact that DMD boys have a retinal abnormality, and get a form of night-blindness, was not appreciated until the early 1990s (136).

It is well recognised that there is a non-progressive intellectual problem in DMD and the average IQ is shifted down one standard deviation from the general population, giving an average of about 85 for full scale IQ score. Approximately 20% of patients have an IQ score of less than 70, classifying them as retarded, and 3% have IQ scores of less than 50 (45). Most studies have shown that boys perform less well on verbal and reading tasks, and a high rate of emotional/behavioural disturbances are associated with the condition (101). Impairment of productive language has been correlated with defects of short-term memory (20). Pursuing the problems in more detail, Billard et al (16) reported that DMD boys exhibited a reading age that was significantly lower than children with spinal muscular atrophy of the chronological age. These learning disabilities were related to a deficit in verbal intelligence, with the DMD boys having particular difficulty with reading non-words, suggesting a processing disability similar to dysphonic dyslexia, the most frequent subtype of developmental dyslexia (16). Other tests indicate that verbal working memory skills are selectively impaired in DMD (79).

The disease process continues, and death may occur from the mid to late teens to the mid 20s. Sometimes this is due to cardiomyopathy, but often the precipitating factor is respiratory failure or pneumonia, and the increased use of home ventilation may both prolong and improve the quality of life for a few years (156).

Becker muscular dystrophy. Becker muscular dystrophy (BMD) is essentially a milder version of Duchenne MD. The age of onset is usually later and the rate of progression is slower, but exactly the same muscles are preferentially involved (44). In some mildly affected patients the first clinical symptoms might not appear until 30 to 60 years of age (171). While the classical Becker phenotype was fairly distinctive, the advent of molecular diagnoses revealed that many patients had been misdiagnosed, due to atypical presentations. A particularly underrated symptom appears to be calf pain, provoked by exercise and relieved by rest, which had been experienced at some stage of the disease by 81% of the individuals in one cohort of 67 BMD patients (24).

Patients with BMD show a high incidence of clinical cardiac involvement despite their milder skeletal muscle disease, and some may require heart transplants. Intellectual problems are much less marked than in DMD, but may still be present. Sporadic cases of BMD, who appear at the outpatient clinical at an unusually early age, might present with problems (eg, late walking) which seem to be related more to intellectual or behavioural difficulties than to problems of muscle function (131). Cognitive dysfunction has even been reported as a major presenting feature in BMD (135). Compared to Limb-Girdle MD with similar physical disability, reproductive fitness is lower than might be expected in BMD (42).

X-Linked dilated cardiomyopathy. X-linked dilated cardiomyopathy (XLDC) is a clinical phenotype of dystrophinopathy characterised by preferential myocardial involvement without any overt signs of skeletal myopathy. However, elevated serum creatine kinase is almost invariably found in affected individuals and the skeletal muscle biopsy shows myopathic changes (114). Typical patients are young males in their teens or early 20s, who present with lethal congestive heart failure; or middle aged female carriers with atypical chest pain. In male patients the disease course is rapidly progressive and results in heart transplant operations or death with 1 or 2 years of presentation. Heart failure in females progresses over several years and is frequently fatal. A significant proportion of patients have shown mutations in the dystrophin gene and abnormal protein expression in heart muscle (122).

Manifesting carriers. Skeletal muscle weakness in manifesting DMD carriers is characteristically asymmetrical, perhaps including hypertrophy of one calf. Weakness in BMD carriers is more rare, but has certainly been recorded. Among a cohort of confirmed DMD/BMD carriers examined in the Netherlands, some clinical symptoms were found in 22% (28/129). Of these, 22 (17%) of 129 had skeletal muscle weakness ranging from mild to moderately severe, and evidence of dilated cardiomyopathy was found in 7 (8%)

of 85 DMD carriers (83). In a UK study of DMD/BMD carriers, the prevalence of skeletal muscle weakness was found to be 12% (7/56) with mild cardiomyopathy present in 4 (7%) of 56 (71). Several reports have commented that carriers with skeletal muscle involvement do not necessarily have cardiac symptoms, and vice versa.

Atypical presentations. When dystrophin gene and protein analysis became available for routine diagnosis, it became obvious that a number of BMD patients had been misdiagnosed in the past. Some patients were advised that they had spinal muscular atrophy on the basis of a neurogenic muscle biopsy with a bimodal distribution of fibre sizes. Other BMD patients were first diagnosed as having Limb-Girdle MD with distal weakness (55), and at the other end of the severity spectrum, DMD patients who appeared floppy at birth were diagnosed as having a form of congenital muscular dystrophy (143). Similarly, others were investigated for metabolic muscle disease because of pain and cramps on exercise (24). Patients presenting with symptoms restricted to exertional cramps and myoglobinuria have been regularly reported, sometimes in combination with normal serum CK levels (154). Indeed, a family with non-progressive myalgia and cramps has been reported with a deletion in the dystrophin gene (68).

Occasionally, some patients with mild and slowly progressive muscle wasting and weakness that was limited to the quadriceps were designated as having "quadriceps myopathy." Subsequent analysis revealed that the patients all had abnormalities of dystrophin expression; a confirmatory gene mutation was identified in one (152). Similarly, a lady with progressive weakness and wasting of only her left calf was undiagnosed until immunoanalysis of her muscle biopsy revealed her to be a carrier with dystrophin-deficiency (113). Asymptomatic individuals with dystrophin gene mutations have occasionally been described (121); howev-

er, in other reports the relatively young age of the patients suggests that it would be more accurate to describe the state as "presymptomatic," bearing in mind that some Becker patients have been 50 to 60 years old before they became aware of any symptoms. In a group of 104 Becker patients, 28 were identified as having mild sub-clinical symptoms at ages ranging from 4 to 41 years (8).

Molecular genetics

Dystrophin. In 1983-1984, Peter Harper's group in Cardiff indicated that Becker MD was allelic to Duchenne MD (95), and in 1986-1987, the dystrophin gene was finally cloned (80, 97). Credit for that feat belongs to Lou Kunkel's team in Boston although other groups (particularly those of Ron Worton in Toronto and Kay Davies in Oxford) contributed earlier data for gene mapping (46). The gene encoding dystrophin is the largest identified to date, covering up to 3 Mb of DNA, and its 79 exons are interspersed by some enormous introns, eg, intron 44 is about 170 kb long (134). The dispersal of the coding regions may predispose the gene to new mutations and to exon skipping. The transcribed mRNA is 14kb and the full-size protein is 427 kDa in molecular mass (80). It is thought that the human dystrophin gene requires 16 hours to be transcribed and is cotranscriptionally spliced (159). The abundance of dystrophin is roughly the same in both fast and slow muscle fibre types, and expression is not affected by electro-stimulation (34). After the dystrophin gene was cloned, an autosomal homologue of similar size to dystrophin was identified and named utrophin (102), while the dystrobrevin family represent smaller dystrophin-related (and -associated) proteins (82).

As shown in Figure 1, the dystrophin molecule has an N-terminal actin binding domain consisting of two calponin homology (or CH) domains followed by 24 spectrin-like triple helical repeats forming the rod domain,

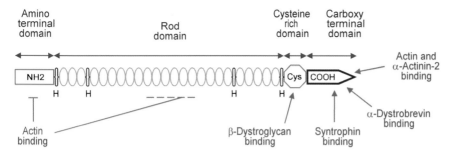

Figure 1. Schematic diagram of a dystrophin molecule showing the domains and protein binding sites. H = hinge.

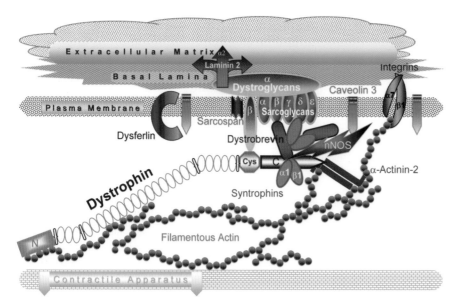

Figure 2. Schematic diagram of dystrophin and other proteins at the muscle plasma membrane. Not drawn to scale.

with four non-helical "hinge regions." In addition to the N-terminal interaction, dystrophin binds F-actin electrostatically through a series of basically charged repeats in the rod domain not present on utrophin (4). The C-terminus of dystrophin contains a domain relatively rich in cysteine residues, that binds to β-dystroglycan, followed by a region that associates with dystrobrevin and the syntrophins (34). Initially, dystrophin molecules were thought to self-associate as antiparallel dimers like α-actinin, but this is not currently thought to be correct (150) although there is evidence for the N-terminal CH domains of two utrophin molecules overlapping as antiparallel dimers (94).

The asssociated complex of proteins. The group of dystrophin-associated proteins or glycoproteins (DAPs, DAGs) (Chapter 2.2) is also known as the dystrophin glycoprotein complex (DGC), and the groups of Kevin Campbell in Iowa (49) and Eijiro Ozawa in Tokyo (172) have been major contributors to this field. The DGC contains several sub-complexes: the dystroglycans (α- and β-, that are products of a single gene), the sarcoglycans (α-, β-, γ-, δ- and ε-) and sarcospan, the syntrophins (α1- and β1- in nonjunctional regions), and α-dystrobrevin. Syntrophin and dystrobrevin bind to each other as well as to dystrophin, and thereby maintain connections to other DGC members in the absence of the dystrophin C-terminus (33). More peripheral members of the complex include neuronal nitric oxide synthase (nNOS), caveolin 3, and the laminin α2 chain of merosin (168) (Chapter 2. 3). F-actin, via linkage to α-actinin-2, may bind to the C-terminus of dystrophin and the β1-integrin subunit (77). The

main proteins involved in these systems are shown diagrammatically in Figure 2.

Although mRNA levels of the dystrophin-associated proteins may appear normal (29), protein expression is altered as a "knock-on" effect of dystrophin deficiency, and this generates secondary effects that contribute to the overall pathology. Levels of the dystroglycans, sarcoglycans, sarcospan, syntrophins, dystrobrevin and nNOS are decreased, whereas expression of caveolin 3 and integrin α7β1 are increased, together with the dystrophin homologue, utrophin. In addition to their various functions in skeletal muscle, there is growing evidence for the dystroglycans to form complexes with different proteins in epithelial cells, and the dystroglycans, sarcoglycans, and sarcospan having important roles in vascular smooth muscle where ε-sarcoglycan replaces α-sarcoglycan (14).

Caveolin 3 levels are increased in muscle from DMD patients, with a concomitant increase in the numbers of caveolae in the plasma membrane (146). Transgenic mice overexpressing caveolin 3 show an increase in the number of caveolae, together with a dystrophic phenotype: a preponderance of hypertrophic, necrotic, and immature/regenerating skeletal muscle fibers with characteristic central nuclei; and down-regulation of dystrophin expression (61). Conversely, caveolin-deficient mice show loss of caveolae, but also develop a milder degenerative myopathy with changes in the distribution of the dystrophin-glycoprotein complex, and abnormalities in the organization of the T-tubule system, with dilated and longitudinally-oriented T-tubules (60, 76). This is compatible with caveolin 3 competing with dystrophin for binding to β-dystroglycan (157). Mutations in the caveolin 3 gene in humans cause a form of limb-girdle muscular dystrophy and may be associated with reduced protein expression (116). Clearly there is an optimum level for caveolin 3 expression and any alteration to its regulation, up or down, may contribute to the pathogenesis of muscular dystrophy.

Dystrophin isoforms in brain and retina. In addition to variation produced by alternative exon splicing, particularly at the C-terminus (54), a number of dystrophin isoforms have now been identified, generated by different promoters that are controlled in a tissue-specific manner. In addition to different full-length isoforms expressed in brain cortex, muscle and brain Purkinje fibres, the promoters also drive transcription of a series of smaller molecules in various tissues and organs. An excellent summary of the generation and expression of dystrophin isoforms is available on the Leiden Muscular Dystrophy Pages© on the internet (*http://www.dmd.nl/isoforms.html*). Different isoforms lack various domains, and it is reasonable to suppose that their interacting proteins and functions vary in different tissues. Each may contribute to the pathogenesis of dystrophinopathy. Figure 3 illustrates the diverse range of dystrophin isoforms that occur in different tissues.

The brain promoter for full-length dystrophin has been excluded from major involvement with the intellectual problems (38), but there does appear to be an association with a deficiency of the smaller Dp140 brain isoform and Dp71 (13, 118). Memory and learning appear to be related to synaptic plasticity, and brain dystrophins (together with particular non-muscle versions of the associated proteins) may participate in a number of cellular signalling pathways that are involved in modelling synapses (17). Increasing experimental evidence suggests that in adult life, dystrophin normally modulates synaptic terminal integrity, distinct forms of synaptic plasticity, and regional cellular signal integration. At a systems level, dystrophin may regulate essential components of an integrated sensorimotor attentional network (111).

Duchenne boys have a form of night blindness that produces an altered response to flashes of light in the dark adapted state, and electroretinogram

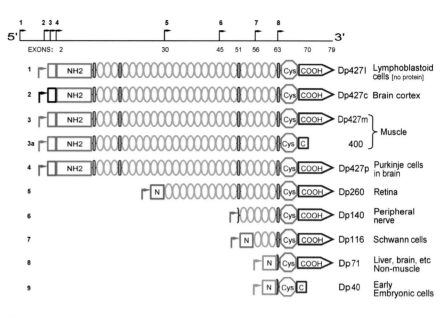

Figure 3. Schematic diagram of dystrophin isoforms and the tissues they are expressed in. The most 5′ promoter (initiating isoform Dp427l) was identified in lymphoblastoid cells, although dystrophin protein is not detected there. The next promoter is active in brain and transcripts for this isoform, Dp427c, have been localized to cortical and hippocampal neurons. The brain promoter appears to be quite restricted in its activity compared with the next promoter (initiating the major Dp427m isoform), which is active in skeletal, cardiac and smooth muscle and, to a lesser extent, in some neurones and cultured glial cells. Dystrophin is normally observed as a doublet of bands on western blots of muscle tissue labelled with antibodies to epitopes away from the C-terminus. These bands represent the 427kDa protein plus a smaller (400kDa) isoform, which probably utilises the alternative polyadenylation site. The fourth 5′ promoter (initiating Dp427p) is located in the first intron of the Dp427m gene and controls expression in the cerebellum, particularly in Purkinje cells. Among the smaller isoforms, Dp260 is initiated with a promoter located in intron 29 of the major muscle isoform, and was first identified in retina. The Dp140 transcript is expressed from a promoter located within intron 44 of Dp427m, yet the first translated exon is number 51: so unlike the other isoforms it has no unique N-terminus. Dp140 is found throughout the central nervous system and in kidney, but not in skeletal or cardiac muscle. Dp116 is expressed from a promoter in intron 55 of Dp427m, and appears exclusively in adult peripheral nerve, along the Schwann cell membrane. The Dp71 isoform promoter is located in intron 62 of Dp427m and is not found in adult skeletal muscle, but may be more abundant than Dp427m in brain, tissues containing smooth muscle (stomach, lung, skin and testis) and many foetal tissues. It is also found in tissues where the full-length protein is not generally synthesized: liver, kidney and spleen, plus hepatoma, lymphoblastoid and Schwannoma cell lines. Dp40 uses the Dp71 promoter and an alternative polyadenylation site located after exon 70. This isoform is expressed in the same tissues as Dp71, but the specific Dp40 transcript has also been uniquely identified in early embryonic stem cells.

measurements reveal a markedly reduced amplitude for the b-wave (139). Immunoanalysis of dystrophin indicates that it is localised to the outer plexiform layer in the retina, a region of synaptic activity. Dp260 is a specific isoform of dystrophin expressed in retina which, together with Dp71, associates with particular groups of interacting proteins. These are differentially distributed in the retina and mounting evidence suggests that the dystrophin complex could have both structural and signalling functions (85, 140).

Mutations and the open reading frame. *Duchenne versus Becker muscular dystrophy.* Dystrophinopathies cover a wide range of clinical severity (presenting symptoms, age of onset and rate of progression), yet the simplest explanation for the phenotypic variation between DMD and BMD lies in the effect that mutations have on the open reading frame for protein translation (120). By far the most frequent type of mutations are exonic or multi-exonic deletions (60-65% in DMD, <80% in BMD (15, 96), although duplications (5-10%) may also occur (86), the remaining mutations are presumed to be missense changes that generate stop codons (DMD) or alter critical amino acids (BMD) (148). The reader is also directed towards the Leiden Muscular Dystrophy Pages© database for point mutations at *http://www.dmd.nl/dmd_dis.html*.

of the milder Becker-like disease is about one fifth that, or 1 in 17500 live male births (43). The prevalence in the general population is roughly equal for both diseases (eg, DMD = 2.48/100 000, BMD = 2.38/100000 in the north east of England) because BMD patients live longer (26). The Becker phenotype covers a wide range of presenting symptoms and this diagnostic confusion led to under-ascertainment of the condition in pre-molecular times. Since the discovery of the gene in 1987, genetic counselling and the increasing sophistication of carrier testing has led to fewer boys with DMD being born in known families. However, the high rate of new mutations in the huge dystrophin gene results in the continual emergence of new carriers and patients. Thus, while up to a third of new DMD cases may have a family history of the disease, one third are caused by a new mutation arising in the mother, and one third by a new mutation in the affected boy. It is also worth noting that in northeast England, the average age of diagnosis for new DMD patients has been no earlier in the 10+ years that molecular diagnostic techniques have been applied. Further affected sons are still being born before the first boy appears at a specialist clinic for diagnosis (25).

Dilated cardiomyopathy. Mutations in the dystrophin gene have been identified in a significant proportion of X-linked dilated cardiomyopathy (XLDC) patients, with one hotspot at the front of the gene (including the promoter region and exons 1-7) and another around exons 48-51 (Figure 5). In several families the dystrophin mutations show a different pattern of expression in cardiac compared to skeletal muscle, and splicing appears to play a relevant role in the 5' end mutations. The pathogenesis of the isolated cardiac phenotype of patients with mutations in the rod domain is not clear, but some introns may contain sequences relevant for the regulation of gene expression (56). In patients with the most severe cardiac phenotype, the cardiac muscle is usually unable to pro-

duce any dystrophin, due to the effect of mutations on gene transcription in that tissue. The skeletal muscle escapes the dystrophic changes by maintaining dystrophin synthesis via exon skipping or alternative splicing that the heart is not able achieve (56). In some female carriers of dystrophin mutations, cardiac symptoms may be the only clinical manifestation, again reflecting the inflexibility of gene expression in cardiac tissue (117).

Pathophysiology

In the early 1970s, there were two divergent theories about the underlying pathogenesis of DMD: *i)* that the primary abnormality resided in the muscle microcirculation, and that the dystrophy was a consequence of repeated small infarctions of muscle (112), or *ii)* that the primary cause was neurogenic and there was an irreversible loss of motor units from muscle (109). Engel's group sought ultrastructural support for the hypotheses and concluded that there was no strong morphological evidence that either microvasculature or sick motor neurons were the primary cause of the disease (90). They did find, however, that DMD neuromuscular junctions (NMJs) were often abnormal with focal atrophy of the postsynaptic regions. Typically, one or more regions of most end-plates demonstrated degeneration of the post-synaptic folds. The folds became atrophic, and collapsed residues of pre-existing folds accumulated within the widened synaptic clefts. Some of the NMJs appeared immature with abundant junctional sarcoplasm, and shallow and poorly-developed junctional folds (90). Despite the focal degeneration and simplification of the postsynaptic region in DMD, the postsynaptic acetylcholine receptors were preserved, with no extrajunctional spreading. The amplitude and frequency of miniature end-plate potentials and the number of transmitter quanta released by nerve impulse were normal although the resting membrane potential is lower than normal. The findings indicated that transmitter release and the postsynaptic

responsiveness to acetylcholine were intact in Duchenne dystrophy (153).

These observations are interesting in the current day context of dystrophin-related and -associated proteins with altered expression in DMD: utrophin, the dystroglycans, the syntrophins, and the dystrobrevins. Thus, it has been suggested that dystrophin is involved in organising small AChR clusters into large AChR aggregates during muscle regeneration although it is not required for initiating the original AChR clustering activity (98). Alternatively, it may be dystroglycan that plays a role in the clustering of acetylcholine receptors at the neuromuscular junction (89). Now α1-syntrophin seems to have an important role in synapse formation and in the organization of utrophin, acetyl-choline receptor, and acetyl cholin-esterase at the neuromuscular synapse (2), and α-dystrobrevin acts via the dystrophin glycoprotein complex to aid maturation and stability of the synapse (70).

Cardiac muscle. Echocardiographic (ECG) abnormalities in DMD reflect selective atrophy and scarring of the posterobasal region and adjacent lateral wall of the left ventricle, rather than actual right ventricle hypertrophy (32). During the second decade, conduction system abnormalities (heart block, bundle branch block, arrhythmias) and overt signs of cardiomyopathy (hypertrophic and dilated) develop. Whereas the incidence of conduction defects remains low, the incidence of cardiomyopathy increases steadily, affecting one third of patients by 14 years, and all patients over 18 years. Dilated cardiomyopathy was the most common type at all ages, and often develops after a period of hypertrophy. Despite the high incidence of cardiac involvement, many patients with DMD remain asymptomatic so that only 57% of patients over 18 years have overt cardiac involvement (132).

In BMD, dilated cardiomyopathy is more common than hypertrophic cardiomyopathy. Cardiomyopathy rarely occurs under 16 years, but may affect

As illustrated in Figure 4, in-frame deletions produce a smaller-than-normal, semi-functional protein (=missing an internal section), while frame shifting deletions generally produce a few incorrect amino acids (= that don't make sense) before a premature stop codon (= END) is generated. In theory, protein could be synthesised up to the new stop codon, but in practice this is rarely detected. Frameshift mutations or stop codons tend to result in nonsense-mediated decay of mutant mRNA, and any grossly abnormal protein that might be produced is usually degraded rapidly (59).

Interestingly, patients with intermediate D/BMD-type severity have mutations that are frame-shifting or in-frame. The in-frame mutations probably delete a more functionally important region than the typical BMD deletions (eg, exon 3 versus exons 45-47) whereas the frame-shifting mutations in these patients may show a higher level of somatic restoration of the reading frame via exon skipping (see later) (131).

Mutations in the dystrophin gene are not randomly distributed. There are two particular hotspots and about 30% occur at a proximal hotspot. Many are associated with breakpoints in the large intron after exon 2, and 70% occur at a distal hotspot particularly associated with breakpoints in intron 44. Interestingly, it has been observed that the ratio of proximal to distal deletions was 1:3 in isolated cases and 1:1 in familial cases, suggesting that proximal deletions probably occur early in embryonic development, causing them to have a higher chance of becoming familial. Distal deletions occur later and have a higher chance of causing only isolated cases (137). Mutations causing DMD are fairly variable in size but those causing BMD are more conservative with a very high proportion of patients bearing the in-frame deletions of exons 45-47, 45-48, or 45-49 (Figure 5).

The incidence of mutations causing Xp21-linked muscular dystrophy of Duchenne-like severity is about 1 in 3500 live male births, whereas the incidence

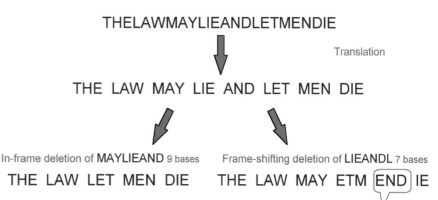

Figure 4. Illustration of the effect of deletions on the open reading frame.

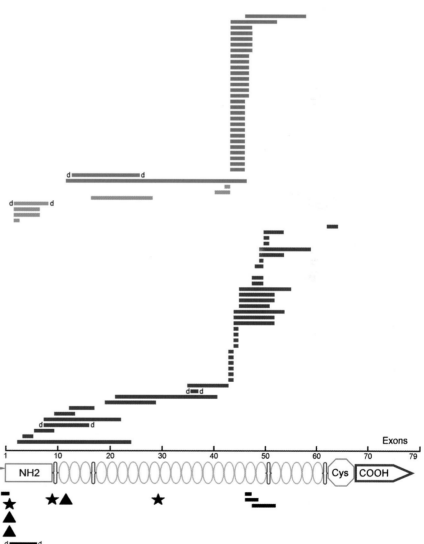

Figure 5. Diagram to illustrate the distribution and extent of deletions in patients with BMD (red bars), intermediate D/BMD (green bars) and DMD (blue bars). The locations of mutations in patients with XLDC are shown in black below the schematic of the dystrophin molecule. d = duplication, stars represent point mutations and arrow heads represent insertions.

70% of patients over 40 years (133). Mitral valve regurgitation may occur in BMD, and probably indicates that cardiac disease progresses at a different rate in BMD (compared to DMD) due to the ability of BMD patients to perform strenuous muscular exertion, with its associated cardiac workload, for longer. In both DMD and BMD, the rate of progression slowed when patients became confined to a wheelchair (32).

The proportion of DMD/BMD carriers with echocardiological evidence of left-ventricle dilation has been reported as 40% (83), and an even higher incidence (up to 90%) of abnormal ECGs was recorded in an Italian study (141). However, in a recent UK study of carriers and controls that was conducted "blind," a much lower incidence of clinical symptoms was recorded. Cardiomyopathic features were present in only 4 (7%) of 56, with an additional 10 (18%) of 56 having previously unrecognised cardiac abnormalities on ECG, with none needing urgent treatment (71).

Musculo-skeletal changes. The selectivity of muscle involvement in the early stages produces an imbalance in muscle strength at most joints, leading to contractures. The stronger muscles shorten, the muscles and their surrounding connective tissues become tight and the joint's range of movement is decreased. Contractures, rather than muscle weakness per se, may cause boys with DMD to lose the ability to walk prematurely. Hip extensor weakness leads to muscle contractures at the hip and increased lumbar lordosis. Stronger calf muscles encourage toe-walking and lead to worsening of ankle contractures. At least 90% of DMD boys develop scoliosis, and spinal curvature is a serious problem since the progressive thoracic deformity restricts adequate pulmonary ventilation and aggravates respiratory problems (11, 45). Other musculoskeletal features include an increased head circumference (9), and altered dental features due to differential weakness of facial mus-

cles (41). None of the cranial abnormalities correlate with intellectual ability.

Mechanical support and structural integrity. The most obvious function to suggest for dystrophin is a structural one, and evidence for structural abnormalities in the membrane had been reported long before dystrophin was identified (119). Loss of dystrophin and a variable reduction in the expression of the other members of the complex would presumably lead to reduced strength, flexibility, and stability of the muscle membrane during contraction (138). Furthermore, the linkage from cytoskeletal F-actin outside the myofibrillar contractile apparatus, through the dystrophin glycoprotein complex, to nNOS may be of significance for vascular control during muscle contraction and exercise (155). As shown in Figure 2, dystrophin is part of two separate linkage systems from the actin cytoskeleton, out through the plasma membrane and basal lamina, to the extracellular matrix (168). One route is via the N-terminus of dystrophin and repeats in the rod domain, through β- and α-dystroglycan; while the other is through the C-terminus of dystrophin via α-actinin-2, to the integrin adhesion system. Enhanced expression of integrin $\alpha7\beta1$-mediated linkage of the extracellular matrix is seen in DMD and may help to compensate for the absence of the dystrophin-mediated linkage (23). In keeping with the role of the DGC in maintaining the alignment and orientation of the contractile apparatus relative to the basal lamina, was the discovery that dystrophin (and other associated proteins including β-spectrin, β-dystroglycan and nNOS) assumed a rib-like or "costameric" distribution around muscle fibres (115). More recently, it has been demonstrated that the dystrophin complex forms a mechanically strong link between the sarcolemma and the costameric cytoskeleton through interaction with γ-actin filaments. Destabilisation of costameric actin filaments may also be an important precursor to

the costamere disarray observed in dystrophin-deficient muscle (151).

Dystrophin in cellular communication and signalling. It has been suggested that the dystrophin glycoprotein complex has signalling as well as structural roles, and that α-dystrobrevin plays a pivotal role in this function (70). Dystrophin and α1-syntrophin interact with calmodulin, a regulator of calcium-dependent kinases (6, 126), and β-dystroglycan binds to Grb2, a signal-transducting adaptor protein (149). α1-Syntrophin contains a PDZ domain (a protein-protein interaction motif) that interacts with at least three sarcolemmal proteins involved in signal transduction: nNOS, voltage-gated sodium channels, and the stress-activated protein kinase ERK6 (19, 63, 78). α-Dystrobrevin binds the syntrophins and dystrophin, and is a substrate for tyrosine kinases (12).

Primary mouse muscle cultures treated with a monoclonal antibody, which blocked α-dystroglycan binding to laminin, induced a dystrophic phenotype in vitro. The phenotype was inducible in differentiated cultures only, and was characterised by reduced myotube size, myofibril disorganisation, loss of contractile activity and reduced spontaneous clustering of acetylcholine receptors. It was reversed by the addition of excess exogenous laminin-2 (merosin). The authors concluded that α-dystroglycan may be part of a signalling pathway for the maturation and maintenance of skeletal myofibres (21).

Mechler et al (110) studied blood flow in BMD patients and concluded that the α-adrenergic receptor responses were abnormal. Recently, evidence has accumulated for the DGC being involved in regulating intramuscular blood flow through the production or transmission of an intercellular signal from muscle fibres to the vascular endothelium (69). While the loss of the extreme C-terminus of dystrophin (which contains the binding sites for the syntrophins and dystrobrevin) does not result in the loss of nNOS, syntrophin, or dystrobrevin (158), syntrophin knock-out mice fail to localise nNOS correctly, and the enzyme remains in the cytosol (91). Nitric oxide (NO), produced by nNOS in a calcium-dependent manner, is thought to regulate blood flow by opposing α-adrenergic vasoconstriction. Absence of nNOS at the sarcolemma appears to impede NO-mediated regulation of vasodilation, and nNOS-null mice, which express normal levels of the DGC at the sarcolemma, are unable to control blood flow and oxygen delivery to skeletal muscle during exercise (160). Similarly, a recent study on boys with DMD concluded that unopposed sympathetic vasoconstriction in exercising skeletal muscle led to functional muscle ischaemia and that this contributed directly and indirectly (via resultant fibre necrosis) to the pathogenesis of this condition (155).

There is plenty of evidence that calcium homeostasis is disturbed in Duchenne muscular dystrophy. Increased intracellular calcium has been found in dystrophin-deficient muscle and cells in culture, and the elevated free Ca^{2+} concentrations result in enhanced protein degradation (163). Abnormal calcium homeostasis may be due to increased activity of calcium leak channels and other stretch-activated ion channels (57), leading to Ca^{2+} overload at the subsarcolemmal level (106). More recently it was suggested that the abnormal Ca^{2+} influx in dystrophin-deficient myofibres could lead to altered developmental programming in regenerating fibres (29). Support for this model comes from evidence that altering the pattern of Ca^{2+} influx in differentiating myogenic cells can determine the developmental pathway that the cells will take (125).

Regeneration, differentiation and maturation. Loss of structural integrity, combined with local ischaemia due to impaired nNOS signalling and disruptions to the microvasculature (via the particular DGC found in smooth muscle), leads to small areas of muscle fibre necrosis (segmental necrosis in

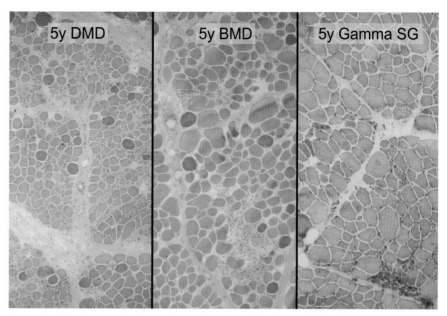

Figure 6. Sections from muscle biopsies taken from patients with Duchenne MD, Becker MD and α-sarcoglycanopathy at the same age. H & E. Magnification ×66.

longitudinal section). Degeneration of muscle fibres follows, and with the limited number of replication cycles available to the satellite cells, regeneration is less than fully effective (145). Unfortunately, by the time the first clinical symptoms become apparent, there is a decline in regenerative capacity since the muscle has already undergone extensive regeneration (as indicated by the rate of telomere loss). The satellite cells are prematurely senescent, having already undergone excessive proliferation during previous bouts of muscle repair (36, 47). Nitric oxide is also known to mediate satellite cell activation, and reduced synthesis may contribute to the impaired regeneration in dystrophin-deficient muscle (5). Fibrous connective tissue quickly grows, and together with fat replaces muscle tissue. Thus, the pattern for progressive muscle weakness is set.

It is clear, however, that the extent of regeneration does not explain the prolonged expression of many developmentally regulated proteins. The proportion of fibres expressing neonatal or developmental myosin heavy chain, for example, may be 25% or more, but this appears to reflect a failure of the fibres to reach maturity, rather than evidence that a quarter of the fibres are currently regenerating (29, 51). As has been

noted previously, the neuromuscular junctions in DMD are immature and poorly developed (90). Dystrophin-deficient *mdx* mouse muscle is highly successful at regeneration and it has been proposed that the generation of a stable population of maturationally arrested centronucleated fibers which express the mature adult myosin isoforms is the main strategy of *mdx* muscle to minimise apoptosis. Thus, it has been suggested that the major element that determines the susceptibility of most human muscles to the dystrophic process is their inability to arrest the maturation of regenerated fibres at the centronucleated stage with a concomitant expression of the adult myosins (88, 124).

Mitochondria and energy regulation. Chronic calcium influx due to the poor integrity of the plasma membrane, amongst other factors, leads to calcium overloading of the mitochondrial matrix, as well as decreased mitochondrial function. Mitochondrial dysfunction has been reported in dystrophin-deficient muscle (100), and in a recent study, the mRNAs from 26 genes involved in mitochondrial function and energy metabolism were found to be downregulated in DMD (29). These data suggest that there is a widespread

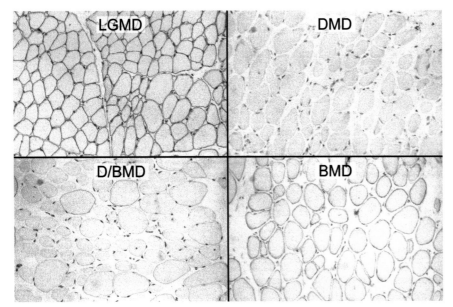

Figure 7. Unfixed frozen sections labelled with monoclonal antibody Dy8/6C5 to the C-terminus of dystrophin. Indirect peroxidase visualised with H$_2$O$_2$ and diaminobenzidine (DAB). Magnification ×76.

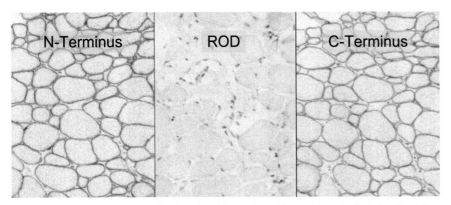

Figure 8. Serial sections from a severe Becker patient with an in-frame deletion of exons 13-47. Dystrophin labelling can be seen with monoclonal antibodies to the N-terminus (Dy10/12B2, exon 10) and C-terminus (Dy8/6C5, exon 78), but no labelling is seen with the rod domain antibody (Dy4/6D3, exon 29), because the deletion removes the antibody binding site. Indirect peroxidase visualised with H$_2$O$_2$ and diaminobenzidine (DAB). Magnification ×80.

disorder of both aerobic and anaerobic energy metabolism in dystrophic muscle. The generalised mitochondrial dysfunction and metabolic crisis is compatible with the finding that performance-enhancing metabolic agents such as creatine, coenzyme Q, and carnitine have a beneficial effect on dystrophin-deficient muscle function (73).

Immune system. Complement follows the entry of calcium in to muscle fibres and heralds the onset of muscle fibre lysis and destruction. Cellular necrosis may be accentuated by T cell-mediated injury and the invasion of macrophages. Extensive mast cell proliferation and degranulation occurs in dystrophin-deficient muscle, and the fibres are very sensitive to mast cell inflammatory mediators and proteases (48, 67). Mast cells in the skin are closely associated with XIIIa+ and HLA-DR+ dendritic cells, and infiltration by this subpopulation of activated dermal dendritic cells has recently been demonstrated in dystrophic muscle (29). Interestingly, it has been found that prednisone prevents activation of dendritic cells (108), which may contribute to the beneficial effects that have been reported for this drug in DMD(35), although the inflammatory cell target of prednisone has not been identified, and drugs that inhibit T and B cell functions do not seem to help patients (75).

Structural changes

A typical dystrophic biopsy has increased variation in fibre size, evidence of fibre necrosis with phagocytosis, hypercontracted eosinophilic hyaline fibres, some centrally nucleated fibres, and an increase in fat and fibrous connective tissue that makes the fibres appear more rounded than angular in outline (Figure 6). In the early stages of the disease process, regenerating fibres may also be seen: these are generally smaller with basophilic cytoplasm and large nuclei with prominent nucleoli. In BMD, muscle histopathology is corresponding milder with a predominance of chronic characteristics (eg, gross fibre size variation, fibre splitting) rather than acute features (eg, hyaline fibres, necrosis). Foci of regenerating fibres are more frequently seen in young patients with Becker muscular dystrophy, or in patients with one of the sarcoglycanopathies (Figure 6). In the later stages of DMD, almost all the fibres become replaced by fat and connective tissue.

In 1975, Mokri and Engel (104) reported electron microscopic findings that pointed to "a basic or early abnormality in the plasma membrane of muscle fibres" in patients with DMD. Further evidence for a primary problem with the muscle membrane came from the elevated serum levels of enzymes normally located inside muscle. Serum creatine kinase (CK) levels may be more than 100 times the normal upper limits in the early years, peaking before loss of independent mobility, and declining thereafter as the muscle bulk decreases. Elevated serum CK has also been used for many years as a basis for carrier detection, although modern molecular techniques are now the first choice (45).

Selective muscle involvement is a feature of the muscular dystrophies in general, and in DMD, certain muscles never seem to be clinically affected. Extraocular muscles are well preserved and have been particularly studied in this context (7). It has been suggested that the sparing may be due to, among other unknown factors, combinations of four features: *i)* the fibres have a fast speed of contraction and high activity levels but this may be compensated for by their diminutive size and the small loads they work against (92), *ii)* extraocular muscles normally require a substantial calcium handling capacity and have enhanced calcium homeostasis, *iii)* they exhibit constitutively high antioxidant activity, and have substantial free radical scavenging mechanisms, and *iv)* extraocular muscles appear to have an inherent facility to increase utrophin expression greatly in response to dystrophin deficiency (and lack of both proteins causes extensive pathology) (142).

Immunohistochemistry and western blot. *Duchenne muscular dystrophy.* Given the size of the dystrophin gene and the possibility of point mutations, diagnosis may be more quickly achieved by labelling sections from a muscle biopsy with antibodies to different dystrophin domains. While patients with non-Xp21-linked forms of muscular dystrophy show clear, uniform labelling at the periphery of all fibres; DMD muscle shows an absence or very little labelling; intermediate D/BMD muscle demonstrates weak labelling on the majority of fibres, possibly with a few more clearly labelled; and BMD sections are characterised by variation in labelling intensity, both between and within fibres (Figure 7). On western blots, no dystrophin labelling may be observed in DMD, although faint bands in various places might be detectable and these may indicate particular mutations (18, 22). A very exceptional case of a patient with Duchenne-type severity, but dystrophin of normal size and near-normal abundance on blots, and a missense mutation (Asp3335His) in the C-terminal domain has been reported (66). Dystrophin labelling of fetal autopsies has also proved to be an effective diagnostic procedure for future pregnancies

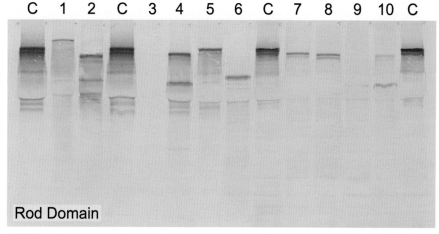

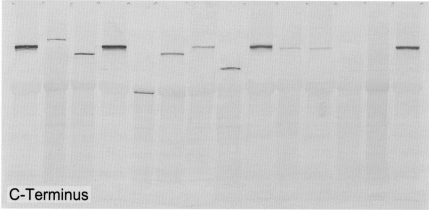

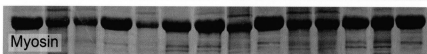

Figure 9. Western blots demonstrating the effect that different mutations have on dystrophin protein expression in muscle. Upper blot is labelled with rod domain antibody (Dy4/6D3), lower blot is labelled with the C-terminal antibody (Dy8/6C5). Lowest panel shows the myosin heavy chain band on the post-blotted gel. This is used to indicate how much 'muscle' protein (as opposed to fat and fibrous connective tissue) was loaded in each lane. C = normal control; lane 1 = severe BMD (duplication of exons 14-26); 2 = BMD (deletion of exons 45-53); 3 = severe BMD (deletion of exons 13-47); 4 = BMD (deletion of exons 45-47; 5 = BMD (no deletion detected: dystrophin normal size but reduced abundance); 6 = DMD (in-frame deletion of exons 3-25, 7 = intermediate D/BMD (in-frame deletion of exon 3); 8 = intermediate D/BMD (frame-shifting deletion of exons 3-7); 9 = DMD (frame-shifting deletion of exon 50); 10 = DMD (frame-shifting deletion of exon 44). Note that the complete loss of all the bands in lane 3 of the upper blot (binding site deleted) is evidence that the multitude of bands seen the control lanes are dystrophin metabolites and not products of other genes. Indirect peroxidase visualised with H_2O_2 and diaminobenzidine (DAB).

(30), and diagnosis of fetal muscle biopsies taken in utero has proved to be possible, even if it is not a widespread practice (50).

Becker muscular dystrophy. Because the absence of dystrophin labelling is pathognomic of DMD, care must be taken to use antibodies to different regions of the dystrophin molecule to avoid false-negative results in a BMD patient. If one antibody binding site is deleted, no labelling will be observed with that particular antibody, although it will be seen with others to different

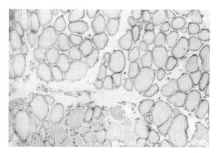

Figure 10. Becker-like dystrophin labelling in a DMD patient with an in-frame deletion of exons 3-25. Indirect peroxidase labelling of an antibody (Dy8/6C5) to the C-terminus of dystrophin, visualised with H_2O_2 and diaminobenzidine (DAB). Magnification ×80.

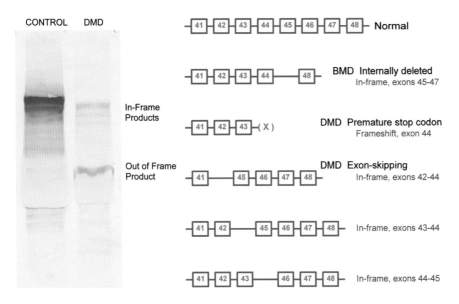

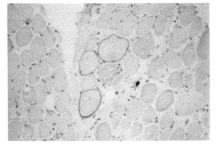

Figure 11. Western blot lanes from a normal control and a DMD patient with a frame-shifting mutation of exon 44. To the right are the various patterns of exon skipping that were found in this patient. The muscle mRNA analysis was undertaken by Dr Jamel Chelly while he was at Oxford in 1992.

Figure 12. "Revertant fibres" in a DMD patient with frame-shifting deletion of exon 51. Indirect peroxidase labelling of an antibody (Dy8/6C5) to the C-terminus of dystrophin, visualised with H_2O_2 and diaminobenzidine (DAB). Magnification ×80.

epitopes (Figure 8, and lane 3 in Figure 9).

Dystrophin labelling on blots is particularly useful in BMD patients because bands of abnormal size and abundance are easily detected (Figure 9). Although a single band (427 kDa) is detected with the C-terminal antibody, the antibody to the rod domain typically recognises a doublet (427 kDa and 400 kDa) plus lower molecular mass metabolites. The presence of a fuzzy degradation band at 220-240 kDa is characteristic of a deletion that commences in exon 45, and may indicate that the internally deleted protein molecules are unstable and susceptible to cleavage at that point (eg, lanes 2 and 4 on Figure 9). The migration distance of the uppermost dystrophin band can then be used to suggest the most likely extent of the gene deletion (eg, exons 45-53, 45-47) for subsequent molecular confirmation (18).

Genotype-phenotype correlations

Frame-shifting BMDs. Although the mutations in most patients obey the reading frame hypothesis (96, 120), it was appreciated very early on that there were some notable exceptions. In particular, the frame-shifting deletion of exons 3-7 was noted in patients classified on the grounds of clinical severity as having Becker MD (62, 105). Initially, it was suggested that alternative initiation sites in exon 8 might be utilised (105), but examination of muscle mRNA revealed various patterns of exon skipping which restored the open reading frame. At protein level, it was clear that the underlying mutation had been modified so that C-terminal dystrophin labelling was detectable (28).

In-frame DMDs. Patients with Duchenne-type clinical severity and confirmed in-frame deletions are quite rare (53, 170). Figure 10 illustrates the Becker-like dystrophin immunohistochemical labelling from one such patient, and his blot may be seen as lane 6 in Figure 9. This patient had an in-frame deletion spanning exons 3-25. The immunolabelling results indicate that he makes quite a lot of dystrophin, but the fuzzy nature of his protein band on the blot labelled with the rod domain antibody indicates that the protein may not have been very stable. This mutation removes most of the region now considered essential for dystrophin function (the N-terminal actin binding domain, the first hinge and the first two rod domain repeats) (167). This patient was wheelchair bound at 9.3 years and died at 17.9 with cardiac and respiratory problems (128).

Somatic variation and exon skipping in DMDs. The vast majority of DMD boys have frame-shifting mutations that should result in no dystrophin protein being produced beyond the position of the new stop codon. Nevertheless, while most fibres in DMD biopsies appear negative for dystrophin antibody labelling there may be a few fibres that are clearly dystrophin-positive with antibodies directed to the extreme C-terminus, but these very rarely represent more than 1% of the fibre population (52). Some biopsies may even show very weak labelling on a high proportion of fibres (130), and western blot analysis reveals protein species of BMD-like size (129). It appears that the underlying frame shifting mutation is being modified at a somatic level in the muscle tissue. As shown in Figure 11 the frame-shifting deletion of single exon 44 may become an in-frame deletion of exons 44-45, 43-44 or 42-44, while the reading frame of an exon 3-7 deletion can be restored by skipping additional exons from 3-9 or 2-7 (127). The dystrophin-positive fibres are generally known as "revertants" (Figure 12), although it is actually low levels of a Becker-like protein that is being produced rather than a return to wild-type protein (81). While the few clearly dystrophin-positive fibres do not seem to have any clinical importance, there is evidence that the weak labelling on many fibres does have some functional significance and this pattern of labelling is a characteristic of patients with milder DMD and intermediate D/BMD (130, 131).

Exon skipping may explain the lack of skeletal muscle symptoms in patients with X-linked dilated cardiomyopathy: the reading frame is restored in skeletal muscle but not heart (56). Furthermore, a nonsense mutation was identified in exon 29 of one XLDC family and, while exon skipping did rescue the reading frame in both cardiac and skeletal muscle, immunohistochemical analysis of the dystrophin-associated proteins revealed a reduction of β-sarcoglycan and δ-sarcoglycan in the sarcolemma of cardiac muscle but not skeletal muscle tissue. It seems as though there was a conformational change in exon-29-deleted dystrophin, resulting in disruption of the sarcoglycan assembly in heart muscle but not skeletal muscle (58).

Manifesting and non-manifesting carriers. Women have two X-chromosomes, but at an early stage of development, one X-chromosome in each cell is inactivated, leaving only a single X transcriptionally active (10). In a heterozygote carrier of a mutation in the dystrophin gene, either the wild-type or mutant X might be active in the fibre segment controlled by any particular nucleus. As shown in Figure 13, the result is a mosaic of dystrophin-positive and -negative nuclei and fibre segments. When the two types of nuclei are very intimately mixed, dystrophin spreads to adjacent segments (99) resulting in a non-manifesting carrier (165). This may also be an age-related phenomenon in skeletal muscle, with its capacity for regeneration, but not in heart (93). If the clonal nature of the inactivation was such that dystrophin-negative nuclei are in large groups together, a female heterozygote may manifest clinical symptoms of dystrophin-deficiency. It follows that *i*) muscle weakness is often asymmetrical in manifesting carriers (45), and *ii*) protein analysis can produce rather variable results depending on the biopsy

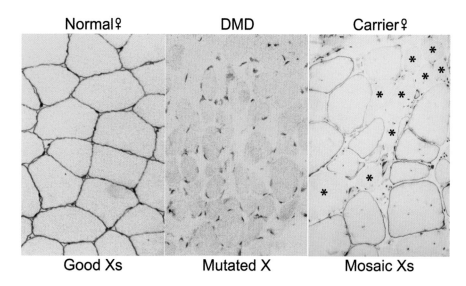

Figure 13. Dystrophin labelling on sections from a normal control, a DMD patient, and a manifesting carrier of DMD, illustrating the mosaic of dystrophin-positive and –negative fibres that arise from X-chromosome inactivation in the muscle tissue.

sample site (39, 123). Furthermore, in a pair of monozygotic girl twins, one may be clinically asymptomatic while the other is quite severely affected, due to skewed X-inactivation (103, 147). The relative abundance of normal sized and internally deleted dystrophin molecules may be estimated from blots of BMD carrier muscle (164).

Future perspectives

Treatments and therapies. The use of orthopaedic assistance with braces, splints and callipers; surgery for contractures; and night ventilation, all have their place in the management of boys with Duchenne muscular dystrophy. The use of steroid drugs has its supporters, and clinicians are now much more aware of the cardiac problems that may occur in carriers or patients with DMD/BMD. However, in the wake of the molecular genetic revolution, there has come an awareness of the need to understand the pathophysiological processes that underlie the newly-identified gene defects. Even in monogenic diseases like the dystrophinopathies, the picture is extremely complex, and some of the physiological features mentioned in the course of this chapter have potential application in treatment or therapy.

For example, the dystrophin homologue, utrophin, is normally localised to the junctional regions of the plasma membrane (72), but in dystrophin-deficiency, it is upregulated to the extrajunctional membrane (as shown in Figure 14). Extrajunctional utrophin forms complexes with normal members of the DGC, and it has been suggested that a significant increase in utrophin expression could be of therapeutic value (161). Utrophin has been overexpressed in the dystrophin-deficient *mdx* mouse by transgenesis technology. The results of a battery of functional tests (ie, mechanical responses, intracellular calcium homeostasis, metabolic reaction to muscle activity) demonstrated that, for most parameters tested, recovery amounted to 80% (65). The caveat to these data is that most muscles in the *mdx* mouse do not suffer the same degenerative changes that occur in DMD: the diaphragm is the only muscle that is really comparable (158).

Two potential forms of therapy derive from the type of mutation in the dystrophin gene that are associated with Duchenne muscular dystrophy. A significant number of these mutations (<15%) are nonsense mutations producing premature stop codons. Exposure of *mdx* cultured myotubes to high doses of the antibiotic gentamicin pro-

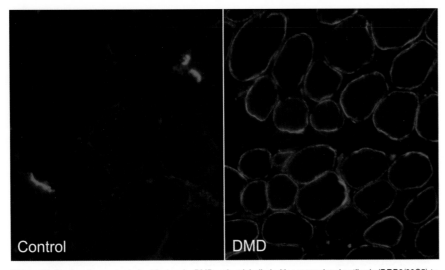

Figure 14. Sections from a control subject and a DMD patient labelled with a monoclonal antibody (DRP3/20C5) to the N-terminus of utrophin. Neuromuscular junctions may be seen in the control whereas the extrajunctional membrane is also labelled in the DMD patient. Indirect rhodamine labelling. Magnification ×237.

duced translation with read-through of the nonsense codon and localised expression of dystrophin at the cell membrane (84). Secondly, the dystrophin gene is prone to exon skipping, and it has been shown that this phenomenon can be beneficial. Antisense oligonucleotides have been used to induce skipping of the exon bearing the *mdx* mutation; consequently, in-frame synthesis of dystrophin is restored, together with the potential to bind members of the all-important DGC (40, 107).

Other therapeutic approaches involve the delivery of normal dystrophin-synthesising nuclei to dystrophin-deficient muscle. Limited migration from the site of injection is one major problem with myoblast transfer; however, the intravenous injection of either normal haematopoietic stem cells or a novel population of muscle-derived stem cells into *mdx* mice has resulted in the incorporation of donor-derived nuclei into muscle, and the partial restoration of dystrophin expression. Initially, the stem cells attached to the capillaries of the muscles, and then participated in regeneration after muscle degeneration (162). Another approach has been the direct intramuscular injection of plasmid DNA, which has also enjoyed some success although inflammatory responses may be a problem, as they are in whole myoblast transfer (1). The great size of the dystrophin gene has dictated approaches to gene therapy, and the use of dystrophin "minigenes" (based on an in-frame deletion of exons 17-48 in a family with mild BMD) has been extensive. More recently, small molecules have been designed with great success (167). The currently held view is that adeno-associated viruses (AAV) are the most effective vectors for future development. They are the only vector system that is based on a nonpathogenic, replication-defective virus, and the safety is matched by good gene transfer efficiency and longevity (74).

Animal models. Studies on the pathophysiology, and for testing potential therapies for dystrophinopathy, have relied for a good part on both naturally occurring and genetically modified animal models (3). Among these, the *mdx* mouse has been the most extensively employed, although it does not clinically manifest a progressive muscular dystrophy (64). The disease-causing nonsense mutation in the *mdx* mouse is in exon 23, so the smaller isoforms of dystrophin would still be expressed. Transgenic variants have therefore been generated which differ in their expression of dystrophin isoforms (31, 87). The Golden Retriever dog (GRMD or CXMD) is the only other spontaneously arising dystrophin-deficient animal that has received much attention, and it does reproduce a more severe myopathic phenotype (166).

The generation of genetically modified mice has been used extensively to examine the physiological effects of "knocking out" specific genes that encode dystrophin-related and -associated proteins. First single, then double and triple (70) genes have been inactivated in increasingly sophisticated attempts to dissect the physiological interactions between gene products (144). This approach has demonstrated that some proteins, like dystroglycan, are essential for development, and their lack is embryonic lethal (169): other strains of transgenic mice like those with a double dystrophin/utrophin knock out, or those which overexpress caveolin 3, might be considered better models of Duchenne MD than the original *mdx* mice (37, 61).

Expression profiling with picroarrays. The technology now exists for high-throughput analysis of gene expression, and in a landmark set of experiments undertaken by Hoffman and his colleagues (29), the muscle mRNA profiles from 6000 genes were compared and contrasted in controls, patients with Duchenne MD, and patients with α-sarcoglycanopathy. This huge undertaking raised almost as many questions as it answered, but this kind of global approach was necessary to start to address the identity of downstream pathophysiological cascades arising from the primary gene defects. The expression profiling was undertaken using mixed tissue samples of multiple patients and iterative (repeated) comparisons of duplicate datasets. Certain categories of mRNA differences were defined and then supported by analysis of representative proteins. A critical aspect of the profiling was to limit the number of variables under study, and the subjects were age-matched (5 DMD, 4 α-sarcoglycanopathy, 5 controls). Each muscle biopsy was divided in half and the mRNA extracted separately from each half.

One half from each individual in the group was then pooled and subjected to analysis on a gene chip.

This method generated two sets for each group, which were then compared (ie, Control1 v DMD1, Control1 v DMD2, Control2 v DMD1, Control2 v DMD2). Only the differences that appeared consistently more than 2 fold in all possible combinations were considered significant. Four categories of pathophysiological pathways were identified using this method: i) evidence was found for persistent expression of developmentally regulated genes suggesting that the muscle may assume a chronically dedifferentiated state, ii) there appeared to be a general metabolic crisis with widespread mitochondrial dysfunction, iii) novel proteins were identified (eg, thrombospondin 4) that were involved in early stages of myofibre necrosis, and iv) novel cells and proteins involved in local inflammatory and bystander responses (eg, dermal dendritic cell infiltrates) were also identified. These results provide a fascinating first glimpse into the disease processes that underlie dystrophinopathy, and it is clear that this sort of global approach is one we will be seeing much more of in the future. Nevertheless, the very nature of this powerful technique means that the results obtained are likely to be open to disagreements of various kinds (technical, interpretational). Thus, Chang et al (27) found that in the *mdx* mouse, nNOS mRNA was reduced while α1-syntrophin levels were normal, but this is the opposite situation to that reported for DMD using expression profiling methods (29).

Concluding remarks. In this chapter, I have attempted to provide a snapshot picture of what we know and understand of the dystrophinopathies at this moment in time. Although we are now in a molecular era, it is fascinating to review some of the observations made many years ago because they suddenly make a whole lot of sense when put in a current context. The last few years have seen huge changes in the way we think about diseases caused by defects in single genes. The picture is a complex one, but we are now moving from diagnosis to the jigsaw puzzle of pathogenesis—each piece of circumstantial evidence fits somewhere, but we seem to be well on the way to identifying all the edge pieces!

References

1. Acsadi G, Dickson G, Love DR, Jani A, Walsh FS, Gurusinghe A, Wolff JA, Davies KE (1991) Human dystrophin expression in mdx mice after intramuscular injection of DNA constructs. *Nature* 352(6338): 815-818

2. Adams ME, Kramarcy N, Krall SP, Rossi SG, Rotundo RL, Sealock R, Froehner SC (2000) Absence of alpha-syntrophin leads to structurally aberrant neuromuscular synapses deficient in utrophin. *J Cell Biol* 150: 1385-1398

3. Allamand V, Campbell KP (2000) Animal models for muscular dystrophy: valuable tools for the development of therapies. *Hum Mol Genet* 9: 2459-2467

4. Amann KJ, Guo AW, Ervasti JM (1999) Utrophin lacks the rod domain actin binding activity of dystrophin. *J Biol Chem* 274: 35375-35380

5. Anderson JE (2000) A role for nitric oxide in muscle repair: nitric oxide-mediated activation of muscle satellite cells. *Mol Biol Cell* 11: 1859-1874

6. Anderson JT, Rogers RP, Jarrett HW (1996) Ca2+-calmodulin binds to the carboxyl-terminal domain of dystrophin. *J Biol Chem* 271: 6605-6610

7. Andrade FH, Porter JD, Kaminski HJ (2000) Eye muscle sparing by the muscular dystrophies: lessons to be learned? *Microsc Res Tech* 48: 192-203

8. Angelini C, Fanin M, Pegoraro E, Freda MP, Cadaldini M, Martinello F (1994) Clinical-molecular correlation in 104 mild X-linked muscular dystrophy patients: characterization of sub-clinical phenotypes. *Neuromuscul Disord* 4: 349-358

9. Appleton RE, Bushby K, Gardner-Medwin D, Welch J, Kelly PJ (1991) Head circumference and intellectual performance of patients with Duchenne muscular dystrophy. *Dev Med Child Neurol* 33: 884-890

10. Avner P, Heard E (2001) X-chromosome inactivation: counting, choice and initiation. *Nat Rev Genet* 2: 59-67

11. Bach JR (1999) *Guide to the Evaluation and Management of Neuromuscular Disease.* Hanley & Belfus: Philadelphia

12. Balasubramanian S, Fung ET, Huganir RL (1998) Characterization of the tyrosine phosphorylation and distribution of dystrobrevin isoforms. *FEBS Lett* 432: 133-140

13. Bardoni A, Felisari G, Sironi M, Comi G, Lai M, Robotti M, Bresolin N (2000) Loss of Dp140 regulatory sequences is associated with cognitive impairment in dystrophinopathies. *Neuromuscul Disord* 10: 194-199

14. Barresi R, Moore SA, Stolle CA, Mendell JR, Campbell KP (2000) Expression of gamma -sarcoglycan in smooth muscle and its interaction with the smooth muscle sarcoglycan-sarcospan complex. *J Biol Chem* 275: 38554-38560

15. Beggs AH, Hoffman EP, Snyder JR, Arahata K, Specht L, Shapiro F, Angelini C, Sugita H, Kunkel LM (1991) Exploring the molecular basis for variability among patients with Becker muscular dystrophy: dystrophin gene and protein studies. *Am J Hum Genet* 49: 54-67

16. Billard C, Gillet P, Barthez M, Hommet C, Bertrand P (1998) Reading ability and processing in Duchenne muscular dystrophy and spinal muscular atrophy. *Dev Med Child Neurol* 40: 12-20

17. Blake DJ, Kroger S (2000) The neurobiology of Duchenne muscular dystrophy: learning lessons from muscle? *Trends Neurosci* 23: 92-99

18. Bornemann A, Anderson LV (2000) Diagnostic protein expression in human muscle biopsies. *Brain Pathol* 10: 193-214

19. Brenman JE, Chao DS, Gee SH, McGee AW, Craven SE, Santillano DR, Wu Z, Huang F, Xia H, Peters MF, Froehner SC, Bredt DS (1996) Interaction of nitric oxide synthase with the postsynaptic density protein PSD-95 and alpha1-syntrophin mediated by PDZ domains. *Cell* 84: 757-767

20. Bresolin N, Castelli E, Comi GP, Felisari G, Bardoni A, Perani D, Grassi F, Turconi A, Mazzucchelli F, Gallotti D, et al. (1994) Cognitive impairment in Duchenne muscular dystrophy. *Neuromuscul Disord* 4: 359-369

21. Brown M, Fisher JS, Salsich G (1999) Stiffness and muscle function with age and reduced muscle use. *J Orthop Res* 17: 409-414

22. Bulman DE, Gangopadhyay SB, Bebchuck KG, Worton RG, Ray PN (1991) Point mutation in the human dystrophin gene: identification through western blot analysis. *Genomics* 10: 457-460

23. Burkin DJ, Wallace GQ, Nicol KJ, Kaufman DJ, Kaufman SJ (2001) Enhanced expression of the alpha 7 beta 1 integrin reduces muscular dystrophy and restores viability in dystrophic mice. *J Cell Biol* 152: 1207-1218

24. Bushby KM, Gardner-Medwin D (1993) The clinical, genetic and dystrophin characteristics of Becker muscular dystrophy. I. Natural history. *J Neurol* 240: 98-104

25. Bushby KM, Hill A, Steele JG (1999) Failure of early diagnosis in symptomatic Duchenne muscular dystrophy. *Lancet* 353: 557-558

26. Bushby KM, Thambyayah M, Gardner-Medwin D (1991) Prevalence and incidence of Becker muscular dystrophy. *Lancet* 337: 1022-1024

27. Chang WJ, Iannaccone ST, Lau KS, Masters BS, McCabe TJ, McMillan K, Padre RC, Spencer MJ, Tidball JG, Stull JT (1996) Neuronal nitric oxide synthase and dystrophin-deficient muscular dystrophy. *Proc Natl Acad Sci U S A* 93: 9142-9147

28. Chelly J, Gilgenkrantz H, Lambert M, Hamard G, Chafey P, Recan D, Katz P, de la Chapelle A, Koenig M, Ginjaar IB, et al. (1990) Effect of dystrophin gene dele-

tions on mRNA levels and processing in Duchenne and Becker muscular dystrophies. *Cell* 63: 1239-1248

29. Chen YW, Zhao P, Borup R, Hoffman EP (2000) Expression profiling in the muscular dystrophies: identification of novel aspects of molecular pathophysiology. *J Cell Biol* 151: 1321-1336

30. Clerk A, Sewry CA, Dubowitz V, Strong PN (1992) Characterisation of dystrophin in fetuses at risk for Duchenne muscular dystrophy. *J Neurol Sci* 111: 82-91

31. Cox GA, Phelps SF, Chapman VM, Chamberlain JS (1993) New mdx mutation disrupts expression of muscle and nonmuscle isoforms of dystrophin. *Nat Genet* 4: 87-93

32. Cox GF, Kunkel LM (1997) Dystrophies and heart disease. *Curr Opin Cardiol* 12: 329-343

33. Crawford GE, Faulkner JA, Crosbie RH, Campbell KP, Froehner SC, Chamberlain JS (2000) Assembly of the dystrophin-associated protein complex does not require the dystrophin COOH-terminal domain. *J Cell Biol* 150: 1399-1410

34. Culligan KG, Mackey AJ, Finn DM, Maguire PB, Ohlendieck K (1998) Role of dystrophin isoforms and associated proteins in muscular dystrophy (review). *Int J Mol Med* 2: 639-648

35. De Silva S, Drachman DB, Mellits D, Kuncl RW (1987) Prednisone treatment in Duchenne muscular dystrophy: Long-term benefit. *Arch Neurol* 44: 818-822

36. Decary S, Hamida CB, Mouly V, Barbet JP, Hentati F, Butler-Browne GS (2000) Shorter telomeres in dystrophic muscle consistent with extensive regeneration in young children. *Neuromuscul Disord* 10: 113-120

37. Deconinck AE, Rafael JA, Skinner JA, Brown SC, Potter AC, Metzinger L, Watt DJ, Dickson JG, Tinsley JM, Davies KE (1997) Utrophin-dystrophin-deficient mice as a model for Duchenne muscular dystrophy. *Cell* 90: 717-727

38. Den Dunnen JT, Casula L, Kakover A, Bakker E, Yaffe D, Nudel U, van Ommen G-JB (1991) Mapping of dystrophin brain promoter: a deletion of this region is compatible with normal intellect. *Neuromusc Disord* 1: 327-331

39. Doriguzzi C, Palmucci L, Mongini T, Chiado-Piat L, Saggiorato C, Ugo I, Hoffman EP (1999) Variable histological expression of dystrophinopathy in two females. *Acta Neuropathol (Berl)* 97: 657-660

40. Dunckley MG, Manoharan M, Villiet P, Eperon IC, Dickson G (1998) Modification of splicing in the dystrophin gene in cultured Mdx muscle cells by antisense oligoribonucleotides. *Hum Mol Genet* 7: 1083-1090

41. Eckardt L, Harzer W (1996) Facial structure and functional findings in patients with progressive muscular dystrophy (Duchenne). *Am J Orthod Dentofacial Orthop* 110: 185-190

42. Eggers S, Lauriano V, Melo M, Takata RI, Akiyama J, Passos-Bueno MR, Gentil V, Frota-Pessoa O, Zatz M (1995) Why is the reproductive performance lower in Becker (BMD) as compared to limb girdle (LGMD) muscular dystrophy male patients? *Am J Med Genet* 60: 27-32

43. Emery AE (1991) Population frequencies of inherited neuromuscular diseases — a world survey. *Neuromuscul Disord* 1: 19-29

44. Emery AE, Skinner R (1976) Clinical studies in benign (Becker type) X-linked muscular dystrophy. *Clin Genet* 10: 189-201

45. Emery AEH (1993) *Duchenne Muscular Dystrophy.* Oxford University Press: New York

46. Emery AEH, Emery MLH (1995) *The History of a Genetic Disease: Duchenne Muscular Dystrophy or Meryon's Disease.* Royal Society of Medicine Press: London

47. Endesfelder S, Krahn A, Kreuzer KA, Lass U, Schmidt CA, Jahrmarkt C, von Moers A, Speer A (2000) Elevated p21 mRNA level in skeletal muscle of DMD patients and mdx mice indicates either an exhausted satellite cell pool or a higher p21 expression in dystrophin-deficient cells per se. *J Mol Med* 78: 569-574

48. Engel AG, Arahata K (1986) Mononuclear cells in myopathies: quantitation of functionally distinct subsets, recognition of antigen-specific cell-mediated cytotoxicity in some diseases, and implications for the pathogenesis of the different inflammatory myopathies. *Hum Pathol* 17: 704-721

49. Ervasti JM, Campbell KP (1991) Membrane organization of the dystrophin-glycoprotein complex. *Cell* 66: 1121-1131

50. Evans MI, Hoffman EP, Cadrin C, Johnson MP, Quintero RA, Golbus MS (1994) Fetal muscle biopsy: collaborative experience with varied indications. *Obstet Gynecol* 84: 913-917

51. Fanin M, Angelini C (1999) Regeneration in sarcoglycanopathies: expression studies of sarcoglycans and other muscle proteins. *J Neurol Sci* 165: 170-177

52. Fanin M, Danieli GA, Vitiello L, Senter L, Angelini C (1992) Prevalence of dystrophin-positive fibers in 85 Duchenne muscular dystrophy patients. *Neuromuscul Disord* 2: 41-45

53. Fanin M, Freda MP, Vitiello L, Danieli GA, Pegoraro E, Angelini C (1996) Duchenne phenotype with in-frame deletion removing major portion of dystrophin rod: threshold effect for deletion size? *Muscle Nerve* 19: 1154-1160

54. Feener CA, Koenig M, Kunkel LM (1989) Alternative splicing of human dystrophin mRNA generates isoforms at the carboxy terminus. *Nature* 338: 509-511

55. Felice KJ (1996) Distal weakness in dystrophin-deficient muscular dystrophy. *Muscle Nerve* 19: 1608-1610

56. Ferlini A, Sewry C, Melis MA, Mateddu A, Muntoni F (1999) X-linked dilated cardiomyopathy and the dystrophin gene. *Neuromuscul Disord* 9: 339-346

57. Fong PY, Turner PR, Denetclaw WF, Steinhardt RA (1990) Increased activity of calcium leak channels in myotubes of Duchenne human and mdx mouse origin. *Science* 250: 673-676

58. Franz WM, Muller M, Muller OJ, Herrmann R, Rothmann T, Cremer M, Cohn RD, Voit T, Katus HA (2000) Association of nonsense mutation of dystrophin gene with disruption of sarcoglycan complex in X-linked dilated cardiomyopathy. *Lancet* 355: 1781-1785

59. Frischmeyer PA, Dietz HC (1999) Nonsense-mediated mRNA decay in health and disease. *Hum Mol Genet* 8: 1893-1900

60. Galbiati F, Engelman JA, Volonte D, Zhang XL, Minetti C, Li M, Hou H, Kneitz B, Edelmann W, Lisanti MP (2001) Caveolin-3 null mice show a loss of caveolae, changes in the microdomain distribution of the dystrophin-glycoprotein complex, and T- tubule abnormalities. *J Biol Chem* 276: 21425-21433

61. Galbiati F, Volonte D, Chu JB, Li M, Fine SW, Fu M, Bermudez J, Pedemonte M, Weidenheim KM, Pestell RG, Minetti C, Lisanti MP (2000) Transgenic overexpression of caveolin-3 in skeletal muscle fibers induces a Duchenne-like muscular dystrophy phenotype. *Proc Natl Acad Sci USA* 97: 9689-9694

62. Gangopadhyay SB, Sherratt TG, Heckmatt JZ, Dubowitz V, Miller G, Shokeir M, Ray PN, Strong PN, Worton RG (1992) Dystrophin in frameshift deletion patients with Becker muscular dystrophy. *Am J Hum Genet* 51: 562-570

63. Gee SH, Madhavan R, Levinson SR, Caldwell JH, Sealock R, Froehner SC (1998) Interaction of muscle and brain sodium channels with multiple members of the syntrophin family of dystrophin-associated proteins. *J Neurosci* 18: 128-137

64. Gillis JM (1999) Understanding dystrophinopathies: an inventory of the structural and functional consequences of the absence of dystrophin in muscles of the mdx mouse. *J Muscle Res Cell Motil* 20: 605-625

65. Gillis JM (2000) An attempt of gene therapy in Duchenne muscular dystrophy: overexpression of utrophin in transgenic mdx mice. *Acta Neurol Belg* 100: 146-150

66. Goldberg LR, Hausmanowa-Petrusewicz I, Fidzianska A, Duggan DJ, Steinberg LS, Hoffman EP (1998) A dystrophin missense mutation showing persistence of dystrophin and dystrophin-associated proteins yet a severe phenotype. *Ann Neurol* 44: 971-976

67. Gorospe JR, Nishikawa BK, Hoffman EP (1996) Recruitment of mast cells to muscle after mild damage. *J Neurol Sci* 135: 10-17

68. Gospe SM, Jr., Lazaro RP, Lava NS, Grootscholten PM, Scott MO, Fischbeck KH (1989) Familial X-linked myalgia and cramps: a nonprogressive myopathy associated with a deletion in the dystrophin gene. *Neurology* 39: 1277-1280

69. Grady RM, Grange RW, Lau KS, Maimone MM, Nichol MC, Stull JT, Sanes JR (1999) Role for alpha-dystrobrevin in the pathogenesis of dystrophin-dependent muscular dystrophies. *Nat Cell Biol* 1: 215-220

70. Grady RM, Zhou H, Cunningham JM, Henry MD, Campbell KP, Sanes JR (2000) Maturation and maintenance of the neuromuscular synapse: genetic evidence for roles of the dystrophin-glycoprotein complex. *Neuron* 25: 279-293

71. Grain L, Cortina-Borja M, Forfar C, Hilton-Jones D, Hopkin J, Burch M (2001) Cardiac abnormalities and skeletal muscle weakness in carriers of Duchenne and

Becker muscular dystrophies and controls. *Neuromuscul Disord* 11: 186-191

72. Gramolini AO, Wu J, Jasmin BJ (2000) Regulation and functional significance of utrophin expression at the mammalian neuromuscular synapse. *Microsc Res Tech* 49: 90-100

73. Granchelli JA, Pollina C, Hudecki MS (2000) Preclinical screening of drugs using the mdx mouse. *Neuromuscul Disord* 10: 235-239

74. Greelish JP, Su LT, Lankford EB, Burkman JM, Chen H, Konig SK, Mercier IM, Desjardins PR, Mitchell MA, Zheng XG, Leferovich J, Gao GP, Balice-Gordon RJ, Wilson JM, Stedman HH (1999) Stable restoration of the sarcoglycan complex in dystrophic muscle perfused with histamine and a recombinant adeno-associated viral vector. *Nat Med* 5: 439-443

75. Griggs RC, Moxley RT, 3rd, Mendell JR, Fenichel GM, Brooke MH, Pestronk A, Miller JP, Cwik VA, Pandya S, Robison J, *et al.* (1993) Duchenne dystrophy: randomized, controlled trial of prednisone (18 months) and azathioprine (12 months). *Neurology* 43: 520-527

76. Hagiwara Y, Sasaoka T, Araishi K, Imamura M, Yorifuji H, Nonaka I, Ozawa E, Kikuchi T (2000) Caveolin-3 deficiency causes muscle degeneration in mice. *Hum Mol Genet* 9: 3047-3054

77. Hance JE, Fu SY, Watkins SC, Beggs AH, Michalak M (1999) alpha-actinin-2 is a new component of the dystrophin-glycoprotein complex. *Arch Biochem Biophys* 365: 216-222

78. Hasegawa M, Cuenda A, Spillantini MG, Thomas GM, Buee-Scherrer V, Cohen P, Goedert M (1999) Stress-activated protein kinase-3 interacts with the PDZ domain of alpha1-syntrophin. A mechanism for specific substrate recognition. *J Biol Chem* 274: 12626-12631

79. Hinton VJ, De Vivo DC, Nereo NE, Goldstein E, Stern Y (2001) Selective deficits in verbal working memory associated with a known genetic etiology: the neuropsychological profile of duchenne muscular dystrophy. *J Int Neuropsychol Soc* 7: 45-54

80. Hoffman EP, Brown RH, Jr., Kunkel LM (1987) Dystrophin: the protein product of the Duchenne muscular dystrophy locus. *Cell* 51: 919-928

81. Hoffman EP, Morgan JE, Watkins SC, Partridge TA (1990) Somatic reversion/suppression of the mouse mdx phenotype in vivo. *J Neurol Sci* 99: 9-25

82. Holzfeind PJ, Ambrose HJ, Newey SE, Nawrotzki RA, Blake DJ, Davies KE (1999) Tissue-selective expression of alpha-dystrobrevin is determined by multiple promoters. *J Biol Chem* 274: 6250-6258

83. Hoogerwaard EM, Bakker E, Ippel PF, Oosterwijk JC, Majoor-Krakauer DF, Leschot NJ, Van Essen AJ, Brunner HG, van der Wouw PA, Wilde AA, de Visser M (1999) Signs and symptoms of Duchenne muscular dystrophy and Becker muscular dystrophy among carriers in The Netherlands: a cohort study. *Lancet* 353: 2116-2119

84. Howard MT, Shirts BH, Petros LM, Flanigan KM, Gesteland RF, Atkins JF (2000) Sequence specificity of aminoglycoside-induced stop condon readthrough:

potential implications for treatment of Duchenne muscular dystrophy. *Ann Neurol* 48: 164-169

85. Howard PL, Dally GY, Wong MH, Ho A, Weleber RG, Pillers DM, Ray PN (1998) Localization of dystrophin isoform Dp71 to the inner limiting membrane of the retina suggests a unique functional contribution of Dp71 in the retina. *Hum Mol Genet* 7: 1385-1391

86. Hu XY, Ray PN, Murphy EG, Thompson MW, Worton RG (1990) Duplicational mutation at the Duchenne muscular dystrophy locus: its frequency, distribution, origin, and phenotypegenotype correlation. *Am J Hum Genet* 46: 682-695

87. Im WB, Phelps SF, Copen EH, Adams EG, Slightom JL, Chamberlain JS (1996) Differential expression of dystrophin isoforms in strains of mdx mice with different mutations. *Hum Mol Genet* 5: 1149-1153

88. Infante JP, Huszagh VA (1999) Mechanisms of resistance to pathogenesis in muscular dystrophies. *Mol Cell Biochem* 195: 155-167

89. Jacobson C, Cote PD, Rossi SG, Rotundo RL, Carbonetto S (2001) The dystroglycan complex is necessary for stabilization of acetylcholine receptor clusters at neuromuscular junctions and formation of the synaptic basement membrane. *J Cell Biol* 152: 435-450

90. Jerusalem F, Engel AG, Gomez MR (1974) Duchenne dystrophy. II. Morphometric study of motor end-plate fine structure. *Brain* 97: 123-130

91. Kameya S, Miyagoe Y, Nonaka I, Ikemoto T, Endo M, Hanaoka K, Nabeshima Y, Takeda S (1999) alpha1-syntrophin gene disruption results in the absence of neuronal- type nitric-oxide synthase at the sarcolemma but does not induce muscle degeneration. *J Biol Chem* 274: 2193-2200

92. Karpati G, Carpenter S (1986) Small-caliber skeletal muscle fibers do not suffer deleterious consequences of dystrophic gene expression. *Am J Med Genet* 25: 653-658

93. Karpati G, Zubrzycka-Gaarn EE, Carpenter S, Bulman DE, Ray PN, Worton RG (1990) Age-related conversion of dystrophin-negative to -positive fiber segments of skeletal but not cardiac muscle fibres in heterozygote mdx mice. *J Neuropath Exp Neurol* 49: 96-105

94. Keep NH, Winder SJ, Moores CA, Walke S, Norwood FL, Kendrick-Jones J (1999) Crystal structure of the actin-binding region of utrophin reveals a head-to-tail dimer. *Structure Fold Des* 7: 1539-1546

95. Kingston HM, Sarfarazi M, Thomas NS, Harper PS (1984) Localisation of the Becker muscular dystrophy gene on the short arm of the X chromosome by linkage to cloned DNA sequences. *Hum Genet* 67: 6-17

96. Koenig M, Beggs AH, Moyer M, Scherpf S, Heindrich K, Bettecken T, Meng G, Muller CR, Lindlof M, Kaariainen H, et al. (1989) The molecular basis for Duchenne versus Becker muscular dystrophy: correlation of severity with type of deletion. *Am J Hum Genet* 45: 498-506

97. Koenig M, Hoffman EP, Bertelson CJ, Monaco AP, Feener C, Kunkel LM (1987) Complete cloning of the Duchenne muscular dystrophy (DMD) cDNA and pre-

liminary genomic organization of the DMD gene in normal and affected individuals. *Cell* 50: 509-517

98. Kong JM, Anderson JE (1999) Dystrophin is required for organizing large acetylcholine receptor aggregates. *Brain Res* 839: 298-304

99. Kong JM, Anderson JE (2001) Dynamic restoration of dystrophin to dystrophin deficient myotubes. *Muscle Nerve* 24: 77-88

100. Kuznetsov AV, Winkler K, Wiedemann FR, von Bossanyi P, Dietzmann K, Kunz WS (1998) Impaired mitochondrial oxidative phosphorylation in skeletal muscle of the dystrophin-deficient mdx mouse. *Mol Cell Biochem* 183: 87-96

101. Leibowitz D DV (1981) Intellect and behaviour in Duchenne muscular dystrophy. *Dev Med Child Neurol* 23: 577-590

102. Love DR, Hill DF, Dickson G, Spurr NK, Byth BC, Marsden RF, Walsh FS, Edwards YH, Davies KE (1989) An autosomal transcript in skeletal muscle with homology to dystrophin. *Nature* 339: 55-58

103. Lupski JR, Garcia CA, Zoghbi HY, Hoffman EP, Fenwick RG (1991) Discordance of muscular dystrophy in monozygotic female twins: evidence supporting asymmetric splitting of the inner cell mass in a manifesting carrier of Duchenne dystrophy. *Am J Med Genet* 40: 354-364

104. Ma H, Shih M, Fukiage C, Azuma M, Duncan MK, Reed NA, Richard I, Beckmann JS, Shearer TR (2000) Influence of specific regions in Lp82 calpain on protein stability, activity, and localization within lens. *Invest Ophthalmol Vis Sci* 41: 4232-4239

105. Malhotra SB, Hart KA, Klamut HJ, Thomas NST, Bodrug SE, Burghes AHM, Bobrow M, Harper PS, Thompson MW, Ray PN, Worton RG (1988) Frameshift deletions in patients with Duchenne and Becker muscular dystrophy. *Science* 242: 755-759

106. Mallouk N, Jacquemond V, Allard B (2000) Elevated subsarcolemmal Ca2+ in mdx mouse skeletal muscle fibers detected with Ca2+-activated K+ channels. *Proc Natl Acad Sci U S A* 97: 4950-4955

107. Mann CJ, Honeyman K, Cheng AJ, Ly T, Lloyd F, Fletcher S, Morgan JE, Partridge TA, Wilton SD (2001) Antisense-induced exon skipping and synthesis of dystrophin in the mdx mouse. *Proc Natl Acad Sci U S A* 98: 42-47

108. Matasic R, Dietz AB, Vuk-Pavlovic S (1999) Dexamethasone inhibits dendritic cell maturation by redirecting differentiation of a subset of cells. *J Leukocyte Biol* 66: 909-914

109. McCormas AJ, Sica REP, Currie SJ (1970) Muscular dystrophy: evidence for a neural factor. *Nature* 226: 1263-1264

110. Mechler F, Mastaglia FL, Haggith J, Gardner-Medwin D (1980) Adrenergic receptor responses of vascular smooth muscle in Becker muscular dystrophy. A muscle blood flow study using the 133Xe clearance method. *J Neurol Sci* 46: 291-302

111. Mehler MF (2000) Brain dystrophin, neurogenetics and mental retardation. *Brain Res Rev* 32: 277-307

112. Mendel JR, Engel WK, Derrer EC (1971) Duchenne muscular dystrophy: functional ischemia

reproduces its charcteristic lesions. *Science* 172: 1143-1145

113. Merlini L (1994) Calf myopathy with a twist. *Neuromusc Disord* 4: 13-15

114. Mestroni L, Giacca M (1997) Molecular genetics of dilated cardiomyopathy. *Curr Opin Cardiol* 12: 303-309

115. Minetti C, Beltrame F, Marcenaro G, Bonilla E (1992) Dystrophin at the plasma membrane of human muscle fibres shows a costameric localization. *Neuromusc Disord* 2: 99-109

116. Minetti C, Sotgia F, Bruno C, Scartezzini P, Broda P, Bado M, Masetti E, Mazzocco M, Egeo A, Donati MA, Volonte D, Galbiati F, Cordone G, Bricarelli FD, Lisanti MP, Zara F (1998) Mutations in the caveolin-3 gene cause autosomal dominant limb-girdle muscular dystrophy. *Nat Genet* 18: 365-368

117. Mirabella M, Servidei S, Manfredi G, Ricci E, Frustaci A, Bertini E, Rana M, Tonali P (1993) Cardiomyopathy may be the only clinical manifestation in female carriers of Duchenne muscular dystrophy. *Neurology* 43: 2342-2345

118. Moizard MP, Toutain A, Fournier D, Berret F, Raynaud M, Billard C, Andres C, Moraine C (2000) Severe cognitive impairment in DMD: obvious clinical indication for Dp71 isoform point mutation screening. *Eur J Hum Genet* 8: 552-556

119. Mokri B, Engel AG (1975) Duchenne dystrophy: electron microscopic findings pointing to a basic or early abnormality in the plasma membrane of the muscle fiber. *Neurology* 25: 1111-1120

120. Monaco AP, Bertelson CJ, Liechti-Gallati S, Moser H, Kunkel LM (1988) An explanation for the phenotypic differences between patients bearing partial deletions of the DMD locus. *Genomics* 2: 90-95

121. Morrone A, Zammarchi E, Scacheri PC, Donati MA, Hoop RC, Servidei S, Galluzzi G, Hoffman EP (1997) Asymptomatic dystrophinopathy. *Am J Med Genet* 69: 261-267

122. Muntoni F, Cau M, Ganau A, Congiu R, Arvedi G, Mateddu A, Marrosu MG, Cianchetti C, Realdi G, Cao A, Melis MA (1993) Deletion of the dystrophin muscle-promoter region associated with X-linked dilated cardiomyopathy. *New Engl J Med* 329: 921-925

123. Muntoni F, Mateddu A, Marrosu MG, Cau M, Congiu R, Melis MA, Cao A, Cianchetti C (1992) Variable dystrophin expression in different muscles of a Duchenne muscular dystrophy carrier. *Clin Genet* 42: 35-38

124. Narita S, Yorifuji H (1999) Centrally nucleated fibers (CNFs) compensate the fragility of myofibers in mdx mouse. *NeuroReport* 10: 3233-3235

125. Naya FJ, Mercer B, Shelton J, Richardson JA, Williams RS, Olson EN (2000) Stimulation of slow skeletal muscle fiber gene expression by calcineurin in vivo. *J Biol Chem* 275: 4545-4548

126. Newbell BJ, Anderson JT, Jarrett HW (1997) Ca2+-calmodulin binding to mouse a1 syntrophin: Syntrophin is also a Ca2+-binding protein. *Biochemistry* 36: 1295-1305

127. Nicholson LVB (1993) The "rescue" of dystrophin synthesis in boys with Duchenne muscular dystrophy. *Neuromusc Disord* 3: 525-532

128. Nicholson LVB, Bushby KMD, Johnson MA, Gardner-Medwin D, Ginjaar HB (1993b) Dystrophin expression in Duchenne patients with "in frame" gene deletions. *Neuropediatrics* 24: 93-97

129. Nicholson LVB, Bushby KMD, Johnson MA, Ginjaar HB, Den Dunnen JT, van Ommen G-JB (1992) Predicted and observed sizes of dystrophin in some patients with gene deletions that disrupt the open reading frame. *J Med Genet* 29: 892-896

130. Nicholson LVB, Johnson MA, Bushby KMD, Gardner-Medwin D (1993c) The functional significance of dystrophin-positive fibres in Duchenne muscular dystrophy. *Arch Dis Child* 68: 632-636

131. Nicholson LVB, Johnson MA, Bushby KMD, Gardner-Medwin D, Curtis A, Ginjaar HB, Den Dunnen JT, Welch JL, Butler TJ, Bakker E, van Ommen G-J, Harris JB (1993a) (Trilogy) Integrated study of 100 patients with Xp21-linked muscular dystrophy using clinical, genetic, immunochemical, and histopathological data. Part 1 Trends across the clinical groups. Part 2 Correlations within individual patients. Part 3 Differential diagnosis and prognosis. *J Med Genet* 30: 728-736, 737-744, 745-751

132. Nigro G, Comi LI, Politano L, Bain RJI (1990) The incidence and evolution of cardiomyopathy in Duchenne muscular dystrophy. *Int J Cardiol* 26: 271-277

133. Nigro G, Comi LI, Politano L, Limogelli FM, Nigro V, De Rimini ML, Giugliano MAM, Petretta VR, Passamano L, Restucci B, Fattore L, Tebloev K, De Luca F, Raia P, Esposito MG (1995) Evaluation of the cardiomyopathy in Becker muscular dystrophy. *Muscle & Nerve* 18: 283-291

134. Nobile C, Marchi J, Nigro V, Roberts RG, Danieli GA (1997) Exon-intron organization of the human dystrophin gene. *Genomics* 45: 421-424

135. North KN, Miller G, Iannaccone ST, Clemens PR, Chad DA, Bella I, Smith TW, Beggs AH, Specht LA (1996) Cognitive dysfunction as the major presenting feature of Becker's muscular dystrophy (1). *Neurology* 46: 61-465

136. Pages M, Echenne B, Pages AM, Dimeglio A, Sires A (1985) Multicore disease and Marfan's syndrome: a case report. *Eur Neurol* 24: 170-175

137. Passos-Bueno MR, Bakker E, Kneppers ALJ, Takata RI, Rapaport D, Den Dunnen JT, Zatz M, G-J.B. vO (1992) Different mosaicism frequencies for proximal and distal Duchenne muscular dystrophy (DMD) mutations indicate difference in etiology and recurrence risk. *Am J Hum Genet* 51: 1150-1155

138. Petrof BJ (1998) The molecular basis of activity-induced muscle injury in Duchenne muscular dystrophy. *Mol Cell Biochem* 179: 111-123

139. Pillers D-AM BD, Weleber RG, Sigesmund DA, Musarella MA, Powell BR, Murphey WH, Westall C, Panton C, Becker LE, Worton RG, Ray PN. (1993) Dystrophin expression in the human retina is required for normal function as defined by electroretinography. *Nature Genet* 4: 82-86

140. Pillers DAH, Fitzgerald KM, Duncan NM, Rash SM, White RA, Dwinnell SJ, Powell BR, Schnur RE, Ray PN, Cibis GW, Weleber RG (1999) Duchenne/Becker muscular dystrophy: correlation of phenotype by electroretinography with sites of dystrophin mutations. *Hum Genet* 105: 2-9

141. Politano L, Nigro V, Nigro G, Petretta VR, Passamano L, Papparella S, Di Somma S, Comi LI (1996) Development of cardiomyopathy in female carriers of Duchenne and Becker muscular dystrophies. *JAMA* 275: 1335-1338

142. Porter JD, Rafael JA, Ragusa RJ, Brueckner JK, Trickett JI, Davies KE (1998) The sparing of extraocular muscle in dystrophinopathy is lost in mice lacking utrophin and dystrophin. *J Cell Sci* 111: 1801-1811

143. Prelle A, Medori R, Moggio M, Chan HW, Gallanti A, Scarlato G, Bonilla E (1992) Dystrophin deficiency in a case of congenital myopathy. *J Neurol* 239: 76-78

144. Rafael JA, Brown SC (2000) Dystrophin and utrophin: genetic analyses of their role in skeletal muscle. *Microsc Res Tech* 48: 155-166

145. Reimann J, Irintchev A, Wernig A (2000) Regenerative capacity and the number of satellite cells in soleus muscles of normal and mdx mice. *Neuromusc Disord* 10: 276-282

146. Repetto S, Bado M, Broda P, Lucania G, Masetti E, Sotgia F, Carbone I, Pavan A, Bonilla E, Cordone G, Lisanti MP, Minetti C (1999) Increased number of caveolae and caveolin-3 overexpression in Duchenne muscular dystrophy. *Biochem Biophys Res Commun* 261: 547-550

147. Richards CS, Watkins SC, Hoffman EP, Schneider NR, Milsark IW, Katz KS, Cook JD, Kunkel LM, Cortada JM (1990) Skewed X inactivation in a female MZ twin results in Duchenne muscular dystrophy. *Am J Hum Genet* 46: 672-681

148. Roberts RG, Gardner RJ, Bobrow M (1994) Searching for the 1 in 2,400,000: A review of dystrophin gene point mutations. *Hum Genet* 4: 1-11

149. Russo K, Di Stasio E, Macchia G, Rosa G, Brancaccio A, Petrucci TC (2000) Characterization of the b-dystroglycan-growth factor receptor 2 (Grb2) interaction. *Biochem Biophys Res Commun* 274: 93-98

150. Rybakova IN, Ervasti JM (1997) Dystrophin-glycoprotein complex is monomeric and stabilizes actin filaments in vitro through lateral association. *J Biol Chem* 272: 28771-28778

151. Rybakova IN, Patel JR, Ervasti JM (2000) The dystrophin complex forms a mechanically strong link between the sarcolemma and costameric actin. *J Cell Biol* 150: 1209-1214

152. Sabatelli P, Squarzoni S, Petrini S, Capanni C, Ognibene A, Cartegni L, Cobianchi F, Merlini L, Toniolo D, Maraldi NM (1998) Oral exfoliative cytology for the non-invasive diagnosis in X-linked Emery-Dreifuss muscular dystrophy patients and carriers. *Neuromuscul Disord* 8: 67-71.

153. Sakakibaram H, Engelm AG, Lambertm EH (1977) Duchenne dystrophy: ultrastructural localization of the acetylcholine receptor and intracellular micro-

electrode studies of neuromuscular transmission. *Neurology* 27: 741-7457

154. Samaha FJ, Quinlan JG (1996) Myalgia and cramps: Dystrophinopathy with wide-ranging laboratory findings. *J Child Neurol* 11: 21-24

155. Sander M, Chavoshan B, Harris SA, Iannaccone ST, Stull JT, Thomas GD, Victor RG (2000) Functional muscle ischemia in neuronal nitric oxide synthase-deficient skeletal muscle of children with Duchenne muscular dystrophy. *Proc Natl Acad Sci USA* 97: 13818-13823

156. Simonds AK, Muntoni F, Heather S, Fielding S (1998) Impact of nasal ventilation on survival in hypercapnic Duchenne muscular dystrophy. *Thorax* 53: 949-952

157. Sotgia F, Lee JK, Das K, Bedford M, Petrucci TC, Macioce P, Sargiacomo M, Bricarelli FD, Minetti C, Sudol M, Lisanti MP (2000) Caveolin-3 directly interacts with the C-terminal tail of b-dystroglycan - Identification of a central WW-like domain within caveolin family members. *J Biol Chem* 275: 38048-38058

158. Stedman HH, Sweeney HL, Shrager JB, Maguire HC, Panettieri RA, Petrof B, Narusawa M, Leferovich JM, Sladky JT, Kelly AM (1991) The mdx mouse diaphragm reproduces the degenerative changes of Duchenne muscular dystrophy. *Nature* 352: 536-539

159. Tennyson CN, Klamut HJ, Worton RG (1995) The human dystrophin gene requires 16 hours to be transcribed and is contranscripturally spliced. *Nature Genet* 9: 184-190

160. Thomas GD, Sander M, Lau KS, Huang PL, Stull JT, Victor RG (1998) Impaired metabolic modulation of a-adrenergic vasoconstriction in dystrophin-deficient skeletal muscle. *Proc Natl Acad Sci USA* 95: 15090-15095

161. Tinsley J, Deconinck N, Fisher R, Kahn D, Phelps S, Gillis JM, Davies K (1998) Expression of full-length utrophin prevents muscular dystrophy in mdx mice. *Nature Med* 4: 1441-1444

162. Torrente Y, Tremblay J, Pisati F, Belicch M, Rossi B, Sironi M, Fortunato F, El Fahime M, D'Angelo M, Caron N, Constantin G, Paulin D, Scarlato G, Bresolin N (2001) Intraarterial injection of muscle-derived CD34(+)Sca-1(+) stem cells restores dystrophin in mdx mice. *J Cell Biol* 152: 335-348

163. Turner PR, Westwood T, Regen CM, Steinhardt RA (1988) Increased protein degradation results from elevated free calcium levels found in muscle from mdx mice. *Nature* 335: 735-738

164. Vainzof M, Passos-Bueno MR, Pavanello RCM, Schreiber R, Zatz M (1992) A model to estimate the expression of the dystrophin gene in muscle from female Becker muscular dystrophy carriers. *J Med Genet* 29: 476-479

165. Vainzof M, Pavanello RCM, Pavanello I, Tsanaclis AM, Levy JA, Passos-Bueno MR, Rapaport D, Zatz M (1991) Dystrophin immunofluorescence pattern in manifesting and asymptomatic carriers of Duchenne's and Becker muscular dystrophies of different ages. *Neuromusc Disord* 1: 177-183

166. Valentine BA, Winand NJ, Pradhan D, Moise NS, de Lahunta A, Kornegay JN, Cooper BJ (1992) Canine X-linked muscular dystrophy as an animal model of Duchenne muscular dystrophy: a review. *Am J Med Genet* 42: 352-356

167. Wang B, Li J, Xiao X (2000) Adeno-associated virus vector carrying human minidystrophin genes effectively ameliorates muscular dystrophy in mdx mouse model. *Proc Natl Acad Sci USA* 97: 13714-13719

168. Watkins SC, Cullen MJ, Hoffman EP, Billington L (2000) Plasma membrane cytoskeleton of muscle: a fine structural analysis. *Microsc Res Tech* 48: 131-141

169. Williamson RA, Henry MD, Daniels KJ, Hrstka RF, Lee JC, Sunada Y, Ibraghimov-Beskrovnaya O, Campbell KP (1997) Dystroglycan is essential for early embryonic development: Disruption of Reichert's membrane in Dag1-null mice. *Hum Mol Genet* 6: 831-841

170. Winnard AV, Klein CJ, Coovert DD, Prior T, Papp A, Snyder P, Bulman DE, Ray PN, McAndrew P, King W, Moxley RT, Mendell JR, Burghes AHM (1993) Characterization of translational frame exception patients in Duchenne/Becker muscular dystrophy. *Hum Mol Genet* 2: 737-744

171. Yazaki M, Yoshida K, Nakamura A, Koyama J, Nanba T, Ohori N, Ikeda S (1999) Clinical characteristics of aged Becker muscular dystrophy patients with onset after 30 years. *Eur Neurol* 42: 145-149

172. Yoshida M, Ozawa E (1990) Glycoprotein complex anchoring dystrophin to sarcolemma. *J Biochem* (Tokyo) 108: 748-752

Sarcoglycanopathies

Eric P. Hoffman

AAV	adeno-associated viruses
AchR	acetyl choline receptor
nNos	neuronal nitric oxide synthase
SCARMD	severe chlidhood autosomal recessive muscular dystrophy

Definition of entities

The sarcoglycans are a group of 4 distinct integral membrane proteins, each from a distinct gene, that associate in a tetrameric complex (the sarcoglycan complex). The sarcoglycan complex associates directly with the dystroglycans and indirectly with dystrophin, and is considered a part of the dystrophin-based membrane cytoskeleton of muscle fibres. Recessive, loss-of-function mutations in any one of the 4 genes result in a muscular dystrophy that is indistinguishable from primary dystrophinopathies, and is grouped under the "limb-girdle muscular dystrophies." North African severe childhood autosomal recessive muscular dystrophy (SCARMD) and recessive muscular dystrophy of European gypsies are sarcoglycanopathies that are common in restricted populations.

Molecular genetics and pathogenesis

There are 4 sarcoglycan genes and corresponding proteins: α-sarcoglycan, β-sarcoglycan, γ-sarcoglycan, and δ-sarcoglycan. These proteins range in size from 35 to 50 kD, and each has a single transmembrane domain. The majority of the coding sequence of each protein is on the extracellular face of the membrane, and each protein is glycosylated (Figure 1). The 4 sarcoglycans associate as a tetrameric complex in the Golgi apparatus, with transition to the membrane occurring as a complete, assembled structure (15). The α/β/γ/δ sarcoglycan complex is muscle-specific; however, a fifth protein, ε-sarcoglycan, replaces α-sarco-

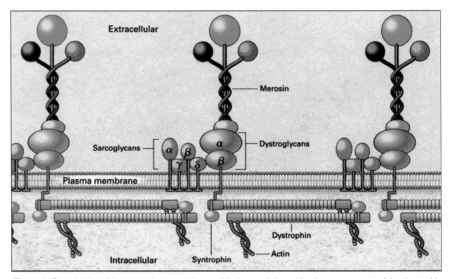

Figure 1. *Organization of the sarcoglycan proteins, and their association with other components of the dystrophin membrane cytoskeleton.* Shown is a schematic of the myofibre plasma membrane cytoskeleton, with the tetrameric sarcoglycan complex stabilizing the association of dystrophin with β-dystroglycan (9). Reprinted with permission of *New England Journal of Medicine* (9).

glycan in some non-striated muscle tissues.

Mutations in any one of the sarcoglycan genes cause a disorder which is clinically indistinguishable from dystrophinopathies (4, 8, 9, 14, 16, 27, 20, 22-25). Importantly, loss-of-function mutations of one of the sarcoglycan genes leads to secondary loss of the other 3 due to failure of the tetrameric complex to assemble and transport to the membrane. For example, homozygous mutations in γ-sarcoglycan show primary loss of γ-sarcoglycan, and also dramatic secondary reductions in α, β, and δ sarcoglycan proteins. The RNA levels of these genes have been found to be normal (5), indicating that the secondary loss of the sarcoglycans occurs at the protein level.

The function of the sarcoglycan complex appears, at least in part, to stabilise the association of the transmembrane β dystroglycan protein with sub-sarcolemmal dystrophin (Figure 1). Destabilization of any part of the dystrophin/dystroglycan association leads to secondary loss of many of the com-

ponents, and subsequent membrane instability. This is particularly true with the sarcoglycans, where loss-of-function mutations of one sarcoglycan leads to dramatic secondary biochemical loss of the other three sarcoglycans. The secondary deficiencies of the sarcoglycans, both in primary sarcoglycanopathies and primary dystrophinopathies, are due to degradation of the proteins as they are unable to assemble at the plasma membrane (sarcolemma) correctly.

The pathogenesis of the sarcoglycanopathies is likely very similar to that of dystrophin-deficiency (Duchenne muscular dystrophy, chapter 2.1), as both involve loss of the integrity of the dystrophin-based membrane cytoskeleton (Figure 2). Loss of the sarcoglycans or dystrophin leads to membrane instability, with consequent efflux of cytoplasmic components, such as serum creatine kinase, out of the myofibre, and influx of calcium and other material into the cell (27). The "leaky membranes" mimic sub-cytotoxic membrane damage during eccentric exercise in normal muscle; however, the damage to the dystrophic muscle is constant and persistent. Functional ischaemia is likely present due to loss of nNOS at the membrane; the ischaemia exacerbates calcium influx and membrane damage, leading to myofibre degeneration and regeneration either in isolated fibres or in groups of myofibres. Inflammatory cells (T cells, mast cells, and dendritic cells) serve to further exacerbate the membrane damage via toxic mediators (proteases and cytokines), leading to eventual failure of regeneration and muscle wasting (Figure 2) (5). It is important to note that there are other membrane cytoskeletal networks, particularly the vinculin/integrin/laminin network, which are partially redundant with the dystrophin-based membrane cytoskeleton. Each network has distinct signal transduction roles.

Structural changes

Patient muscle shows a dystrophic myopathy, indistinguishable from Duchenne/Becker muscular dystrophies, with evidence of degeneration and regeneration of myofibres, both singly and in groups (Figure 3). Light microscopic features include myofibre size variation, increased number of central nuclei, and endomysial fibrosis. The pathological changes, like the clinical symptoms, are progressive, with end-stage muscle showing fibrofatty replacement and failed regeneration.

Diagnosis is typically done by protein analyses of patient muscle biopsy, using either immunohistochemistry or immunoblotting for the sarcoglycan proteins (Figure 3). The sarcoglycan proteins show secondary deficiency in primary dystrophinopathies, so interpretation of sarcoglycan immunostaining or immunoblotting must be done in the context of dystrophin protein studies (Table 1). Gene mutation studies are encouraged to confirm the biochemical findings, and localize the primary defect to a specific sarcoglycan gene.

Primary sarcoglycanopathy patients typically show a dramatic reduction in all four sarcoglycan proteins. Dys-

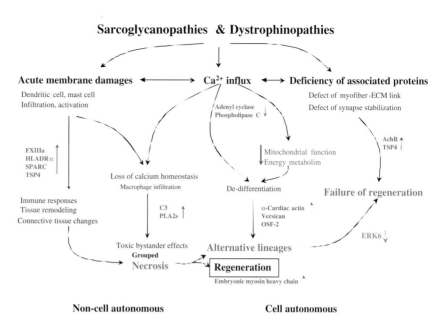

Sarcoglycanopathies & Dystrophinopathies

Figure 2. *Pathogenesis of the sarcoglycanopathies and dystrophinopathies.* Shown is a schematic flow-chart, showing the primary and secondary (downstream) consequences of defects of loss of any one of the sarcoglycan proteins, or dystrophin. This model is based upon both the literature, and expression profiling results (5). Reprinted with permission of the Journal of Cell Biology (5).

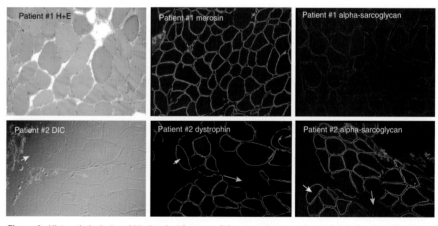

Figure 3. *Histopathological and biochemical features of the sarcoglycans and associated disorders.* Shown are muscle biopsy sections from a primary sarcoglycanopathy patient (Patient #1, top panels), and a female manifesting carrier of Duchenne muscular dystrophy (Patient #2, bottom panels). The primary sarcoglycanopathy patient (Patient #1) shows a dystrophic muscle biopsy by H & E staining, although the dystrophic process is relatively mild in nature, with only minor fibrotic changes. Merosin (laminin α2) immunostaining shows a normal pattern, while immunostaining for α-sarcoglycan shows dramatic reduction of the protein.
The sarcoglycan proteins show secondary biochemical deficiency in primary dystrophinopathies, as exemplified by the manifesting carrier of Duchenne dystrophy (Patient #2). The white arrows point to the same dystrophin-positive muscle fibre in each of the three panels, which shows strong immunostaining for both dystrophin and α-sarcoglycan. The pale red arrow shows the same dystrophin-negative muscle fibre in each panel. This fibre shows secondary loss of α-sarcoglycan, consequent to primary dystrophin-deficiency.

trophin immunostaining can be normal or "Becker-like" (weak and variable), but this is due to poor localization of dystrophin at the plasma membrane; immunoblotting typically shows normal size and amount of dystrophin in primary sarcoglycanopathy patients. Merosin immunostaining is normal (Figure 3).

Mutations in any single sarcoglycan gene result in secondary biochemical reductions of the other three sarcoglycans (Table 1). Thus, immunostaining with a single sarcoglycan antibody is reported to be sufficient to detect all primary sarcoglycanopathy patients (9). In other words, routine use of α-sarcoglycan antibodies (the most com-

	Chromosome; Gene Symbol	Limb-girdle subtype; Common mutations	Sub-population?	Secondary deficiency in primary dystrophinopathy?	Secondary deficiency in other sarcoglycanopathies?	Animal model
α-sarcoglycan	17q12-21 SGCA	LGMD2D R77C (50% alleles)	None Most common of sarcoglycanopathies	Yes	Yes	knock-out mouse
β-sarcoglycan	4q12 SGCB	LGMD2E	None	Yes	Yes	knock-out mouse
γ-sarcoglycan	13q13 SGCG	LGM2DC del645T (North Africa) C283Y (Gypsies)	North Africa (SCARMD); Western European Gypsies	Yes	Yes	knock-out mouse
δ-sarcoglycan	5q33 SGCD	LGMD2F	Brazil Least common of the sarcoglycanopathies	Yes	Yes	cardiomyopathic hamster (Bio14.6)
ε-sarcoglycan	7q21-22 SGCE	no disease association; replaces α-sarcoglycan in smooth muscle				

Table 1. The sarcglycanopathies.

mon of the sarcoglycanopathies) will detect patients with β-, γ-, or δ-sarcoglycan mutations. Many patients will show the greatest reductions in the specific sarcoglycan protein, which harbors mutations. For example, patients with γ-sarcoglycan gene mutations typically show complete absence of γ-sarcoglycan protein, and partial loss of α-, β-, and δ-sarcoglycan proteins. Thus, it is possible in some cases to predict the specific sarcoglycan gene which harbors the causative mutations. However, such correlations are not perfect (ie, completely sensitive and specific), and some laboratories test for only a single sarcoglycan protein as this will still detect all primary sarcoglycanopathies. Many laboratories prefer to test for all four sarcoglycan proteins so that better targeting of mutation studies can be accomplished.

Most patients with complete absence of one or more sarcoglycan proteins (with normal dystrophin) will show mutations in 1 of the 4 sarcoglycan genes (9). However, many sarcoglycanopathy patients show partial reductions in immunostaining patterns, and this finding is less specific for primary sarcoglycanopathies. Thus, in all cases, it is important to follow biochemical studies with gene mutation studies so that a specific diagnosis can

be made. Mutation studies are complicated as each sarcoglycan gene contains around 20 exons. In some subpopulations, a specific mutation is seen in a specific sarcoglycan gene; North Africans typically show a single base deletion in γ-sarcoglycan, while European Gypsies typically show a γ-sarcoglycan missense mutation (Table 1) (23). There is also a relatively common α-sarcoglycan mutation in Caucasians that accounts for approximately 50% of alleles (R77C) (24).

Genotype–phenotype correlations

The shared pathogenesis between the sarcoglycanopathies and dystrophinopathies fits well with the clinical pictures of these disorders, which are indistinguishable from each other. The sarcoglycans show a wide spectrum of clinical severity, much as the dystrophinopathies, from severe (Duchenne-like) to asymptomatic hyperCKemia (1, 2, 9, 19, 24). The severity of the sarcoglycanopathy correlates with the type of mutation (deletion vs. missense) and residual protein present. Alpha-sarcoglycanopathy patients typically show missense mutations, and these can vary from Duchenne-like to asymptomatic. The other sarcoglycanopathies (β, γ, δ) show a higher frequency of deletion mutations, which lead to complete loss

of the corresponding protein, and a more severe phenotype (Duchenne-like). All patients present with primarily proximal weakness, and all show striking elevations of serum creatine kinase.

Cardiac involvement is variable, and typically sub-clinical (detectable through EKG and/or echocardiography) (11, 18).

Future perspectives

Patient management is done as for primary dystrophinopathies. Corticosteroids have been reported to show similar efficacy in primary sarcoglycanopathies, as they do in dystrophinopathies (6). As membrane instability likely has a central role in pathogenesis, activities that put excessive stress on the muscle, such as eccentric exercise, should be avoided.

The low incidence of the primary sarcoglycanopathies makes it difficult to establish large-scale clinical trials; however, it is expected that any treatment that proves effective in the primary dystrophinopathies will also show efficacy in the primary sarcoglycanopathies. A series of clinical trials in Duchenne dystrophy patients have begun based on emerging pathophysiological data, and there is promise that these will lead to more effective treatments which slow the progression of both the dystrophinopathies and sarcoglycanopathies (5, 10).

The primary sarcoglycanopathies have become a major focus for gene delivery experimentation (ie, "gene therapy"). Indeed, there is considerably more success reported for gene delivery in animal models of the sarcoglycanopathies than there is for the much more common dystrophinopathies. This is because the sarcoglycan genes are much easier to work with and rodent animal models exist for each of the 4 sarcoglycanopathies (3). The sarcoglycan coding sequences (cDNAs) are only about 1.5 kb in size, in contrast to the dystrophin cDNA which is nearly 10-times larger (11 kb).

Particularly encouraging have been a series of reports using recombinant adeno-associated virus (AAV) as a vehicle to deliver the sarcoglycan genes to sarcoglycan-deficient dystrophic rodent muscle. AAV is a virus that infects up to 80% of normal individuals, and muscle tissue appears to be a major tissue site for infection (28). The virus is considered "non-pathogenic," as it causes no known untoward tissue pathology or clinical symptoms. It requires a helper virus to undergo its life cycle, and probably attenuates other pathogenic viruses; it may be considered a parasite of other more harmful viruses. Indeed, the virus may be beneficial in some instances, with reports of the virus protecting from HPV-induced cervical carcinoma, and polymyositis (28). Thus, AAV seems ideal as a gene delivery vehicle for muscle and the muscular dystrophies. A major limitation of recombinant AAV is the fact that it can only package genes of 5 kb or less. This precludes use of the virus for delivery of the full-length dystrophin cDNA; however, the sarcoglycan genes easily fit within the packaging constraints of AAV.

A series of impressive reports of sarcoglycan gene delivery have been published, with up to 80% of large muscle groups showing complete histological and functional rescue by single injections of recombinant AAV con-taining specific sarcoglycan genes (7, 12, 13, 27, 29). The most success has been reported for δ-sarcoglycan, due to the pre-existence of the cardiomyopathic hamster (Bio 14.6) which has a sporadically occurring mutation of the δ-sarcoglycan gene (21, 27).

Intramuscular injections in the tibialis anterior of the dystrophic hamster have shown complete functional recovery of the muscle (29), and delivery via permeabilised vascular route has led to high scale transduction of the entire leg of the hamster (12). δ-sarcoglycan human patients are exceedingly rare, and no human trials have yet been attempted in these patients. More recent studies of gene delivery in γ- and α-sarcoglycan in knock-out mouse models also show promise, although there is concern that appropriate levels of protein expression must be attained. A human clinical trial for recombinant AAV in sarcoglycanopathies was begun in 1999 (26), but then halted due to concerns about the safety of gene therapy trials in general. Given the apparent lack of toxicity of AAV vectors, it is hoped that new trials can begin in the near future.

References

1. Angelini C, Fanin M, Freda MP, Duggan DJ, Siciliano G, Hoffman EP (1999) The clinical spectrum of sarcoglycanopathies. *Neurology* 52: 176-179

2. Angelini C, Fanin M, Menegazzo E, Freda MP, Duggan DJ, Hoffman EP (1998) Homozygous α-sarcoglycan mutation in two siblings: one asymptomatic and one steroid-responsive mild limb-girdle muscular dystrophy patient. *Muscle Nerve* 21: 769-775

3. Araishi K, Sasaoka T, Imamura M, Noguchi S, Hama H, Wakabayashi E, Yoshida M, Hori T, Ozawa E (1999) Loss of the sarcoglycan complex and sarcospan leads to muscular dystrophy in β-sarcoglycan-deficient mice. *Hum Mol Genet* 8: 1589-1598

4. Bonnemann CG, Modi R, Noguchi S, Mizuno Y, Yoshida M, Gussoni E, McNally EM, Duggan DJ, Angelini C, Hoffman EP, Kunkel LM (1995) B-sarcoglycan (A3b) mutations cause autosomal recessive muscular dystrophy with loss of the sarcoglycan complex. *Nat Genet* 11: 266-273

5. Chen YW, Zhao P, Borup R, Hoffman EP (2000) Expression profiling in the muscular dystrophies: identification of novel aspects of molecular pathophysiology. *J Cell Biol* 151: 1321-1336

6. Connolly AM, Pestronk A, Mehta S, Al-Lozi M (1998) Primary a-sarcoglycan deficiency responsive to immunosuppression over three years. *Muscle Nerve* 21: 1549-1553

7. Cordier L, Hack AA, Scott MO, Barton-Davis ER, Gao G, Wilson JM, McNally EM, Sweeney HL (2000) Rescue of skeletal muscles of γ-sarcoglycan-deficient mice with adeno-associated virus-mediated gene transfer. *Mol Ther* 1: 119-129

8. Duggan DJ, Manchester D, Stears KP, Mathews DJ, Hart C, Hoffman EP (1997) Mutations in the δ-sarcoglycan gene are a rare cause of autosomal recessive limb-girdle muscular dystrophy (LGMD2). *Neurogenetics* 1: 49-58

9. Duggan DJ, Gorospe JR, Fanin M, Hoffman EP, Angelini C (1997) Mutations in the sarcoglycan genes in patients with myopathy. *N Engl J Med* 336: 618-624

10. Escolar DM, Henricson EK, Mayhew J, Florence J, Leshner R, Patel K, Clemens PR, and the CINRG Investigators (2001) Clinical evaluator reliability for quantitative and manual muscle testing measures of strength in children. *Muscle Nerve*, in press

11. Gnecchi-Ruscone T, Taylor J, Mercuri E, Paternostro G, Pogue R, Bushby K, Sewry C, Muntoni F, Camici PG (1999) Cardiomyopathy in Duchenne, Becker, and sarcoglycanopathies: a role for coronary dysfunction? *Muscle Nerve* 22: 1549-1556

12. Greelish JP, Su LT, Lankford EB, Burkman JM, Chen H, Konig SK, Mercier IM, Desjardins PR, Mitchell MA, Zheng XG, Leferovich J, Gao GP, Balice-Gordon RJ, Wilson JM, Stedman HH (1999) Stable restoration of the sarcoglycan complex in dystrophic muscle perfused with histamine and a recombinant adeno-associated viral vector. *Nat Med* 5: 439-443

13. Li J, Dressman D, Tsao YP, Sakamoto A, Hoffman EP, Xiao X (1999) rAAV vector-mediated sarcogylcan gene transfer in a hamster model for limb girdle muscular dystrophy. *Gene Ther* 6: 74-82

14. Lim LE, Duclos F, Broux O, Bourg N, Sunada Y, Allamand V, Meyer J, Richard I, Moomaw C, Slaughter C, *et al.* (1995) B-sarcoglycan: characterization and role in limb-girdle muscular dystrophy linked to 4q12. *Nat Genet* 11: 257-265

15. Liu LA, Engvall E (1999) Sarcoglycan isoforms in skeletal muscle. *J Biol Chem* 274: 38171-38176

16. Ljunggren A, Duggan D, McNally E, Boylan KB, Gama CH, Kunkel LM, Hoffman EP (1995) Primary adhalin deficiency as a cause of muscular dystrophy in patients with normal dystrophin. *Ann Neurol* 38: 367-372

17. McNally EM, Duggan D, Gorospe JR, Bonnemann CG, Fanin M, Pegoraro E, Lidov HG, Noguchi S, Ozawa E, Finkel RS, Cruse RP, Angelini C, Kunkel LM, Hoffman EP (1996) Mutations that disrupt the carboxyl-terminus of γ-sarcoglycan cause muscular dystrophy. *Hum Mol Genet* 5: 1841-1847

18. Melacini P, Fanin M, Duggan DJ, Freda MP, Berardinelli A, Danieli GA, Barchitta A, Hoffman EP, Dalla Volta S, Angelini C (1999) Heart involvement in muscular dystrophies due to sarcoglycan gene mutations. *Muscle Nerve* 22: 473-479

19. Merlini L, Kaplan JC, Navarro C, Barois A, Bonneau D, Brasa J, Echenne B, Gallano P, Jarre L, Jeanpierre M, Kalaydjieva L, Leturcq F, Levi-Gomes A,

Toutain A, Tournev I, Urtizberea A, Vallat JM, Voit T, Warter JM (2000) Homogeneous phenotype of the gypsy limb-girdle MD with the γ-sarcoglycan C283Y mutation. *Neurology* 54: 1075-1079

20. Nigro V, de Sa Moreira E, Piluso G, Vainzof M, Belsito A, Politano L, Puca AA, Passos-Bueno MR, Zatz M (1996) Autosomal recessive limb-girdle muscular dystrophy, LGMD2F, is caused by a mutation in the δ-sarcoglycan gene. *Nat Genet* 14: 195-198

21. Nigro V, Okazaki Y, Belsito A, Piluso G, Matsuda Y, Politano L, Nigro G, Ventura C, Abbondanza C, Molinari AM, Acampora D, Nishimura M, Hayashizaki Y, Puca GA (1997) Identification of the Syrian hamster cardiomyopathy gene. *Hum Mol Genet* 6: 601-607

22. Noguchi S, McNally EM, Ben Othmane K, Hagiwara Y, Mizuno Y, Yoshida M, Yamamoto H, Bonnemann CG, Gussoni E, Denton PH, et al (1995) Mutations in the dystrophin-associated protein γ-sarcoglycan in chromosome13 muscular dystrophy. *Science* 270: 819-822

23. Piccolo F, Jeanpierre M, Leturcq F, Dode C, Azibi K, Toutain A, Merlini L, Jarre L, Navarro C, Krishnamoorthy R, Tome FM, Urtizberea JA, Beckmann JS, Campbell KP, Kaplan JC (1996) A founder mutation in the γ-sarcoglycan gene of gypsies possibly predating their migration out of India. *Hum Mol Genet* 5: 2019-2022

24. Piccolo F, Roberds SL, Jeanpierre M, Leturcq F, Azibi K, Beldjord C, Carrie A, Recan D, Chaouch M, Reghis A, et al (1995) Primary adhalinopathy: a common cause of autosomal recessive muscular dystrophy of variable severity. *Nat Genet* 10: 243-245

25. Roberds SL, Leturcq F, Allamand V, Piccolo F, Jeanpierre M, Anderson RD, Lim LE, Lee JC, Tome FM, Romero NB, et al (1994) Missense mutations in the adhalin gene linked to autosomal recessive muscular dystrophy. *Cell* 78: 625-633

26. Stedman H, Wilson JM, Finke R, Kleckner AL, Mendell J (2000) Phase I clinical trial utilizing gene therapy for limb girdle muscular dystrophy: α-, β-, γ-, or δ-sarcoglycan gene delivered with intramuscular instillations of adeno-associated vectors. *Hum Gene Ther* 11: 777-790

27. Straub V, Duclos F, Venzke DP, Lee JC, Cutshall S, Leveille CJ, Campbell KP (1998) Molecular pathogenesis of muscle degeneration in the δ-sarcoglycan-deficient hamster. *Am J Pathol* 153: 1623-1630

28. Tezak Z, Nagaraju K, Plotz P, and Hoffman EP (2000) Adeno-associated virus in normal and myositis human skeletal muscle. *Neurology* 55: 1913-1917

29. Xiao X, Li J, Tsao YP, Dressman D, Hoffman EP, Watchko JF (2000) Full functional rescue of a complete muscle (TA) in dystrophic hamsters by adeno-associated virus vector-directed gene therapy. *J Virol* 74: 1436-1442

Dysferlinopathies

Mengfatt Ho
Anthony Amato
Robert H. Brown

DGC	dystrophin glycoprotein complex
DYSF	human dysferlin gene
LGMD 2B	limb girdle muscular dystrophy type 2B
MM	Miyoshi myopathy

Definition of entities

Miyoshi myopathy and limb girdle muscular dystrophy type 2B. Autosomal recessive forms of muscular dystrophies constitute a genetically heterogeneous group of disorders (9). Although proximal muscles of the extremities are predominantly affected, there are rare cases that preferentially involve the distal muscles. Recently, two forms of muscular dystrophy, limb girdle muscular dystrophy type 2B (LGMD 2B) and a form of distal myopathy known as Miyoshi myopathy (MM), have been reported to arise from defects in the same genetic locus (4, 15). This was particularly intriguing because MM and LGMD 2B were considered to be distinct clinical entities as different muscle groups are preferentially involved in each disorder.

MM is a young adult onset disease characterized by weakness that initially affects the distal parts of the legs, most commonly in the gastrocnemius muscles. Thus, inability to stand on tiptoe is a common early symptom. Proximal lower and upper limb weakness often develops as the disease progresses, and some patients become non-ambulant 10 to 20 years after onset of the disease (14). In contrast, individuals with LGMD 2B develop weakness in the proximal muscles at onset, involving predominantly the lower limbs. Interestingly, the distal muscles of the arms and legs are relatively spared even at late stages of the disease. Despite these differences, MM and LGMD 2B share several common features. Both disorders have an autosomal recessive mode of inheritance. Onset is typically in the late teens or early adulthood, with no previous history of muscle weakness. The initial symptoms in both diseases are difficulty in climbing stairs and in running. Both are characterized by marked elevations in the levels of the muscle enzyme creatine kinase, typically 10 to 150 times above normal levels. Cardiac muscles and respiratory muscles are not involved in either disorder.

Molecular genetics and pathogenesis

In previous studies, two groups have mapped the gene for MM and LGMD 2B to the same genetic region on chromosome 2p13 (5, 6). This has fueled speculation that two apparently distinct muscle diseases might be allelic variants of the same gene. Support for this idea came from the description of two large inbred kindreds whose members include both MM and LGMD 2B patients (13, 22). This concept was eventually confirmed by reports that MM and LGMD2B both arise from defects in the gene encoding the protein "dysferlin." (4, 15).

The human dysferlin gene, designated *DYSF*, is relatively large and complex. *DYSF* spans a genomic region of at least 150 kb (3). It is composed of 55 exons whose sizes range from 30 bp to 461 bp. Northern blot analysis reveals that *DYSF* is highly expressed in skeletal muscles, heart, and placenta. Remarkably, an equally abundant but shorter transcript of about 3.5 kb is detected exclusively in brain. Further analysis shows that this transcript is widely expressed in all regions of the human brain. However, there have been no reports of cognitive impairment or mental retardation in MM or LGMD 2B patients.

The translated sequence of *DYSF* is predicted to encode the 237 kDa dysferlin protein, composed of 2080 amino acids. This protein had no homology to any known mammalian protein at the time of its cloning. However, it does show significant homology to *fer-1*, a *Caenorhabditis elegans* protein required for the fusion of membranous organelles with the plasma membrane of sperm to produce fertile spermatozoa (1). Like *fer-1*, dysferlin is predicted to have a single transmembrane segment at its carboxyl terminus and is thought to be a type II membrane protein where most of the protein would be placed within the cytoplasm and it is anchored to the membrane at its C-terminus. Support for this proposed topology came from recent immunohistochemical studies that showed dysferlin expression at the plasma membrane of muscle cells (2, 16). Moreover, the distribution of dysferlin in myofibres is strikingly similar to that of dystrophin. However, the expression and localization of dystrophin and components of the dystrophin glycoprotein complex (DGC) are unaffected in MM and LGMD 2B patients, suggesting that dysferlin is unlikely to be an integral part of the DGC (2).

The predicted cytoplasmic portion of dysferlin contains between four to six motifs that are homologous to so-called C2 domains (10, 15). C2 domains are typically found in proteins that function in signal transduction or in membrane trafficking, such as protein kinase C and synaptotamins. These domains interact with multiple targets including calcium, phospholipids, or other proteins, to mediate signaling events or membrane fusions (18). These findings, together with the membrane fusion function of *fer-1* in *C. elegans*, suggest that muscle degeneration in the absence of dysferlin may reflect defects in one or more processes of muscle membrane fusion or trafficking.

Following the cloning of dysferlin, two additional human genes with

Ferlin Family

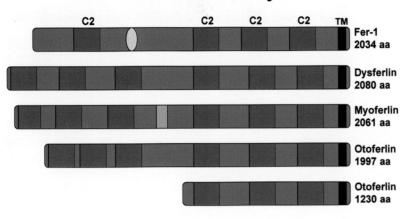

Figure 1. *Ferlin family.* Schematic representation of members of the ferlin family showing the sites of common structural motifs such as C2 domains (shaded box) and the putative transmembrane segment (TM) found in all *fer-1* related proteins. Otoferlin is predicted to encode both long and short forms of the protein via alternative splicing. In addition, myoferlin and fer-1 are predicted to have a SH3 domain (green box) and a saposin B domain (yellow oval) respectively.

strong homology to *fer-1* were identified, indicating the existence of a family of *fer-1* related proteins (Figure 1). While members of this family share common structural features, such as multiple C2 domains and a putative transmembrane segment at its carboxyl-terminus, they differ in their expression profiles. *Otoferlin*, showing 55% similarity to dysferlin, is predominantly expressed in cells of the inner ear and has been implicated in an autosomal recessive form of non-syndromic deafness, DFNB9 (23, 24). On the other hand, *myoferlin* or *Fer-1L3* is the most closely related member to dysferlin showing 68% similarity at the amino acid level. It is abundantly expressed in heart, lung, and the placenta, and is localized at the nuclear and plasma membranes of skeletal muscles (8, 10). To date, there are no mutant phenotypes associated with mutations in myoferlin. Nevertheless, it is noteworthy that myoferlin expression is upregulated in *mdx* mice: a mouse model for Duchenne muscular dystrophy. These findings suggest that myoferlin might be a candidate gene for muscular dystrophy and cardiomyopathy, or as a modifier gene in the selective patterning of muscle involvement in dysferlinopathies (10).

Recently, a splice site mutation in the dysferlin gene has been identified in the *SJL* mouse, making it a natural mouse model for dysferlinopathies (7, 20). These animals develop a progressive muscle weakness with dystrophic pathology. Interestingly, this highly inbred strain also has a number of immune and inflammatory phenotypes not commonly seen in human dysferlinopathies.

Structural changes

Histopathology. As with the other forms of LGMD, muscle biopsy from LGMD 2B and MM patients shows non-specific myopathic changes that include marked variations in fibre size, centrally situated nuclei, fibre splitting, scattered necrotic and regenerating fibres, and an occasional perivascular infiltrate comprising lymphocytes and macrophages. There is increased connective tissue in the endomysium and perimysium. Fibre type distribution is normal and rimmed vacuoles and ragged red fibres are absent.

Immunohistochemistry. In healthy muscle, dysferlin immunoreactivity is localized along the plasma membrane of muscle fibres (Figure 2). This pattern of immunostaining is either completely absent or markedly reduced in LGMD 2B and MM patients, depending on the nature of the genetic mutation (Figure 2). Moreover, in some partially dysferlin-deficient cases, a clear cytoplasmic staining was observed (17). It is noteworthy that a recent study has found reduced dysferlin immunoreactivity in about half of sacroglycanopathies and 20% of dystrophinopathies examined, indicating that diminished dysferlin expression could be due to secondary processes related to muscle cell degeneration (17).

Electron microscopy. Ultrastructural analysis of dysferlin-deficient muscle reveals extensive plasma membrane defects in necrotic fibres characterized by membrane discontinuities and deep invaginations (Figure 3). Small membrane discontinuities (ranging from 0.11-1.8 μm), are seen in non-necrotic fibres as well (19). In addition, an increased number of small vesicles can be found close to the plasma membrane defects. Also seen are apparent exophytic projections of the surface membrane (papillary projections). Also, the basement membrane is altered in dysferlin-deficient muscle fibres, showing thickening as well as focal duplication along the plasma membrane (Figure 3) (19).

Genotype-phenotype correlations

Despite its relatively large size, the mutations identified in the dysferlin gene have been predominantly single nucleotide changes, involving substitutions or deletions leading to reduced levels or complete absence of the protein. The only exception to this observation is the report of a 23 bp duplication in a large kindred of Palestinian-Arabic origin (4).

Unlike Duchenne muscular dystrophy, there is no apparent mutation hotspot in the dysferlin gene. In addition, there is no correlation between the site of mutation or its type, with the clinical phenotype (3). Therefore, it remains unexplained why mutations in the dysferlin gene can give rise to either a predominantly proximal or distal phenotype. Furthermore, the same mutation in a family can lead to variable phenotypes among affected members; differing either in severity or in the distribution of muscle weakness (11, 12, 21). These findings indicate that mutations in the dysferlin gene do not solely determine the phenotype, and additional factors, genetic or environmental, may contribute to modify the phenotype.

Future perspectives

In the past decade, the identification of novel skeletal muscle genes has provided new insights and understanding into the molecular pathogenesis of muscular dystrophies. These studies have identified several pathogenic mechanisms in muscular dystrophies, namely *i)* loss of integrity of the muscle cell membrane, for example, defects in dystrophin and dystrophin-associated proteins (chapter 2), *ii)* mitochondrial disorders affecting energy production (chapter 10.3), and *iii)* altered enzymatic activity of the muscle enzyme calpain (chapter 8.2.1). Defects in dysferlin do not fall into any of the above categories, and therefore, may define a novel pathogenic mechanism in muscular dystrophy.

To better understand the molecular basis in dysferlinopathies, it is essential to determine the normal biological function of dysferlin. This knowledge will be useful not only to understand how dysferlin deficiency causes myofibre degeneration, but also for the future development of effective therapies. In addition, it would be helpful to identify proteins that normally interact with dysferlin to evaluate their roles and their contribution, if any, to the variable phenotypes. One approach is to use gene chips to compare expression profiles of normal and diseased muscles. Such a study could provide valuable information to define the pathophysio-

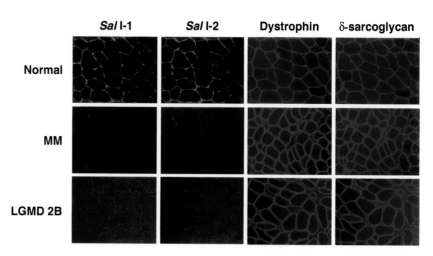

Figure 2. Immunofluorescent staining of Miyoshi myopathy (MM), LGMD2B, and normal muscle for dysferlin (using Sal I-1 and Sal I-2 anti-dysferlin antibodies), dystrophin and δ-sarcoglycan. In the normal muscle dysferlin as well as dystrophin and δ-sarcoglycan are expressed at the plasma membrane. By contrast in MM and LGMD2B dysferlin protein is not expressed in contrast to the normal staining of dystrophin and δ-sarcoglycan. Modified from Matsuda et al. (16).

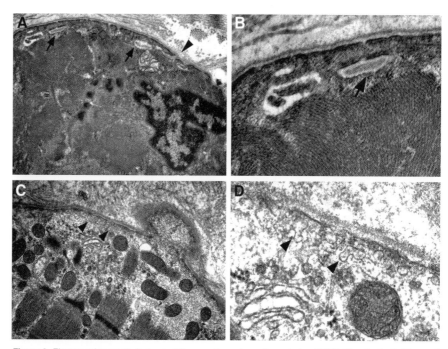

Figure 3. Electron microscopic features of the sarcolemmal membrane in two LGMD 2B patients. **A.** Biopsy of patient #1 shows a highly convoluted sarcolemma with deep invaginations (arrowhead) into the sarcoplasm. **B.** At higher magnification, these invaginations appear as cytoplasmic vesicles (arrow) that contain electron dense basement membrane material. **C, D.** Biopsy of patient #2 shows an abundance of pinocytotic vesicles (arrowheads) beneath the sarcolemmal membrane that are scattered throughout the sarcoplasm. Figure C illustrates in addition a papillary exophytic defects in the sarcolemma with thickening of the basement membrane. Electron micrographs kindly provided by Dr Keith L. Ligon and Dr Jennifer A. Chan.

logical pathways involved in muscle cell degeneration. This strategy may be particularly useful to help identify factors that influence muscle patterning in dysferlinopathies. Thus, comparative analysis of gene expression from affected individuals with the same mutations but different distributions of muscle weakness may yield clues to the identity of the modifying factors.

References

1. Achanzar WE, Ward S (1997) A nematode gene required for sperm vesicle fusion. *J Cell Sci* 110: 1073-1081

2. Anderson LV, Davison K, Moss JA, Young C, Cullen MJ, Walsh J, Johnson MA, Bashir R, Britton S, Keers S (1999) Dysferlin is a plasma membrane protein and is expressed early in human development. *Hum Mol Genet* 8: 855-861

3. Aoki M, Liu J, Richard I, Bashir R, Britton S, Keers SM, Oeltjen J, Brown HEV, Marchand S, Bourg N, Beley C, McKenna-Yasek D, Arahata A, Bohlega S, Cupler E, Illa I, Mahjneh I, Barohn RJ, Urtizberea JA, Fardeau M, Amato A, Angelini C, Bushby K, Beckmann JS, Brown RH, Jr (2001) Genomic organization of the dysferlin gene and novel mutations in Miyoshi myopathy. *Neurology* 57: 271-278

4. Bashir R, Britton S, Strachan T, Keers S, Vafiadaki E, Lako M, Richard I, Marchand S, Bourg N, Argov Z, Sadeh M, Mahjneh I, Marconi G, Passos-Bueno MR, Moreira E, Zatz M, Beckmann JS, Bushby K (1998) A gene related to Caenorhabditis elegans spermatogenesis factor fer-1 is mutated in limb-girdle muscular dystrophy type 2B. *Nat Genet* 20: 37-42

5. Bashir R, Strachan T, Keers S, Stephenson A, Mahjneh I, Marconi G, Nashef L, Bushby KM (1994) A gene for autosomal recessive limb-girdle muscular dystrophy maps to chromosome 2p. *Hum Mol Genet* 3: 455-457

6. Bejaoui K, Hirabayashi K, Hentati F, Haines JL, Ben Hamida C, Belal S, Miller RG, McKenna-Yasek D, Weissenbach J, Rowland LP (1995) Linkage of Miyoshi myopathy (distal autosomal recessive muscular dystrophy) locus to chromosome 2p12-14. *Neurology* 45: 768-772

7. Bittner RE, Anderson LV, Burkhardt E, Bashir R, Vafiadaki E, Ivanova S, Raffelsberger T, Maerk I, Hoger H, Jung M (1999) Dysferlin deletion in SJL mice (SJL-Dysf) defines a natural model for limb girdle muscular dystrophy 2B. *Nat Genet* 23: 141-142

8. Britton S, Freeman T, Vafiadaki E, Keers S, Harrison R, Bushby K, Bashir R (2000) The third human FER-1-like protein is highly similar to dysferlin. *Genomics* 68: 313-321

9. Brown RJ (1997) Dystrophin-associated proteins and the muscular dystrophies. *Annu Rev Med 48*: 457-466

10. Davis DB, Delmonte AJ, Ly CT, McNally EM (2000) Myoferlin, a candidate gene and potential modifier of muscular dystrophy. *Hum Mol Genet* 9: 217-226

11. Illa I, Serrano-Munuera C, Gallardo E, Lasa A, Rojas-Garcia R, Palmer J, Gallano P, Baiget M, Matsuda C, Brown RH (2001) Distal anterior compartment myopathy: a dysferlin mutation causing a new muscular dystrophy phenotype. *Ann Neurol* 49: 130-134

12. Illarioshkin SN, Ivanova-Smolenskaya IA, Greenberg CR, Nylen E, Sukhorukov VS, Poleshchuk VV, Markova ED, Wrogemann K (2000) Identical dysferlin mutation in limb-girdle muscular dystrophy type 2B and distal myopathy. *Neurology* 55: 1931-1933

13. Illarioshkin SN, Ivanova-Smolenskaya IA, Tanaka H, Vereshchagin NV, Markova ED, Poleshchuk VV, Lozhnikova SM, Sukhorukov VS, Limborska SA, Slominsky PA (1996) Clinical and molecular analysis of a large family with three distinct phenotypes of progressive muscular dystrophy. *Brain* 119: 1895-1909

14. Linssen WH, Notermans NC, Van der Graaf Y, Wokke JH, Van Doorn PA, Howeler CJ, Busch HF, De Jager AE, De Visser M (1997) Miyoshi-type distal muscular dystrophy. Clinical spectrum in 24 Dutch patients. *Brain* 120: 1989-1996

15. Liu J, Aoki M, Illa I, Wu C, Fardeau M, Angelini C, Serrano C, Urtizberea JA, Hentati F, Hamida MB, Bohlega S, Culper EJ, Amato AA, Bossie K, Oeltjen J, Bejaoui K, McKenna-Yasek D, Hosler BA, Schurr E, Arahata K, de Jong PJ, Brown RH, Jr. (1998) Dysferlin, a novel skeletal muscle gene, is mutated in Miyoshi myopathy and limb girdle muscular dystrophy. *Nat Genet* 20: 31-36

16. Matsuda C, Aoki M, Hayashi YK, Ho MF, Arahata K, Brown RH, Jr. (1999) Dysferlin is a surface membrane-associated protein that is absent in Miyoshi myopathy. *Neurology* 53: 1119-1122

17. Piccolo F, Moore SA, Ford GC, Campbell KP (2000) Intracellular accumulation and reduced sarcolemmal expression of dysferlin in limb-girdle muscular dystrophies. *Ann Neurol* 48: 902-912

18. Rizo J, Sudhof TC (1998) C2-domains, structure and function of a universal Ca2+-binding domain. *J Biol Chem* 273: 15879-15882

19. Selcen D, Stilling G, Engel AG (2001) The earliest pathologic alterations in dysferlinopathy. *Neurology* 56: 1472-1481

20. Vafiadaki E, Reis A, Keers S, Harrison R, Anderson LV, Raffelsberger T, Ivanova S, Hoger H, Bittner RE, Bushby K, Bashir R (2001) Cloning of the mouse dysferlin gene and genomic characterization of the SJL-Dysf mutation. *Neuroreport* 12: 625-629

21. Weiler T, Bashir R, Anderson LV, Davison K, Moss JA, Britton S, Nylen E, Keers S, Vafiadaki E, Greenberg CR (1999) Identical mutation in patients with limb girdle muscular dystrophy type 2B or Miyoshi myopathy suggests a role for modifier gene(s). *Hum Mol Genet* 8: 871-877

22. Weiler T, Greenberg CR, Nylen E, Halliday W, Morgan K, Eggertson D, Wrogemann K (1996) Limb-girdle muscular dystrophy and Miyoshi myopathy in an aboriginal Canadian kindred map to LGMD2B and segregate with the same haplotype. *Am J Hum Genet* 59: 872-878

23. Yasunaga S, Grati M, Chardenoux S, Smith TN, Friedman TB, Lalwani AK, Wilcox ER, Petit C (2000) OTOF encodes multiple long and short isoforms: genetic evidence that the long ones underlie recessive deafness DFNB9. *Am J Hum Genet* 67: 591-600

24. Yasunaga S, Grati M, Cohen-Salmon M, El-Amraoui A, Mustapha M, Salem N, El-Zir E, Loiselet J, Petit C (1999) A mutation in OTOF, encoding otoferlin, a FER-1-like protein, causes DFNB9, a nonsyndromic form of deafness. *Nat Genet* 21: 363-369

Caveolinopathies

Mengfatt Ho
Robert H. Brown

CK	creatine kinase
DCG	dystrophin glycoprotein complex
LGMD	limb girdle muscular dystrophies
nNOS	neuronal nitric oxide synthase
RMD	rippling muscle disease

Definition of entities

Limb-girdle muscular dystrophy type 1C, HyperCKemia, Rippling muscle disease. Caveolin-3 is a recently identified member of the caveolin family of proteins, which includes caveolin-1 and –2. Unlike the latter 2 members, caveolin-3 is a muscle-specific protein that is expressed in cardiac, skeletal, and smooth muscle cells. Mutations in the caveolin-3 gene (*cav-3*) were first identified in patients with an autosomal dominant form of limb-girdle muscular dystrophy (LGMD) known as LGMD 1C (12, 15). Patients with LGMD 1C are characterized by an early age of onset (at around 5 years of age), calf hypertrophy, mild to moderate proximal muscle weakness, and cramping muscle pains after exercise. In addition, the levels of the muscle enzyme creatine kinase are typically elevated 4 to 25 fold above normal (12, 15).

A novel mutation in *cav-3* was recently reported in 2 unrelated children with a muscle disorder that is distinct from LGMD 1C. The affected children (ages 4 and 6 years) have persistent elevated levels of serum creatine kinase (hyperCKemia) without muscle weakness or other symptoms of myopathy (3).

Remarkably, the mutations in *cav-3* that are associated with LGMD 1C and hyperCKemia, were recently found to cause a third form of muscle disorder known as hereditary rippling muscle disease (RMD) (2). RMD is a rare autosomal dominant disorder characterized by electrically silent, percussion-induced muscular contractions. Muscle stiffness, cramps, and pain, especially during or following exercise, are the prominent features of this disorder. Thus, identical mutations in *cav-3* can give rise to 3 distinct muscle disorders (Table 1).

Molecular genetics and pathogenesis

Caveolae are flask-shaped plasma membrane invaginations that participate in membrane trafficking, sorting, transport, and signal transduction (13). They are found in many cell types but are especially abundant in fibroblasts, adipocytes, endothelial cells, and in smooth and striated muscle cells (5). Caveolin, a family of 21-24 kDa membrane proteins, is the principal component of caveolae membranes (17). They are thought to play an important structural role in the formation of caveolae membranes by acting as scaffolding proteins to organize and concentrate specific caveolin-interacting lipids and proteins (1).

The mammalian caveolin gene family consists of caveolins -1, -2, and -3. Caveolins -1 and -2 are expressed predominantly in endothelial cells and adipocytes where they form multivalent homo- and hetero-oligomers (4, 18, 19). In contrast, caveolin-3 expression is restricted to muscle cell types. The human caveolin-3 gene maps to chromosome 3p25. It consists of 2 exons and encodes a protein of 150 amino acids (14, 15).

All caveolins share a similar overall structure characterized by a hydrophilic N-terminal domain, a 33 amino acid membrane spanning segment, and a 43-44 amino acid hydrophilic C-terminal (22). The transmembrane segment is thought to form a hairpin loop within the cell membrane so that both the N- and C- terminal domains are in the cytoplasm (22). A "caveolin signature" composed of an invariant sequence of FEDVIAEP is found at the N-terminal region in all 3 caveolins, suggesting an essential but as yet, unknown function. Adjacent to this sequence is a common

Caveolin-3 mutant	Disease	Clinical features
(TFT)$_{63-65}$ deletion	1. LGMD 1C	1. Early age of onset (5 year), proximal muscle weakness, muscle cramps, non-specific myopathic changes and elevated CK levels (15).
P104L	1. LGMD 1C	1. Similar clinical findings as described for (TFT) deletion. No evidence of mechanical hyperirritability (15).
	2. Rippling muscle disease	2. Mechanical hyperirritability (2).
A45T	1. LGMD 1C	1. Early age of onset (3.5 year), elevated CK levels, muscle cramps, myalgia & dystrophic muscle biopsy without muscle weakness or signs of mechanical hyperirritability (12).
	2. Rippling muscle disease	2. Mechanical hyperirritability (2).
A45V	1. Rippling muscle disease	1. Mechanical hyperirritability (2).
R26Q	1. HyperCKemia	1. Elevated CK levels without muscle weakness or mechanical hyperirritability in two unrelated children with normal muscle biopsy (3).
	2. Rippling muscle disease	2. Mechanical hyperirritability (2).

Table 1. Caveolin-3 mutations in LGMD 1C, hyperCKemia, and hereditary rippling muscle disease.

Caveolin-3 Protein

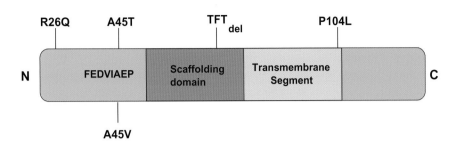

Figure 1. *Schematic representation of the caveolin-3 protein.* The caveolin-3 protein is characterized by a signature of eight amino acids (FEDVIAEP) that is highly conserved in all caveolins, a scaffolding domain and a transmembrane segment. The distribution of mutations in the caveolin-3 protein is shown.

domain, the caveolin-scaffolding domain, involved in the self-assembly of caveolins into high molecular mass oligomers and in the interaction with caveolin signaling molecules (16) (Figure 1).

Expression of caveolin-3 is induced during the differentiation of skeletal myoblasts. It is localized to the sarcolemma, where it forms a complex with dystrophin and its associated glycoproteins (20). However, caveolin-3 is not thought to be an integral component of the dystrophin glycoprotein complex (DGC) as it can be physically separated from the DGC under certain biochemical conditions (6). Support for this hypothesis can be found in patients with primary defects in either dystrophin or the sarcoglycans, but show normal expression of caveolin-3 (6). Caveolin-3 also interacts with and negatively regulates the catalytic activity of nNOS in skeletal muscles (23).

To date, there are only 3 mutations in *cav-3* known to cause autosomal dominant LGMD 1C (Figure 1, Table 1). Two missense changes, G55S and C71W, previously thought to cause LGMD 1C were recently found to be rare polymorphisms in the Brazilian population (7, 14). Interestingly, the 3 mutations linked to LGMD 1C are all found within putative functional domains: *i)* a missense mutation in the transmembrane segment that changed a proline to a leucine (P104L), *ii)* a 9-bp deletion in the scaffolding domain that

removes 3 amino acids without disrupting the open reading frame (15), and *iii)* a G to A substitution in the caveolin signature, that changed an alanine to threonine (A45T) (12). By contrast, the mutation associated with hyperCKemia is a missense change at the N-terminus that substituted an arginine for a glutamine at amino acid position 26 (R26Q) (3). Remarkably, three of the above mutations (R26Q, A45T and P104L) are also found in patients with hereditary rippling muscle disease (RMD) (Table 1).

Consistent with a dominant mode of transmission in caveolinopathies, all *cav-3* mutations identified to date are heterozygous and they cause a marked reduction of the caveolin-3 protein. The near complete loss of caveolin-3 in patients with heterozygous mutations suggests that mutant caveolin-3 might behave in a dominant negative manner. This hypothesis is supported by recent studies that show mutant caveolin-3 proteins forming unstable, high molecular mass aggregates that are retained within the Golgi complex and are not targeted to the plasma membrane (10). These findings suggest that mutant caveolin-3 proteins might interfere with the formation of normal homo-oligomers, which in turn, leads to an accelerated degradation of the misfolded caveolin-3 proteins.

The recent production of transgenic mice expressing the P104L mutant caveolin-3 protein provides further

support for a dominant negative mechanism in LGMD 1C (21). The transgenic animals show myopathic changes in muscles and a marked reduction in caveolin-3. In addition, these mice show poor growth and are significantly smaller than the wild-type littermates. The expression levels of dystrophin and β-dystroglycan are unaffected in these transgenic mice, indicating that caveolin-3 deficiency is specific and it is not due to secondary processes related to muscle cell degeneration. However, nNOS activity is elevated in these animals, suggesting that disturbance in nNOS signaling may also contribute to muscle fiber degeneration (21). Interestingly, overexpression of wild-type caveolin-3 in mouse skeletal muscle fibers can also induce dystrophic changes, involving dramatic increase in sarcolemmal caveolae and down-regulation of dystrophin and β-dystroglycan expression. These findings indicate that tight regulation of caveolin-3 expression is required to maintain normal muscle homeostasis (9).

To gain further insights into the normal biological function of caveolin-3, 2 groups have recently generated caveolin-3 null (*cav-3 -/-*) mice using standard gene targeting methods (8, 11). Unlike transgenic animals expressing mutant caveolin-3, *cav-3 -/-* mice show normal growth rates and only mild myopathic changes in skeletal muscles. The heterozygous mice do not show any pathological changes in their muscles, indicating that partial caveolin-3 deficiency on its own is not sufficient to cause muscle cell degeneration.

While the expression and the macroscopic localization of dystrophin and its associated proteins are not affected in *cav-3 -/-* mice, they are not properly targeted to the lipids rafts in the caveolae (8). In addition, electron microscopic studies reveal abnormalities in the organization of T-tubule system in *cav-3 -/-* muscles. Taken together, these findings indicate that caveolin-3 may be required for the proper targeting of the dystrophin glycoprotein complex to lipid rafts, and for the proper organiza-

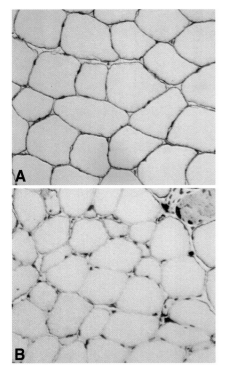

Figure 2. *Caveolin 3 immunolabelling of muscle biopsies.* **A.** Normal control biopsy showing the expected distribution of immunoreactivity at the surface of muscle fibres. **B.** Biopsy from a patient with a progressive limb girdle syndrome and immunohistochemical signs of caveolin-3 deficiency. Labelling is reduced in virtually all muscle fibres. This case may represent a primary caveolin deficiency since reduced labelling like this has not been seen in more than 300 normal and disease controls. However, the mutation in this patient was not confirmed since it was impossible to obtain material for molecular genetic investigations. Sections counterstained with haematoxyline. Illustration kindly provided by Dr Louise Anderson.

tion of the T-tubule system in the muscle cell (8).

Structural changes

Muscle biopsies of LGMD 1C and RMD patients show mild and non-specific myopathic changes. By contrast, there are no dystrophic changes in the muscle fibers of hyperCKemia patients with *cav-3* mutations. Despite these differences, all 3 muscle disorders show a marked reduction in the levels of caveolin-3 protein by immunohistochemical and immunoblot analyses (Figure 2). It is noteworthy that patients with LGMD 1C show the greatest reduction (over 90%) in caveolin-3 expression while the reduction in hyperCKemia patients range from 71% to 84% (3, 12, 15).

Genotype-phenotype correlations

As with dysferlinopathies, identical mutations in the caveolin-3 gene can lead to distinct muscle diseases (LGMD 1C, hyperCKemia or rippling muscle disease). To date, there are only 5 documented mutations in the caveolin-3 gene (Table 1). Three of these mutations (R26Q, A45T, and P104L) are associated with more than one type of muscle disease. Therefore, mutations in *cav-3* do not solely determine the type of the muscle disease and additional factors (genetic and non-genetic) contribute to modify the phenotype.

Future perspectives

While the pathogenic mechanism underlying caveolinopathies remains to be defined, the combination of biochemical data and the availability of different animal models for caveolin-3 defects have provided valuable clues and insights for the normal biological function of caveolin-3. These studies have also provided compelling evidence that caveolinopathies are caused by the dominant negative effects of mutant caveolin-3 proteins. However, very little is known about their role in muscle cell degeneration. For instance, it is not known why a single amino acid substitution in caveolin-3 confers dominant negative adverse properties. A parallel question is whether all caveolin-3 mutant proteins will behave in a dominant negative fashion. Still unknown, are the identities of proteins that normally interact with caveolin-3 and whether these are abnormally expressed or distributed when caveolin-3 is mutated. Equally intriguing is whether these interacting proteins may have a role in determining the type of muscle disease in caveolinopathies. Thus, the definition of caveolin-3 interacting proteins may provide insight into muscular dystrophies other than just LGMD 1C, hyperCkemia, and RMD.

Ultimately, the greatest challenge for research in caveolin myopathies is the development of effective therapy. Here, we need to devise strategies that will allow correction of the dominant negative cytotoxicity of the mutant caveolin-3 proteins.

References

1. Anderson RGW (1998) The caveolae membrane system. *Annu Rev Biochem* 67: 199-225

2. Betz RC, Schoser BG, Kasper D, Ricker K, Ramirez A, Stein V, Torbergsen T, Lee YA, Nothen MM, Wienker TF, Malin JP, Propping P, Reis A, Mortier W, Jentsch TJ, Vorgerd M, Kubisch C (2001) Mutations in CAV3 cause mechanical hyperirritability of skeletal muscle in rippling muscle disease. *Nat Genet* 28: 218-219

3. Carbone I, Bruno C, Sotgia F, Bado M, Broda P, Masetti E, Panella A, Zara F, Bricarelli FD, Cordone G, Lisanti MP, Minetti C (2000) Mutation in the CAV3 gene causes partial caveolin-3 deficiency and hyperCKemia. *Neurology* 54: 1373-1376

4. Couet J, Li S, Okamoto T, Ikezu T, Lisanti MP (1997a) Identification of peptide and protein ligands for the caveolin- scaffolding domain. Implications for the interaction of caveolin with caveolae-associated proteins. *J Biol Chem* 272: 6525-6533

5. Couet J, Li S, Okamoto T, Scherer PS, Lisanti MP (1997b) Molecular and cellular biology of caveolae: Paradoxes and plasticities. *Trends in Cardiovascular Medicine* 7: 103-110

6. Crosbie RH, Yamada H, Venzke DP, Lisanti MP, Campbell KP (1998) Caveolin-3 is not an integral component of the dystrophin glycoprotein complex. *FEBS Lett* 427: 279-282

7. de Paula F, Vainzof M, Bernardino AL, McNally E, Kunkel LM, Zatz M (2001) Mutations in the caveolin-3 gene: When are they pathogenic? *Am J Med Genet* 99: 303-307

8. Galbiati F, Engelman JA, Volonte D, Zhang XL, Minetti C, Li M, Hou H, Kneitz B, Edelmann W, Lisanti MP (2001) Caveolin-3 null mice show a loss of caveolae, changes in the microdomain distribution of the dystrophin-glycoprotein complex, and T- tubule abnormalities. *J Biol Chem* 276: 21425-21433

9. Galbiati F, Volonte D, Chu JB, Li M, Fine SW, Fu M, Bermudez J, Pedemonte M, Weidenheim KM, Pestell RG, Minetti C, Lisanti MP (2000) Transgenic overexpression of caveolin-3 in skeletal muscle fibers induces a Duchenne-like muscular dystrophy phenotype. *Proc Natl Acad Sci U S A* 97: 9689-9694

10. Galbiati F, Volonte D, Minetti C, Chu JB, Lisanti MP (1999) Phenotypic behavior of caveolin-3 mutations that cause autosomal dominant limb girdle muscular dystrophy (LGMD-1C). Retention of LGMD-1C caveolin-3 mutants within the golgi complex. *J Biol Chem* 274: 25632-25641

11. Hagiwara Y, Sasaoka T, Araishi K, Imamura M, Yorifuji H, Nonaka I, Ozawa E, Kikuchi T (2000) Caveolin-3 deficiency causes muscle degeneration in mice. *Hum Mol Genet* 9: 3047-3054

12. Herrmann R, Straub V, Blank M, Kutzick C, Franke N, Jacob EN, Lenard HG, Kroger S, Voit T (2000) Dissociation of the dystroglycan complex in caveolin-3-deficient limb girdle muscular dystrophy. *Hum Mol Genet* 9: 2335-2340

13. Lisanti MP, Tang Z, Scherer PE, Kubler E, Koleske AJ, Sargiacomo M (1995) Caveolae, transmembrane signalling and cellular transformation. *Mol Membr Biol* 12: 121-124

14. McNally EM, de Sa Moreira E, Duggan DJ, Bonnemann CG, Lisanti MP, Lidov HG, Vainzof M, Passos-Bueno MR, Hoffman EP, Zatz M, Kunkel LM (1998) Caveolin-3 in muscular dystrophy. *Hum Mol Genet* 7: 871-877

15. Minetti C, Sotgia F, Bruno C, Scartezzini P, Broda P, Bado M, Masetti E, Mazzocco M, Egeo A, Donati MA, Volonte D, Galbiati F, Cordone G, Bricarelli FD, Lisanti MP, Zara F (1998) Mutations in the caveolin-3 gene cause autosomal dominant limb-girdle muscular dystrophy. *Nat Genet* 18: 365-368

16. Okamoto T, Schlegel A, Scherer PE, Lisanti MP (1998) Caveolins, a family of scaffolding proteins for organizing "preassembled signaling complexes" at the plasma membrane. *J Biol Chem* 273: 5419-5422

17. Rothberg KG, Heuser JE, Donzell WC, Ying YS, Glenney JR, Anderson RG (1992) Caveolin, a protein component of caveolae membrane coats. *Cell* 68: 673-682

18. Sargiacomo M, Scherer PE, Tang Z, Kubler E, Song KS, Sanders MC, Lisanti MP (1995) Oligomeric structure of caveolin: implications for caveolae membrane organization. *Proc Natl Acad Sci U S A* 92: 9407-9411

19. Scherer PE, Lewis RY, Volonte D, Engelman JA, Galbiati F, Couet J, Kohtz DS, van Donselaar E, Peters P, Lisanti MP (1997) Cell-type and tissue-specific expression of caveolin-2. Caveolins 1 and 2 co-localize and form a stable hetero-oligomeric complex i*n vivo. J Biol Chem* 272: 29337-29346

20. Song KS, Scherer PE, Tang Z, Okamoto T, Li S, Chafel M, Chu C, Kohtz DS, Lisanti MP (1996) Expression of caveolin-3 in skeletal, cardiac, and smooth muscle cells. Caveolin-3 is a component of the sarcolemma and co-fractionates with dystrophin and dystrophin-associated glycoproteins. *J Biol Chem* 271: 15160-15165

21. Sunada Y, Ohi H, Hase A, Hosono T, Arata S, Higuchi S, Matsumura K, Shimizu T (2001) Transgenic mice expressing mutant caveolin-3 show severe myopathy associated with increased nNOS activity. *Hum Mol Genet* 10: 173-178

22. Tang Z, Scherer PE, Okamoto T, Song K, Chu C, Kohtz DS, Nishimoto I, Lodish HF, Lisanti MP (1996) Molecular cloning of caveolin-3, a novel member of the caveolin gene family expressed predominantly in muscle. *J Biol Chem* 271: 2255-2261

23. Venema VJ, Ju H, Zou R, Venema RC (1997) Interaction of neuronal nitric-oxide synthase with caveolin-3 in skeletal muscle. Identification of a novel caveolin scaffolding/inhibitory domain. *J Biol Chem* 272: 28187-28190

Laminin α2 (merosin) gene mutations

Eric P. Hoffman
Elena Pegoraro

CK	creatine kinase
CVS	chorionic villus sample
MRI	magnetic resonance imaging

Definition of entities

Congenital muscular dystrophy refers to a dystrophic myopathy present from birth. As such, the disease is associated with floppy muscle tone, grossly elevated serum creatine kinase levels, and dystrophic changes in muscle biopsies. The congenital muscular dystrophies have been segregated into a number of different types, which show varying frequencies in different world populations. Congenital muscular dystrophy is considered a relatively rare condition; incidences typically quoted are 1:10 000 to 1:50 000. For further information, see *www.geneclinics.org*, "congenital muscular dystrophy").

The most common single form of congenital muscular dystrophy is caused by loss-of-function mutations of the laminin α2 (merosin) gene, leading to a complete absence of this protein in the myofibre basal lamina (13). The disease shows no common mutations, and is not endemic to any particular world population. Patients have normal cognition and high serum creatine kinase levels. They do not achieve any motor milestones, yet have a relatively stable clinical course. All mutation-positive patients show white matter changes on MRI, and some of these patients show cortical cysts with associated epilepsy and cognitive dysfunction. The majority of patients present at birth, and show complete laminin α2-deficiency by both immunostaining of

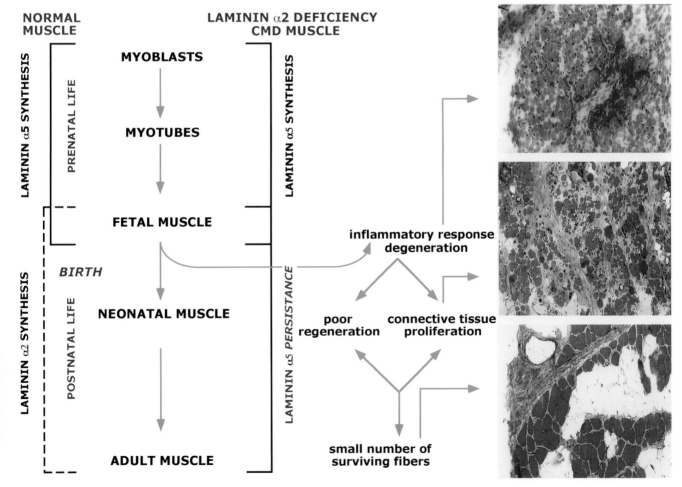

Figure 1. *The pathophysiology of laminin α2 (merosin) deficiency.* Shown is a schematic of the isoform switch from laminin α4 and α5 to laminin α2 around the time of birth. Normal development is shown on the left, while the consequences of laminin α2 (merosin) deficiency is shown in the center. The histopathological consequences of the misdirected isoform switches are shown to the right; each microscopical picture is from a merosin-deficient congenital muscular dystrophy patient at different ages. The top right one shows a dramatic inflammatory infiltrate characteristic of laminin α2-deficient newborn muscle, the center picture shows the more "dystrophic" pathology of the infant, while the lower picture shows the end-stage myopathic features typically seen in older patients.

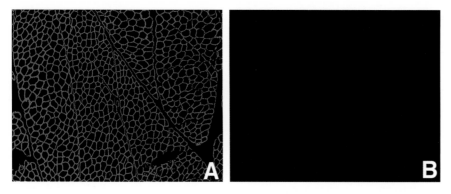

Figure 2. *Immunostaining of muscle biopsies for laminin α2.* Shown is immunofluorescence microscopy of laminin α2 using cryosections. **A.** Normal laminin α2 immunostaining is seen in control, where the basal lamina of all muscle fibres stains brightly red. **B.** To the right a biopsy from a patient with congenital muscular dystrophy and complete lack of laminin α2 immunostaining. This patient also showed dramatic white matter abnormalities by MRI, but normal intelligence.

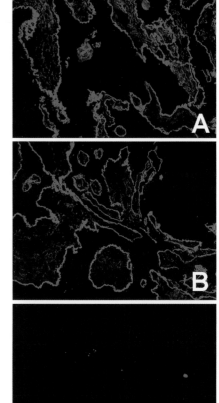

Figure 3. *Prenatal diagnosis of a foetus with congenital muscular dystrophy by immunostaining of chorionic villus sample.* **A.** Immunostaining for laminin α2 in a normal control chorionic villus sample (CVS). **B** and **C** show two foetuses of unknown affected status. In both, an older affected relative had laminin α2 deficient congenital muscular dystrophy by immunostaining of muscle biopsy (Figure 2). CVS sampling of both foetuses was done at about 15 weeks gestational age, the maternal and foetal components of the CVS sample were separated and flash frozen. Immunostaining of cryosections showed normal laminin α2 in one foetus (**B**). This was given the diagnosis "unaffected" and was born as a normal child. The sample from the second foetus (**C**) showed complete laminin α2 deficiency, and was given the diagnosis "congenital muscular dystrophy."

frozen sections and immunoblot analyses. The disease is autosomal recessive, and both males and females are affected.

There are a limited number of reports of patients with *partial* laminin α2 deficiency on muscle biopsy. About 10% show mutations in the corresponding gene (usually missense mutations). Two spontaneous murine models have been characterized, which faithfully reproduce much of the clinical picture of the human disease (15).

Molecular genetics and pathophysiology

The laminin α2 gene is located at 6q2, and is a large and complex gene with 64 exons (16). There are no common mutations, and thus considerable effort must be expended to identify causative gene changes (1, 8). The clinical findings of severe congenital muscular dystrophy with high serum creatine kinase levels, white matter changes by MRI, and the biochemical finding of complete laminin α2 deficiency on muscle biopsy by immunostaining is considered diagnostic, and nearly all such patients studied to date have shown gene mutations (8).

Laminin α2 is a major component of the myofibre basal lamina, where it interacts with the myofibre plasma membrane both through the dystrophin membrane cytoskeleton (via dystroglycan), and with the vinculin/integrin membrane cytoskeleton (via integrin).

It mediates interactions between the basal lamina and extracellular matrix (endomysial connective tissue) via perlecan, nidogen, and a series of other proteins. The mature myofibre laminin molecule is a heterotrimer, composed of α2, β1, and γ1 proteins (each from a different gene). In the literature, some authors use the term "merosin" to describe the complete (α2, β1, γ1) heterotrimer, while others use the term "merosin" for only the α2 chain. As most antibodies used for immunostaining are directed against the α2 chain, and mutations in the corresponding gene are the cause of congenital muscular dystrophy, it is more accurate to use the term "laminin α2" rather than "merosin."

There are many isoforms of heterotrimeric laminin in different cell types and tissues, produced by utilization of different combinations of different genes α1, α2 or α3; β1, β2; γ1, γ2), and also alternative splicing. The basal lamina of capillaries in muscle uses the α1 gene (α1, β1, γ1). Developing embryonic and fetal myofibres use different isoforms as well, with both the α4 and α5 genes utilized in the basal lamina (Figure 1) (2, 5, 10). Around the time of birth, the α2 gene is expressed more highly, and the α1 protein is replaced by the α2 protein. For this reason, muscle in patients with laminin α2 gene mutations probably forms normally during fetal life; however, the muscle fails to transition from

the α1 chain to the α2 chain at birth, with pathology and functional disability ensuing (Figure 1).

Structural changes

The structural changes of laminin α2-deficient patient muscle biopsies varies dramatically both between and within patients (7, 8) (Figure 1). The biopsies of neonates can show striking inflammatory cell infiltration (T cell and B cell), and most patients given the morphological diagnosis of infantile polymyositis probably have laminin α2-deficient congenital muscular dystrophy. Soon after birth, the biopsy findings change to a more dystrophic picture, and then to an end-stage myopathic alteration.

The lack of this transition in muscle leads to a series of events (Figure 1). First, there appears to be a response of the immune system, such that muscle can be seen to be infiltrated with both T and B cells. This has led to some patients initially being given the diagnosis of "infantile polymyositis" at birth (7). There is then an abnormal *persistence* of *laminin* α4 and α5, which appears able to functionally rescue remaining myofibres, and possibly protect them from subsequent immune attack and degeneration (10). However, this abnormal basal lamina is likely a poor scaffold for regeneration, and there is little or no evidence of successful myofibre regeneration in patients older than 1 year of age (2, 5) (Figures 1, 2).

Testing for laminin a2 is typically done by immunostaining of frozen sections of muscle biopsy, but skin biopsy and fetal chorionic villus samples can also be used (4, 11). Thus, prenatal diagnosis can be done by testing chorionic villus samples for the presence of laminin α2 immunostaining (4) (Figure 3).

Genotype - phenotype correlations

All laminin α2-deficient patients show dramatic white matter changes of the brain. Though detectable by MRI, there is no clinical evidence of a demyelinating CNS disease (3). This is in contrast to *laminin α2-positive* cases which generally show normal MRI scans. It is thought that the imaging changes are due to altered water distribution in the brain, secondary to blood-brain barrier dysfunction. The MRI findings may not be present at birth, but always develop by 6 months of age. Laminin α2-negative patients generally

show very high serum creatine kinase levels, while laminin α2-positive cases do not.

There is slowed nerve conduction consistent with a peripheral demyelinating process, but the profound skeletal muscle involvement obscures any clinical evidence of this (12). Most patients never achieve any functional mobility, and some do not survive the neonatal period (8, 9). Surviving patients show normal intellectual function and a relatively stable clinical course, although a few patients have shown more severe CNS involvement (6).

All patients showing complete deficiency of laminin α2 on muscle biopsy show a consistent, severe phenotype caused by "loss-of-function" mutations (nonsense, frameshift) of the corresponding gene. Partial merosin deficiency patients show much more variability in phenotype; however, there are too few patients reported to date to provide genotype/phenotype correlations.

Future perspectives

Patient care is currently palliative, with consideration of respiratory support and spinal fusions as with any patient with profound muscle weakness. The availability of the mouse model for laminin α2 should promote the development of experimental therapeutics. Gene delivery is problematic due to the large size of the gene. Cellular transplantation has been used to deliver laminin α2 to deficiency mice (14). However, cellular transplantation suffers from a number of hurdles before being expected to show efficacy in human patients; namely, survival of implanted cells, sufficient delivery methods, adequate numbers of donor cells, and immune responses against laminin α2.

References

1. Helbling-Leclerc A, Zhang X, Topaloglu H, Cruaud C, Tesson F, Weissenbach J, Tome FM, Schwartz K, Fardeau M, Tryggvason K, et al. (1995) Mutations in the laminin alpha 2-chain gene (LAMA2) cause merosin- deficient congenital muscular dystrophy. *Nat Genet* 11: 216-218

2. Kuang W, Xu H, Vilquin JT, Engvall E (1999) Activation of the lama2 gene in muscle regeneration: abortive regeneration in laminin alpha2-deficiency. *Lab Invest* 79: 1601-1613

3. Mercuri E, Muntoni F, Berardinelli A, Pennock J, Sewry C, Philpot J, Dubowitz V (1995) Somatosensory and visual evoked potentials in congenital muscular dystrophy: correlation with MRI changes and muscle merosin status. *Neuropediatrics* 26: 3-7

4. Naom I, D'Alessandro M, Sewry C, Ferlini A, Topaloglu H, Helbling-Leclerc A, Guicheney P, Schwartz K, Akcoren Z, Dubowitz V, Muntoni F (1997) The role of immunocytochemistry and linkage analysis in the prenatal diagnosis of merosin-deficient congenital muscular dystrophy. *Hum Genet* 99: 535-540

5. Patton BL, Connoll AM, Martin PT, Cunningham JM, Mehta S, Pestronk A, Miner JH, Sanes JR (1999) Distribution of ten laminin chains in dystrophic and regenerating muscles. *Neuromuscul Disord* 9(6-7): 423-433

6. Pegoraro E, Fanin PM, Trevisan CP, Angelini C, Hoffman EP (2000) A novel laminin alpha2 isoform in severe laminin alpha2 deficient congenital muscular dystrophy [In Process Citation]. *Neurology* 55: 1128-1134

7. Pegoraro E, Mancias P, Swerdlow SH, Raikow RB, Garcia C, Marks H, Crawford T, Carver V, Di Cianno B, Hoffman EP (1996) Congenital muscular dystrophy with primary laminin alpha2 (merosin) deficiency presenting as inflammatory myopathy. *Ann Neurol* 40: 782-791

8. Pegoraro E, Marks H, Garcia CA, Crawford T, Mancias P, Connolly AM, Fanin M, Martinello F, Trevisan CP, Angelini C, Stella A, Scavina M, Munk RL, Servidei S, Bonnemann CC, Bertorini T, Acsadi G, Thompson CE, Gagnon D, Hoganson G, Carver V, Zimmerman RA, Hoffman EP (1998) Laminin alpha2 muscular dystrophy: genotype/phenotype studies of 22 patients [see comments]. *Neurology* 51: 101-110

9. Philpot J, Sewry C, Pennock J, Dubowitz V (1995) Clinical phenotype in congenital muscular dystrophy: correlation with expression of merosin in skeletal muscle. *Neuromuscul Disord* 5: 301-305

10. Sewry CA, Chevallay M, Tome FM (1995) Expression of laminin subunits in human fetal skeletal muscle. *Histochem J* 27: 497-504

11. Sewry CA, D'Alessandro M, Wilson LA, Sorokin LM, Naom I, Bruno S, Ferlini A, Dubowitz V, Muntoni F (1997) Expression of laminin chains in skin in merosin-deficient congenital muscular dystrophy. *Neuropediatrics* 28: 217-222

12. Shorer Z, Philpot J, Muntoni F, Sewry C, Dubowitz V (1995) Demyelinating peripheral neuropathy in merosin-deficient congenital muscular dystrophy. *J Child Neurol* 10: 472-475

13. Tome FM, Evangelista T, Leclerc A, Sunada Y, Manole E, Estournet B, Barois A, Campbell KP, Fardeau M (1994) Congenital muscular dystrophy with merosin deficiency. *C R Acad Sci* III 317: 351-357

14. Vilquin JT, Guerette B, Puymirat J, Yaffe D, Tome FM, Fardeau M, Fiszman M, Schwartz K, Tremblay JP (1999) Myoblast transplantations lead to the expression of the laminin alpha 2 chain in normal and dystrophic (dy/dy) mouse muscles. *Gene Ther* 6: 792-800

15. Xu H, Christmas P, Wu XR, Wewer UM, Engvall E (1994) Defective muscle basement membrane and lack of M-laminin in the dystrophic dy/dy mouse. *Proc Natl Acad Sci USA* 91: 5572-5576

16. Zhang X, Vuolteenaho R, Tryggvason K (1996) Structure of the human laminin alpha2-chain gene (LAMA2), which is affected in congenital muscular dystrophy. *J Biol Chem* 271: 27664-27669

Collagen VI gene mutations. Bethlem myopathy/Limb-girdle muscular dystrophy

Eric P. Hoffman
Elena Pegoraro

Definition of entities

Bethlem myopathy is a congenital myopathy. The age of onset varies considerably, from birth to the second decade, depending on the extent of contractures present and the extent of weakness seen. Typical cases show non-progressive congenital flexion contractures of the ankles, elbows, and interphalangeal joints of the fingers. Contractures of the neck and back are generally not observed. Patients have normal serum creatine kinase levels, and plantar flexion contractures of the ankles are constant findings. The disease is autosomal dominant with complete penetrance. No "new mutations" in isolated cases have yet been described, but this may be due to difficulty in molecular diagnosis. Both males and females are affected equally.

Linkage studies, with subsequent candidate gene mutation screening, found all families with Bethlem to harbor missense or splice-site mutations of 1 of the 3 collagen VI genes (α1, α2, or α3) (1-3). To date a total of 6 different mutations have been described (3 in COL6A1, 1 in COL6A2, and 2 in COL6A3).

Recent studies have found some families carrying the diagnosis of autosomal dominant "limb-girdle muscular dystrophy" to similarly show mutations of the 3 collagen VI genes (5). These can occur in any of the 3 collagen VI genes, but the mutations are distinct from those seen in Bethlem myopathy families (4, 5). In these families, contractures are not a consistent feature of the disorder, and the histopathology is more "dystrophic" in nature.

There are only about a dozen families reported in the literature, and molecular characterisation of the underlying biochemical defect has only recently been accomplished. Further studies are needed to delineate the incidence and world distribution of this disorder.

Molecular genetics and pathophysiology

Collagen VI is a heterotetramer composed of 3 different chains, each from a different gene. The collagen VI α1 and VI α2 genes (COL6A1, COL6A2) are located on chromosome 21q22.3, while the collagen VI α3 gene (COL6A3) is on chromosome 2q37. Each of the genes has a large number (~30) exons, and there are no common mutations. There is also no biochemical test for the disorder, with all patient biopsies reported to date showing normal collagen VI immunostaining and immunoblot findings. Thus, each family suspected of having a disorder related to collagen VI (Bethlem myopathy, limb-girdle muscular dystrophy) must be tested for mutations of each of the collagen VI genes.

Collagen VI has a major role in connecting the endomysial connective tissue to the myofibre basal lamina (Figure 1). Thus, abnormalities of this heterotetramer likely disrupt the ability of muscle fibres to appropriate connect with the endomysium. However, there remain a number of unresolved questions concerning the pathophysiology of this disease. First and foremost, collagen VI is a ubiquitously expressed protein, yet patient symptoms appear to be limited to muscle and tendon. Second, unpublished results from our laboratory have found normal levels of the collagen VI protein and mRNA isoforms in samples of patient muscle, suggesting that the defect is not a defi-

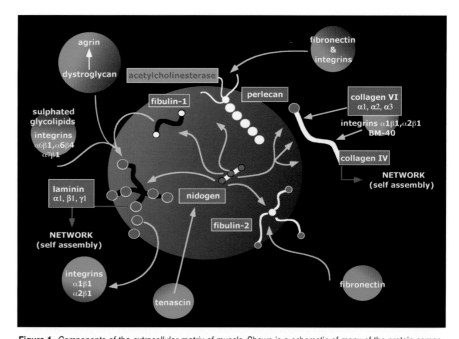

Figure 1. *Components of the extracellular matrix of muscle.* Shown is a schematic of many of the protein components of the extracellular matrix and basal lamina of muscle. The proteins indicated with a red box are those discussed in Chapter 2.3 as inducing specific neuromuscular conditions. Dominant missense mutations of collagen VI cause a clinically variable muscle disease, which can present as either a relatively benign congenital myopathy with contractures, or as a limb-girdle muscular dystrophy. The consequence of perlecan deficiency (Chapter 2.3.3) is loss of acetylcholinesterase from the neuromuscular junctions, with subsequent inability to clear acetylcholine, and faulty relaxation of muscle (myotonia) (Schwartz-Jampel syndrome). The consequences of laminin α2 (merosin) deficiency is presented in Chapter 2.3.1.

ciency of this heterotetramer. Finally, different missense mutations lead to either a "myopathic" picture, or a "dystrophic" phenotype; the reasons underlying the different response of muscle to different missense mutations is not known.

Structural changes

Muscle biopsies show fibre size variation, increased endomysial connective tissue, and rounded fibres, without considerable evidence of overt degeneration/regeneration of fibres. In our experience, the muscle can be difficult to section on a cryostat, as if there is considerable fatty replacement of the tissue; however, there is usually little light microscopic evidence of this. Possibly, this reflects a poor anchoring of the myofibres to the endomysial connective tissue. Immunostaining for collagen VI shows apparently normal quantities of this protein in the extracellular connective tissue adjacent to the basal lamina, suggesting that dominant missense mutations of the different collagen VI genes do not lead to a deficiency (dominant-negative) loss of the protein in muscle. There are no other reported histological or histochemical methods that are sensitive or specific for patients harboring collagen VI mutations.

Genotype-phenotype correlations

Clinical symptoms of patients are highly variable both within, and between, families. There are 3 different genes in which mutations occur (collagen VI $\alpha 1$, VI $\alpha 2$, and VI $\alpha 3$ genes). To date, there are no consistent clinical features that can distinguish between the 3 different genetic causes, suggesting that the pathogenesis (namely poor assembly of the complete collagen VI trimer) is identical for all 3 proteins. Whether a patient presents with a congenital myopathy phenotype (with contractures), or with a later onset limb-girdle muscular dystrophy phenotype, appears to depend on the location of the mutations within the domain structure of the protein. However, more patients need to be studied before clear geno-type-phenotype correlations will emerge.

Future perspectives

The most bewildering feature of collagen VI disorders is why a protein expressed throughout the body shows such muscle-specific symptoms. Future studies will need to address the fate of the collagen VI proteins containing the missense mutations, and the sister molecules that are structurally normal but likely are unable to form appropriate larger order oligomeric structures. In addition, the effect of different mutations in different regions of the gene, and their effects on the contracture and dystrophic subphenotypes need further investigation.

Most dominant disorders result from the production of a toxic protein, and therapeutics must be targeted towards abrogating the deleterious effects of the toxic protein, or decreasing its abundance. This remains a challenge for most dominant disorders, including those involving collagen VI subunits.

References

1. Jobsis GJ, Boers JM, Barth PG, de Visser M (1999) Bethlem myopathy: a slowly progressive congenital muscular dystrophy with contractures. *Brain* 122: 649-655

2. Jobsis GJ, Keizers H, Vreijling JP, de Visser M, Speer MC, Wolterman RA, Baas F, Bolhuis PA (1996) Type VI collagen mutations in Bethlem myopathy, an autosomal dominant myopathy with contractures. *Nat Genet* 14: 113-115

3. Pan TC, Zhang RZ, Pericak-Vance MA, Tandan R, Fries T, Stajich JM, Viles K, Vance JM, Chu ML, Speer MC (1998) Missense mutation in a von Willebrand factor type A domain of the alpha 3(VI) collagen gene (COL6A3) in a family with Bethlem myopathy. *Hum Mol Genet* 7: 807-812

4. Pepe G, Bertini E, Giusti B, Brunelli T, Comeglio P, Saitta B, Merlini L, Chu ML, Federici G, Abbate R (1999) A novel *de novo* mutation in the triple helix of the COL6A3 gene in two-generation Italian family affected by Bethlem myopathy. A diagnostic approach in the mutations' screening of type VI collagen. *Neuromuscul Disord* 9: 264-271

5. Scacheri PC, Gillanders EM, Subramoney S, Vedanarayanan V, Crowe CA, Engvall E, Watkins S, Bingler M, Trent JM, Hoffman EP. Novel mutations in Collagen genes (COL6A1, COL6A2): A pathogenic model for muscle-specific symptoms of a ubiquitously-expressed protein. *Neurology* in press.

Heparin sulfate proteoglycan (perlecan) deficiency. Schwartz-Jampel syndrome

Eric P. Hoffman
Elena Pegoraro

EMG	electro myography
HSPG	heparin sulfate proteoglycan

Definition of entity

Schwartz-Jampel syndrome has myotonia as a major clinical feature, and is often discussed together with other myotonic syndromes. This disorder is due to *partial* loss-of-function, recessively inherited mutations of the major heparin sulfate proteoglycan gene, often called "perlecan" (2, 7). Thus, it is an autosomal recessive condition although there can be EMG abnormalities in carriers. Both males and females are affected equally.

The causative mutations are consistent with secretion of a partially functional protein, much as is the case with dystrophin in Becker muscular dystrophy patients. Patients showing *complete* biochemical deficiency of perlecan due to loss-of-function (null) mutations have a lethal neonatal disorder termed "dyssegmental dysplasia, Silverman-Handmaker type" due to severe lack of bone growth (1).

Patients with Schwartz-Jampel syndrome have problems with osteous growth (short stature and pigeon chest deformities), abnormalities of epiphyseal cartilage, and joint contractures. Immunostaining for perlecan reveals that perlecan is present in the matrix, but mutations show in-frame deletions and insertions which likely perturb the normal function of the protein, both during bone development and growth, and in maintenance of the neuromuscular junction. The disorder is considered very rare, although a number of clinical variants will most likely be presented as genotype/phenotype studies evolve over the next few years.

Molecular genetics and pathophysiology

The perlecan (*HSPG2*) gene, has been mapped to chromosome 1p36.1-35 (4, 6). The gene is large (>100 kb) and contains 94 exons (1). To date, molecular findings in 6 Schwartz-Jampel families have been reported, and all 6 show missense, or *in-frame* insertion, deletion, or splice site mutations of the perlecan gene, leading to production of semi-functional protein (2, 7). The mutations permit secretion of the protein into the extracellular matrix; however, the partially functional protein does not direct correct formation of cartilage, bone, or the neuromuscular junction. The causative gene is extremely large and difficult to screen for mutations. The enigmatic association of skeletal and muscle symptoms in this disease can provide a tentative diagnosis, with subsequent testing done in research laboratories.

Heparin sulfate proteoglycan (perlecan) (Figure 1) is a very large, multifunctional protein, with large regions of homology to low density lipoprotein receptor, laminin, neural cell adhesion molecules, and epidermal growth factor. It includes domains known to regulate fibroblast growth factor release and activity (8), and many of the bone growth abnormalities in Schwartz-Jampel patients resemble those seen in fibroblast growth factor receptor gene defects, such as thanatophoric dysplasia and achondroplastic dwarfism. Perlecan also plays a role in connecting the basal lamina to the plasma membrane via interactions with integrins. However, the integrin-based cytoskeleton of muscle does not seem as important for muscle homeostasis as the dystrophin-based cytoskeleton (5). Deficiency of perlecan does not prevent the formation of basal lamina, but it causes increased

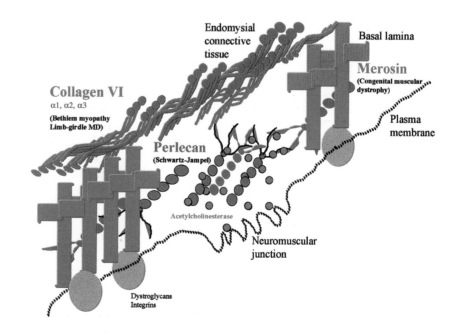

Figure 1. *Schematic presentation of the muscle fibre basal lamina bordering the plasma membrane of the muscle fibre.* Perlecan has a major role in the clustering of acetylcholine esterase to the neuromuscular junctions.

stress-induced fragility of this structure (3).

Most important for muscle biology are the defects of the neuromuscular junction. Recent studies have shown that perlecan has a major role in the clustering of acetylcholinesterase to the neuromuscular junction (9). Thus, the severe and constant myotonia characteristic of Schwartz-Jampel is the result of loss of acetylcholine esterase at the neuromuscular junction. The lack of acetylcholinesterase causes persistent depolarization of the myofibre due to inability to clear acetylcholine following each nerve-induced contraction.

Future perspectives

Given the clear role of perlecan in localizing acetylcholinesterase, one would expect that pharmacological use of acetylcholinesterase activators would lead to a lessening of the symptoms of myotonia. The blepharophimosis can be particularly disabling to patients, and increasing the activity of acetylcholinesterase is likely to provide some relief to this.

References

1. Arikawa-Hirasawa E, Wilcox WR, Le AH, Silverman N, Govindraj P, Hassell JR, Yamada YM (2001 a) Dyssegmental dysplasia, Silverman-Handmaker type, is caused by functional null mutations of perlecan. Submitted for publication:

2. Arikawa-Hirasawa E, Wilcox WR, Le AH, Silverman N, Govindraj P, Hassell JR, Yamada YM (2001 b) Partial loss-of-function mutations of perlecan cause Schwartz-Jampel syndrome. Submitted for publication:

3. Costell M, Gustafsson E, Aszodi A, Morgelin M, Bloch W, Hunziker E, Addicks K, Timpl R, Fassler R (1999) Perlecan maintains the integrity of cartilage and some basement membranes. *J Cell Biol* 147: 1109-1122

4. Dodge GR, Kovalszky I, Chu ML, Hassell JR, McBride OW, Yi HF, Iozzo RV (1991) Heparan sulfate proteoglycan of human colon: partial molecular cloning, cellular expression, and mapping of the gene (HSPG2) to the short arm of human chromosome 1. *Genomics* 10: 673-680

5. Hayashi YK, Chou FL, Engvall E, Ogawa M, Matsuda C, Hirabayashi S, Yokochi K, Ziober BL, Kramer RH, Kaufman SJ, Ozawa E, Goto Y, Nonaka I, Tsukahara T, Wang JZ, Hoffman EP, Arahata K (1998) Mutations in the integrin alpha7 gene cause congenital myopathy. *Nat Genet* 19: 94-97

6. Kallunki P, Eddy RL, Byers MG, Kestila M, Shows TB, Tryggvason K (1991) Cloning of human heparan sulfate proteoglycan core protein, assignment of the gene (HSPG2) to 1p36.1—p35 and identification of a BamHI restriction fragment length polymorphism. *Genomics* 11: 389-396

7. Nicole S, Davoine CS, Topaloglu H, Cattolico L, Barral D, Beighton P, Hamida CB, Hammouda H, Cruaud C, White PS, Samson D, Urtizberea JA, Lehmann-Horn F, Weissenbach J, Hentati F, Fontaine B (2000) Perlecan, the major proteoglycan of basement membranes, is altered in patients with schwartz-jampel syndrome (chondrodystrophic myotonia) [In Process Citation]. *Nat Genet* 26: 480-483

8. Nugent MA, Nugent HM, Iozzo RV, Sanchack K, Edelman ER (2000) Perlecan is required to inhibit thrombosis after deep vascular injury and contributes to endothelial cell-mediated inhibition of intimal hyperplasia. *Proc Natl Acad Sci U S A* 97: 6722-6727

9. Peng HB, Xie H, Rossi SG, Rotundo RL (1999) Acetylcholinesterase clustering at the neuromuscular junction involves perlecan and dystroglycan. *J Cell Biol* 145: 911-921

Muscular dystrophy caused by α7 integrin deficiency

Maggie C. Walter
Hanns Lochmüller

> **OMIM** Online Mendelian Inheritance in Man
> (*http://www.ncbi.nlm.nih.gov/omim*)

Definition of entity

Patients with a new form of congenital muscular dystrophy caused by *α7 integrin (ITGA7) deficiency* were described in 1998 by Hayashi et al (4) (OMIM 600536). In this study, 117 muscle biopsies from patients with laminin α2-positive congenital myopathies were surveyed by immunhistochemistry. Three unrelated Japanese patients were found to have complete α7 integrin deficiency in skeletal muscle. So far, no additional patients have been described in the literature. Therefore, a detailed description of the originally communicated patients is given below.

The first patient is a 4-year-old boy with a compound heterozygous 21-bp in-frame insertion and a 98-bp frame shift deletion of the *ITGA* gene. The patient exhibited delayed psychomotor milestones, acquiring the ability to roll over at 9 months, and walking at $2^{1}/_{2}$ years. At 4 years of age he was unable to jump and run, and he exhibited mental retardation and limited verbal abilities. EEG and brain MRI were normal, CK levels were mildly elevated. Muscle biopsy confirmed congenital myopathy at 15 months of age. The second patient, an 11-year-old girl, had the same 98-bp deletion as patient 1 and a 1-bp chain termination deletion at the second allele of the *ITGA* gene. At 2 months she was diagnosed with congenital dislocation of the hip and torticollis that required surgery. She acquired independent ambulation at a little over 2 years of age and exhibited Gower's sign and waddling gait. She was never able to run or climb stairs without assistance. Mental retardation was not observed. CK levels were mildly elevated. Muscle biopsy revealed congenital myopathy with fatty replacement and fibre size variation. The third patient, a 5-year-old boy, exhibited reduced *ITGA7* mRNA; so far, the underlying mutation of the *ITGA7* gene has not been identified. He showed hypotonia and torticollis from birth. He was unable to walk without support and exhibited delayed motor milestones. Biopsy revealed congenital myopathy with fibre size variation (4). Clinical symptoms and histopathological changes exhibited by all 3 patients are consistent with the putative role for α7 integrin in the formation and integrity of the plasmalemmal membrane (1, 4).

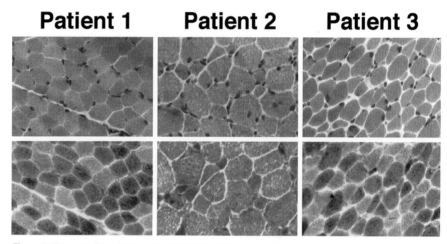

Figure 1. Haematoxylin and eosin (HE) and NADH staining of skeletal muscles from three patients with primary integrin α7 deficiency showing mild myopathic changes with variation of muscle fibre diameter. Figure kindly provided by Dr Y. K. Hayashi, Department of Neuromuscular Research, National Institute of Neuroscience, NCNP, Ogawa-Higashi, Kodaira, Tokyo, Japan.

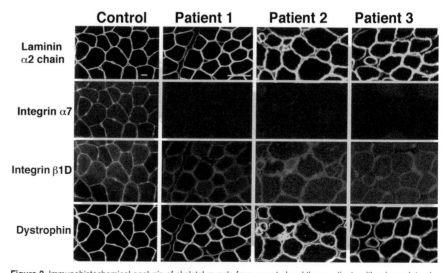

Figure 2. Immunohistochemical analysis of skeletal muscle from a control and three patients with primary integrin α7 deficiency. Consecutive cryosections are immunostained for laminin α2 chain, integrin α7, integrin β1D and dystrophin. In the patients, immunostaining of integrin α7 is negative. Reduced immunoreaction for the β1D is also seen. Laminin α2 chain and dystrophin are normal in all samples. Bar = 25 micrometer. Illustration: Dr Y. K. Hayashi, Tokyo, Japan.

Similarly, α7 integrin knockout mice develop muscular dystrophy and exhibit a shortened life span. Major structural changes include the myotendinous junction (6). More detailed analysis of these animals may reveal whether the expression of other laminin-binding integrins (for example, α3β1 and α6β1) has been altered to compensate for the decrease in α7β1 during myogenic development and in adult muscle.

Molecular genetics and pathophysiology

The integrins are a family of heterodimeric membrane glycoproteins that mediate a wide spectrum of cell-cell and cell-matrix interactions. In humans, the *ITGA7* gene is located on chromosome 12q13 between D12S312 and D12S90 (8). Vignier et al (7) determined the genomic structure of the *ITGA7* gene, which is composed of at least 27 exons spanning a region of about 22.5 kb. Investigation of the different splicing forms showed 2 major cytoplasmic variants α7A and α7B, which are developmentally regulated and tissue specific, as well as the extracellular isoforms X1 and X2. The recently described D variant was detected in adult tissues by RT-PCR but not the C variant (7).

Expression of *ITGA7* is developmentally regulated during the formation of skeletal muscle. Increased levels of expression and production of isoforms containing different cytoplasmic and extracellular domains accompany myogenesis (8). In adult muscle, the α7 subunit is concentrated at the myotendinous junctions, but is also detected at the neuromuscular junctions and along the sarcolemmal membrane. α7β1 integrin is a specific cellular receptor for the basement membrane protein laminin-1, as well as for the laminin isoforms –2 and –4 (6). Cohn et al (3) investigated the expression of 2 alternative splice variants, the α7B and β1D integrin subunits, in normal human skeletal muscle, as well as in various forms of muscular dystrophy. In normal human skeletal muscle the expression of the α7 integrin subunit appeared to be developmentally regulated: it was first detected at 2 years of age. In contrast, the β1D integrin could be detected in immature and mature muscle in the sarcolemma of normal fetal skeletal muscle at 18 weeks gestation.

Structural changes

Altered expression of α7β1 integrin in various human and murine muscular dystrophies was described by Hodges et al (5). Immunofluorescence demonstrated an increase in α7β1 integrin in dystrophin deficiency, ie, patients with Duchenne muscular dystrophy (DMD) and in mdx mice. RNA analysis indicated that the increase of α7β1 integrin is regulated at the level of transcription. Interestingly, in human dystrophinopathies expression of α7B was upregulated irrespective of the level of dystrophin expression. Increased expression of α7β1 integrin in the absence of dystrophin may compensate for the reduced dystrophin-mediated linkage of fibres with the basal lamina and may modulate the development of pathology associated with these diseases. Conversely, the level of α7β1 integrin is severely diminished in patients with congenital muscular dystrophy and in *dy/dy* mice due to α2 laminin mutations. The decrease of α7β1 integrin in the absence of laminin may likely contribute to the severe myopathy that results from laminin α2 chain deficiency (3, 5). However, this reduction was not correlated with the amount of laminin α2 chain expressed (3).

In contrast, the expression of the laminin α2 chain was not altered in the skeletal muscle of α7 integrin knockout mice. Sarcolemmal expression of β1D integrin was significantly reduced, whereas the expression of the components of the DGC was not altered. Similarly, Hayashi et al (4) detected a mild reduction of integrin β1D in patients described above, but normal expression of the laminin α2 chain, dystrophin, β-dystroglycan, and α-sarcoglycan. These findings reinforce the hypothesis that α7B integrin is an important laminin receptor within the plasma membrane which plays a significant role in skeletal muscle function and stability (3).

Future perspectives

Human congenital muscular dystrophy caused by α7 integrin (*ITGA7*) deficiency appears to be rare, so far solely detected in few Japanese patients. However, the functional roles of α7β1 integrin in the formation and stability of the neuromuscular and myotendinous junctions suggest that altered expression or function of this integrin may have a widespread, secondary involvement in other myopathies. Moreover, increased expression of α7 integrin may open new avenues for the molecular treatment of other muscular dystrophies such as dystrophin deficiency (2).

References

1. Burkin DJ, Kaufman SJ (1999) The α7β1 integrin in muscle development and disease. *Cell Tissue Res* 296: 183-190

2. Burkin DJ, Wallace GQ, Nicol KJ, Kaufman DJ, Kaufman SJ (2001) Enhanced expression of the α7β1 integrin reduces muscular dystrophy and restores viability in dystrophic mice. *J Cell Biol* 152: 1207-1218

3. Cohn RD, Mayer U, Saher G, Herrmann R, van der Flier A, Sonnenberg A, Sorokin L, Voit T (1999) Secondary reduction of α7B integrin in laminin α2 deficient congenital muscular dystrophy supports an additional transmembrane link in skeletal muscle. *J Neurol Sci* 163: 140-152

4. Hayashi YK, Chou FL, Engvall E, Ogawa M, Matsuda C, Hirabayashi S, Yokochi K, Ziober BL, Kramer RH, Kaufman SJ, Ozawa E, Goto Y, Nonaka I, Tsukahara T, Wang JZ, Hoffman EP, Arahata K (1998) Mutations in the integrin α7 gene cause congenital myopathy. *Nat Genet* 19: 94-97

5. Hodges BL, Hayashi YK, Nonaka I, Wang W, Arahata K, Kaufman SJ (1997) Altered expression of the α7β1 integrin in human and murine muscular dystrophies. *J Cell Sci* 110: 2873-2881

6. Mayer U, Saher G, Fassler R, Bornemann A, Echtermeyer F, von der Mark H, Miosge N, Poschl E, von der Mark K (1997) Absence of integrin α7 causes a novel form of muscular dystrophy. *Nat Genet* 17: 318-323

7. Vignier N, Moghadaszadeh B, Gary F, Beckmann J, Mayer U, Guicheney P (1999) Structure, genetic localization, and identification of the cardiac and skeletal muscle transcripts of the human integrin α7 gene (*ITGA7*). *Biochem Biophys Res Commun* 260: 357-364

8. Wang W, Wu W, Desai T, Ward DC, Kaufman SJ (1995) Localization of the α7 integrin gene (*ITGA7*) on human chromosome 12q13: clustering of integrin and Hox genes implies parallel evolution of these gene families. *Genomics* 26: 568-570

CHAPTER 3

Diseases associated with myonuclear abnormalities

3.1 Defects of nuclear membrane related proteins (emerin, lamins A/C)   48
3.2 Abnormalities in nuclear positioning (centronuclear myopathies)   57

There has been a tendency to ignore myonuclei in the pathology and biology of the muscle fibre, even though the nucleus contains an overwhelmingly large part of the genome of the cell. Traditionally, descriptions of myonuclear abnormality were limited to their internal position either as a non-specific feature or a distinct entity in centronuclear myopathies, as well as their typical alterations in regenerating muscle fibres.

Recently, novel molecules of myonuclei have been identified whose genetically determined deficiency or abnormality was linked to specific muscle diseases. These molecules include emerin, lamin A/C and poly(A) binding protein 2 (PAB2). Although PAB2 deficiency in oculopharyngeal muscular dystrophy (OPMD) could logically belong to this chapter, we have chosen to place it in chapter 6 on account of the unusual type of mutation that occurs in that gene in OPMD.

In other instances, abnormal filaments accumulate as a distinct disease marker in myonuclei of sporadic inclusion body myositis. These may represent abnormal nuclear matrix molecules. Distinctive myonuclear changes may occur in rare instances of muscle cell apoptosis. Specific microscopic techniques have been designed to demonstrate major gene rearrangements or chromosomal abnormalities that can be useful for pathological diagnosis (fluorescent in situ hybridization, FISH). Further disease-related discoveries are expected regarding the myonuclear matrix and putative myonuclear anchoring elements that ensure their normal subsarcolemmal position.

Defects of nuclear membrane related proteins (emerin, lamins A/C)

Gisèle Bonne

This chapter is dedicated to Dr. Kiichi Arahata, Tokyo, Japan who did such outstanding work in the field of Emery-Dreifuss muscular dystrophy and was one of the experts in the study of emerin.

AD-EDMD	autosomal dominant form of Emery-Dreifuss muscular dystrophy
BMD	Becker muscular dystrophy
DCM-CD	dilated cardiomyopathy with conduction defects
DMD	Duchenne muscular dystrophy
ER	endoplasmic reticulum
FPLD	Dunnigan-type familial partial lipodystrophy
LMNA	lamin A/C gene
LAP	lamina-associated protein
LBR	lamin B receptor
LGMD	limb-girdle muscular dystrophy
XL-EDMD	X-linked Emery-Dreifuss muscular-dystrophy

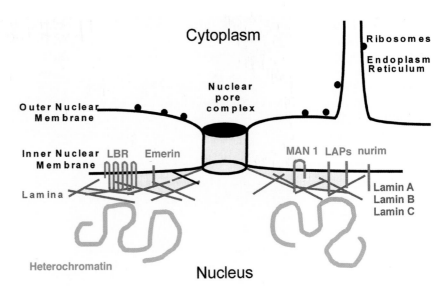

Figure 1. *Schematic view of the nuclear envelope.* The nuclear envelope is composed of two lipid bilayer membranes, nuclear pore complexes and nuclear lamina. The outer nuclear membrane is continuous with the endoplasmic reticulum. The inner nuclear membrane is separated from the outer nuclear membrane by the perinuclear space, except at the nuclear pore complexes, where the outer nuclear membrane and the inner nuclear membrane are connected. Underlying the inner membrane is the fibrous nuclear lamina. It is composed of two types of lamin proteins: A-type lamins (lamins A/C) and B-type lamins (lamin B). They interact with chromatin as well as with other proteins of the inner nuclear membrane (Lamin B receptor (LBR), lamina-associated proteins (LAPs), emerin, MAN1, Nurim). Image kindly provided by M. R. Barton and H. Worman, Columbia University, New York, NY. Adapted with permission from Roberts and Schwartz, 2000 (60).

Background

Eukaryotic cells have a nuclear envelope (Figure 1) that separates nucleoplasm from cytoplasmic compartment, and organises nuclear structure. The nuclear envelope is composed of outer and inner nuclear membranes, nuclear pore complexes and nuclear lamina. The outer and inner nuclear membranes fuse at the nuclear pore complexes which perforate the double nuclear membranes and participate in nuclear-cytoplasmic molecular transport. The outer nuclear membrane is directly continuous with the rough endoplasmic reticulum (ER). Thus, the lumen of the endoplasmic reticulum has continuity with the perinuclear cistern or space; diffusion or trafficking of molecules from the endoplasmic reticulum to Golgi apparatus uses the envelope as an intermediary compartment (68). The inner nuclear membrane faces the nuclear lamina and nucleoplasm, and integral membrane proteins of the inner nuclear envelope bind to lamins and chromatin in the initial events of nuclear envelope reassembly during the cell cycle (26).

Six integral inner nuclear membrane proteins have been identified: lamina-associated protein LAP1 (43), LAP2 (26, 28), lamin B receptor (LBR) (81), MAN1 (39), emerin (2, 44, 55) and nurim (61) (Figure 1). Emerin is anchored to the inner nuclear membrane via a carboxy-terminal tail with remainder of the molecule projecting within the nucleoplasm (16, 46). This protein presents several serine protein kinase sites (44, 55). Emerin appears to be important in the organisation of the nuclear membrane during cell division (21). The targeting of integral proteins to the inner membrane is thought to involve lateral diffusion along the ER and the "pore membrane domain," followed by retention at the inner membrane mediated by binding to lamins or chromosomes. The functions of these integral proteins of the inner nuclear membrane are poorly understood; however, their attachment to lamins, and in many cases to chromatin, suggest that they might link chromatin and lamins to the membrane (79). A subset of nuclear membrane proteins including LAP2, emerin, and MAN1, belong to the newly defined "LEM domain" family since they shared a distinct ~43-residue motif called LEM domain (LEM = LAP2, Emerin and MAN1) (39). The exact function of this LEM domain is still unknown (79). In LAP2, the LEM domain mediates binding to a ubiquitous, highly conserved and novel DNA-bridging protein named BAF (27).

Lamins are the principal components of the nuclear lamina, a quasi-regular network forming the major structural framework of the nuclear envelope of all eucaryotic cells (68). Lamins are type V intermediate filaments. They are classified as A- or B-type, according to homology in sequence, expression pattern, biochemical properties and their cellular localisation in mitosis (68). In humans, two A-type lamins (lamins A and C) and two B-type lamins (B1 and B2) have been described (7, 40). Lamins display a central-α-helical rod domain characterised by a heptad repeat of hydrophobic amino acids, flanked by non-α-helical domains at the amino and carboxy-terminal ends. A prominent feature that distinguishes lamins from other cytoplasmic intermediate filaments proteins is a nuclear localisation signal. Located early in the tail past the carboxyl end of the rod domain, the signal is necessary for nuclear import of the lamins (41). Lamins can interact with themselves, lamina-associated proteins, and chromatin.

The role of lamins has been extensively studied. There is compelling evidence that lamins play a role in DNA replication, chromatin organisation, spatial arrangement of nuclear pore complexes, nuclear growth, mechanical stabilisation of the nucleus, and anchorage of the nuclear envelope proteins (31, 68). Direct interaction between emerin and lamin A has been demonstrated by biomolecular interaction analysis on a BIAcore sensor and by immunoprecipitation analysis (12, 63).

The nuclear envelope has structural interactions with the cytoskeletal filaments that may participate in determining the position of the nucleus, movement of cytoplasmic molecules, and presumably, linkage between extracellular matrix and nucleus (47). Possible connections between the surface membrane integrins, cytoskeletal filaments and nuclear envelope imply a structural role for these proteins.

Clinical phenotypes

In 1994 mutations in a new gene were identified by positional cloning in patients with X-linked Emery-Dreifuss muscular-dystrophy (XL-EDMD) (2). The corresponding protein was therefore called "emerin" and described as an integral membrane protein of the nuclear envelope (2, 44, 55). An unexpected breakthrough came with the discovery in 1999, that mutations in the gene of two other nuclear envelope proteins, the lamin A/C gene (*LMNA*), cause the autosomal dominant form of Emery-Dreifuss muscular dystrophy (AD-EDMD). In some patients, the disease was confined exclusively to the heart and associated with a high incidence of sudden death (1, 3). This set the stage for analysing other hereditary diseases. Within a few months, it was demonstrated that naturally occurring mutations within the *LMNA* gene underlie AD-EDMD, the autosomal recessive form of EDMD and three other diseases: limb-girdle muscular dystrophy type 1B (LGMD1B), dilated cardiomyopathy with conduction defects (DCM-CD), and Dunnigan-type familial partial lipodystrophy (FPLD) (9, 14, 22, 53, 66).

Emery-Dreifuss muscular dystrophy. Emery-Dreifuss muscular dystrophy (EDMD) is an inherited disorder described by Cestan and Lejonne in 1902 (11). A detailed clinical characterisation of the disorder was reported in the 1960s by Emery and Dreifuss (20). EDMD is a clinically and genetically heterogeneous condition. It is typically characterised by a triad of *i*) early contractures, often before there is any significant weakness of the Achilles tendons, elbows and post cervical muscles, *ii*) slowly progressive muscle wasting and weakness with a distinctive humero-peroneal distribution early during the course of the disease, and *iii*) by adult life, affected individuals invariably develop a cardiomyopathy, usually presenting as conduction defects ranging from sinus bradycardia, prolongation of the PR interval on ECG, to complete block requiring pacing. Thus, affected individuals may die suddenly from heart block, or develop progressive heart failure. The latter may occur subsequent to the insertion of a pacemaker to correct an arrhythmia (1, 19, 78).

Two major modes of inheritance exist, X-linked (XL-EDMD) and autosomal dominant (AD-EDMD). Rare cases of autosomal recessive transmission (AR-EDMD) have been reported (14, 70, 72). Defects in emerin are responsible of XL-EDMD (2), whereas mutations in lamin A/C gene cause AD and AR-EDMD (3, 14). Overall, the three forms are clinically identical (24, 50, 78) although some slight differences occur between XL and AD forms of EDMD (4). AD-EDMD patients have more severe and progressive wasting of the biceps brachii compared to what is typically present in XL-EDMD (18, 82). Hypertrophy of the quadriceps muscle, and of the extensor digitorum brevis muscles, was present in several AD-EDMD patients but not in XL-EDMD. Contractures, the first symptoms in XL-EDMD, might appear after weakness and difficulty while running in AD-EDMD patients. Loss of ambulation due to a combination of increasing joint stiffness and weakness is observed in AD-EDMD, but is extremely rare in XL-EDMD (33, 78).

Limb-girdle muscular dystrophy associated with atrioventricular conduction disturbances (LGMD1B). Limb girdle muscular dystrophies (LGMD) represent a genetically heterogeneous group of myogenic disorders with a limb girdle distribution of weakness (8). The inheritance pattern in LGMD is heterogeneous. Four dominant (LGMD1) and eight recessive forms (LGMD2) have been defined to date. Van der Kooi et al (75) have described the LGMD1B form, inherited as an autosomal dominant trait. It is characterised by symmetrical weakness starting in the proximal lower limb muscles. Gradually, upper limb muscles become affected. Early contractures of the spine are absent, and contractures of elbows or Achilles tendons are either minimal or late. These features led the authors to conclude that this disorder differs from EDMD.

Cardiological abnormalities including dysarrhythmias and atrioventricular conduction disturbances were found in

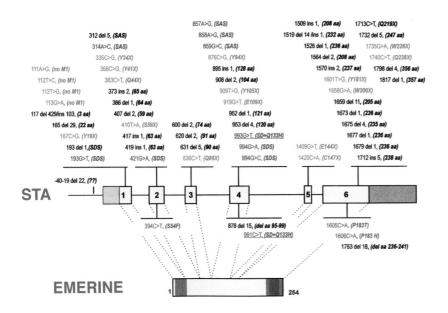

Figure 2. *Emerin gene (STA) mutations identified in XL-EDMD and their consequences on the protein structure of emerin.* Mutations identified in XL-EDMD are presented (83). The number of nucleotide affected refers to the genomic sequence (83). Each mutation is depicted by its nucleotide number, its nucleotide change and in bracket and bold the corresponding protein modifications. **Above** the gene are mutations leading to truncated emerin: insertions/deletions are in black, splice acceptor site (SAS) and splice donor site (SDS) mutations are in blue, nonsense point mutation suppressing ATG or introduction a stop codon are in green. **Below** the gene are mutations leading to mutated emerin: in frame deletions are in black, missense point mutations are in red, splice donor site (SDS) mutations are in blue. The underlined mutation affects a slice donor site and produce either a missense mutation (Q133H), either an aberrant slicing (51). Blue box on emerin structure corresponds to the transmembrane domain; orange boxes correspond to part of emerin that are homologous to LAP2 domains (2). Kindly provided by Dr Dominique Recan, Cochin Hospital, Paris, France.

	Emerin gene (*STA*)	Lamins A and C gene (*LMNA*)
Large gene deletion	3	None
Promoter	1	None
Nonsense (STOP or no ATG)	22	1
Deletion with frameshift + STOP	22	2
Insertion with frameshift + stop	6	None
Splice site mutation	11*	2*
Missense	4*	35*
In frame deletion	2	3

Table 1. *Type of mutations identified in STA encoding emerin and in LMNA encoding lamins A/C. STA* mutations have been reported in one publication (83) and *LMNA* mutations in several papers (4, 6, 14, 22, 23, 29, 36, 53, 66, 67, 77). *One *STA* mutation (83) and one *LMNA* mutation (4) lead potentially to two mutants proteins, one with a missense mutation and one with an aberrant splicing.

the majority of the patients; they presented as bradycardia and syncopal attacks necessitating pacemaker implantation, and sudden cardiac death. In the families analysed by van der Kooi et al, (75) there was a significant relationship between the severity of atrioventricular conduction disturbances and age; the neuromuscular symptoms preceded heart involvement. Because the locus of LGMD1B had been mapped to chromosome 1q11-21 (76) where *LMNA* is located, this became a good candidate gene for this muscular disease. Mutation analysis of *LMNA* in the three LGMD1B families described by van der Kooi et al (75) identified three different *LMNA* mutations, thus demonstrating that LGMD1B and AD-EDMD are allelic disorders (53).

Dilated cardiomyopathy and conduction defects (DCM-CD). Car-

diomyopathies are defined as diseases of the myocardium associated with cardiac dysfunction (59). The most common types are the dilated forms, responsible for approximately 60% of cases of cardiomyopathy, with an annual incidence estimated to be 5 to 8 cases per 100 000 population (13). Dilated cardiomyopathy (DCM) is characterised by dilatation and impaired contraction of either the left or both ventricles. Structural changes are non-specific. Presentation is usually with heart failure, which is often progressive. Arrhythmias, thromboembolism and sudden death are common and may occur at any stage. Many causes for DCM have been described, but most commonly this disease is considered idiopathic. Familial DCM accounts for 20 to 30% of all DCM (49).

That *LMNA* could be involved in DCM was completely unexpected. In the majority of affected members of one French family with AD-EDMD, the disease was confined exclusively to the heart and associated with arrhythmias, left ventricular dysfunction, dilated cardiomyopathy and a high incidence of sudden death (1, 3). These patients could easily have been diagnosed as DCM with conduction defects (DCM-CD). This showed *i)* that the variability of the AD-EDMD phenotype is wider than originally thought, and *ii)* that *LMNA* is one of the disease genes of familial DCM-CD. Mutations in *LMNA* were subsequently found in unrelated families with DCM-CD (22). In addition, a *LMNA* mutation was identified in a family in which three phenotypes were described: DCM with EDMD-like skeletal muscle abnormalities, DCM with LGMD-like skeletal muscle abnormalities, and pure DCM-CD (6).

Dunnigan-type of familial partial lipodystrophy. Dunnigan-type familial partial lipodystrophy (FPLD) is a rare autosomal dominant disease that is part of a heterogeneous group of disorders characterised by the absence or reduction of subcutaneous adipose tissue (37). Patients with FPLD have a nor-

mal fat distribution in early childhood, but with the onset of puberty almost all subcutaneous adipose tissue from the upper and lower extremities and gluteal and truncal areas gradually disappears, causing prominence of muscles and superficial veins. Adipose tissue accumulates in the face and neck, causing a double chin, fat neck or Cushing-like appearance. Affected patients are insulin-resistant and may develop glucose intolerance and diabetes mellitus after the age of 20 years. The FPLD locus was mapped to chromosome 1q21-22 (58). The elegant rationale to consider *LMNA* as a candidate gene for this disease was that there is an analogy between the highly specific anatomical involvement in AD-EDMD and FPLD. Indeed, *LMNA* mutations have been identified in families with FPLD (9, 66, 67, 77). So far, no cardiac or skeletal defects have been reported in FPLD patients with *LMNA* mutation.

Molecular genetics and pathophysiology

Mutations of emerin gene (STA). *STA* is very small; only 2kb long and composed of 6 exons. Emerin is its 32 kDa protein product of 254 amino acids (2). To date, 70 mutations in *STA* have been reported (Table 1, Figure 2). A mutation database is maintained (83). The distribution of the mutations is homogeneous along the gene, with no evidence of "hot spot" of mutation. They are composed approximately by 40% of small deletions or insertions, 31% of nonsense mutations, 16% of mutations in splice sites, 4% of large deletion of a part or the totality of the gene, 8% of missense mutations and 1% of mutation in the promoter.

Almost all mutations (88%) potentially lead to truncated emerin, which lack the C-terminal transmembrane sequence. These mutations actually result in lack of emerin on Western blotting and immunocytochemistry (45). Since emerin mRNA levels are usually normal, absence of emerin suggests that truncated emerin mutants are unstable under normal conditions. In

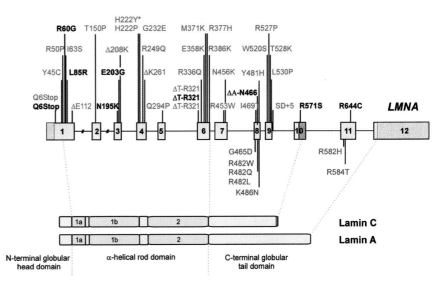

Figure 3. *Lamin A/C gene (LMNA) mutations identified in AD-EDMD, LGMD1B, CMD and FPLD, and their position on the protein structure of lamins A and C.* Mutations identified in AD-EDMD are presented in red (3, 4, 6, 14, 23). The AR-EDMD mutation is depicted by an asterisk (*) (14). LGMD 1B mutations are in green (6, 53). Black mutations correspond to DCM mutations (1, 6, 22). The blue mutations are report in FPLD (9, 66, 67, 77). Image adapted with permission from Roberts and Schwartz, 2000 (60).

patients presenting a frameshift in the sixth exon, a new hydrophobic tail was synthesised, compatible in amino acid composition and length with a nuclear envelope transmembrane domain. In one of these patients, Western blot analysis revealed the presence of the truncated form of the protein, and the immunocytochemical analysis on muscle sections demonstrated reduced amounts of the protein in correct regions (10). In another patient, in whom mutated emerin was predicted to have a new transmembrane domain with a larger tail, immunocytochemical studies showed mutated emerin localised only in the cytoplasm of muscle fibres and lymphoblastoid cells (15).

Only 6 missense mutations have been reported: S54F, Q133H, P183W, P183H, and two in frame deletion (83). The Q133H mutation had a double effect; this point mutation at the last nucleotide of exon 4 causes a change of glutamine to histamine, but also interfered with splicing by reducing the amount of correctly processed RNA (51).

Mutations in lamins A/C gene (LMNA). Lamins A and C (664 and 572 amino acids, respectively) are

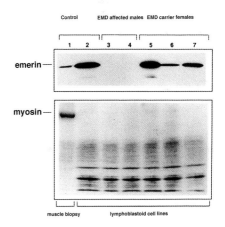

Figure 4. *Western blot analysis of emerin carried out lymphoblastoid cell lines of XL-EDMD cases.* Emerin is absent in the lymphoblastoid cell line of affected males (line 3 and 4), and shows variable expression levels in female carriers (lines 5-7). Figure kindly given by Dr D. Recan, Cochin Hospital, Paris, France.

encoded by *LMNA* through alternative splicing within exon 10. *LMNA* contains 12 exons, which are spread over approximately 24 kilobases of genomic DNA (40) (Figure 3). Since the first description of *LMNA* mutations in AD-EDMD, a total of 42 different mutations were reported (Table 1, Figure 3): 1 nonsense mutation, 2 deletions with frameshift, 1 splice site mutation, 3 in-frame deletions, and 35 missense mutations. As in *STA* gene, one of the missense mutation affects the last

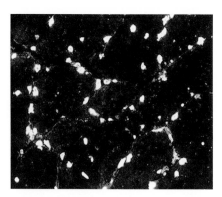

Figure 5. *Emerin detection on tissue sections of XL-EDMD patient shown in Figure 5-8. Originally published by Muntoni et al. (1998) (54) and reproduced by kind permission from Elsevier Science. Illustration provided by Dr Caroline Sewry, London, UK. Cryostat sections immunolabelled with a monoclonal antibody to emerin showing normal nuclear labelling in control muscle.*

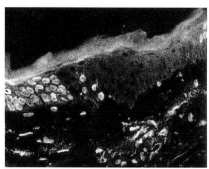

Figure 7. A mosaic pattern of groups of emerin-positive and emerin-negative nuclei in the skin of the patient's mother compared with his aunt shown in Figure 8.

nucleotide of *LMNA* exon 6, leading to 2 possible mutants, a missense (R386K) and a splice site mutation. The latter results in the retention of intron 6 within the mRNA and the potential production of truncated lamins A/C (4).

The mutations are distributed along the gene between exons 1 and 10 in the region common to lamins A and C; except for 2 missense mutations, which are located in exon 10 specific of lamin C and in exon 11 specific of lamin A (22, 30). Two "hot spot" mutations have been observed: among the 66 reported laminopathy cases, 14% carry the R453W missense mutation (4, 14) and 12% have a missense mutation at R482, this latter being modified in three different amino acids (R482W, R482Q and R482L) (9, 66, 67, 77).

Figure 6. Absence of emerin immunoreactivity in all nuclei of the muscle biopsy of a XL-EDMD patient.

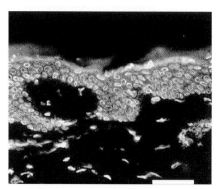

Figure 8. The aunt has a normal expression of emerin and is not a carrier. Bar = 50 μm.

Twenty-eight mutations have been identified in 14 AD-EDMD families, 27 sporadic EDMD cases and 4 LGMD1B families (3, 4, 14, 23, 36, 53). *LMNA* is also responsible for AR-EDMD since in a consanguineous family where a patient carries a homozygote missense mutation (H222Y), the parents who are heterozygotes for the mutation are not affected by the disease (14). Nine mutations have been reported in patients with isolated DCM (1, 6, 22, 29, 30). It was initially suggested that mutations in either the rod domain or the tail domain of lamin C might underlie the DMC-CD phenotype (22).

However, two reports demonstrated that within a family, the same *LMNA* mutation gives rise to various phenotypes ranging from an isolated DCM to LGMD1B or EDMD (1, 6). Among all the reported cases with cardiac and/or skeletal disorders (EDMD, LGMD1B and DCM) due to *LMNA* mutation, there is no clear correlation between the phenotype and type or localisation of the mutation in the gene (1, 4, 6, 36,

53). In contrast, the majority of mutations (90%) described in FPLD affect the same codon of exon 8, ie, the arginine 482 is mutated in 28 of 32 FLPD reported cases. Besides this "hot spot," 4 other mutations have been reported in FPLD families: 2 located in exon 8 and 2 in exon 11 that encodes only the tail domain of lamin A (9, 66, 67, 77).

Structural changes

Light microscopy. Skeletal muscle biopsies from patients with EDMD show dystrophic changes with a few necrotic and regenerating fibres; however, this is not specific to this muscular disease. Fibre necrosis is usually less prominent than in Duchenne muscular dystrophy (DMD) or Becker muscular dystrophy (BMD) (35). Skeletal muscles show marked variations in fibre diameter associated with an increased number of hypertrophic fibres and internal nuclei (32, 34, 65). Myocardial changes with focal degeneration and increased endomysial fatty and fibrous connective tissues are also present (85). Muscle biopsies from patients with LGMD1B show non-specific myopathic changes similar to those observed in XL and AD-EDMD (75).

Immunohistochemistry. If morphological changes observed in muscle biopsies of EDMD and LGMD1B patients are non-specific, immunocytochemical analysis could at least give some clue for XL-EDMD cases. Indeed, the fact that almost all *STA* mutations result in the absence of emerin enables rapid diagnosis of most X-linked cases. This could be achieved either by immunocytochemistry (Figures 4-7) on muscle biopsies—but more easily on skin biopsies or buccal smears—or by Western blotting (Figure 8) of white blood cells (46, 62). Immunocytochemistry of skin fibroblasts or exfoliative buccal cell reveals a mosaic pattern of expression of emerin in carriers, and thus provides a valuable test for identifying clinically unaffected female carriers who requests genetics counselling. On Western blot analysis, this mosaic pattern of expression of emerin in carriers is revealed by a reduction of emerin (45, 46) (Figure 8). Rare cases with reduced amount of emerin—due to a missense mutation—could also be observed and may have a milder phenotype (17).

Regarding lamin A/C gene mutations, all but one are inherited on an autosomal dominant trait (see above), ie, one normal and one mutant gene are expressed in the various tissues of the patients. Immunocytochemical analysis of lamin A/C and emerin on skeletal muscle biopsies of nine AD-EDMD patients carrying missense *LMNA* mutation showed no detectable differences from control muscles (64, 65). The same analysis performed on a cardiac biopsy of an AD-EDMD patient with a non-sense mutation showed the same results, indicating that the mutation does not significantly alter the structure of the nuclear envelope (3). This latter mutation potentially leads to the production of truncated lamins A/C of only five amino acids. Such small peptides are most likely degraded and only lamins A/C produced by the intact allele are expressed in the patients. This hypothesis was confirmed by the Western-blot analysis of the explanted myocardial tissue that showed a decreased expression of lamins A/C as compared to that of a control heart tissue (1). A secondary reduction of laminin β1 in the extracellular matrix of muscle fibres was observed in some cases of AD-EDMD (65). Expression of laminin β1 on blood vessels is normal and the reduction was seen only on the muscle fibres. This is an age-related phenomenon and has only been observed in adult and adolescent cases. However, it is not a specific marker of the laminopathies since it has been observed in cases of Bethlem myopathy (48), other dominant myopathies (5, 73), and forms of limb-girdle muscular dystrophy (38).

Electron microscopy. Ultrastructure analyses have been performed on emerinopathy and laminopathy muscle biopsies (25, 56, 65). Nuclear changes were observed in the nuclei of skeletal muscle and cultured fibroblasts of a XL-EDMD patient with a frequency of 10% and 18%, respectively. Nuclear envelope associated heterochromatin was affected, whereas the pore complexes appeared preserved and the cytoplasm of the same cells were normal (56). Another study of nine emerinopathy muscle biopsies revealed different degrees of abnormalities in the sarcolemmal nuclei ranging from marked condensation of the chromatin to complete damage of the nuclear component. Other nuclei in the same muscle cell very often appeared normal. The extrusion of nuclear chromatin into sarcoplasm as a consequence of the nuclear membrane disintegration was observed in numerous nuclei (25). Finally, the first results of ultrastructure analysis of laminopathy cases revealed alterations in the chromatin distribution in 2 out of 3 cases analysed (65).

Genotype–phenotype correlations

In both emerinopathies and laminopathies, a wide clinical variability both at intra and inter familial levels is reported (1, 4, 6, 14, 19, 22, 52, 75). This is completely independent of the type or localisation of the mutation. Indeed, in the majority of XL-EDMD cases, the same defect, namely the absence of emerin, leads to a wide range of phenotype severity from very early and severe EDMD to very mild EDMD (19, 78). Similarly, among the reported cases of laminopathy with cardiac and/or skeletal defects (EDMD, LGMD1B and DCM), the same mutation leads to various phenotypes (1, 6).

No correlation is observed between the gene defect and the structural abnormalities present in the muscle biopsies since they are mainly non specific dystrophic or myopathic features. At the immunohistochemical level, there is a good correlation between the defects of *STA* gene and the expression of emerin, ie, absence of the protein for the nonsense mutation, possible reduction for missense mutation, and mosaic

pattern of expression in female carriers (17, 45, 46). Such correlation has not yet been found in laminopathies due to the autosomal dominant inheritance of the gene defects. Indeed, lamins A/C produced by the intact allele are expressed in the patient tissues, and a variation in the quantity of the proteins is difficult to detect at the immunohistochemical level. Western-blot analysis might help in certain cases (1), but is not yet currently used.

Finally, ultrastructural changes are observed in both emerinopathy and laminopathy but not in a large extent , and only a small proportion of muscle nuclei exhibit abnormalities (25, 56, 65). Thus, the abnormalities in heterochromatin distribution are not a consistent feature and might be secondary to other pathological factors. In the few cases reported, the nuclear abnormalities were slightly different—possibly related to their different mutations—which might affect nuclear envelope organisation in a different manner (65). Additional cases are needed before any conclusion can be drawn.

Future perspectives

The involvement of nuclear envelope proteins, emerin and lamins A/C, implicated in tissue-specific diseases (cardiac and/or skeletal muscle or adipose tissue) raises a certain number of unanswered questions. Emerin and lamins A/C have a quasi-ubiquitous expression (2, 7). Therefore, it could be asked why only striated muscle tissues are affected in EDMD, LGMD1B, and DCM. The most probable hypothesis is that mechanical constraints induced during muscle contraction heighten the fragility of muscle cell nucleus (74). Lamins A/C, as well as emerin could thus constitute a nucleo-cytoskeletal network (74) to protect muscle cell nucleus from stress. Recently, a murine model that exhibits a loss of expression of lamins A/C has been published supporting this notion of the disorder of the nuclear architecture (69). At birth, the homozygous mice *lmna*-/- are no different from normal mice, but develop a skeletal and cardiac myopathy similar to AD-EDMD towards the fourth week. However, it is surprising to see that the heterozygous mice present no muscular phenotype. It would seem that these murine muscle cells are less sensitive to the loss of lamins A/C expression than human cells.

However, an increased fragility of the muscle cell nucleus cannot by itself explain the very selective damage to certain muscles in the three muscular pathologies. Why is it that only humeroperoneal skeletal muscles, the scapular and pelvic girdle, and/or the cardiac muscle are particularly damaged? A tissue-specific gene regulation model has been suggested by Östlund et al (57). Emerin and lamins A/C—which directly or indirectly interact with the chromatin proteins, transcription factors, or the DNA sequences involved in the regulation of the genes (12, 42, 63, 71, 84)—could also play a role in gene expression. Therefore, a modulation of the tissue-specific gene sequences could be at the origin of these three muscles pathologies associated with lamins A/C (80). An emerin or a lamin A/C deficiency would prevent the correct anchorage of chromatin in the nuclear envelope.

All these hypotheses are based on the functionality of emerin and lamins A/C, of which still little is known or explored. Hopefully, future research into the roles of these nuclear membrane proteins, as well as those of their partners, will lead to a better comprehension of the molecular and/or cellular mechanisms responsible for the pathologies concerned. The characterisation of the interactions between emerin, lamins A/C, and other nuclear proteins will be important in determining the exact sites of their domains of interaction with these proteins. The identification of new mutations in EDMD, LGMD1B, DCM, and FLPD will permit the validation of such domains. Another line of investigation, which seems to be emerging, is based on a better knowledge of the interactions between emerin, lamins A/C, and chromatin, as the latter is disorganized in the muscles of EDMD patients and

in the murine inactivation model of the *LMNA* gene (25, 56, 64, 69). We also believe that research into the role of lamins A/C in the regulation of the expression of genes will open the way to confirming or disproving the hypothesis of tissue-specific gene regulation.

References

1. Becane HM, Bonne G, Varnous S, Muchir A, Ortega V, Hammouda EH, Urtizberea JA, Lavergne T, Fardeau M, Eymard B, Weber S, Schwartz K, Duboc D (2000) High incidence of sudden death with conduction system and myocardial disease due to lamins A and C gene mutation. *Pacing Clin Electrophysiol* 23: 1661-1666

2. Bione S, Maestrini E, Rivella S, Mancini M, Regis S, Romeo G, Toniolo D (1994) Identification of a novel X-linked gene responsible for Emery-Dreifuss muscular dystrophy. *Nat Genet* 8: 323-327

3. Bonne G, Di Barletta MR, Varnous S, Becane HM, Hammouda EH, Merlini L, Muntoni F, Greenberg CR, Gary F, Urtizberea JA, Duboc D, Fardeau M, Toniolo D, Schwartz K (1999) Mutations in the gene encoding lamin A/C cause autosomal dominant Emery- Dreifuss muscular dystrophy. *Nat Genet* 21: 285-288

4. Bonne G, Mercuri E, Muchir A, Urtizberea A, Becane HM, Recan D, Merlini L, Wehnert M, Boor R, Reuner U, Vorgerd M, Wicklein EM, Eymard B, Duboc D, Penisson-Besnier I, Cuisset JM, Ferrer X, Desguerre I, Lacombe D, Bushby K, Pollitt C, Toniolo D, Fardeau M, Schwartz K, Muntoni F (2000) Clinical and molecular genetic spectrum of autosomal dominant Emery-Dreifuss muscular dystrophy due to mutations of the lamin A/C gene. *Ann Neurol* 48: 170-180

5. Bornemann A, Anderson LV (2000) Diagnostic protein expression in human muscle biopsies. *Brain Pathol* 10: 193-214

6. Brodsky GL, Muntoni F, Miocic S, Sinagra G, Sewry C, Mestroni L (2000) Lamin A/C gene mutation associated with dilated cardiomyopathy with variable skeletal muscle involvement. *Circulation* 101: 473-476

7. Broers JL, Machiels BM, Kuijpers HJ, Smedts F, van den Kieboom R, Raymond Y, Ramaekers FC (1997) A- and B-type lamins are differentially expressed in normal human tissues. *Histochem Cell Biol* 107: 505-517

8. Bushby KM (1999) The limb-girdle muscular dystrophies-multiple genes, multiple mechanisms. *Hum Mol Genet* 8: 1875-1882

9. Cao H, Hegele RA (2000) Nuclear lamin A/C R482Q mutation in Canadian kindreds with Dunnigan- type familial partial lipodystrophy. *Hum Mol Genet* 9: 109-112

10. Cartegni L, di Barletta MR, Barresi R, Squarzoni S, Sabatelli P, Maraldi N, Mora M, Di Blasi C, Cornelio F, Merlini L, Villa A, Cobianchi F, Toniolo D (1997) Heart-specific localization of emerin: new insights into Emery-Dreifuss muscular dystrophy. *Hum Mol Genet* 6: 2257-2264

11. Cestan R, LeJonne S (1902) Une myopathie avec rétractions familiales. *Nouvelle iconographie de la Salpétrière* 15: 38-52

12. Clements L, Manilal S, Love DR, Morris GE (2000) Direct interaction between emerin and lamin A. *Biochem Biophys Res Commun* 267: 709-714

13. Codd MB, Sugrue DD, Gersh BJ, Melton LJ (1989) Epidemiology of idiopathic dilated and hypertrophic cardiomyopathy. A population-based study in Olmsted County, Minnesota, 1975-1984. *Circulation* 80: 564-572

14. di Barletta MR, Ricci E, Galluzzi G, Tonali P, Mora M, Morandi L (2000) Different mutations in the LMNA gene cause autosomal dominant and autosomal recessive Emery-Dreifuss muscular dystrophy. *Am J Hum Genet* 66: 1407-1412

15. Di Blasi C, Morandi L, Raffaele di Barletta M, Bione S, Bernasconi P, Cerletti M, Bono R, Blasevich F, Toniolo D, Mora M (2000) Unusual expression of emerin in a patient with X-linked Emery-Dreifuss muscular dystrophy. *Neuromuscul Disord* 10: 567-571

16. Ellis JA, Craxton M, Yates JR, Kendrick-Jones J (1998) Aberrant intracellular targeting and cell cycle-dependent phosphorylation of emerin contribute to the Emery-Dreifuss muscular dystrophy phenotype. *J Cell Sci* 111: 781-792

17. Ellis JA, Yates JR, Kendrick-Jones J, Brown CA (1999) Changes at P183 of emerin weaken its protein-protein interactions resulting in X-linked Emery-Dreifuss muscular dystrophy. *Hum Genet* 104: 262-268

18. Emery AE (1987) X-linked muscular dystrophy with early contractures and cardiomyopathy (Emery-Dreifuss type). *Clin Genet* 32: 360-367

19. Emery AE (2000) Emery-Dreifuss muscular dystrophy - a 40 year retrospective. *Neuromuscul Disord* 10: 228-232

20. Emery AE, Dreifuss FE (1966) Unusual type of benign x-linked muscular dystrophy. *J Neurol Neurosurg Psychiatry* 29: 338-342

21. Fairley EA, Kendrick-Jones J, Ellis JA (1999) The Emery-Dreifuss muscular dystrophy phenotype arises from aberrant targeting and binding of emerin at the inner nuclear membrane. *J Cell Sci* 112: 2571-2582

22. Fatkin D, MacRae C, Sasaki T, Wolff MR, Porcu M, Frenneaux M, Atherton J, Vidaillet HJ, Jr., Spudich S, De Girolami U, Seidman JG, Seidman C, Muntoni F, Muehle G, Johnson W, McDonough B (1999) Missense mutations in the rod domain of the lamin A/C gene as causes of dilated cardiomyopathy and conduction-system disease. *N Engl J Med* 341: 1715-1724

23. Felice KJ, Schwartz RC, Brown CA, Leicher CR, Grunnet ML (2000) Autosomal dominant Emery-Dreifuss dystrophy due to mutations in rod domain of the lamin A/C gene. *Neurology* 55: 275-280

24. Fenichel GM, Sul YC, Kilroy AW, Blouin R (1982) An autosomal-dominant dystrophy with humeropelvic distribution and cardiomyopathy. *Neurology* 32: 1399-1401

25. Fidzianska A, Toniolo D, Hausmanowa-Petrusewicz I (1998) Ultrastructural abnormality of sarcolemmal nuclei in Emery-Dreifuss muscular dystrophy (EDMD). *J Neurol Sci* 159: 88-93

26. Foisner R, Gerace L (1993) Integral membrane proteins of the nuclear envelope interact with lamins and chromosomes, and binding is modulated by mitotic phosphorylation. *Cell* 73: 1267-1279

27. Furukawa K (1999) LAP2 binding protein 1 (L2BP1/BAF) is a candidate mediator of LAP2-chromatin interaction. *J Cell Sci* 112: 2485-2492

28. Furukawa K, Pante N, Aebi U, Gerace L (1995) Cloning of a cDNA for lamina-associated polypeptide 2 (LAP2) and identification of regions that specify targeting to the nuclear envelope. *Embo J* 14: 1626-1636

29. Genschel J, Baier P, Kuepferling S, Proepsting MJ, Buettner C, Ewert R, Hetzer R, Lochs H, Schmidt HH (2000) A new frameshift mutation at codon 466 (1397delA) within the LMNA gene. *Hum Mutat* 16: 278

30. Genschel J, Bochow B, Kuepferling S, Ewert R, Hetzer R, Lochs H, Schmidt H (2001) A R644C mutation within lamin A extends the mutations causing dilated cardiomyopathy. *Hum Mutat* 17: 154

31. Gruenbaum Y, Wilson KL, Harel A, Goldberg M, Cohen M (2000) Review: nuclear lamins--structural proteins with fundamental functions. *J Struct Biol* 129: 313-323

32. Hausmanowa-Petrusewicz I (1988) The Emery-Dreifuss disease. *Neuropatol Pol* 26: 265-281

33. Hoeltzenbein M, Karow T, Zeller JA, Warzok R, Wulff K, Zschiesche M, Herrmann FH, Grosse-Heitmeyer W, Wehnert MS (1999) Severe clinical expression in X-linked Emery-Dreifuss muscular dystrophy. *Neuromuscul Disord* 9: 166-170

34. Hopkins LC, Jackson JA, Elsas LJ (1981) Emery-dreifuss humeroperoneal muscular dystrophy: an x-linked myopathy with unusual contractures and bradycardia. *Ann Neurol* 10: 230-237

35. Hopkins LC, Warren S (1992) Emery-Dreifuss muscular dystrophy. In *Handbook of Clinical Neurology: Myopathies*, LP Rowland, S DiMauro: pp. 145-160

36. Kitaguchi T, Matsubara S, Sato M, Miyamoto K, Hirai S, Schwartz Kea (2001) A missense mutation in the exon 8 of lamin A/C gene in a Japanese case of autosomal dominant limb-girdle muscular dystrophy and cardiac conduction block. *Neuromusc Disord* in press

37. Kobberling J, Dunnigan MG (1986) Familial partial lipodystrophy: two types of an X linked dominant syndrome, lethal in the hemizygous state. *J Med Genet* 23: 120-127

38. Li M, Dickson DW, Spiro AJ (1997) Abnormal expression of laminin beta 1 chain in skeletal muscle of adult- onset limb-girdle muscular dystrophy. *Arch Neurol* 54: 1457-1461

39. Lin F, Blake DL, Callebaut I, Skerjanc IS, Holmer L, McBurney MW, Paulin-Levasseur M, Worman HJ (2000) MAN1, an inner nuclear membrane protein that shares the LEM domain with lamina-associated polypeptide 2 and emerin. *J Biol Chem* 275: 4840-4847

40. Lin F, Worman HJ (1993) Structural organization of the human gene encoding nuclear lamin A and nuclear lamin C. *J Biol Chem* 268: 16321-16326

41. Loewinger L, McKeon F (1988) Mutations in the nuclear lamin proteins resulting in their aberrant assembly in the cytoplasm. *Embo J* 7: 2301-2309

42. Luderus ME, den Blaauwen JL, de Smit OJ, Compton DA, van Driel R (1994) Binding of matrix attachment regions to lamin polymers involves single-stranded regions and the minor groove. *Mol Cell Biol* 14: 6297-6630

43. Maison C, Pyrpasopoulou A, Theodoropoulos PA, Georgatos SD (1997) The inner nuclear membrane protein LAP1 forms a native complex with B- type lamins and partitions with spindle-associated mitotic vesicles. *Embo J* 16: 4839-4850

44. Manilal S, Nguyen TM, Sewry CA, Morris GE (1996) The Emery-Dreifuss muscular dystrophy protein, emerin, is a nuclear membrane protein. *Hum Mol Genet* 5: 801-808

45. Manilal S, Recan D, Sewry CA, Hoeltzenbein M, Llense S, Leturcq F, Deburgrave N, Barbot J, Man N, Muntoni F, Wehnert M, Kaplan J, Morris GE (1998) Mutations in Emery-Dreifuss muscular dystrophy and their effects on emerin protein expression. *Hum Mol Genet* 7: 855-864

46. Manilal S, Sewry CA, Man N, Muntoni F, Morris GE (1997) Diagnosis of X-linked Emery-Dreifuss muscular dystrophy by protein analysis of leucocytes and skin with monoclonal antibodies. *Neuromuscul Disord* 7: 63-66

47. Maniotis AJ, Chen CS, Ingber DE (1997) Demonstration of mechanical connections between integrins, cytoskeletal filaments, and nucleoplasm that stabilize nuclear structure. *Proc Natl Acad Sci USA* 94: 849-854

48. Merlini L, Villanova M, Sabatelli P, Malandrini A, Maraldi NM (1999) Decreased expression of laminin beta 1 in chromosome 21-linked Bethlem myopathy. *Neuromuscul Disord* 9: 326-329

49. Michels VV, Moll PP, Miller FA, Tajik AJ, Chu JS, Driscoll DJ, Burnett JC, Rodeheffer RJ, Chesebro JH, Tazelaar HD (1992) The frequency of familial dilated cardiomyopathy in a series of patients with idiopathic dilated cardiomyopathy. *N Engl J Med* 326: 77-82

50. Miller RG, Layzer RB, Mellenthin MA, Golabi M, Francoz RA, Mall JC (1985) Emery-Dreifuss muscular dystrophy with autosomal dominant transmission. *Neurology* 35: 1230-1233

51. Mora M, Cartegni L, Di Blasi C, Barresi R, Bione S, Raffaele di Barletta M, Morandi L, Merlini L, Nigro V, Politano L, Donati MA, Cornelio F, Cobianchi F, Toniolo D (1997) X-linked Emery-Dreifuss muscular dystrophy can be diagnosed from skin biopsy or blood sample. *Ann Neurol* 42: 249-253

52. Morris GE, Manilal S (1999) Heart to heart: from nuclear proteins to Emery-Dreifuss muscular dystrophy. *Hum Mol Genet* 8: 1847-1851

53. Muchir A, Bonne G, van der Kooi AJ, van Meegen M, Baas F, Bolhuis PA, de Visser M, Schwartz K (2000) Identification of mutations in the gene encoding lamins A/C in autosomal dominant limb girdle muscular dystrophy with atrioventricular conduction disturbances (LGMD1B). *Hum Mol Genet* 9: 1453-1459

54. Muntoni F, Lichtarowicz-Krynska EJ, Sewry CA, Manilal S, Recan D, Llense S (1998) Early presentation of X-linked Emery-Dreifuss muscular dystrophy resembling limb-girdle muscular dystrophy. *Neuromuscul Disord* 8: 72-76

55. Nagano A, Koga R, Ogawa M, Kurano Y, Kawada J, Okada R, Hayashi YK, Tsukahara T, Arahata K (1996) Emerin deficiency at the nuclear membrane in patients with Emery- Dreifuss muscular dystrophy. *Nat Genet* 12: 254-259

56. Ognibene A, Sabatelli P, Petrini S, Squarzoni S, Riccio M, Santi S, Villanova M, Palmeri S, Merlini L, Maraldi NM (1999) Nuclear changes in a case of X-linked Emery-Dreifuss muscular dystrophy. *Muscle Nerve* 22: 864-869

57. Ostlund C, Ellenberg J, Hallberg E, Lippincott-Schwartz J, Worman HJ (1999) Intracellular trafficking of emerin, the Emery-Dreifuss muscular dystrophy protein. *J Cell Sci* 112: 1709-1719

58. Peters JM, Barnes R, Bennett L, Gitomer WM, Bowcock AM, Garg A (1998) Localization of the gene for familial partial lipodystrophy (Dunnigan variety) to chromosome 1q21-22. *Nat Genet* 18: 292-295

59. Richardson P, McKenna W, Bristow M, Maish B, Mautner B, O'Connell J (1995) Report of the 1995 World Health Organisation/International Society and Federation of Cardiology task force on the definition and classification of cardiomyopathies. *Circulation* 93: 841-842

60. Roberts R, Schwartz K (2000) Myocardial diseases. *Circulation* 102: IV 34-39

61. Rolls MM, Stein PA, Taylor SS, Ha E, McKeon F, Rapoport TA (1999) A visual screen of a GFP-fusion library identifies a new type of nuclear envelope membrane protein. *J Cell Biol* 146: 29-44

62. Sabatelli P, Squarzoni S, Petrini S, Capanni C, Ognibene A, Cartegni L, Cobianchi F, Merlini L, Toniolo D, Maraldi NM (1998) Oral exfoliative cytology for the non-invasive diagnosis in X-linked Emery-Dreifuss muscular dystrophy patients and carriers. *Neuromuscul Disord* 8: 67-71

63. Sakaki M, Koike H, Takahashi N, Sasagawa N, Tomioka S, Arahata K, Ishiura S (2001) Interaction between Emerin and Nuclear Lamins. *J Biochem* (Tokyo) 129: 321-327

64. Sewry C, Brown S, Feng L, Morris G, Muntoni F (2000) Skeletal pathology in patients with mutations in the lamin A/C gene. *Neuromusc Disord* 10: 361

65. Sewry CA, Brown SC, Mercuri E, Bonne G, Feng L, Camici Gea (2001) Skeletal muscle pathology in autosomal dominant Emery-Dreifuss muscular dystrophy with lamin A/C mutations. *Neuropathology and Applied Neurobiology* in press

66. Shackleton S, Lloyd DJ, Jackson SN, Evans R, Niermeijer MF, Singh BM, Schmidt H, Brabant G, Kumar S, Durrington PN, Gregory S, O'Rahilly S, Trembath RC (2000) LMNA, encoding lamin A/C, is mutated in partial lipodystrophy. *Nat Genet* 24: 153-156

67. Speckman RA, Garg A, Du F, Bennett L, Veile R, Arioglu E, Taylor SI, Lovett M, Bowcock AM (2000) Mutational and haplotype analyses of families with familial partial lipodystrophy (Dunnigan variety) reveal recurrent missense mutations in the globular C-termi-

nal domain of lamin A/C. *Am J Hum Genet* 66: 1192-1198

68. Stuurman N, Heins S, Aebi U (1998) Nuclear lamins: their structure, assembly, and interactions. *J Struct Biol* 122: 42-66

69. Sullivan T, Escalante-Alcalde D, Bhatt H, Anver M, Bhat N, Nagashima K, Stewart CL, Burke B (1999) Loss of A-type lamin expression compromises nuclear envelope integrity leading to muscular dystrophy. *J Cell Biol* 147: 913-920

70. Takamoto K, Hirose K, Uono M, Nonaka I (1984) A genetic variant of Emery-Dreifuss disease. Muscular dystrophy with humeropelvic distribution, early joint contracture, and permanent atrial paralysis. *Arch Neurol* 41: 1292-1293

71. Taniura H, Glass C, Gerace L (1995) A chromatin binding site in the tail domain of nuclear lamins that interacts with core histones. *J Cell Biol* 131: 33-44

73. Taylor J, Sewry CA, Dubowitz V, Muntoni F (1998) Early onset, autosomal recessive muscular dystrophy with Emery-Dreifuss phenotype and normal emerin expression. *Neurology* 51: 1116-1120

74. Tsuchiya Y, Hase A, Ogawa M, Yorifuji H, Arahata K (1999) Distinct regions specify the nuclear membrane targeting of emerin, the responsible protein for Emery-Dreifuss muscular dystrophy. *Eur J Biochem* 259: 859-865

75. van der Kooi AJ, Ledderhof TM, de Voogt WG, Res CJ, Bouwsma G, Troost D, Busch HF, Becker AE, de Visser M (1996) A newly recognized autosomal dominant limb girdle muscular dystrophy with cardiac involvement. *Ann Neurol* 39: 636-642

76. van der Kooi AJ, van Meegen M, Ledderhof TM, McNally EM, de Visser M, Bolhuis PA (1997) Genetic localization of a newly recognized autosomal dominant limb- girdle muscular dystrophy with cardiac involvement (LGMD1B) to chromosome 1q11-21. *Am J Hum Genet* 60: 891-895

77. Vigouroux C, Magre J, Vantyghem MC, Bourut C, Lascols O, Shackleton S, Lloyd DJ, Guerci B, Padova G, Valensi P, Grimaldi A, Piquemal R, Touraine P, Trembath RC, Capeau J (2000) Lamin A/C gene: sex-determined expression of mutations in Dunnigan-type familial partial lipodystrophy and absence of coding mutations in congenital and acquired generalized lipoatrophy. *Diabetes* 49: 1958-1962

78. Wehnert M, Muntoni F (1999) 60th ENMC International Workshop: non X-linked Emery-Dreifuss Muscular Dystrophy 5-7 June 1998, Naarden, The Netherlands. *Neuromuscul Disord* 9: 115-121

79. Wilson KL, Zastrow MS, Lee KK (2001)Lamins and disease: insights into nuclear infrastructure. *Cell* 104: 647-650

80. Wilson KL (2000) The nuclear envelope, muscular dystrophy and gene expression. *Trends Cell Biol* 10: 125-129

81. Worman HJ, Evans CD, Blobel G (1990) The lamin B receptor of the nuclear envelope inner membrane: a polytopic protein with eight potential transmembrane domains. *J Cell Biol* 111: 1535-1542

82. Yates JR (1997) 43rd ENMC International Workshop on Emery-Dreifuss Muscular Dystrophy, 22 June 1996, Naarden, The Netherlands. *Neuromuscul Disord* 7: 67-69

83. Yates JR, Wehnert M (1999) The Emery-Dreifuss Muscular Dystrophy Mutation Database. *Neuromuscul Disord* 9: 199

84. Ye Q, Callebaut I, Pezhman A, Courvalin JC, Worman HJ (1997) Domain-specific interactions of human HP1-type chromodomain proteins and inner nuclear membrane protein LBR. *J Biol Chem* 272: 14983-14989

85. Yoshioka M, Saida K, Itagaki Y, Kamiya T (1989) Follow up study of cardiac involvement in Emery-Dreifuss muscular dystrophy. *Arch Dis Child* 64: 713-715

Abnormalities in nuclear positioning (centronuclear myopathies)

Stirling Carpenter

Definition of entity

Centronuclear myopathy is defined histologically as a myopathy in which a significant number of myonuclei are in the geographic centre of muscle fibres. This feature is shared by the X-linked neonatal-onset myopathy which is due to mutation in the myotubularin gene at Xq28, and which, in this book, is discussed separately in chapter 7.1 under the name of myotubular myopathy. In the past, however, including the recent past, the terms myotubular myopathy and centronuclear myopathy have both been applied to both types of myopathy.

Clinical picture. A distinction is often made between an early childhood-onset form and an adult-onset form. In the neonatal period, there may be hypotonia, reduced activity, weak sucking and crying (16) although signs are generally much less severe than in myotubular myopathy, which typically presents at this age. Delayed motor development usually follows. When onset is in childhood or adolescence it is insidious, with hypotonia, limb weakness, usually more marked proximally, while there may also be axial weakness, ptosis, ophthalmoplegia, facial and masticatory weakness. Tendon reflexes are reduced or absent. There is considerable variation in the degree of disability.

Biopsy of these patients often occurs some years after onset. Periods of improvement in strength are reported in some patients (16). High-arched palate and a long thin triangular face may be present (16). Central nervous system abnormality, reported in some patients, is probably secondary to anoxia rather than being part of the genetic disease.

Adult onset may occur in the second decade (8) or as late as the 6th decade (6). Ophthalmoplegia and bulbar signs

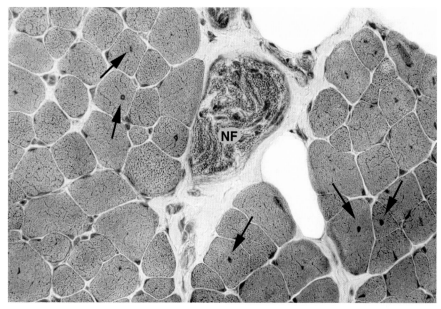

Figure 1. About 30% of the muscle fibres in this field contain a single nucleus in their exact centre. They are uniformly small. Examples are indicated by arrows. A small nerve fascicle (NF) appears normal. Modified trichrome.

are usually lacking in patients with adult onset, and the picture is that of a limb-girdle syndrome. A facioscapulohumeral syndrome has been described in one family (4). Pseudohypertrophy of calves can be present. Serum creatine kinase is almost always normal.

Molecular genetics

The gene responsible is still unknown, and to date no information on linkage studies is available. It is conceivable that a causal mutation lies in one of the eight autosomal analogues of the myotubularin gene.

An autosomal dominant form of the disease is proven by male to male inheritance. Families with adult onset of symptoms particularly tend to show this pattern. Autosomal recessive inheritance is probable in other families (15). A controversial point is whether a positive biopsy in an asymptomatic parent of a patient (12) indicates incomplete penetrance of an autosomal dominant mutation, or a manifesting heterozygote of an autosomal recessive

gene (3). In several patients, the disease has appeared to be sporadic.

Structural changes

General tissue stains. The most essential feature is the presence of rounded or polygonal fibres with one or more nuclei in their geographic centre on transverse sections (Figure 1). Most commonly it is a single nucleus, but especially in patients with later onset a clump of central nuclei is found in some fibres (11). Often there appears to be a halo around central nuclei on H&E stains. The proportion of centronucleated fibres varies from up to at least 95% down to about 25%, although it is difficult to specify a lower limit since considerable variation in the number of central nuclei from muscle to muscle and from the same muscle from right and left limbs is described (1). Below 20% some doubt attaches to the diagnosis. The centronucleated fibres are usually small, although occasional central nuclei can be seen in normal sized or hypertrophied fibres. On longitudi-

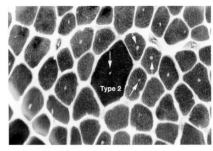

Figure 2. Myosin ATPase with preincubation at 9.4. All fibres except one are small in calibre as well as being of histochemical type 1. Central nuclei are visible as small nonstaining areas. Examples are indicated by arrows. The hypertrophic type 2 fibre also contains a central nucleus, although most of the type 2 fibres in this biopsy did not.

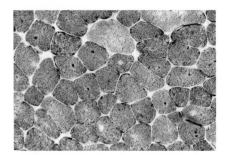

Figure 3. Clusters of mitochondria in the centre of several fibres show as dark reaction product. Longitudinal sections would show that they are located at the poles of central nuclei. Cytochrome oxidase.

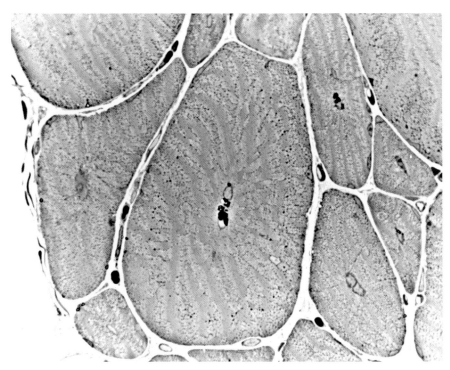

Figure 4. In this semithin resin section, there is a fibre with a radial arrangement of the intermyofibrillar network as well as a ring of dark lysosomes. Patient with adult onset. Paraphenylene diamine, phase optics.

nal sections the central nuclei form chains.

Active necrosis and phagocytosis of muscle fibres is almost never seen, nor is regeneration. On the other hand, depletion of muscle fibres from fascicles occurs, and adipose substitution is often present if the disease has been manifest for a number of years

A few typically centronucleated fibres can be encountered in a variety of biopsies which preclude a diagnosis of centronuclear myopathy. Possibly the most common occasion is in small infants with central nervous system damage and histochemical type 2 smallness. In infantile myotonic dystrophy (chapter 6.1.1), there is smallness of type 1 fibres, and many fibres have nuclei which are separated from the sarcolemma; however, these nuclei are almost never in the exact centre of the fibre. They may be associated with sarcoplasmic masses. Acid phosphatase activity is prominent in many fibres

before the age of 4 years. The mother usually shows myotonia.

Histochemistry. ATPase reactions show the central nuclei as empty spaces and may also show a central absence of myofibrils that extends between the enchained nuclei. The extent of centronucleation may thus be clearer on ATPase reactions than on general tissue stains. The majority of cases also show smallness of the type 1 fibres (Figure 2). This may be combined with predominance of the type 1 fibres, and/or hypertrophy of the type 2 fibres. A few large type 1 fibres may be present. Type 2B fibres are absent in some cases (11). A few type 2C fibres may be present. The central nuclei are much more common in the type 1 fibres and may be confined to them.

Oxidative enzyme often shows a clump of reaction product in the centre of some fibres, corresponding to mitochondria at the poles of central nuclei (Figure 3). PAS staining may show positivity of glycogen surrounding the central nuclei in areas which would appear as halos on H and E. Acid phosphatase may show some reaction prod-

uct in the centre of fibres, representing lipofuscin. This is particularly marked in some adult cases.

An abnormal radial organization of the intermyofibrillar network may be seen in scattered fibres (11). This is best seen with oxidative enzyme reactions, PAS staining, desmin antibodies, or on semithin sections (Figure 4).

Immunocytochemistry. Immunostaining for desmin shows increased activity, especially in the centre of many fibres, encircling and trailing central nuclei (5). Vimentin was diffusely present in a few fibres in 2 adult-onset patients but was absent in 2 others (5, 9). Developmental myosin heavy chain was demonstrated in rare fibres, which also expressed slow myosin heavy chains. Most of them also displayed the embryonic form of NCAM (5). A patient with childhood onset had no evidence of developmental myosin heavy chains (10).

Electron microscopy. Smaller average size of the myofibrils in centre of fibres than on their periphery has been demonstrated in several biopsies (7).

The central nuclei show normal ultra-structure. Occasional fibres may contain some large dense bodies, probably lysosomal (11). Myofibrillar lesions such as Z disc streaming are sometimes seen.

Molecular pathogenesis

In the absence of knowledge of the responsible protein and its functions, theories of pathogenesis are speculative. It is not known what determines the position of nuclei in skeletal muscle cells, although desmin filaments probably have a role in maintaining it. In avian smooth muscle cells, desmin-containing filaments appeared to form linkages with the nuclear envelope (13). In centronuclear myopathies, a disturbance of maturation has most often been evoked to explain the position of nuclei, which recalls that in fetal myocytes. If so, the disturbance is highly selective.

It is not clear whether the central nuclei are, in fact, residues of fetal development, or whether postnatal migration of nuclei to the centre of fibres occurs. One male infant showed only nonspecific abnormality on biopsy at 11 months, but definite centronuclear myopathy at 9 years (14). Another male on biopsy at 7 months showed only fibre type disproportion, while repeat biopsy at 2 and 4 years showed numerous central nuclei (2). In one adult-onset patient, some sarcolemmal nuclei had their long axis pointing towards the interior of the fibre, as if they were on the point of moving inwards.

Patients in some families with mutations in the myotubularin gene survive into adult life with relatively few muscle symptoms. Biopsy distinction of these patients from those with centronuclear myopathy may prove difficult.

References

1. Bradley WG, Price DL, Watanabe CK (1970) Familial centronuclear myopathy. *J Neurol Neurosurg Psychiatry* 33: 687-693

2. Danon MJ, Giometti CS, Manaligod JR, Swisher C (1997) Sequential muscle biopsy changes in a case of congenital myopathy. *Muscle Nerve* 20: 561-569

3. De Angelis MS, Palmucci L, Leone M, Doriguzzi C (1991) Centronuclear myopathy: clinical, morphological and genetic characters. A review of 288 cases. *J Neurol Sci* 103: 2-9

4. Felice KJ, Grunnet ML (1997) Autosomal dominant centronuclear myopathy: report of a new family with clinical features simulating facioscapulohumeral syndrome. *Muscle Nerve* 20: 1194-1196

5. Figarella-Branger D, Calore EE, Boucraut J, Bianco N, Rougon G, Pellissier JF (1992) Expression of cell surface and cytoskeleton developmentally regulated proteins in adult centronuclear myopathies. *J Neurol Sci* 109: 69-76

6. Harriman DG, Haleem MA (1972) Centronuclear myopathy in old age. *J Pathol* 108: 237-247

7. Headington JT, McNamara JO, Brownell AK (1975) Centronuclear myopathy: histochemistry and electron microscopy. Report of two cases. *Arch Pathol* 99: 16-24

8. McLeod JG, Baker W, Lethlean AK, Shorey CD (1972) Centronuclear myopathy with autosomal dominant inheritance. *J Neurol Sci* 15: 375-387

9. Misra AK, Menon NK, Mishra SK (1992) Abnormal distribution of desmin and vimentin in myofibers in adult onset myotubular myopathy. *Muscle Nerve* 15: 1246-1252

10. Sawchak JA, Sher JH, Norman MG, Kula RW, Shafiq SA (1991) Centronuclear myopathy heterogeneity: distinction of clinical types by myosin isoform patterns. *Neurology* 41: 135-140

11. Serratrice G, Pellissier JF, Faugere MC, Gastaut JL (1978) Centronuclear myopathy: possible central nervous system origin. *Muscle Nerve* 1: 62-69

12. Sher JH, Rimalovski AB, Athanassiades TJ, Aronson SM (1967) Familial myotubular myopathy: a clinical, pathological, histochemical, and ultrastructural study. *J Neuropathol Exp Neurol* 26: 132-133

13. Stromer MH, Bendayan M (1990) Immunocytochimical identification of cytoskeletal linkages to smooth muscle cell nuclei and mitochondria. *Cell Motility and the Cytoskeleton* 17: 11-18

14. van der Ven PF, Jap PH, Wetzels RH, ter Laak HJ, Ramaekers FC, Stadhouders AM, Sengers RC (1991) Postnatal centralization of muscle fibre nuclei in centronuclear myopathy. *Neuromuscul Disord* 1: 211-220

15. Wallgren-Pettersson C, Clarke A, Samson F, Fardeau M, Dubowitz V, Moser H, Grimm T, Barohn RJ, Barth PG (1995) The myotubular myopathies: differential diagnosis of the X linked recessive, autosomal dominant, and autosomal recessive forms and present state of DNA studies. *J Med Genet* 32: 673-679

16. Zanoteli E, Oliveira AS, Schmidt B, Gabbai AA (1998) Centronuclear myopathy: clinical aspects of ten Brazilian patients with childhood onset. *J Neurol Sci* 158: 76-82

CHAPTER 4

Myofibrillar and internal cytoskeletal proteins

4.1 Actinopathies   62
4.2 Core diseases
    4.2.1 Central core disease   65
    4.2.2 Multiminicore disease   68
4.3 Desmin-related myopathies   70
4.4 Nemaline myopathies   74
4.5 Plectin deficiency   78
4.6 Telethonin deficiency   81
4.7 Myotilinopathy   82
4.8 Myosin heavy chain depletion disease   83
4.9 Autosomal dominant myosin heavy chain IIa myopathy   85

Myofibrillar proteins represent the largest constituents of the muscle fibre. Genetically determined defects of the myofibrillar and internal cytoskeletal genes are relatively rare. The affected molecules include α-actin, desmin, α-actinin, and β-tropomyosin. A particular missense mutation of myosin heavy chain occurring in type 2a fibres (MHCIIa) causes a peculiar dominant progressive myopathy with a myopathology reminiscent of that in inclusion body myopathy. For this reason it is also mentioned in chapter 15.3.

Actinopathies

Hans H. Goebel
Nigel G. Laing

Definition of entities

Actinopathies are marked by mutations in the gene for sarcomeric actin, *ACTA 1* (10), one member of the nemaline myopathy group. Muscle tissue may show aggregates of actin filament (3).

Clinical symptoms in patients with actinopathy conform to those seen in patients with nemaline myopathy, ie, with early onset, a rapid course and often with early death (1, 3) or of a benign type (3). Muscle weakness, at early onset, combined with respiratory insufficiency, is the major feature. Cardiomyopathy has not been documented. As almost all the different *ACTA 1* missense mutations are isolated ones, genotype phenotype correlation is not yet consistent. Since actinopathy has only recently been described, no data of frequency are available. However, that more than 30 mutations have already been discovered within some 2 years by a single genetic centre (9, 10) suggests that actinopathy, with or without aggregates of actin filaments, may not be a rare condition among the congenital myopathies.

Molecular genetics and pathogenesis

The *ACTA 1* gene is located on chromosome 1q42.1 (12) and consists of 7 exons, only 6 of which are coding exons (11). The protein product of the gene, sarcomeric alpha-actin, has a molecular weight of 43 kD and is the principal component of muscle thin filaments, interacting with myosin to generate the force which makes muscles contract. It is thus a crucial protein in muscle function.

In 1997, Goebel et al (3) described three patients with a phenotype that on muscle biopsy showed excess accumulation of actin thin filaments. Mutations in the *ACTA1* gene were subsequently identified in all 3 of these patients (10). Since 2 of them having a mutation in

Dominant

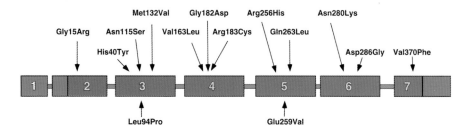

Recessive

Figure 1. Genomic structure of the skeletal muscle alpha-actin gene ACTA1 and the published mutations in ACTA1 associated with muscle disease.

the *ACTA 1* gene also had intranuclear rod bodies or sarcoplasmic nemaline bodies, other patients diagnosed with nemaline myopathy were tested for *ACTA 1* gene mutations. Twelve mutations in nemaline myopathy patients were identified and described in the original publication (10) on diseases causing mutations in the *ACTA1* gene (Figure 1).

The mutations were distributed throughout the 6 coding exons of *ACTA1*. The *ACTA1* mutations were associated with either dominant or recessive phenotypes, but in many cases were de novo dominant mutations since tested parents did not have the mutations present in their affected offspring (10). This high new mutation rate is to be expected in what is most frequently a severe, genetically lethal condition.

Until mid-year 2000, 30 different mutations in the *ACTA1* gene had been discovered (9) and now, in early 2001, there is a total of close to 50 known different ACTA1 mutations (Laing, Beggs, unpublished). The unpublished mutations are also distributed throughout all the 6 coding exons.

In 2 families, a mildly affected parent appears to be a somatic mosaic for the mutation in their 2 severely affected children (10) (Laing unpublished).

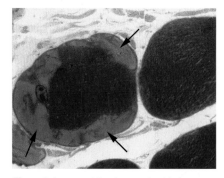

Figure 2. Large peripheral areas devoid of sarcomeres within muscle fibres containing actin filament aggregates (arrows). 1 μm thick methylene blue stained resin section.

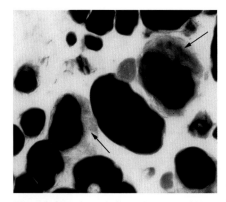

Figure 3. Several muscle fibres show reduced histochemical enzyme activity containing actin filament aggregates (arrows), ATPase reaction.

ACTA1 mutations may be associated with a range of disease severity from severe nemaline myopathy, fatal during the first few days after birth (10) to mild nemaline myopathy (7). *ACTA1* mutations appear to account for 10 to 20% of nemaline myopathy cases (Laing, Beggs, unpublished) and, thus, form a significant group of patients. Mutations in the *ACTA1* gene have not been identified in all cases with the phenotype of excess accumulation of thin filaments (Laing, unpublished) suggesting genetic heterogeneity for this condition.

Also, since *ACTA1* mutations are frequently associated with a severe, fatal phenotype, the parents of *ACTA1* cases are frequently interested in prenatal diagnosis, and a number of prenatal diagnoses have been performed for at risk couples. Since so many of the *ACTA1* mutations are de novo dominant mutations, the recurrence risk is much less than the one fourth for a couple carrying a recessive disorder.

The mutated amino-acid residues in the *ACTA1* gene are involved in a number of the known protein/protein interactions of skeletal muscle alpha actin, including myosin binding and DNase I binding (10). However, the pathophysiology of how the mutations lead to disease is uncertain.

Structural changes

Aggregation of thin filaments suggesting actin was earlier mentioned in context with nemaline myopathy (8) as a peculiar muscle finding in an infant (2) and subsequently as a major pathological feature (1).

The morphological spectrum of actinopathies (Figures 2-6), a member of the emerging "protein surplus myopathies" (5, 6) can be divided into 3 groups based on the definition of actinopathy as a condition with mutations in the *ACTA1* gene: *i)* muscle tissues with aggregates of thin or actin filaments only (Figures 4-6), *ii)* muscle specimens containing both aggregates of thin or actin filaments and rods, and *iii)* muscle specimens containing rods only with, so far, no detected actin aggregates. The rods may be sarcoplasmic or intranuclear only, or both (4). The degree of thin or actin filament aggregation may vary (Figure 2).

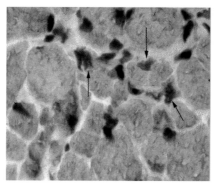

Figure 4. Actin is increased in the periphery of several muscle fibres. Examples of such fibres are indicated by arrows. Immunohistochemical reaction against sarcomeric actin, immunoperoxidase technique.

Two separate biopsies taken several years apart in one patient showed consistent actin aggregates in both biopsied muscles (3). In another patient, large aggregates of actin filaments were encountered in the diaphragm at autopsy, but only few small aggregates in biopsied muscle (3). Thus, little is known about the distribution of actin aggregates and whether there is increase in number and size during the course of the actinopathy. Patients with mutations in the *ACTA 1* gene but with nemaline bodies in their muscle fibres, only, may therefore have had aggregates of actin outside of the biopsied site or may develop them at a later stage of their disease. Aggregates of actin show defects in the histochemical oxidative enzyme and adenosine triphosphatase preparations (Figure 3).

Future perspectives

As a newly discovered congenital myopathy, actinopathy requires designation of its complete genetic spectrum. The consistency of the 2 structural hallmarks, aggregates of actin filaments and nemaline bodies also needs to be further explored. Genotype phenotype correlation is in its infancy. The relationship of the actin filament aggregates to the formation of rods as well as the impairment of muscle fibre function, ie, pathogenesis, await explanation. Identification of mutant and normal actin proteins and their submicroscopic location will be another target of future research.

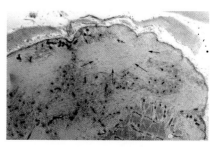

Figure 5. Electron microscopy shows large confluent areas of fine (actin) filaments under the sarcolemma.

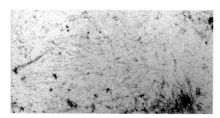

Figure 6. Immunoelectron microscopically, the actin filaments are labelled with gold grain antibodies against sarcomeric actin.

References

1. Bornemann A, Petersen MB, Schmalbruch H (1996) Fatal congenital myopathy with actin filament deposits. *Acta Neuropathol (Berl)* 92: 104-108

2. Dubowitz V (1985) *Muscle Biopsy: A Practical Approach.* London: Baillière Tindal. 664-667

3. Goebel HH, Anderson JR, Hubner C, Oexle K, Warlo I (1997) Congenital myopathy with excess of thin myofilaments. *Neuromuscul Disord* 7: 160-168

4. Goebel HH, Piirsoo A, Warlo I, Schofer O, Kehr S, Gaude M (1997) Infantile intranuclear rod myopathy. *J Child Neurol* 12: 22-30

5. Goebel HH, Warlo I (2000) Gene-related protein surplus myopathies. *Mol Genet Metab* 71: 267-275

6. Goebel HH, Warlo IA (2001) Surplus protein myopathies. Neuromuscul Disord 11: 3-6

7. Jungbluth H, Sewry CA, Brown SC, Nowak KJ, Laing NG, Wallgren-Pettersson C, Pelin K, Manzur AY, Mercuri E, Dubowitz V, Muntoni F (2001) Mild phenotype of nemaline myopathy with sleep hypoventilation due to a mutation in the skeletal muscle alpha-actin (ACTA1) gene. *Neuromuscul Disord* 11: 35-40

8. Karpati G, Carpenter S. Skeletal muscle pathology in neuromuscular diseases, in *Handbook of Clinical Neurology. Myopathies,* Rowland LP, DiMauro S, Editors, Elsevier Science Publishers B.V: Amsterdam. 1-48

9. Laing NG, Nowak K, Durling H, North K, Nonaka I, Hutchinson DO, von Kaisenberg C, Muntoni F, Pelin K, Wallgren-Pettersson C (2000) Actin and nemaline-related myopathy. *Brain Pathol* 10: 595 (abstract W502-503)

10. Nowak KJ, Wattanasirichaigoon D, Goebel HH, Wilce M, Pelin K, Donner K, Jacob RL, Hubner C, Oexle K, Anderson JR, Verity CM, North KN, Iannaccone ST, Muller CR, Nurnberg P, Muntoni F, Sewry C,

Hughes I, Sutphen R, Lacson AG, Swoboda KJ, Vigneron J, Wallgren-Pettersson C, Beggs AH, Laing NG (1999) Mutations in the skeletal muscle alpha-actin gene in patients with actin myopathy and nemaline myopathy. *Nat Genet* 23: 208-212

11. Taylor A, Erba HP, Muscat GE, Kedes L. (1988) Nucleotide sequence and expression of the human skeletal alpha-actin gene: evolution of functional regulatory domains. *Genomics* 3: 323-336.

12. Ueyama H, Inazawa J, Ariyama T, Nishino H, Ochiai Y, Ohkubo I, Miwa T (1995) Reexamination of chromosomal loci of human muscle actin genes by fluorescence *in situ* hybridization. *Jpn J Hum Genet* 40: 145-148.

Central core disease

Hans H. Goebel

CCD	central core diseases
MH	malignant hyperthermia
MYH 7	β-myosin heavy chain gene
RYR	ryanodine receptor

Definition of entity

Central core disease (CCD) was the first congenital myopathy described (24) and ushered in the concept of congenital myopathies originally also called "new myopathies" (6). It was finally designated shortly afterwards (9). Later, it was found that central core disease was strongly associated with malignant hyperthermia (MH) (5, 7). For further reading about MH, see chapter 5.2.

To date, it appears that CCD may be a subgroup of patients and families within the much larger spectrum of MH because CCD patients are susceptible to MH. CCD, in general, is a non-progressive disorder marked by limb weakness, generalized muscle hypotonia and delayed milestones in motor development during infancy and childhood (23). Hip dislocation and scoliosis, as well as flat feet, are skeletal abnormalities. A more severe course has been recorded (13, 14).

Molecular background and pathogenesis

CCD is an autosomal dominant disorder, and only putative autosomal recessive inheritance has been described (14). CCD has been assigned to chromosome 19q12-13.2 and its *RYR 1* gene region (10, 12, 18). All of the mutations in this *RYR 1* receptor gene have been missense mutations, the majority of which affect the N terminus or rod domains of the mutant proteins (11). Only a few missense mutations affect the C terminus region (17). The ryanodine receptor protein is part of the calcium release channel. Patients with mutations in the *RYR 1* gene may also be susceptible to MH (2). Some

Ryanoid Receptor

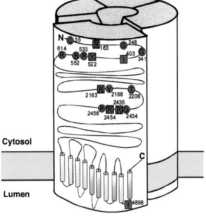

Figure 1. *Ryanodine receptor.* Transmembraneous ryanodine receptor with sites of few mutations for central core disease and numerous mutations for malignant hyperthermia (source Prof. F. Lehmann-Horn, Ulm, Germany).

patients with the same *RYR 1* mutation share CCD and MH, others with MH only have different *RYR 1* mutations and very few patients with *RYR 1* mutations have been found to have CCD (15), but not MH susceptibility (11) (Figure 1).

The pathogenesis of cores in relationship to mutant ryanodine receptor proteins is not yet known, but recently the RYR 1 protein has been identified in core regions by immunohistochemistry (20). Central cores were also found in a soleus muscle biopsy specimen of a patient having familial hypertrophic cardiomyopathy owing to a mutation in the β-myosin heavy chain gene (*MYH 7*) (8), suggesting that CCD might be genetically heterogeneous (3).

Cores and rods/nemaline bodies rarely appear admixed within muscle specimens (1, 19, 22, 26). Recently identified missense mutations in the *RYR 1* gene in this complex myopathy (16) now suggest that such patients

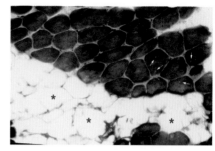

Figure 2. *Central core disease.* There are numerous fat cells within muscle fascicles (stars), increased variation of fibre diameter and pallor within some fibres (cores). Modified trichrome stain.

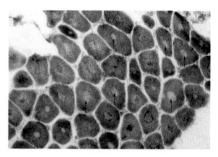

Figure 3. *NADH reaction.* Single round defects in reaction product identify cores (examples indicated by arrow).

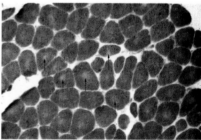

Figure 4. *ATPase staining.* Cores are marked by reduced activity.

genetically have CCD, and for still unexplained reasons, associated rods.

Structural changes

CCD (Figures 2-5) is marked by the formation of cores, large round areas within the muscle fibre devoid of oxidative enzyme activities (Figure 3). Characteristically, cores run along the long axes of the muscle fibres across numerous sarcomeres, often measuring up to 300 μm. Such cores are common-

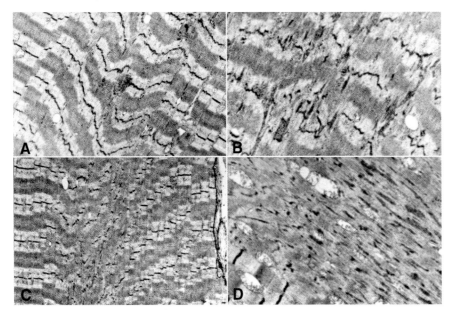

Figure 5. *Ultrastructural features of cores.* Same patient, same biopsied muscle and same time of biopsy. **A.** structured core, **B.** semi-structured core, **C.** partly structured, partly unstructured core, **D.** unstructured core.

ly located in the center, but may also be found in the periphery of the muscle fibre. They may appear solitary or multiple. Smaller lesions of this kind may also be encountered, which gives rise to the confusion of CCD with multi-minicore disease.

The core may also be surrounded by a small rim of enhanced oxidative enzyme activity and, immunohistochemically, both the core and its rim, or one lesion may contain increased amounts of desmin (27), vimentin, developmental myosin heavy chain, and tubulin (4).

A new finding is the immunohistochemical demonstration of an increased RYR 1 protein within cores (20), perhaps suggesting a pathogenetic role in the formation of cores by the RYR 1 protein. A frequent feature is type I fibre predominance or even type I fibre uniformity. Occasionally, there might be type I fibre uniformity without cores (25). An increase with age in cores has been noticed. The significance of cores only, for instance, in a patient tested for hyperthermia susceptibility, remains obscure. In such situations, a neurogenic process associated with targetoid lesions has to be excluded.

By electron microscopy (Figure 5), the core is a circumscribed lesion within the myofibrils which may show structured cores; a different register of sarcomeres compared to their surrounded myofibrils, without any disruption of the intrinsic sarcomeric structure over a considerable length of the myofibril. In unstructured cores, the fine structure of the sarcomeres within the cores is not preserved and excessive Z band streaming may be evident. In both structured and unstructured cores, mitochondria and triads are absent, thus, resulting in histochemical defects in oxidative enzyme preparations. Additional myopathic features, eg, considerable variation in fibre diameters and endomysial fibrosis, may be usually seen in patients with a more severe clinical phenotype (14).

Future perspectives

It appears essential to discover newly arisen mutations in the RYR 1 gene in the spectrum of CCD patients, including sporadic ones, as well as to find out whether mutations in other genes than the RYR 1 one may exist. Genetically, CCD has appeared to be a homogeneous disorder.

Moreover, the relationship between CCD and MH remains to be further elucidated and the significance of cores without a disease should be studied. The pathogenesis and morphogensis in CCD are still little understood. Therefore, the formation of cores should be investigated, perhaps in suitable tissue culture systems to clarify factors that influence the formation of cores and their protein content.

References

1. Afifi AK, Smith JW, Zellweger H (1965) Congenital nonprogressive myopathy: central core disease and nemaline myopathy in one family. *Neurology* 15: 371-381

2. Brandt A, Schleithoff L, Jurkat-Rott K, Klingler W, Baur C, Lehmann-Horn F (1999) Screening of the ryanodine receptor gene in 105 malignant hyperthermia families: novel mutations and concordance with the *in vitro* contracture test. *Hum Mol Genet* 8: 2055-2062

3. Curran JL, Hall WJ, Halsall PJ, Hopkins PM, Iles DE, Markham AF, McCall SH, Robinson RL, West SP, Bridges LR, Ellis FR (1999) Segregation of malignant hyperthermia, central core disease and chromosome 19 markers. *Br J Anaesth* 83: 217-222

4. De Bleecker JL, Ertl BB, Engel AG (1996) Patterns of abnormal protein expression in target formations and unstructured cores. *Neuromuscul Disord* 6: 339-349

5. Denborough MA, Dennett X, Anderson RM (1973) Central-core disease and malignant hyperpyrexia. *Br Med J* 1: 272-273

6. Dubowitz V (1969) The "new" myopathies. *Neuropediatrics* 1: 137-148

7. Eng GD, Epstein BS, Engel WK, McKay DW, McKay R (1978) Malignant hyperthermia and central core disease in a child with congenital dislocating hips. *Arch Neurol* 35: 189-197

8. Fananapazir L, Dalakas MC, Cyran F, Cohn G, Epstein ND (1993) Missense mutations in the beta-myosin heavy-chain gene cause central core disease in hypertrophic cardiomyopathy. *Proc Natl Acad Sci USA* 90: 3993-3997

9. Greenfield G, Cornman T, M. S (1958) The prognostic value of the muscle biopsy in the "floppy infant." *Brain* 81: 461-484

10. Haan EA, Freemantle CJ, McCure JA, Friend KL, Mulley JC (1990) Assignment of the gene for central core disease to chromosome 19. *Hum Genet* 86: 187-190

11. Jurkat-Rott K, McCarthy T, Lehmann-Horn F (2000) Genetics and pathogenesis of malignant hyperthermia. *Muscle Nerve* 23: 4-17

12. Kausch K, Lehmann-Horn F, Janka M, Wieringa B, Grimm T, Muller CR (1991) Evidence for linkage of the central core disease locus to the proximal long arm of human chromosome 19. *Genomics* 10: 765-769

13. Lynch PJ, Tong J, Lehane M, Mallet A, Giblin L, Heffron JJ, Vaughan P, Zafra G, MacLennan DH, McCarthy TV (1999) A mutation in the transmembrane/luminal domain of the ryanodine receptor is associated with abnormal Ca2+ release channel function and severe central core disease. *Proc Natl Acad Sci USA* 96: 4164-4169

14. Manzur AY, Sewry CA, Ziprin J, Dubowitz V, Muntoni F (1998) A severe clinical and pathological variant of central core disease with possible autosomal recessive inheritance. *Neuromuscul Disord* 8: 467-473

15. McCarthy T, Quane KA, Lynch PJ (2000) Ryanodine receptor mutations in malignant hyperthermia and central core disease. *Human Mutat* 15: 410-417

16. Monnier N, Procaccio V, Stieglitz P, Lunardi J (1997) Malignant-hyperthermia susceptibility is associated with a mutation of the alpha 1-subunit of the human dihydropyridine-sensitive L-type voltage-dependent calcium-channel receptor in skeletal muscle. *Am J Hum Genet* 60: 1316-1325

17. Monnier N, Romero NB, Lerale J, Nivoche Y, Qi D, MacLennan DH, Fardeau M, Lunardi J (2000) An autosomal dominant congenital myopathy with cores and rods is associated with a neomutation in the RYR1 gene encoding the skeletal muscle ryanodine receptor. *Hum Mol Genet* 9: 2599-2608

18. Mulley JC, Kozman HM, Phillips HA, Gedeon AK, McCure JA, Iles DE, Gregg RG, Hogan K, Couch FJ, MacLennan DH, et al. (1993) Refined genetic localization for central core disease. *Am J Hum Genet* 52: 398-405

19. Pallagi E, Molnar M, Molnar P, Dioszeghy P (1998) Central core and nemaline rods in the same patient. *Acta Neuropathol (Berl)* 96: 211-214

20. Scacheri PC, Hoffman EP, Fratkin JD, Semino-Mora C, Senchak A, Davis MR, Laing NG, Vedanarayanan V, Subramony SH (2000) A novel ryanodine receptor gene mutation causing both cores and rods in congenital myopathy. *Neurology* 55: 1689-1696

21. Scacheri PC, Gillanders EM, Subramony S, Vedanarayayanan V, Crowe CA, Engvall E, Watkins S, Bingler M, Trent JM, Hoffman EP (2001) Novel mutations in collagen VI genes (COL6A1, COL6A2): A pathogenic model for muscle-specific symptoms of a ubiquitously expressed protein. *Submitted for publication.*

22. Seitz RJ, Toyka KV, Wechsler W (1984) Adult-onset mixed myopathy with nemaline rods, minicores, and central cores: a muscle disorder mimicking polymyositis. *J Neurol* 231: 103-108

23. Shuaib A, Paasuke RT, Brownell KW (1987) Central core disease. Clinical features in 13 patients. *Medicine (Baltimore)* 66: 389-396

24. Shy GM, Magee K (1956) A new congenital nonprogressive myopathy. *Brain* 79: 610-621

25. Tojo M, Ozawa M, Nonaka I (2000) Central core disease and congenital neuromuscular disease with uniform type 1 fibers in one family. Brain Dev 22: 262-264

26. Vallat JM, de Lumley L, Loubet A, Leboutet MJ, Corvisier N, Umdenstock R (1982) Coexistence of minicores, cores, and rods in the same muscle biopsy. A new example of mixed congenital myopathy. *Acta Neuropathol (Berl)* 58: 229-232

27. Vita G, Migliorato A, Baradello A, Mazzeo A, Rodolico C, Falsaperla R, Messina C (1994) Expression of cytoskeleton proteins in central core disease. *J Neurol Sci* 124: 71-76

Multi-minicore disease

Hans H. Goebel

CCD	central core disease
MmD	multi-minicore disease

Definition of entity

This condition is characterized by the formation of multiple small cores, originally reported as multicore disease (6, 7), though later also described as minicore disease (2). The term multi-minicore disease (MmD) may now identify this nosologically separate entity. Its frequency is unknown. In general, MmD is a slowly developing congenital myopathy, marked by generalized weakness and muscle hypotonia. Respiratory insufficiency may be a severe problem, even leading to early death. Cardiomyopathy and ophthalmoplegia may be additional features (10).

Molecular background and pathogenesis

Most patients have a sporadic disease. Autosomal recessive inheritance (16) appears to be more frequent than an autosomal dominant one (13, 19). As there are several clinical variants, it is not clear whether MmD is genetically heterogeneous. No gene locus has been identified. Although one patient reacted to generalized anaesthesia (11), MmD does not seem to link to the CCD locus on chromosome 19.

Structural changes

Minicores (Figures 1-3) detected in oxidative enzyme preparations ought to be verified as in vivo lesions in semithin resin sections and by electron microscopy. Minicores are small lesions of sarcomeric disruption with Z band streaming as well as dissolution of some myofilaments (Figure 3). These lesions are multiple, ill defined and only stretch across a few sarcomeres, thus affecting adjacent sarcomeres. Occasionally they extend across a considerable width of the muscle fibre.

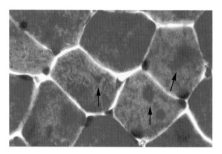

Figure 1. *Modified trichrome stain.* Numerous small patches within muscle fibres. Examples indicated by arrows.

Devoid of mitochondria, these cores are unstructured ones, though structured ones, ie, circumscribed areas with absence of mitochondria and preservation of sarcomeric structures, do exist. Confluence of numerous spatially close minicores may occur, but obviously not to form unstructured central cores. Type 1 fibre predominance, type 1 fibre hypotrophy and a pathological pattern of fibre type disproportion, may be seen as additional pathological features. Immunohistochemically, accumulations of desmin, α-actinin, α-B crystalline, heat shock protein, and dystrophin may be present (4).

The concomitant occurrence of numerous central nuclei within muscle fibres containing minicores (8), even in a familial setting (9) may not be a rare feature. Therefore, classification of such a sporadic or familial congenital myopathy as MmD with central nuclei or centronuclear myopathy with minicores may be a matter of dispute. Minicore lesions have actually been observed both in skeletal muscle fibres and cardiac myocytes in the same patient (3).

Minicores have been seen in Marfan's syndrome (12), the cerebro-retino-muscular syndrome (1), type III glycogenosis (14), short chain acyl-CoA dehydrogenase deficiency (17), and anhidrotic ectodermal dysplasia (5). This indicates that the formations

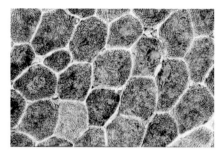

Figure 2. *NADH-tetrazolium reductase.* Multiple minicores are present as irregular defects in this staining.

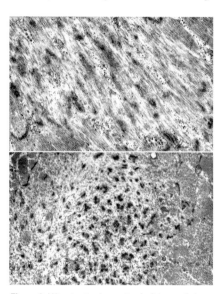

Figure 3. *Ultrastructural aspects of minicores:* **A.** Longitudinal section. Destruction of sarcomeres, **B.** Cross section. Irregular content of the sarcomeres.

of minicores may well be an unspecific feature.

Minicores, when observed together with rods may indicate multiple small cores in CCD (15, 18) and, thus, belong to CCD with rods, rather than representing a variant of MmD.

Future perspectives

Progress in elucidating this rare congenital myopathy requires genetic analysis with identification of a gene(s) and mutations concerning affected protein(s). Such genetic analysis has thus far been hampered by the low incidence of the disorder. Informative MmD families should be investigated to clarify its relationship with CCD, including perhaps the pathogenesis of minicores in comparison to that of central cores. Such studies may provide further genotype phenotype correlations.

References

1. Avoni P, Monari L, Carelli V, Carcangiu R, Barboni P, Donati C, Badiali L, Baruzzi A, Montagna P (2000) Congenital encephalomyopathy with epilepsy, chorioretinitis, basal ganglia involvement, and muscle minicores. *Ann Neurol* 47: 395-399

2. Currie S, Noronha M, Harriman D (1974) "Minicore" disease. *Excerpta Medica: Amsterdam* p 12: abstract no. 27

3. Davis DG, Nelson KR, Markesbery WR (1990) Congenital myopathy and cardiomyopathy with identical ultrastructural changes. *Arch Neurol* 47: 1141-1144

4. De Bleecker JL, Ertl BB, Engel AG (1996) Patterns of abnormal protein expression in target formations and unstructured cores. *Neuromuscul Disord* 6: 339-349

5. Docquier MA, Veyckemans F, Prudhomme S, Rossillon R (2000) Anesthesia in a child presenting a anhydrotic ectodermic dysplasia associated with a multiminicore myopathy. *Can J Anaesth* 47: 449-453

6. Engel AG, Gomez MR (1966) Congenital myopathy associated with multifocal degeneration of muscle fibers. *Trans Am Neurol Assoc* 91: 222-223

7. Engel AG, Gomez MR, Groover RV (1971) Multicore disease. A recently recognized congenital myopathy associated with multifocal degeneration of muscle fibers. *Mayo Clin Proc* 46: 666-681

8. Fitzsimons RB, McLeod JG (1982) Myopathy with pathological features of both centronuclear myopathy and multicore disease. *J Neurol Sci* 57: 395-405

9. Goebel HH, Meinck HM, Reinecke M, Schimrigk K, Mielke U (1984) Centronuclear myopathy with special consideration of the adult form. *Eur Neurol* 23: 425-434

10. Jungbluth H, Sewry C, Brown SC, Manzur AY, Mercuri E, Bushby K, Rowe P, Johnson MA, Hughes I, Kelsey A, Dubowitz V, Muntoni F (2000) Minicore myopathy in children: a clinical and histopathological study of 19 cases. *Neuromuscul Disord* 10: 264-273

11. Koch BM, Bertorini TE, Eng GD, Boehm R (1985) Severe multicore disease associated with reaction to anesthesia. *Arch Neurol* 42: 1204-1206

12. Pages M, Echenne B, Pages AM, Dimeglio A, Sires A (1985) Multicore disease and Marfan's syndrome: a case report. *Eur Neurol* 24: 170-175

13. Paljarvi L, Kalimo H, Lang H, Savontaus ML, Sonninen V (1987) Minicore myopathy with dominant inheritance. *J Neurol Sci* 77: 11-22

14. Pellissier JF, de Barsy T, Faugere MC, Rebuffel P (1979) Type III glycogenosis with multicore structures. *Muscle Nerve* 2: 124-132

15. Seitz RJ, Toyka KV, Wechsler W (1984) Adult-onset mixed myopathy with nemaline rods, minicores, and central cores: a muscle disorder mimicking polymyositis. *J Neurol* 231: 103-108

16. Shuaib A, Martin JM, Mitchell LB, Brownell AK (1988) Multicore myopathy: not always a benign entity. *Can J Neurol Sci* 15: 10-14

17. Tein I, Haslam RH, Rhead WJ, Bennett MJ, Becker LE, Vockley J (1999) Short-chain acyl-CoA dehydrogenase deficiency: a cause of ophthalmoplegia and multicore myopathy. *Neurology* 52: 366-372

18. Vallat JM, de Lumley L, Loubet A, Leboutet MJ, Corvisier N, Umdenstock R (1982) Coexistence of minicores, cores, and rods in the same muscle biopsy. A new example of mixed congenital myopathy. *Acta Neuropathol (Berl)* 58: 229-232

19. Vanneste JA, Stam FC (1982) Autosomal dominant multicore disease. *J Neurol Neurosurg Psychiatry* 45: 360-365

Desmin-related myopathies

Hans H. Goebel
Lev Goldfarb

CRYAB	α-B crystalline gene
DRM	desmin-related myopathy

Definition of entities

Desmin-related myopathies (DRM) are a newly designated group of myopathies marked by the intracellular accumulation of desmin, the intermediate filament specific to muscle fibres as in cytoplasmic bodies (12), sarcoplasmic bodies (5), spheroid bodies (11, 13) and in granulofilamentous material (6, 8). DRM have been termed desminopathies, desmin myopathies, desmin storage myopathies and, recently, in a more generic fashion, myofibrillar myopathy (4, 21). The frequency of DRM is unknown, but the increased awareness of these conditions has led to a growing number of publications.

Clinically, DRM show a predominantly distal muscle weakness. Children may be affected and as a result of autosomal recessive mode of inheritance, mutations in both desmin alleles result in an earlier onset (16). Cardiomyopathy is a frequent feature, especially in patients with granulofilamentous material. DRM belong to the newly emerging group of "protein surplus myopathies" (14, 15).

Molecular genetics and pathogenesis

Desmin is a 53 kD intermediate filament protein organised in three domains. A highly conserved central alpha-helical core domain of 310 amino acids in length is flanked by non-helical amino-terminal head and carboxy-terminal tail domains (Figure 1). The core consists of four alpha-helical rods, 1A, 2A, 1B and 2B, separated by linkers (9). This structure guides two full-size desmin polypeptide chains intertwined in a coiled-coil fashion to form a homodimer by interchain twisting.

Two dimers polymerise in an antiparallel order to form a stable tetramer. Tetramers form protofilaments that assemble into a rope-like 10 nm desmin filament visible in the electron microscope (10). It has been experimentally shown that the integrity of the alpha-helical core domain is essential for desmin assembly and intermediate filament network formation (24, 31). In building an intermediate filament network, desmin interacts with other proteins which cross-link desmin filaments and attach them to the membranes. Desmin is encoded by a single copy gene located in the chromosome 2q35 band (28). The desmin gene, highly conserved among vertebrate species, encompasses nine exons located within an 8.4 kb region (17).

Over the past several years, research activity has been focused upon the identification of gene(s) responsible for DRM. It is probably etiologically heterogeneous, involving at least 2 genes for which mutations have been reported. Eight missense mutations and 2 different type deletions have been described in the desmin gene (3, 16, 20, 23, 25, 26) (Figure 1). In addition, an R120G missense mutation causing DRM was identified in the α-B crystalline gene (CRYAB) that encodes a 20 kD desmin-associated molecular chaperone (27). α-B crystalline, a cytoplasmic small heat shock protein, is implicated in the protective effects of the intermediate filament network against stress-induced damage.

Thus, different types of mutations in the desmin and CRYAB genes are directly responsible for familial cardiac and skeletal myopathy in families with massive desmin immunoreactive deposits. A new category of disease—characterized by ectopic accumulation of desmin in muscle cells and different from other myopathies—was established. The disease caused by desmin and CRYAB mutations may acquire variable clinical features, and, although the pathology is remarkably identical, it is not specific since other types of myopathy may exhibit desmin-reactive deposits (3).

To prove the association of disease with the desmin or CRYAB mutations, SW13 and other types of cells were transfected with patient's cDNA. The results clearly demonstrated that mutant desmin protein was unable to form a functional intracellular network, apparently reflecting inadequate filament assembly.

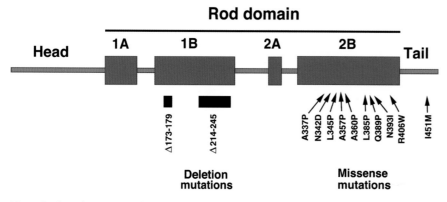

Figure 1. *Secondary structure of human desmin and the location of the mutations associated with cardiac and skeletal myopathy.* Boxes indicate four conserved α-helical subdomains (1A, 1B, 2A, and 2B) that are separated by nonhelical linkers. The helical rods are flanked by a nonhelical amino terminal domain (head) and carboxy terminal domain (tail). Most of the identified point mutations are located in the carboxy terminal part of 2B, whereas both deletion mutations are found in the 1B subdomain.

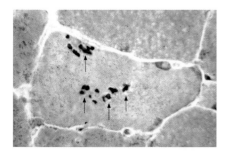

Figure 2. Aggregates of *cytoplasmic* bodies. Examples are indicated by arrows. Modified trichrome stain.

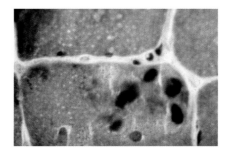

Figure 3. Several *spheroid* bodies. Modified trichrome stain.

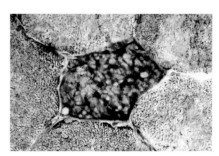

Figure 4. Uneven distribution of enzyme activity around *spheroid bodies*. NADH staining.

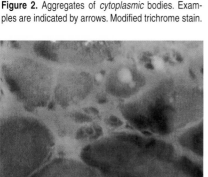

Figure 5. *Patches of granulofilamentous material* within muscle fibres. Modified trichrome stain.

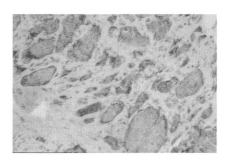

Figure 6. *Granulofilamentous material* in a peripheral muscle fibre is rich in desmin. Immunohistochemistry.

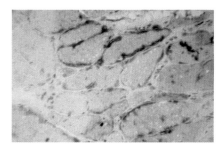

Figure 7. *Granulofilamentous material* is rich in a-B crystalline. Immunohistochemistry.

The type of desmin mutation and its location within the relatively large, structurally and functionally complex desmin molecule may influence the disease severity and outcome. Nine of the 12 mutations identified in patients with desmin myopathy are clustered within the 2B alpha helix at the C-terminal part of the desmin rod domain and are believed to disrupt the alpha-helix and impair desmin filament assembly in the muscle cell. Furthermore, 6 of the 9 mutations in 2B helix introduce proline residues. Mutagenesis experiments with keratin, an intermediate filament of skin cells structurally and functionally similar to desmin, demonstrated that introduction of proline residues resulted in production of short, thick and kinked abnormally looking filaments (24, 31). Genetic heterogeneity of the DRM is further corroborated by having found linkage of other DRM families to chromosomes 2 (19, 30), 10 and 12 (29).

Structural changes

The DRM characteristic accumulation of desmin, by light and electron microscopy, is of 2 types: *i)* the formation of inclusion bodies, *i.e.* cytoplasmic, sarcoplasmic, and spheroid bodies, and patches or "hyaline structures" (Figures 2-4, 9) (4), and *ii)* granulofilamentous material or "dappled dense structures," by electron micro-scopy (21) or "non hyaline structures," by immunohistochemistry (Figures 5-8, 10-12) (4).

Separation into inclusion bodies and granulofilamentous material is not always present, as both morphological features have been observed within the same muscle biopsy and even in the same muscle fibres. This indicates that they are part of a spectrum rather than different entity specific lesions.

By electron microscope, 2 components are present in both types of lesions (Figures 9, 10), *i)* a granular amorphous electron dense component and *ii)* filaments, which are randomly mixed with the granular component in granulofilamentous material, and around the electron dense granular core in cytoplasmic bodies (12, 22).

Spheroid bodies, though distinct at the light microscopic level, are often less well limited at the ultrastructural level (11, 13). While the accumulated desmin is of diagnostic significance,

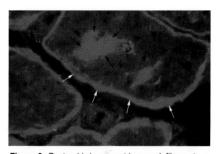

Figure 8. *Dystrophin* is present in granulofilamentous material under the sarcolemma (white arrows) as well as within muscle fibres. One example indicated with light arrows. Immunohistochemistry with fluorescent Texas Red.

the functional deficit may actually be related to the impaired non-aggregated desmin network.

While the presence of desmin is consistently found, a large and diverse number of other proteins have been found to co-aggregate with desmin. These include cytoskeletal proteins, myofibrillar or sarcomeric proteins, chaperone proteins, and proteins usually associated with amyloid formation such as β-A amyloid, gelsolin and others (4). By immunoelectron microscopy, such associated proteins as α-B crystalline (Figure 12) and dystrophin, may be located to filaments.

Oxidative and adenosine triphosphatase enzyme histochemical prepara-

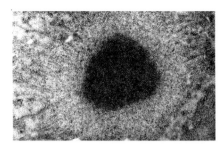

Figure 9. *Ultrastructure of a cytoplasmic body.* There is a central granular core surrounded by a halo of fine filaments.

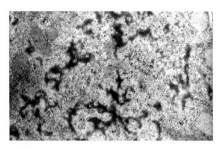

Figure 10. Ultrastructure of *granulofilamentous* material. There is a patchy network of granular electron dense material whereas the filamentous component is rather inconspicuous.

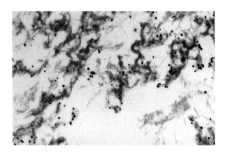

Figure 11. By immunoelectron microscopy, fine filaments are labelled (dark spheres) located close to, but outside the granular electron dense material. Immunogold technique.

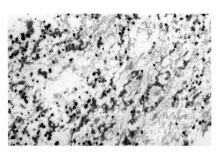

Figure 12. By immunoelectron microscopy, fine filaments outside of the granular electron dense material are also labelled (dark spheres) for α-B crystallin. Immunogold technique with silver enhancement.

tions reveal absence of staining from the desmin containing aggregates, which therefore have been termed "rubbed out" lesions (7). By light microscopy, the muscle specimen reveals a myopathic pattern with variation in fibre diameters with an occasional necrotic fibre and endomysial fibrosis. Cardiac pathology resembles that of skeletal muscle pathology in that abnormal desmin may occur in both types of muscle fibres (18). In a few instances, abnormalities have also been seen in gastrointestinal smooth muscle cells (1, 2).

Future perspectives

The DRM have only recently been separated among the congenital myopathies and several major topics are to be explored: *i)* more precise genotype phenotype correlation among desminopathies, ie, with mutations in the desmin gene including more precise correlation with types of desmin aggregates, *ii)* demonstration of mutant desmin by immunomorphology and immunoblot techniques, *iii)* identification of other mutant proteins in mutated non-desmin genes, ie, located on chromosomes 2 (30) 10 (19), and 12 (29), *iv)* mechanisms that result in the aggregation of desmin and other proteins and *v)* more precise details of the desmin network within muscle fibres of patients affected by a desmin mutation and formation of mutant desmin.

References

1. Abraham SC, DeNofrio D, Loh E, Minda JM, Tomaszewski JE, Pietra GG, Reynolds C (1998) Desmin myopathy involving cardiac, skeletal, and vascular smooth muscle: report of a case with immunoelectron microscopy. *Hum Pathol* 29: 876-882

2. Ariza A, Coll J, Fernandez-Figueras MT, Lopez MD, Mate JL, Garcia O, Fernandez-Vasalo A, Navas-Palacios JJ (1995) Desmin myopathy: a multisystem disorder involving skeletal, cardiac, and smooth muscle. *Hum Pathol* 26: 1032-1037

3. Dalakas MC, Park KY, Semino-Mora C, Lee HS, Sivakumar K, Goldfarb LG (2000) Desmin myopathy, a skeletal myopathy with cardiomyopathy caused by mutations in the desmin gene. *N Engl J Med* 342: 770-780

4. De Bleecker JL, Engel AG, Ertl BB (1996) Myofibrillar myopathy with abnormal foci of desmin positivity. II. Immunocytochemical analysis reveals accumulation of multiple other proteins. *J Neuropathol Exp Neurol* 55: 563-577

5. Edstrom L, Thornell LE, Eriksson A (1980) A new type of hereditary distal myopathy with characteristic sarcoplasmic bodies and intermediate (skeletin) filaments. *J Neurol Sci* 47: 171-190

6. Fardeau M, Godet-Guillain J, Tome FM, Collin H, Gaudeau S, Boffety C, Vernant P (1978) A new familial muscular disorder demonstrated by the intrasarcoplasmic accumulation of a granulofilamentous material which is dense on electron microscopy. *Rev Neurol (Paris)* 134: 411-425

7. Fardeau M, Tomé FMS. Congenital myopathies, in *Myology*, Engel AG Franzini-Armstrong C, Editors. 1994, McGraw-Hill Inc.: New York. p. 1487-1532

8. Fardeau M, Vicart P, Caron A, Chateau D, Chevallay M, Collin H, Chapon F, Duboc D, Eymard B, Tome FM, Dupret JM, Paulin D, Guicheney P (2000) Familial myopathy with desmin storage seen as a granulo-filamentar, electron-dense material with mutation of the alphaB-cristallin gene. *Rev Neurol* (Paris) 156: 497-504

9. Fuchs E, Weber K (1994) Intermediate filaments: structure, dynamics, function, and disease. *Annu Rev Biochem* 63: 345-382

10. Geisler N, Weber K (1982) The amino acid sequence of chicken muscle desmin provides a common structural model for intermediate filament proteins. *Embo J* 1: 1649-1656

11. Goebel HH, Muller J, Gillen HW, Merritt AD (1978) Autosomal dominant "spheroid body myopathy." *Muscle Nerve* 1: 14-26

12. Goebel HH, Schloon H, Lenard HG (1981) Congenital myopathy with cytoplasmic bodies. *Neuropediatrics* 12: 166-180

13. Goebel HH, D'Agostino AN, Wilson J, Cole G, Foroud T, Koller D, Farlow M, Azzarelli B, Muller J (1997) Spheroid body myopathy revisited. *Muscle Nerve* 20: 1127-1136

14. Goebel HH, Warlo I (2000) Gene-related protein surplus myopathies. *Mol Genet Metab* 71: 267-275

15. Goebel HH, Warlo IA (2001) Surplus protein myopathies. *Neuromuscul Disord* 11: 3-6

16. Goldfarb LG, Park KY, Cervenakova L, Gorokhova S, Lee HS, Vasconcelos O, Nagle JW, Semino-Mora C, Sivakumar K, Dalakas MC (1998) Missense mutations in desmin associated with familial cardiac and skeletal myopathy. *Nat Genet* 19: 402-403

17. Li ZL, Lilienbaum A, Butler-Browne G, Paulin D (1989) Human desmin-coding gene: complete nucleotide sequence, characterization and regulation of expression during myogenesis and development. *Gene* 78: 243-254

18. Lobrinus JA, Janzer RC, Kuntzer T, Matthieu JM, Pfend G, Goy JJ, Bogousslavsky J (1998) Familial cardiomyopathy and distal myopathy with abnormal desmin accumulation and migration. *Neuromuscul Disord* 8: 77-86

19. Melberg A, Oldfors A, Blomstrom-Lundqvist C, Stalberg E, Carlsson B, Larsson E, Lidell C, Eeg-Olofsson KE, Wikstrom G, Henriksson KG, Dahl N (1999) Autosomal dominant myofibrillar myopathy with arrhythmogenic right ventricular cardiomyopathy linked to chromosome 10q. *Ann Neurol* 46: 684-692

20. Munoz-Marmol AM, Strasser G, Isamat M, Coulombe PA, Yang Y, Roca X, Vela E, Mate JL, Coll J, Fernandez-Figueras MT, Navas-Palacios JJ, Ariza A, Fuchs E (1998) A dysfunctional desmin mutation in a patient with severe generalized myopathy. *Proc Natl Acad Sci USA* 95: 11312-11317

21. Nakano S, Engel AG, Waclawik AJ, Emslie-Smith AM, Busis NA (1996) Myofibrillar myopathy with abnormal foci of desmin positivity. I. Light and electron microscopy analysis of 10 cases. *J Neuropathol Exp Neurol* 55: 549-562

22. Osborn M, Goebel HH (1983) The cytoplasmic bodies in a congenital myopathy can be stained with antibodies to desmin, the muscle-specific intermediate filament protein. *Acta Neuropathol* 62: 149-152

23. Park KY, Dalakas MC, Goebel HH, Ferrans VJ, Semino-Mora C, Litvak S, Takeda K, Goldfarb LG (2000) Desmin splice variants causing cardiac and skeletal myopathy. *J Med Genet* 37: 851-857

24. Raats JM, Henderik JB, Verdijk M, van Oort FL, Gerards WL, Ramaekers FC, Bloemendal H (1991) Assembly of carboxy-terminally deleted desmin in vimentin-free cells. *Eur J Cell Biol* 56: 84-103

25. Sjoberg G, Saavedra-Matiz CA, Rosen DR, Wijsman EM, Borg K, Horowitz SH, Sejersen T (1999) A missense mutation in the desmin rod domain is associated with autosomal dominant distal myopathy, and exerts a dominant negative effect on filament formation. *Hum Mol Genet* 8: 2191-2198

26. Sugawara M, Kato K, Komatsu M, Wada C, Kawamura K, Shindo PS, Yoshioka PN, Tanaka K, Watanabe S, Toyoshima I (2000) A novel de novo mutation in the desmin gene causes desmin myopathy with toxic aggregates. *Neurology* 55: 986-990

27. Vicart P, Caron A, Guicheney P, Li Z, Prevost MC, Faure A, Chateau D, Chapon F, Tome F, Dupret JM, Paulin D, Fardeau M (1998) A missense mutation in the alphaB-crystallin chaperone gene causes a desmin-related myopathy. *Nat Genet* 20: 92-95

28. Viegas-Pequignot E, Li ZL, Dutrillaux B, Apiou F, Paulin D (1989) Assignment of human desmin gene to band 2q35 by nonradioactive in situ hybridization. *Hum Genet* 83: 33-36

29. Wilhelmsen KC, Blake DM, Lynch T, Mabutas J, De Vera M, Neystat M, Bernstein M, Hirano M, Gilliam TC, Murphy PL, Sola MD, Bonilla E, Schotland DL, Hays AP, Rowland LP (1996) Chromosome 12-linked autosomal dominant scapuloperoneal muscular dystrophy. *Ann Neurol* 39: 507-520

30. Xiang F, Nicolao P, Chapon F, Edstrom L, Anvret M, Zhang Z (1999) A second locus for autosomal dominant myopathy with proximal muscle weakness and early respiratory muscle involvement: a likely chromosomal locus on 2q21. *Neuromuscul Disord* 9: 308-312

31. Yu KR, Hijikata T, Lin ZX, Sweeney HL, Englander SW, Holtzer H (1994) Truncated desmin in PtK2 cells induces desmin-vimentin-cytokeratin coprecipitation, involution of intermediate filament networks, and nuclear fragmentation: a model for many degenerative diseases. *Proc Natl Acad Sci USA* 91: 2497-2501

Nemaline myopathies

Hans H. Goebel
Nigel G. Laing

ACTA1	skeletal muscle α-actin gene
CCD	central core disease
NEB	nebulin gene
RYR1	ryanodine receptor gene
TNNT1	slow troponin T gene
TPM2	β-tropomyosin gene
TPM3	slow α-tropomyosin gene

Definition of entities

Nemaline myopathies are now considered as a genetically diverse group of congenital myopathies marked by excessive formation of rods or nemaline bodies within muscle fibres and/or, more rarely, nuclei.

Shy et al (23) as well as Conen et al (2) are usually credited with having first described nemaline myopathy. The latter group named the nemaline bodies "myogranules," a non-specific term, which did not earn full acceptance by the scientific community. However, it is now clear that in 1958 the Australian pathologist Douglas Reye discovered "nemaline bodies" in the muscle biopsy of a boy, who some 40 years later was found to have a mutation in the ACTA1 gene (22).

Four broad clinical types of nemaline myopathy have been described (15, 28): a severe neonatal form, a much milder congenital or "classic" form, a late or adult onset form—all following an autosomal recessive mode of inheritance—and a separate autosomal dominant form commencing in childhood.

Clinically, the nemaline myopathies present with proximal or generalized muscle weakness sparing bulbar muscle innervated by cranial nerves except facial muscles, which may be severely affected. This results in a characteristic long face, a high arched palate, and a tent shaped mouth. Respiratory insufficiency may remain a threat in early onset forms and may be a major feature in the adult form. Occasional arthrogryposis may reflect intrauterine onset

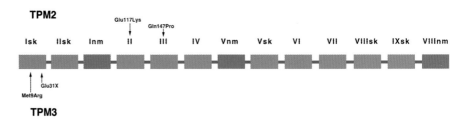

Figure 1. *Genomic structure of the tropomyosin genes.* Mutations in slow-α tropomyosin (TPM3) and β tropomyosin (TPM2) associated with nemaline myopathy. Red-stained exons are alternatively spliced exons in the non-muscle isoforms of the protein.

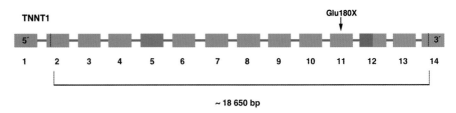

Figure 2. *Genomic structure of the slow troponin T gene (TNNT1).* Position of the nonsense mutation identified in the Amish population. Red-stained exons are alternatively spliced exons.

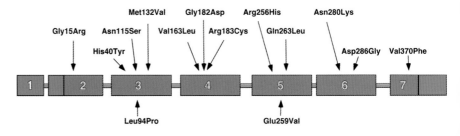

Figure 3. *Genomic structure of the skeletal muscle alpha-actin gene ACTA1 and the published mutations in ACTA1 associated with muscle disease.*

(4, 21). The presence of intranuclear rods may indicate a serious prognosis (1, 6, 19). The heart may occasionally be involved morphologically both in children (24, 27) and adults (13, 25).

Molecular genetics and pathogenesis

The first 2 nemaline myopathy disease genes to be identified, slow α-tropomyosin (*TPM3*) and nebulin (*NEB*) were discovered through positional cloning (12, 18). Both of the encoded proteins are components of the

thin filament, and subsequent candidate gene approaches or positional candidate approaches have been directed at other thin filament proteins. This has resulted in the identification of mutations associated with nemaline myopathy in three other thin filament protein genes—skeletal muscle α-actin (*ACTA1*) (17), β-tropomyosin (*TPM2*) (3) and slow troponin T (*TNNT1*) in the unique autosomal recessive nemaline myopathy seen in the Amish community (10).

In addition, mutations in the ryanodine receptor gene (*RYR1*), more usually associated with either malignant hyperthermia or central core disease (CCD), lead to the production of nemaline bodies (14, 20). Thus, while mutations of five thin filament proteins and one sarcoplasmic reticulum protein have been associated with the formation of nemaline bodies, the major proteins of Z bands and rods, α-actinin 2 and α-actinin 3, have not yet been found as a mutant form in nemaline myopathy. In fact, absence of α-actinin 3 is not associated with disease (16).

Mutations have been identified in *ACTA1* and *TPM3* which lead to both dominant and recessive diseases, while mutations in *NEB* and *TNNT1* have to date been associated with recessive conditions (Figures 1-4).

The dominant mutation first identified in *TPM3*, was a Met9Arg missense mutation (12). The dominant mutations in *TPM2* are missense mutations (3) (Figure 1) and the vast majority of the missense mutations in *ACTA1* are dominant mutations (17) (Figure 3). The published recessive mutation in *TPM3* is a nonsense mutation (26) (Figure 1), as is the recessive mutation identified in *TNNT1* in the Amish nemaline myopathy (10) (Figure 2). In contrast, most of the recessive mutations in NEB are frameshift mutations (18) (Figure 4). Thus, there is a pattern emerging in the thin filament diseases of missense mutations being associated in the main with dominant disease while nonsense, or null mutations, are associated with recessive disease.

To date, close to 50 almost exclusively missense mutations in the *ACTA1* gene have been identified (Laing N, unpublished observations). Most frequently, the patients with *ACTA1* mutations are isolated cases with no previous family history, though the disease is inherited in a dominant fashion in some of the milder forms. In every isolated case examined to date where it has been possible to examine DNA from the parents, the *ACTA1* mutation has been shown to be a de novo mutation. This indicates a very

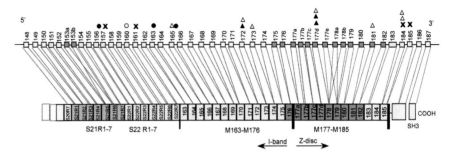

Figure 4. Mutations in the 3′ end of the nebulin gene from exon 148 to exon 187 corresponding to the C-terminal end of the protein, from repeat 7 in superrepeat 29 (S20R7) to the SH3 domain. The exons are shown as boxes numbered from 148 to 187, and the introns are shown as lines, above the protein structure. Alternatively spliced exons are shown as grey boxes. Mutations are indicated by symbols, one for every mutation identified: X, nonsense mutation; open circles, missense mutations; closed circles, splice site mutations; open triangles, small deletions; closed triangles, small insertion. By courtesy of Dr L. Pelin and Dr C. Wallgren-Pettersson, Helsinki, Finland.

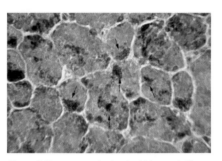

Figure 5. Numerous stained rods within muscle fibres. Examples indicated by arrows. Modified trichrome stain.

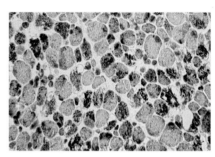

Figure 6. Rods marked by antibody against α-actinin, the chief protein of the Z disk. Immunohistochemistry.

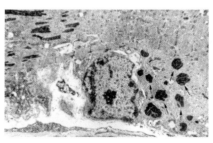

Figure 7. By electron microscopy, rods are situated close to the nucleus under the sarcolemma (arrows) or deeper inside the muscle fibre.

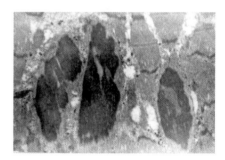

Figure 8. Rods appearing at higher magnification with irregular size and intrinsic structure.

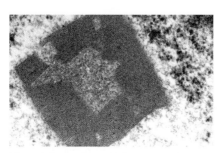

Figure 9. Intranuclear rods. By electron microscopy the intranuclear rod displays the characteristic criss cross pattern of Z disks.

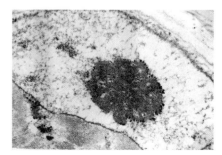

Figure 10. By immunoelectron microscopy, the antibody against α-actinin, the chief protein of the Z disk, labels the intranuclear rod, and the Z disks close to the nucleus as an internal control. Immunogold technique.

high rate of spontaneous new mutations (11). Mutations in the α- and β-tropomyosin genes have been found in only a few families, suggesting that such mutations represent only a minor component within the genetic spectrum of nemaline myopathies whereas mutations in the nebulin gene on chromosome 2q21.2-22 are more numerous (18).

Structural changes

The formation of rods (Figures 5-10) within muscle fibres is the hallmark of nemaline myopathies. These rods often form clusters beneath the sarcolemma and they may occur as large bodies among myofibrils; their long axes often paralleling the long axes of the sar-comeres. Their origin from pre-existing Z bands can occasionally be seen.

The nemaline bodies represent a surplus of Z-band material predominantly composed of α-actinin, the major component of the Z-disc (Figure 6). The pathogenesis of the nemaline bodies is still unclear. The role of the mutant proteins—actin, nebulin, the tropomyosins, troponin T—and the ryanodine receptor in inducing, relating to rod formation, remains to be clarified.

Mutations in the *ACTA1* gene are linked to 2 peculiar morphological phenomena in muscle fibres: *i)* aggregation of actin filaments (5), thus forming an actinopathy and *ii)* the presence of rods within nuclei of muscle fibres: intranuclear rod myopathy. The pathogenesis of these changes is also uncertain. In both adults and in children affected by nemaline myopathy, rods have been seen within nuclei (Figure 9, 10) (7) and these rods usually, though not always, occur singly and have a rather large size. Whether they originate from soluble sarcoplasmic proteins which have entered the nucleus, or merely constitute invaginations and nuclear membrane penetration is still undecided, especially when rods may almost exclusively occur within nuclei (6).

By immunohistochemistry and immunoelectron microscopy, sarco-plasmic and nuclear rods contain α-actinin (Figure 10) and sarcomeric actin, but nebulin, a large sarcomeric protein, has not been found abnormal (8). The formation of rod bodies, which are structured similarly to Z bands, and the presence of both α-actinin and α-actin within both the intranuclear and sarcoplasmic rods, indicate another surplus protein myopathy. However, this surplus protein myopathy is different from other forms. In actinopathy and in desmin-related myopathies containing the mutant proteins, ie, actin and desmin, surplus protein myopathy occurs in a filamentous arrangement, not unlike the Z-band-like structures of the rods.

Trains of rods may occasionally occupy circumscribed areas resembling and, perhaps, even forming cores. Such "rods in cores" now seem to be evidence of CCD (14, 20), rather than that of nemaline myopathies because mutations in the CCD specific gene locus RYR 1 have been identified in such patients.

Cardiac myocytes may occasionally show rod-like abnormalities (9, 13, 25, 27), and these lesions often show electron dense material within cardiac sarcomeres rather than structured rods. Additional features within muscle biopsy specimens are type 1 fibre hypotrophy, often together with type I1fibre predominance, and fulfilling the criteria of fibre type disproportion, the latter phenomenon also occurs in other congenital myopathies.

Future perspectives

Regular studies of families with nemaline myopathy have, surprisingly, opened a new view of this group of disorders documenting genetic heterogeneity which may even encompass additional long identified gene loci. To explain the pathogenetic role of mutant Z band-associated proteins in nemaline myopathies will be a major undertaking. Additional challenges will also present themselves; exploration of the complete composition of rods, both formed within the sarcoplasm as well as within nuclei, and explanation of intranuclear rod appearance.

References

1. Barohn RJ, Jackson CE, Kagan-Hallet KS (1994) Neonatal nemaline myopathy with abundant intranuclear rods. *Neuromuscul Disord* 4: 513-520

2. Conen PE, Murphy EG, Donohue WL (1963) Light and electron microscopic studies of "myogranules" in a child with hypotonia and muscle weakness. *Can Med Assoc J* 89: 983-986

3. Donner K, Ollikainen M, Pelin K, Grönholm M, Carpén O, Wallgren-Pettersson C, Ridanpää M (2000) Mutations in the beta-tropomyosin (TPM2) gene in rare cases of autosomal-dominant nemaline myopathy. *Neuromuscul Disord* 10: 342 (abstract # C.O.341)

4. Fidzianska A, Goebel HH, Kleine M (1990) Neonatal form of nemaline myopathy, muscle immaturity, and a microvascular injury. *J Child Neurol* 5: 122-126

5. Goebel HH, Anderson JR, Hubner C, Oexle K, Warlo I (1997) Congenital myopathy with excess of thin myofilaments. *Neuromuscul Disord* 7: 160-168

6. Goebel HH, Piirsoo A, Warlo I, Schofer O, Kehr S, Gaude M (1997) Infantile intranuclear rod myopathy. *J Child Neurol* 12: 22-30

7. Goebel HH, Warlo I (1997) Nemaline myopathy with intranuclear rods--intranuclear rod myopathy. *Neuromuscul Disord* 7: 13-19

8. Imoto C, Kimura S, Kawai M, Nonaka I (1999) Nebulin is normally expressed in nemaline myopathy. *Acta Neuropathol (Berl)* 97: 433-436

9. Ishibashi-Ueda H, Imakita M, Yutani C, Takahashi S, Yazawa K, Kamiya T, Nonaka I (1990) Congenital nemaline myopathy with dilated cardiomyopathy. *Hum Pathol* 21: 77-82

10. Johnston JJ, Kelley RI, Crawford TO, Morton DH, Agarwala R, Koch T, Schaffer AA, Francomano CA, Biesecker LG (2000) A novel nemaline myopathy in the Amish caused by a mutation in troponin T1. *Am J Hum Genet* 67: 814-821

11. Laing NG, Nowak K, Durling, H., North K, Nonaka I, Hutchinson D, von Kaisenberg C, Muntoni F, Pelin K, Wallgren-Pettersson C (2000) Actin and nemaline-related myopathy. *Brain Pathology* 10: 595 (abstract W502-503)

12. Laing NG, Wilton SD, Akkari PA, Dorosz S, Boundy K, Kneebone C, Blumbergs P, White S, Watkins H, Love DR, et al. (1995) A mutation in the alpha tropomyosin gene TPM3 associated with autosomal dominant nemaline myopathy. *Nat Genet* 9: 75-79

13. Meier C, Voellmy W, Gertsch M, Zimmermann A, Geissbuhler J (1984) Nemaline myopathy appearing in adults as cardiomyopathy. A clinicopathologic study. *Arch Neurol* 41: 443-445

14. Monnier N, Romero NB, Lerale J, Nivoche Y, Qi D, MacLennan DH, Fardeau M, Lunardi J (2000) An autosomal dominant congenital myopathy with cores and rods is associated with a neomutation in the RYR1 gene encoding the skeletal muscle ryanodine receptor. *Hum Mol Genet* 9: 2599-2608

15. North KN, Laing NG, Wallgren-Pettersson C (1997) ENMC International Consortium on Nemaline Myopathy. Nemaline myopathy. Current comcepts. *J Med Genet* 34: 705-713

16. North KN, Yang N, Wattanasirichaigoon D, Mills M, Easteal S, Beggs AH (1999) A common nonsense mutation results in alpha-actinin-3 deficiency in the general population. *Nat Genet* 21: 353-354

17. Nowak KJ, Wattanasirichaigoon D, Goebel HH, Wilce M, Pelin K, Donner K, Jacob RL, Hubner C, Oexle K, Anderson JR, Verity CM, North KN, Iannaccone ST, Muller CR, Nurnberg P, Muntoni F, Sewry C, Hughes I, Sutphen R, Lacson AG, Swoboda KJ, Vigneron J, Wallgren-Pettersson C, Beggs AH, Laing NG (1999) Mutations in the skeletal muscle alpha-actin gene in patients with actin myopathy and nemaline myopathy. *Nat Genet* 23: 208-212

18. Pelin K, Hilpela P, Donner K, Sewry C, Akkari PA, Wilton SD, Wattanasirichaigoon D, Bang ML, Centner T, Hanefeld F, Odent S, Fardeau M, Urtizberea JA, Muntoni F, Dubowitz V, Beggs AH, Laing NG, Labeit S, de la Chapelle A, Wallgren-Pettersson C (1999) Mutations in the nebulin gene associated with autosomal recessive nemaline myopathy. *Proc Natl Acad Sci USA* 96: 2305-2310

19. Rifai Z, Kazee AM, Kamp C, Griggs RC (1993) Intranuclear rods in severe congenital nemaline myopathy. *Neurology* 43: 2372-2377

20. Scacheri PC, Hoffman EP, Fratkin JD, Semino-Mora C, Senchak A, Davis MR, Laing NG, Vedanarayanan V, Subramony SH (2000) A novel ryanodine receptor gene mutation causing both cores and rods in congenital myopathy. *Neurology* 55: 1689-1696

21. Schmalbruch H, Kamieniecka Z, Arroe M (1987) Early fatal nemaline myopathy: case report and review. *Dev Med Child Neurol* 29: 800-804

22. Schnell C, Kan A, North KN (2000) "An artefact gone away": identification of the first case of nemaline myopathy by Dr R.D.K. Reye. *Neuromuscul Disord* 10: 307-312

23. Shy GM, Engel WK, Somers JE, Wanko T (1963) Nemaline myopathy. A new congenital myopathy. *Brain* 86: 793-810

24. Skyllouriotis ML, Marx M, Skyllouriotis P, Bittner R, Wimmer M (1997) Nemaline myopathy and cardiomyopathy. *Pediatr Neurol* 20: 319-321

25. Stoessl AJ, Hahn AF, Malott D, Jones DT, Silver MD (1985) Nemaline myopathy with associated cardiomyopathy. Report of clinical and detailed autopsy findings. *Arch Neurol* 42: 1084-1086

26. Tan P, Briner J, Boltshauser E, Davis MR, Wilton SD, North K, Wallgren-Pettersson C, Laing NG (1999) Homozygosity for a nonsense mutation in the alpha-tropomyosin slow gene TPM3 in a patient with severe infantile nemaline myopathy. *Neuromuscul Disord* 9: 573-579

27. Van Antwerpen CL, Gospe JSM, Dentinger MP (1988) Nemaline myopathy associated with hypertrophic cardiomyopathy. *Pediatr Neurol* 4: 306-308

28. Wallgren-Pettersson C, Pelin K, Hilpela P, Donner K, Porfirio B, Graziano C, Swoboda KJ, Fardeau M, Urtizberea JA, Muntoni F, Sewry C, Dubowitz V, Iannaccone S, Minetti C, Pedemonte M, Seri M, Cusano R, Lammens M, Castagna-Sloane A, Beggs AH, Laing NG, de la Chapelle A (1999) Clinical and genetic heterogeneity in autosomal recessive nemaline myopathy. *Neuromuscul Disord* 9: 564-572

Plectin deficiency

Rolf Schröder
Hans H. Goebel

EBS-MD	epidermolysis bullosa simplex muscular dystrophy
IF	intermediate filament
Plec1	plectin gene

Definition of entity

Epidermolysis bullosa simplex with muscular dystrophy (EBS-MD) is a rare autosomal-recessive disorder caused by mutations of the human plectin gene (Plec1) on chromosome 8q24 (7, 8). As of January 2001, less than 20 cases of EBS-MD have been reported.

While blistering of skin and mucous membranes manifests at birth or shortly thereafter, the age of onset of progressive muscle involvement varies from infancy to the fourth decade. Weakness is usually profound and affects facial, extraocular, limb and trunk muscles. In addition to the classical dermatological and muscular phenotype, a myasthenic syndrome, laryngeal webs, infantile respiratory complications, urethral strictures and brain atrophy have been reported (2, 7, 8).

Molecular genetics and pathogenesis

Plectin, a protein of exceptionally large size (>500 kD), is abundantly expressed in a wide variety of mammalian tissues and cell types. The severe structural changes of skin and muscle tissue in EBS-MD patients and plectin (-,-) mice (1) indicate that plectin has an essential role in mechanical stress bearing tissues. In humans, plectin is encoded by a single copy gene on chromosome 8q24, which contains 32 exons (4) (Figure 1). Apart from a high affinity intermediate filament-binding site in its C-terminal region, plectin has an actin-binding site in its N-terminal region, which shares a high degree of sequence similarity with actin-binding domains in α-actinin, utrophin and dystrophin (9).

Plectin: exon and dominant structures

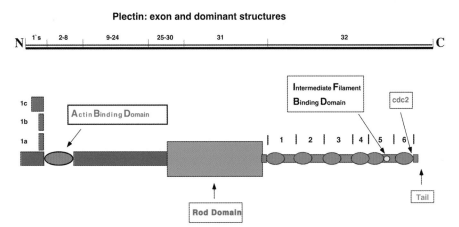

Figure 1. *Exon and domain structure of plectin.* Plectin has a tripartite molecular structure comprising a central α-helical coiled rod domain flanked by large globular domains. The N-terminal globular domain (blue), encoded by over 30 exons including several alternative first coding exons which are all spliced into a common exon 2, contains an actin binding domain that shares a high degree of similarity to actin binding domains found in α-actinin, dystrophin and utrophin. The predominant part of the central rod domain (green) is encoded by exon 31 (> 3 kb) whereas the C-terminal globular domain (brown-red), encoded by the very large exon 32, consists of a tail preceded by 6 repeats (ellipsoids) and a short segment linking it to the rod domain. The IF binding site of plectin has been mapped to a short segment between repeats 5 and 6. Plectin is also a target of p34[cdc2] kinase that regulates the dissociation of plectin molecules from intermediate filaments during mitosis. The majority of Plec1 mutations causing EBS-MD reside in exons 31 and 32.

In human skeletal muscle, plectin is co-localised with desmin at structures forming the intermyofibrillar scaffold and beneath the sarcolemma (5). Furthermore, plectin is thought to play an essential central role in the attachment of the desmin cytoskeleton to the periphery of Z-discs during skeletal muscle development (5, 6). The majority of EBS-MD patients are offsprings of consanguineous marriages. Among 11 EBS-MD patients, 10 had premature termination codon mutations in both Plec1 alleles and only one patient with a particularly mild clinical phenotype had a homozygous 9 bp in-frame deletion that resulted in the elimination of 3 amino acids (3, 7). Most of the Plec1 mutations reported thus far reside within exons 31 and 32 which encode for the rod and C-terminal globular domain of plectin. Genetic alterations in these two exons are thought to interfere with the dimerisation of plectin molecules, as well as with the binding of plectin to intermediate filaments.

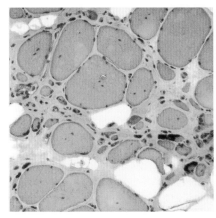

Figure 2. *Skeletal muscle pathology in EBS-MD.* Note severe myopathic changes with increased connective tissue and fat cells, rounded muscle fibres, marked variation of fibre size, centralisation and clustering of myonuclei. Haematoxylin-eosin.

Structural changes

Muscle biopsies from EBS-MD patients (Figures 2-5) reveal severe dystrophic features with increased connective tissue, rounded muscle fibres, marked variation in fibre size, rimmed vacuoles, fibre splitting, increased

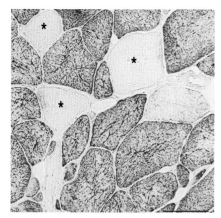

Figure 3. Cytochrome C oxidase (COX) staining demonstrates the presence of multiple COX-negative fibres and muscle fibres displaying a reticular pattern of increased enzymatic activity. Bar = 100 μm.

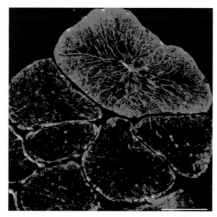

Figure 4. Immunofluorescence staining using mab-D33 directed against desmin. Note the subsarcolemmal accumulation of desmin-positive deposits. Bar = 50 μm.

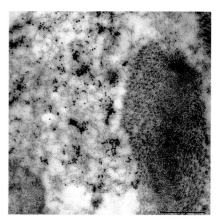

Figure 5. Desmin immunogold electron microscopy. Note the presence of preformed, though highly disordered desmin positive filaments between myofibrils.

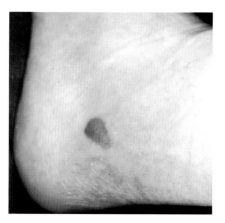

Figure 6. *Skin pathology in EBS-MD.* Superficial skin lesion in response to minor mechanical trauma.

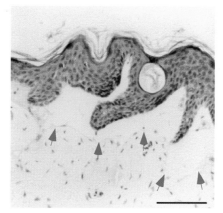

Figure 7. Histopathology demonstrates dermal-epidermal tissue separation (arrows). Haematoxylin-eosin. Bar = 100 μm.

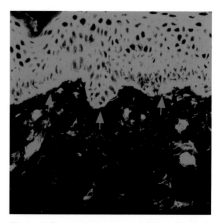

Figure 8. Immunofluorescence staining of normal human skin using P2 antiserum directed against the C-terminal end of plectin. Note the intense labelling at the dermal-epidermal basement membrane zone (arrows) and at the cell surface of keratinocytes in all skin layers.

Figure 9. In contrast, immunolabelling of EBS-MD skin revealed an absence of specific immunoreactivity in basal keratinocytes and at the dermal-epidermal basement membrane zone. Bar = μ100 mm.

numbers of central myonuclei as well as necrotic and regenerating fibres (Figure 2). In addition, there is evidence of mitochondrial dysfunction as indicated by multiple muscle fibres displaying areas of attenuated or even absent cytochrome C oxidase and/or succinate dehydrogenase reactions (Figure 3).

Ultrastructural analysis of skeletal muscle tissue reveals a wide variety of changes: cytoplasmic and nuclear rods, disarrayed myofibrils, thick filament loss, large heterochromatic and lobulated nuclei, and pathological alterations of membranous organelles and neuromuscular endplates (2). Immunogold electron microscopy shows the presence of subsarcolemmal and intermyofibrillar accumulation of highly disordered, normally assembled desmin filaments (Figure 5). The disorganisation of the desmin cytoskeleton may be attributed to impaired desmin binding capability of mutant plectin.

Indirect immunofluorescence shows either reduced or absent plectin staining in skin and muscle tissue of EBS-MD patients (7) (Figures 8, 9). Furthermore, accumulation of cytoplasmic and subsarcolemmal desmin is a prominent feature in skeletal muscle fibres (Figure 4). Electron microscopy of skin samples from EBS-MD patients demonstrates tissue separation in the lower portion of the basal keratinocytes just above the attachment of the hemidesmosomes. In skin, blisters (Figure 6) form at the epidermis-sub-epidermal junction (Figure 7)

Future perspectives

Clinical and molecular genetic analysis of more EBS-MD patients is essential to establishing clear-cut geno-type-phenotype correlations. Furthermore, the identification and functional characterisation of muscle specific plectin isoform is of paramount importance for the understanding of the role of plectin in normal and diseased human skeletal muscle. Since skeletal muscle changes in EBS-MD are associated with marked desmin accumulation, it remains to be seen if certain desmin-related myopathies, without desmin or alpha-B-crystallin mutations, may be attributed to plectin gene defects.

References

1. Andrä K, Lassmann H, Bittner R, Shorny S, Fassler R, Propst F, Wiche G (1997) Targeted inactivation of plectin reveals essential function in maintaining the integrity of skin, muscle, and heart cytoarchitecture. *Genes Dev* 11: 3143-3156.

2. Banwell BL, Russel J, Fukudome T, Shen XM, Stilling G, Engel AG (1999) Myopathy, myasthenic syndrome, and epidermolysis bullosa simplex due to plectin deficiency. *J Neuropathol Exp Neurol* 58: 832-846.

3. Kunz M, Rouan F, Pulkkinen L, Hamm H, Jeschke R, Bruckner-Tuderman L, Brocker EB, Wiche G, Uitto J, Zillikens D (2000) Mutation reports: epidermolysis bullosa simplex associated with severe mucous membrane involvement and novel mutations in the plectin gene. *J Invest Dermatol* 114: 376-380.

4. Liu CG, Maercker C, Castanon MJ, Hauptmann R, Wiche G (1996) Human plectin: organization of the gene, sequence analysis, and chromosome localization (8q24). *Proc Natl Acad Sci USA* 93: 4278-4283.

5. Schröder R, Fürst DO, Klasen C, Reimann J, Herrmann H, van der Ven PF (2000) Association of plectin with Z-discs is a prerequisite for the formation of the intermyofibrillar desmin cytoskeleton. *Lab Invest* 80: 455-464.

6. Schröder R, Warlo I, Herrmann H, van der Ven PF, Klasen C, Blümcke I, Mundegar RR, Furst DO, Goebel HH, Magin TM (1999) Immunogold EM reveals a close association of plectin and the desmin cytoskeleton in human skeletal muscle. *Eur J Cell Biol* 78: 288-295.

7. Shimizu H, Masunaga T, Kurihara Y, Owaribe K, Wiche G, Pulkkinen L, Uitto J, Nishikawa T (1999) Expression of plectin and HD1 epitopes in patients with epidermolysis bullosa simplex associated with muscular dystrophy. *Arch Dermatol Res* 291: 531-537.

8. Smith FJ, Eady RA, Leigh IM, McMillan JR, Rugg EL, Kelsell DP, Bryant SP, Spurr NK, Geddes JF, Kirtschig G, Milana G, de Bono AG, Owaribe K, Wiche G, Pulkkinen L, Uitto J, McLean WH, Lane EB (1996) Plectin deficiency results in muscular dystrophy with epidermolysis bullosa. *Nat Genet* 13: 450-457.

9. Steinböck FA, Wiche G (1999) Role of plectin in cytoskeleton organization and dynamics. *J Cell Sci* 380: 151-158

Telethonin deficiency

Hans H. Goebel
Rolf Schröder

LGMD	limb-girdle muscular dystrophy

Definition of entity

Mutations of the human telethonin gene on chromosome 17q11-12 cause the autosomal recessive limb-girdle muscular dystrophy type 2G (LGMD 2G) (5). As of January 2001, only three families with telethonin mutations have been reported (5).

The age of onset ranges from 2 to 15 years. Difficulty in walking on heels has been reported to be the first symptom. Proximal muscle weakness in the arms, as well as distal and proximal weakness in the legs, are the main clinical findings. Extraocular and facial muscles are spared. In one family, cardiac involvement and calf hypertrophy were present (4, 5).

Molecular genetics and pathogenesis

The human telethonin gene on chromosome 17q11-12 consists of 2 exons encoding a single protein isoform of 19 kD (4, 7). Telethonin, also known as "T-cap," was first identified as one of the most abundant messenger RNAs in striated muscle encoding a sarcomeric protein with a distinct localisation in the central parts of myofibrillar Z-discs (2, 7). Telethonin is exclusively expressed in cardiac and skeletal muscle tissue and is a ligand of the N-terminal immunoglobulin-like domains of the giant muscle protein titin (connectin) (1, 6). Furthermore, titin can phosphorylate the C-terminal domain of telethonin in early differentiating myocytes (3). Although the exact significance of these observations remains to be elucidated, the corroborative data on telethonin indicate that it has a key role in the control of sarcomere assembly and possibly disassembly.

Mutation analysis in 3 Brazilian LGMD 2G families revealed 2 separate mutations, a 157 C→T transition in exon 2 resulting in a premature stop codon (Q53X) and a deletion of 2 guanine nucleotides within 4 guanines (nt 637-640 in the genomic sequence) at the junction of exon 1 and intron 1. The deletion is predicted to induce a frameshift and results in a premature stop codon. While the 157 C→T mutation was homozygous in 2 LGMD 2G kindreds, the third family showed compound heterozygosity with 157 C→T transition in one allele and the deletion mutation in the other (5). Both mutations cause disruption of the functionally relevant C-terminal domain of telethonin, which is phosphorylated by titin kinase in the early events of myofibrillogenesis.

Structural changes

LGMD 2G skeletal muscle tissue shows dystrophic changes. In addition, rimmed vacuoles are a prominent feature (4, 5). Immunohistochemistry and Western blot analysis of skeletal muscle tissue failed to detect telethonin in four LGMD 2G patients (5).

Future perspectives

Since only a small number of families have been described so far, the identification of further patients harbouring telethonin mutations is the central issue for elucidation of the clinical and molecular spectrum of autosomal recessive LGMD 2G.

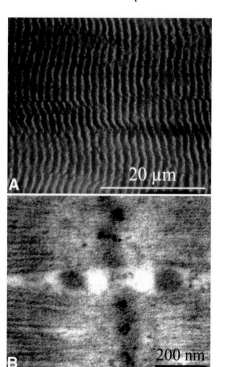

Figure 1. The location of telethonin is at the Z-disk level seen by light microscopy in **A** and by immuno-electron microscopy (gold grains) in **B**.

References

1. Gregorio CC, Trombitas K, Centner T, Kolmerer B, Stier G, Kunke K, Suzuki K, Obermayr F, Herrmann B, Granzier H, Sorimachi H, Labeit S (1998) The NH2 terminus of titin spans the Z-disc: its interaction with a novel 19-kD ligand (T-cap) is required for sarcomeric integrity. *J Cell Biol* 143: 1013-1027.

2. Mason P, Bayol S, Loughna PT (1999) The novel sarcomeric protein telethonin exhibits developmental and functional regulation. *Biochem Biophys Res Commun* 257: 699-703.

3. Mayans O, van der Ven PF, Wilm M, Mues A, Young P, Furst DO, Wilmanns M, Gautel M (1998) Structural basis for activation of the titin kinase domain during myofibrillogenesis. *Nature* 395: 863-869.

4. Moreira ES, Vainzof M, Marie SK, Sertie AL, Zatz M, Passos-Bueno MR (1997) The seventh form of autosomal recessive limb-girdle muscular dystrophy is mapped to 17q11-12. *Am J Hum Genet* 61: 151-159.

5. Moreira ES, Wiltshire TJ, Faulkner G, Nilforoushan A, Vainzof M, Suzuki OT, Valle G, Reeves R, Zatz M, Passos-Bueno MR, Jenne DE (2000) Limb-girdle muscular dystrophy type 2G is caused by mutations in the gene encoding the sarcomeric protein telethonin. *Nat Genet* 24: 163-166.

6. Mues A, van der Ven PF, Young P, Furst DO, Gautel M (1998) Two immunoglobulin-like domains of the Z-disc portion of titin interact in a conformation-dependent way with telethonin. *FEBS Lett* 428: 111-114.

7. Valle G, Faulkner G, De Antoni A, Pacchioni B, Pallavicini A, Pandolfo D, Tiso N, Toppo S, Trevisan S, Lanfranchi G (1997) Telethonin, a novel sarcomeric protein of heart and skeletal muscle. *FEBS Lett* 415: 163-168.

Myotilinopathy

Hans H. Goebel
Rolf Schröder

| LGMD | limb-girdle muscular dystrophy |

Definition of entity

Myotilinopathy is an autosomal dominant limb girdle muscular dystrophy (LGMD 1A) which is assigned to chromosome 5q31 (4), the gene locus that codes for myotilin (2). This LGMD 1A may be allelic to the distal type of myopathy marked by vocal cord and pharyngeal weakness (VPDMD) (1).

Molecular background and pathogenesis

Myotilin is a sarcomeric protein that interacts with actin, α-actinin, and filaments. It can be documented within the Z disk and, thus, within rods or nemaline bodies. It shares a certain homology with the giant sarcomeric protein titin (3). A missense mutation in residue 57 causes an amino acid change, resulting in LGMD 1A (2). This mutation apparently disrupts or compromises interaction of associated sarcomeric proteins, but neither results in a reduction or absence of myotilin nor in an accumulation of myotilin. The mutation in the myotilin gene and the formation of a mutant myotilin do not as easily explain a type of muscular dystrophy as the mutation in a gene that codes for any of the members of the sarcolemmal dystrophin glycoprotein complex.

Structural changes

LGMD 1A is a muscular dystrophy characterised by myopathic changes. It also exhibits rimmed vacuoles, streaming of the Z band and formation of rod like inclusions (2). Immunohistochemically, abnormalities of myotilin may be detected when both alleles are affected, and the resultant mutant protein may not be formed or altered in such a way that it cannot be detected. In the heterozygous state, no immunohistochemical abnormalities of myotilin may be expected. This is similar to the heterozygous mutation in the lamin A/C gene in autosomal dominant Emery Dreifuss muscular dystrophy or LGMD 1B.

Future perspectives

More families with myotilinopathy should be studied to determine the complete clinical and morphological genetic spectrum. Both how the mutation in the myotilin gene is actually expressed at the cellular level, and the role of myotilin among the sarcomeric proteins also require further clarification. The precise significance of intracellular inclusions as observed in LGMD 1A (2), and their relationship to nemaline myopathy, remain to be further studied.

References

1. Feit H, Silbergleit A, Schneider LB, Gutierrez JA, Fitoussi RP, Reyes C, Rouleau GA, Brais B, Jackson CE, Beckmann JS, Seboun E (1998) Vocal cord and pharyngeal weakness with autosomal dominant distal myopathy: clinical description and gene localization to 5q31. *Am J Hum Genet* 63: 1732-1742.

2. Hauser MA, Horrigan SK, Salmikangas P, Torian UM, Viles KD, Dancel R, Tim RW, Taivainen A, Bartoloni L, Gilchrist JR, Vance JM, Pericak-Vance MA, Carpén O, Westbrook CA, Speer MC (2000) Myotilin is mutated in limb girdle muscular dystrophy 1A. *Hum Mol Genet* 9: 2141-2147

3. Salmikangas P, Mykkanen OM, Gronholm M, Heiska L, Kere J, Carpen O (1999) Myotilin, a novel sarcomeric protein with two Ig-like domains, is encoded by a candidate gene for limb-girdle muscular dystrophy. *Hum Mol Genet* 8: 1329-1336.

4. Speer MC, Yamaoka LH, Gilchrist JH, Gaskell CP, Stajich JM, Vance JM, Kazantsev A, Lastra AA, Haynes CS, Beckmann JS, et al. (1992) Confirmation of genetic heterogeneity in limb-girdle muscular dystrophy: linkage of an autosomal dominant form to chromosome 5q. *Am J Hum Genet* 50: 1211-1217.

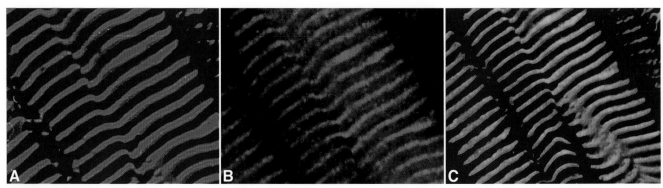

Figure 1. Longitudinal section of skeletal muscle. **A**. a-actinin, the marker protein for the Z-disk red fluorescence colocalizes with myotilin (**B**) showing green flurescence at the Z-disk **C** (yellow fluorescence).

Myosin heavy chain depletion syndrome

George Karpati

AQM	acute quadriplegic myopathy
MHCDS	myosin heavy chain depletion syndrome

Definition of entity

Myosin heavy chain depletion syndrome (MHCDS) is the commonest basis of acute quadriplegic myopathy, which is the most frequent presentation of the so-called "critical illness myopathy" (3). As the name would imply, acute flaccid weakness of limb and respiratory muscles develops in patients who have received high dose intravenous glucocorticoids as well as a neuromuscular blocking agent to facilitate mechanical ventilation (2). The commonest scenario is a patient with severe status asthmaticus who is paralyzed with vecuronium, and put on a mechanical ventilator while receiving high dose of methylprednisolone. This regime terminates the asthmatic attack within a few days but when the neuromuscular blocking agent is stopped, and an attempt to discontinue the respirator is made, the patient is found severely paralyzed and the respirator needs to be continued.

Upon cessation of the administration of corticosteriods and the neuromuscular blocking agent, recovery of muscle strength occurs within days to months. In some severely ill septic patients, the syndrome may develop without receiving corticosteroids or neuromuscular blocking agents. Old age and prior chronically low protein intake, as well as mechanical muscle disuse, tend to predispose patients for this complication in the presence of a severe systemic illness. Genetic predisposition has not been suggested.

Molecular pathogenesis

Microscopic studies and animal experiments revealed that the basis of the muscle paralysis is a severe, acute loss of thick myofilaments from the A band of the myofibrils in many muscle fibres. A similar picture can be produced in acutely denervated plantaris muscles of rats receiving high dose of systemic corticosteroids (6). While in both the patients and in the experimental model, there is a marked paucity of thick myofilaments in the A band of the sarcomeres, immunostaining for myosin heavy chain is still present in the A band, albeit less than normal. This constellation suggests that the myosin monomers, normally held together in the thick myofilaments in the A band by electrostatic molecular forces, disaggregate and form a "pool" in the A band. The disaggregated myosin monomers lose their ATPase activity and, of course, cannot contribute to force generation of the muscle fibres; hence, the paralysis.

The disaggregated myosin monomers are subject to proteolysis and increased calpain activity was demonstrated in such muscles (8). However, since the overall organization of the sarcomere is maintained, the cessation of the triggering factors could relatively rapidly permit the reassembly of the myosin monomers into thick filaments with restoration of muscle force (5). However, if there is substantial loss of the myosin monomers before that can happen, de novo synthesis of new myosin heavy chain molecules needs to occur, which can delay and/or permit only partial restoration of muscle force generation. The precise physicochemical mechanism(s) by which the putative disassembly of myosin monomers occurs is not fully understood. Since in vitro, in fresh muscle strips, high ionic strength of the bathing fluid can give rise to a similar and rapidly reversible picture, we hypothethized that the ultrarapid shrinking of muscle fibres by the combined effect of disuse (denervation) and corticosteroids raises the ionic strength in the myofibrillar com-

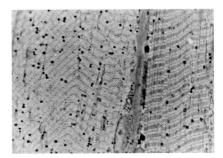

Figure 1. Longitudinal view of an epon section shows on the left a muscle fibre lacking A band density in a case of a typical acute quadriplegic myopathy 23 days after the onset of paralysis. The fibre on the right appears to have normal A band density. ×550

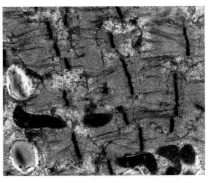

Figure 2. Electron microscopy shows a near total loss of thick myofilaments in a fibre in the same case as shown in Figure 1. ×50000

partment above a threshold level that favors disaggregation of the myosin monomers from the thick myofilaments.

Rich et al (6) have identified an additional mechanism of muscle fibre paralysis in the rat model (5, 7) of acute myopathy with massive thick filament loss. These authors used intracellular recording combined with loose patch voltage clamp of single fibres to show that muscle fibres were unexcitable due to abnormal inactivation of the voltage-regulated sodium channels as a result of an abnormality of the voltage dependence of sodium channel inactivation. It is not clear as to how this change is linked, if at all, to the myosin heavy chain loss and which of the two changes becomes normalized first when steroids are stopped and reinnervation of muscle takes place.

Structural changes

The structural changes have recently been described elsewhere (1). On cryostat sections of muscle biopsies obtained 24 hours after of the onset of symptoms, muscle fibres tend to contain areas of smudgy, purplish staining with the modified trichrome stain. This is due to the preponderance of the purple staining of the Z discs on account of the attenuation of the green staining of the A band. In the same zones, myosin ATPase activity is markedly reduced, but immunostaining for myosin heavy chain shows less attenuation. Resin-embedded longitudinal semithin sections viewed by phase microscopy shows near abolition of the A band density, but otherwise, preservation of the structure of the sarcomere (Figure 1). By electron microscopy on longitudinal view, direct visualization of the massive loss of thick myofilaments is possible in some fibres (Figure 2). There is no fibre type predilection for these changes.

Future perspectives

Further research is needed to determine if there is some genetic predisposition for this change. This is raised in view of the fact that some individuals have recurrent episodes (4). Furthermore, the observed changes permit research into the molecular forces that maintain the myosin monomers assembled in the thick myofilaments. The key to effective therapy is prevention or early recognition of the syndrome.

References

1. Carpenter S, Karpati G (2001) *Pathology of Skeletal Muscle.* Oxford University Press: New York.

2. Danon MJ, Carpenter S (1991) Myopathy with thick filament (myosin) loss following prolonged paralysis with vecuronium during steroid treatment. *Muscle Nerve* 14: 1131-1139

3. Hirano M, Ott BR, Raps EC, Minetti C, Lennihan L, Libbey NP, Bonilla E, Hays AP (1992) Acute quadriplegic myopathy: a complication of treatment with steroids, nondepolarizing blocking agents, or both. *Neurology* 42: 2082-2087

4. Kuntzer T, Schaller MD, Vuadens P, Janzer RC (1998) Recurrent acute quadriplegic myopathy with myosin deficiency. *Muscle Nerve* 21: 266-267

5. Massa R, Carpenter S, Holland P, Karpati G (1992) Loss and renewal of thick myofilaments in glucocorticoid-treated rat soleus after denervation and reinnervation. *Muscle Nerve* 15: 1290-1298

6. Rich MM, Pinter MJ (2001) Sodium channel inactivation in an animal model of acute quadriplegic myopathy. *Ann Neurol* 50: 26-33

7. Rouleau G, Karpati G, Carpenter S, Soza M, Prescott S, Holland P (1987) Glucocorticoid excess induces preferential depletion of myosin in denervated skeletal muscle fibers. *Muscle Nerve* 10: 428-438

8. Showalter CJ, Engel AG (1997) Acute quadriplegic myopathy: analysis of myosin isoforms and evidence for calpain-mediated proteolysis. *Muscle Nerve* 20: 316-322

Autosomal dominant myosin heavy chain IIa myopathy

Anders Oldfors
Niklas Darin
Tommy Martinsson

h-IBM	hereditary inclusion body myopathy
MyHC	myosin heavy chain

Definition of entity

Autosomal dominant myosin heavy chain IIa myopathy is a recently recognized disorder associated with a mutation of the myosin heavy chain type IIa gene in chromosome region 17p13.1 (3, 5, 6). This disorder was previously regarded as a variant of hereditary inclusion body myopathy (h-IBM) (8). Thus far, it has only been described in one Swedish family with 20 affected cases. The inheritance is autosomal dominant with full penetrance. The onset of muscle weakness varies from birth to adulthood. Clinical characteristics are congenital joint contractures, which normalize during early childhood, external ophthalmoplegia, and predominantly proximal muscle weakness and atrophy. The course is frequently progressive in adulthood.

Molecular genetics and pathogenesis

Myosin is an actin-based molecular motor protein, which transduces chemical energy of ATP hydrolysis into mechanical force. Several genes encode myosin heavy chains (MyHC) in striated muscle of mammals. In humans, alfa and slow/beta MyHCs are encoded by genes located on chromosome 14, while the genes encoding embryonic, IIa, IIx/d, IIb, perinatal, and extraocular MyHCs are located in a cluster on chromosome 17 (9) (Figure 1A). Slow/beta MyHC is expressed in the heart and in type 1 muscle fibres in skeletal muscle. Type IIa MyHC is mainly expressed in type 2A muscle fibres while MyHC IIx is the major isoform in type 2B muscle fibres of skeletal muscle. Whereas numerous point mutations in the chromosome 14 group of genes have been reported in associa-

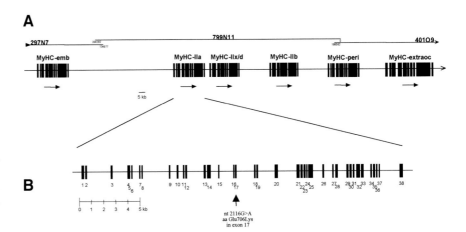

Figure 1. A. Genomic organization of the cluster of 6 MyHC genes in chromosome region 17p13.1. Three completely sequenced BAC clones are shown at the top while the detailed organization of the MyHC IIa gene (MYH2) is shown in **B**: The location of the mutation 2116G>A (Glu706Lys) in exon 17 of MYH2 is depicted with an arrow. Reproduced from *Proc Natl Acad Sci U S A* 2000;97:14614-14619, with permission, Copyright (2000) National Academy of Sciences, U.S.A.

tion with familial hypertrophic cardiomyopathy (FHC)(2), the chromosome 17 group of MyHCs was until recently not linked to any myopathy. However, in a recent report the disease in one family with autosomal dominant hereditary inclusion body myopathy (IBM3) was shown to be caused by a mutation (nt2116G>A) in one of the fast myosins, ie, MyHC type IIa, HGM locus: MYH2 (6). The sequence alteration leads to a missense mutation, Glu706Lys (Figure 1B), in the highly conserved region of the motor domain, the so-called SH1 helix region (Figure 2). By conformational changes, this region communicates activity at the nucleotide-binding site to the neck region, resulting in the lever arm swing. The mutation in this region is likely to result in a dysfunctional myosin, compatible with the disorder in the family.

Several animal model systems presented support the association between myopathy and mutations in the fast myosins. Targeted disruption of fast MyHC genes in mice causes myopathy with muscle weakness and disorganization of myofilaments (1), and point

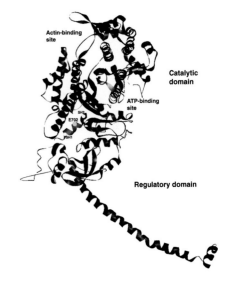

Figure 2. Ribbon model of MyHC subfragment 1 of chicken skeletal muscle. The ATP- and actin-binding sites are indicated. The site of the mutation (Glu-706→Lys) (E107 in chicken) in the SH1 helix (red) is indicated by a yellow sphere. Conformational changes upon binding and hydrolysis of ATP in the catalytic region are transmitter via the SH-1 helix region, which constitutes a joint or fulcrum, to the regulatory domain, which acts as a lever arm. Reproduced from *Proc Natl Acad Sci U S A* 2000;97:14614-14619, with permission, Copyright (2000) National Academy of Sciences, U.S.A.

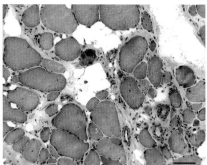

Figure 3. Severe myopathic changes with marked variation in fibre size and increased amount of connective tissue. H&E. Bar = 30 μm

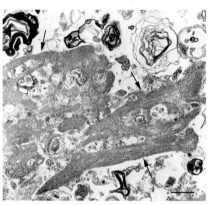

Figure 4. Irregular staining of the intermyofibrillar network and mitochondria in type 2A muscle fibres (arrows). NADH-tetrazolium reductase. Bar = 20 μm

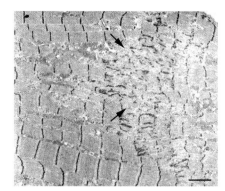

Figure 5. Ultrastruture of focal areas of disorganization of myofilaments (arrows). Bar = 2 μm

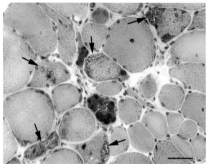

Figure 6. Muscle fibres with rimmed vacuoles (arrows). H&E. Bar = 20 μm

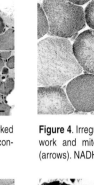

Figure 7. Ultrastructural appearance of inclusions of 15-20 nm tubulofilaments (arrows) in association with rimmed vacuoles. Bar = 1 μm. Reproduced from *Ann Neurol* 1998;44:242-248, with permission, copyright (1998), John Wiley & Sons, Inc.

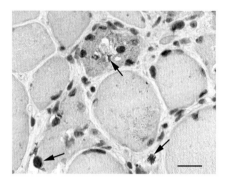

Figure 8. Immunostaining of ubiquitin showing ubiquitin-positive inclusions (arrows) in muscle fibers with rimmed vacuoles. Bar = 15 μm

mutations in MyHC genes result in muscle dysfunction in *Drosophila*, *C.elegans*, and *Dictyostelium* (7).

Structural changes

Muscle biopsies show marked inter-individual variability (3, 4, 6). Young individuals show minor changes including reduced number and hypotrophy/atrophy of type 2A fibres. Adults with a clinically progressive course show severe myopathy with increased interstitial connective tissue, marked variability in fibre size and centrally located nuclei (Figure 3). The most prominent alteration in muscle biopsies with minor changes is a patchy, focal loss of oxidative enzyme activity and disorganization of the intermyofibrillar network in 2A fibres (Figure 4). This alteration apparently corresponds to focal disorganization of myofilaments and focal loss of mitochondria in a minicore-like pattern as disclosed at the ultrastructural level (Figure 5). In

severely affected muscles all fibre types show pathological changes, as demonstrated by myofibrillar ATPase staining.

The occurrence of rimmed vacuoles is variable and they are only present in muscle tissue with marked myopathic changes (Figure 6). The rimmed vacuoles may be frequent and was in one case present in 12% of the muscle fibres in a muscle biopsy from the quadriceps femoris muscle. Collections of tubulofilaments with a diameter of 15 to 20 nm are frequently present in association with the rimmed vacuoles (Figure 7). In one case, intranuclear filaments were reported. By immunohistochemical analysis the rimmed vacuoles are associated with ubiquitin positive inclusions (Figure 8) that are also stained with the SMI-31 antibody.

The histopathological changes in adults with marked myopathic changes include muscle fibres with segmental

loss and cytochrome *c* oxidase activity and occasional ragged red fibres.

Genotype-phenotype correlations

MyHC IIa is the major isoform of MyHCs in type 2A muscle fibres. There is an apparent correlation between the mutation in the gene encoding type IIa MyHC and the involvement of type 2A muscle fibres. This is expressed as structural changes in the muscle fibres as well as a reduction in the number of type 2A fibres in some cases. In severely affected muscles where all fibre types are involved, there is a large proportion of hybrid muscle fibres, which express more than one MyHC isoform, including MyHC IIa. Muscle fibres with rimmed vacuoles consistently express type IIa MyHC. The observed muscle fibres with cyto-chrome *c* oxidase deficiency, which are present in adult patients with progressive course, are associated with accumulation of mitochondrial DNA with large-scale deletions, explaining the reduced respiratory chain activity (4).

Future perspectives

Although this is the first human myopathy that has been shown to be associated with a mutation in a fast MyHC gene, this association put forward the fast MyHC genes as important candidates in similar disorders such as variants of "minicore," "minimal change," and "type-II fibre atrophy" myopathies, in addition to hereditary myopathies with rimmed vacuoles, such as h-IBMs and distal myopathies.

The findings of rimmed vacuoles and filamentous inclusions in adults with progressive muscle weakness, are thought-provoking and suggest a possible relationship between the degradation of sarcomeric proteins and the generation of rimmed vacuoles. Since the expression of MyHC isoforms are influenced by physical training and inactivity, studies on the importance of these factors for the phenotypic expression in this family are another important direction for future studies.

References

1. Acakpo-Satchivi LJ, Edelmann W, Sartorius C, Lu BD, Wahr PA, Watkins SC, Metzger JM, Leinwand L, Kucherlapati R (1997) Growth and muscle defects in mice lacking adult myosin heavy chain genes. *J Cell Biol* 139: 1219-29

2. Bonne G, Carrier L, Richard P, Hainque B, Schwartz K (1998) Familial hypertrophic cardiomyopathy: from mutations to functional defects. *Circ Res* 83: 580-593

3. Darin N, Kyllerman M, Wahlström J, Martinsson T, Oldfors A (1998) Autosomal dominant myopathy with congenital joint contractures, ophthalmoplegia, and rimmed vacuoles. *Ann Neurol* 44: 242-248

4. Jansson M, Darin N, Kyllerman M, Martinsson T, Wahlstrom J, Oldfors A (2000) Multiple mitochondrial DNA deletions in hereditary inclusion body myopathy. *Acta Neuropathol (Berl)* 100: 23-28

5. Martinsson T, Darin N, Kyllerman M, Oldfors A, Hallberg B, Wahlström J (1999) Dominant hereditary inclusion-body myopathy gene (IBM3) maps to chromosome region 17p13.1. *Am J Hum Genet* 64: 1420-1426

6. Martinsson T, Oldfors A, Darin N, Berg K, Tajsharghi H, Kyllerman M, Wahlström J (2000) Autosomal dominant myopathy: Missense mutation (Glu-706 to Lys) in the myosin heavy chain IIa gene. *Proc Natl Acad Sci U S A* 97: 14614-14619

7. Ruppel KM, Spudich JA (1996) Structure-function analysis of the motor domain of myosin. *Annu Rev Cell Dev Biol* 12: 543-573

8. Tomé FM, Fardeau M (1998) Hereditary inclusion body myopathies. *Curr Opin Neurol* 11: 453-459

9. Weiss A, McDonough D, Wertman B, Acakpo-Satchivi L, Montgomery K, Kucherlapati R, Leinwand L, Krauter K (1999) Organization of human and mouse skeletal myosin heavy chain gene clusters is highly conserved. *Proc Natl Acad Sci U S A* 96: 2958-63

CHAPTER 5

Diseases associated with ion channel and ion transporter defects

5.1 Chloride and sodium channel myotonias   90
5.2 Dyskalemic episodic weakness   95
5.3 Malignant hyperthermia and central core disease associated with defects
   in Ca^{2+} channels of the sarcotubular system   99
5.4 Brody disease associated with defects in a Ca^{2+} pump   103

T his field of myology has undergone a spectacular development during the past 15 years. Fundamental new information has accumulated about the biology of cation and anion channels located in the plasma membrane, T tubules, and sarcoplasmic reticulum.

The normal function of these channels is the cornerstone of excitation contraction coupling of the muscle fibre; their malfunction can bring about diverse deleterious consequences including myotonia, paralysis, cramps, and even necrosis. Most of these ion channel disturbances are genetically determined. The analysis of the genetic defects in these disorders has elucidated not only the normal function of these molecules but also the diversity of function of their different domains. These points are discussed in depth in this chapter.

Chloride and sodium channel myotonias

Karin Jurkat-Rott
Josef Müller-Höcker
Dieter Pongratz
Frank Lehmann-Horn

DMC	dominant myotonia congenita
HyperPP	hyperkalemic periodic paralysis
HypoPP	hypokalemic periodic paralysis
PAM	K⁺-aggravated myotonia
PC	paramyotonia congenita
RMC	recessive myotonia congenita

Definition of entities

Muscle excitability is based on ion channel activity. Motoneuron activity is transferred to skeletal muscle in the neuromuscular junction generating an action potential in the muscle that propagates along the sarcolemma and the transverse (T) tubular system: a membrane region projecting deep into the cell to ensure even distribution of the impulse. An action potential is elicited when the endplate potential exceeds the threshold of the voltage-gated tetrodotoxin-sensitive Na^+ channels. The upstroke of the action potential is the result of the rapid activation (opening) of these channels and subsequent influx of the positively charged Na^+ ions along both the electrical and the concentration gradient into the cells. By this, the muscle fibres are depolarised from -80 mV resting potential to an overshoot of +20 mV within one millisecond. Repolarisation back to the resting potential is mainly the result of inactivation (closing) of the Na^+ channels. Additionally, opening of voltage-gated K^+ channels contributes to re-establishing the resting potential because this leads to the efflux of positively charged K^+ ions along the concentration gradient from the cell interior to the extracellular T tubular space.

At specialised junctions in the T tubular systems, the signal is transmitted from the outer membrane to the inside of the muscle cell where calcium ions are released from the sarcoplasmic stores and initiate contraction. This transmission, called excitation-contraction coupling, is initiated by voltage-gated dihydropyridine-sensitive Ca^{2+} channels. Buffering of after-depolarisations following an action potential is achieved by an especially high Cl^- conductance near the resting membrane potential. This conductance results from voltage-gated chloride channels and the Cl^- ions flowing through these electrically neutralise the extracellular K^+ charge accumulation during the repolarisation phase. From this, ion channel malfunctions leading to hyperexcitability can easily be predicted. For example, a reduction of Cl^- conductance will allow supra-threshold after-depolarisation initiating additional action potentials. Re-openings of the Na^+ channels themselves will have the same effect whereas lack of their activation will cause total muscle fibre membrane inexcitability (16).

Ion channelopathies result from disturbed excitability. Primary sarcolemmal and T tubular system ion channel defects generally lead to abnormal muscle fibre excitation. Therefore, the ability to generate action potentials is either enhanced or decreased in these so-called ion channelopathies. Clinically, this results in phenotypes caused by muscle fibre membrane hyperexcitability leading to myotonic stiffness and/or phenotypes associated with sarcolemmal inexcitability resulting in dyskalemic weakness. These disorders belong to the so-called non-dystrophic myotonias and periodic paralyses, a term already indicating that regularly occurring specific morphologic changes are not to be expected in persons under 45 years. One reason may be directly concluded from the fact that symptoms up to this

Disease entity	Gene name Chromosome	Gene product Functional disturbance	Number of mutations % patients with mutations	Symptoms, prevalence, inheritance
Myotonia congenita Becker (RMC)	CLCN1 7q35	Cl⁻ channel ClC1 loss-of-function	>30 missense & nonsense mutations 60% of patients	~1:25 000; autosomal recessive; childhood onset, generalised myotonia, warm-up phenomenon, muscle hypertrophy, transient weakness
Myotonia congenita Thomsen (DMC)	CLCN1 7q35	Cl⁻ channel ClC1 dominant-negative effects	12 missense mutations 35% of patients	~1:400 000; autosomal dominant; teenage onset, generalized myotonia, warm-up phenomenon, mild muscle hypertrophy
K⁺-aggravated myotonia (PAM)	SCN4A 17q23	Na⁺ channel α subunit gain-of-function	7 missense mutations 35% of patients	~1:250 000; autosomal dominant; onset varies from congenital to adult onset, generalised myotonia of variable severity, aggravation by K⁺ administration, no weakness
Paramyotonia congenita (PC)	SCN4A 17q23	Na⁺ channel α subunit gain-of-function	11 missense mutations 50% of patients	~1:250 000; autosomal dominant; childhood onset, paradoxical myotonia, cold-induced muscle stiffness followed by weakness/paralysis

Table 1. Voltage-gated channelopathies of the sarcolemma and the T tubular membrane.

age occur only episodically with varying intervals of normal muscle function and excitation in between. Apparently, the ion channel defects are usually well-compensated and an additional, special endogenous or exogenous trigger is required for malfunction to become apparent. Morphologically, non-dystrophic myotonias and periodic paralyses follow general patterns of myopathic changes depending on the type of excitational disturbance: syndromes with hyperexcitability show muscle fibre type 2B deficiency, whereas syndromes with inexcitability are associated with vacuolar myopathy and tubular aggregates. With increasing age, a portion of the patients develops permanent weakness especially of the hands and the lower extremities and then an additional vacuolar muscle degeneration with fatty replacement may be found morphologically.

Clinical findings. Muscle stiffness, termed myotonia, ameliorates by exercise (warm-up phenomenon) and can be associated with transient weakness during quick movements lasting only for seconds. On the contrary, paradoxical myotonia, or paramyotonia, worsens with exercise and cold, and is followed by long spells of limb weakness lasting from hours to days. Both are associated with muscle hypertrophy especially of the lower limbs. Clinically, they are distinguished according to mode of transmission and K+ sensitivity: dominant K+-aggravated myotonia fluctuans (31, 32) and permanens (20), dominant K+-insensitive myotonia congenita (36), recessive myotonia congenita or recessive generalised myotonia (2), and paramyotonia congenita (7) (Table 1).

Molecular genetics and pathogenesis

Both myotonia and paradoxical myotonia are brought about by uncontrolled repetitive firing of action potentials of the sarcolemma following an initial voluntary activation. This may be noted as a myotonic burst in the electromyogramm. The involuntary

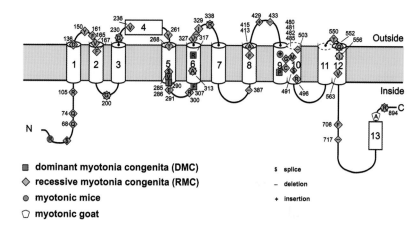

Figure 1. *Membrane topology model of the skeletal muscle chloride channel monomer, CIC-1.* The functional channel is a homodimer. The different symbols used for the known mutations leading to dominant Thomsen-type myotonia and recessive Becker-type myotonia are explained on the left-hand bottom. Conventional 1-letter abbreviations are used for replaced amino acids.

electrical activity prevents the muscle from immediate relaxation after contraction, which the patients experience as muscle stiffness. Basic pathology of the myotonic reaction in Thomsen and Becker myotonia is a reduced chloride conductance that fails to sufficiently buffer the after-depotential and triggers new premature action potentials (1, 22, 33). In paramyotonia and potassium-aggravated myotonia, the increased sarcolemmal excitability is due to inactivation defects of the Na+ channels that mediate the upstroke of the action potential (17, 19). This results in channel re-openings and intracellular Na+ accumulation, which depolarises the muscle cells, and thus, elicits additional action potentials.

Chloride channel myotonias Thomsen and Becker. The Cl- channel consists of a homodimer encoded by the *CLCN1* gene on chromosome 7q (15). Both missense mutations (exchange of single amino acid residues) and nonsense mutations (alternative protein splicing or premature truncation) have been identified (9, 10, 13, 18). While splicing mutations always lead to the recessive phenotype, various truncations and missense muta-

tions are found in the Thomsen and Becker myotonia (Figure 1). A few intermediate mutations are even able to generate both modes of transmission depending on supplemental genetic or environmental factors. Functionally, the dominant mutants exert a so-called dominant negative effect on the dimeric channel complex as shown by co-expression studies meaning that mutant/mutant *and* mutant/wildtype complexes are malfunctional. The most common feature of the thereby resulting Cl- currents is a shift of the activation threshold towards more positive membrane potentials almost out of the physiological range (30, 39). As a consequence of this, the Cl- conductance is drastically reduced in the crucial vicinity of the resting membrane potential. This is not the case for the recessive mutants, which do not functionally hinder the co-associated subunit supplying the explanation as to why 2 mutant alleles are required to reduce Cl- conductance so much that myotonia develops (at least down to 30%) (27).

This knowledge has led to a double-barrel model of the Cl- channel with two independent ion conducting pores each with a fast opening mechanism of its own that is affected by the recessive

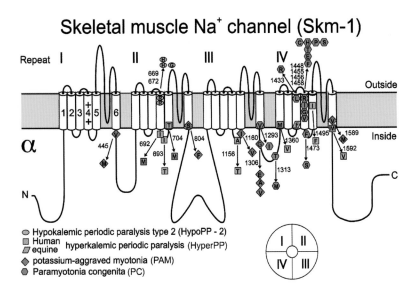

Figure 2. *Membrane topology model of the voltage-gated sodium channel of skeletal muscle.* The α subunit functions as ion-conducting channel and consists of four highly homologous domains (repeats I-IV) containing six transmembrane segments each (S1-S6). The S6 transmembrane segments and the S5-S6 loops form the ion selective pore, and the S4 segments contain positively charged residues conferring voltage dependence to the protein. The repeats are connected by intracellular loops; one of them, the III-IV linker, contains the supposed inactivation particle of the channel. When inserted in the membrane, the four repeats of the protein fold to generate a central pore as schematically indicated on the right-hand bottom of the figure. The different symbols used for the known mutations leading to potassium-aggravated myotonia, paramyotonia congenita or two types of periodic paralysis are explained on the left-hand bottom. Conventional 1-letter abbreviations are used for replaced amino acids.

mutations, but with a common slow additional gate structure shared with the co-associated subunit that is affected by the dominant mutations (34). Intriguingly, this model has been confirmed by cryo-electron microscopy on two-dimensional protein crystals (25).

Sodium channel myotonia and paramyotonia. In K⁺-aggravated myotonia and paramyotonia there is a gating defect of the Na⁺ channels destabilizing the inactivated state, ie, channel inactivation may be slowed or incomplete (5, 19, 20, 26, 41). This results in an increased tendency of the muscle fibres to depolarise, generating action potentials and myotonia (19, 21). It does not necessarily additionally affect channel activation because the pore-occluding gate structures decisive for activation and inactivation are located in different regions of the protein. Because the mutant channels exert an effect on cell excitability, the mutations produce a dominant change or gain-of-function.

One hot spot for the paramyotonia mutations is a special voltage-sensing transmembrane region (3, 21, 28) that couples channel inactivation to channel activation (5); another hot spot is an intracellular protein loop containing the inactivation particle (24). The K⁺-aggravated myotonia mutations are found in intracellular regions of the protein, potentially interfering with the channel inactivation process (Figure 2). Corresponding to the severity of the disruption of the inactivation gate structure on the protein level, there are three clinical severities to be distinguished (20, 26): *i)* myotonia fluctuans where patients may not be aware of their disorder, *ii)* myotonia responsive to acetazolamide (29) with a Thomsen-like clinical phenotype, and *iii)* myotonia permanens with continuous electrical myotonia leading to a generalized muscle hypertrophy including face and neck muscles suggestive of facial dysmorphia. In all 3 types, body exertion or administration of depolarising agents may result in a severe or even

life-threatening myotonic crisis (14, 20, 32, 38).

Structural changes

Chloride channel myotonias Thomsen and Becker. Muscle samples of some patients may have normal appearance. In others, slight myopathic changes with increased occurrence of central nuclei and pathological variation of fibre diameter may be found. Muscle fibre hypertrophy, especially of type 2A fibres, and fibre atrophy may be present. Finally, there may be reduction or complete absence of fibre type 2B (Figure 3) (6, 12).

K⁺-aggravated (Na⁺ channel) myotonia. Despite the seemingly drastic differences in clinical severity, the morphological findings do not systematically differ. In myotonia fluctuans, light microscopy may show a normal appearance or increased central nuclei and fibre diameter variation. Subsarcolemmal vacuoles representing a nonspecific enlargement of the T tubular system may by found by electron microscopy (31). In myotonia permanens, subsarcolemmal myoplasmic space and mitochondria may be increased, focal disarray or interruption of myofibrils and disappearance of Z disks, involving one or more sarcomeres observed (Figure 4). In these areas, glycogen particles and elongated or branched mitochondria can be found. Between the bundles of myofibrils, membrane-bound vacuoles may be visible which are empty or filled with fine granular material or electron dense whorls.

Paramyotonia congenita. Light microscopy may be unremarkable except for unspecific myopathological changes such as occasional central nuclei, variation of fibre diameter with hypertrophic, splitted, rare atrophic and regenerating fibres (23, 40). ATPase type 2A fibres may be hypertrophied and number of type 2B fibres may be decreased as in the Cl- channelopathies (11, 12); however, normal muscle fibre area and distribution of fibre types 1, 2A and 2B have also been described (8). In some areas, there may be focal myofibril degeneration with myelin bodies, lipid deposits, and occasional subsarcolemmal vacuoles without PAS-positive material; (37) and tubular aggregates (35). Muscle fibre degeneration followed by phagocyte invasion and fatty replacement may occur, perhaps induced by the cold-induced attacks of weakness (see also periodic paralysis and structural alterations due to electrolyte shifts or phases of muscle inexcitability).

Genotype-phenotype correlations

For non-dystrophic myotonias, the histological findings are variable, independent of sex, and not specific for the diagnosis. The findings produced by the different genotypes seem to follow a common pattern and may be functionally due to the hyperexcitability. The degree of myopathic changes detected seem to be associated with the severity of the symptoms which vary considerably even among carriers of the same mutation. Even within one family, light cases may show normal morphology, somewhat more severe cases increased nuclei and fibre diameter variation, and the severe cases focal changes in myofibrils, mitochondria, and vacuole formation and/or disturbances of fibre type differentiation with fibre type 2B deficiency.

The slight changes may be interpreted as due to involuntary "myotonic bodybuilding," ie, centralisation of nuclei due to increased shear stress and muscle fibre hypertrophy, as in athletes. The deficiency of fibre type 2B may be the result of transformation into type 2A fibres brought about by the myotonic bursts. Focal changes in myofibril arrangement may be associated with focal lack of mitochondria because fibre type 2B have much less of these organelles than fibre type 2A. Corresponding to the lack of progression of the hyperexcitability episodes is the lack of progression of these unspecific changes. This may not hold true for the fibre degeneration, atrophy, and fatty replacement, which could indicate

permanent weakness and is a process independent of the frequency and severity of the myotonic episodes.

Future perspectives and therapy

Many myotonia patients can manage their disease without medication. Should treatment be necessary, myotonic stiffness responds well to drugs that reduce the increased excitability of the cell membrane by interfering with the Na$^+$ channels, ie, local anaesthetics, antifibrillar and antiarrhythmic drugs, and related agents. These drugs suppress myotonic runs by decreasing the number of available Na$^+$ channels and have no known effect on Cl$^-$ channels. Of the many drugs tested that can be administered orally, mexiletine is the drug of choice. It is also very effective in preventing weakness in paramyotonia congenita, probably by stabilizing the inactivated channel state. The effect of treatment on the histological findings has not been studied.

Given a clinical diagnosis of myotonia by electromyographic examination, the first step is to exclude myotonic dystrophy. This can be performed by a genetic test from EDTA whole blood because the underlying mutation is known: an unphysiological expansion of a trinucleotide CTG repeat in the 3′ untranslated region of the gene encoding a serine/threonine kinase on chromosome 19q. If exclusion is successful, usually there is no need for a muscle biopsy because *i)* the diagnosis can be less invasively confirmed by a genetic blood test, *ii)* an effective therapy exists, *iii)* the prognosis, ie, especially the development of permanent weakness cannot be influenced by therapy, and *iv)* no specific changes are to be expected that influence therapy or prognosis.

From the pathogenetic viewpoint, several clinical phenomena are not yet fully understood indicating that there could be secondary alterations in muscle of myotonic patients functionally and subsequently morphologically: *i)* the warm-up phenomenon, ie, amelioration of the myotonia with exercise is

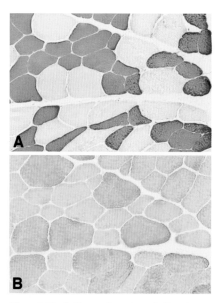

Figure 3. Myofibrillar reactions of muscle fibres from a myotonia congenita patient. **A.** All type 2 fibres are dark in this ATPase preparation at pH 9.4. **B.** Type 2A fibres in the same biopsy show light staining at pH 4.3 suggesting complete absence of type 2B fibres. Magnification: ×100.

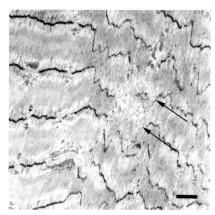

Figure 4. Myofibrillar architecture of a muscle fibre from a myotonia permanens patient. Note the focal disarray of myofibrils and the disappearance of Z disks (arrows). Bar = 1 μm.

not explainable by the Cl$^-$ or Na$^+$ channel dysfunction (4), *ii)* exactly which factors decide what mode of inheritance the four Cl$^-$ channel mutations that can produce either the Thomsen or Becker phenotype will follow, *iii)* what pathomechanism underlies the few recessive mutations that do not lead to Cl$^-$ conductance reduction when functionally expressed, and *iv)* what generates the temperature dependence in paramyotonia congenita (but not in the allelic K$^+$-aggravated myotonia)?

References

1. Adrian RH, Bryant SH (1974) On the repetitive discharge in myotonic muscle fibres. *J Physiol* 240: 505-515

2. Becker PE (1977) *Myotonia Congenita and Syndromes Associated with Myotonia.* Georg Thieme Verlag: Stuttgart.

3. Bendahhou S, Cummins TR, Kwiecinski H, Waxman SG, Ptacek LJ (1999) Characterization of a new sodium channel mutation at arginine 1448 associated with moderate Paramyotonia congenita in humans. *J Physiol* 518: 337-344

4. Birnberger KL, Klepzig M (1979) Influence of extracellular potassium and intracellular pH on myotonia. *J Neurol* 222: 23-35

5. Chahine M, George AL, Jr., Zhou M, Ji S, Sun W, Barchi RL, Horn R (1994) Sodium channel mutations in paramyotonia congenita uncouple inactivation from activation. *Neuron* 12: 281-294

6. Crews J, Kaiser KK, Brooke MH (1976) Muscle pathology of myotonia congenita. *J Neurol Sci* 28: 449-457

7. Eulenburg A (1886) Über eine familiäre durch 6 Generationen verfolgbare Form kongenitaler Paramyotonie. *Neurol Zentralbl* 5: 265-272

8. Friis ML, Johnsen T, Saltin B, Paulson OB (1985) Skeletal muscle in paramyotonia congenita: biochemistry, histochemistry and morphology. *Acta Neurol Scand* 71: 62-68

9. George AL, Jr., Crackower MA, Abdalla JA, Hudson AJ, Ebers GC (1993) Molecular basis of Thomsen's disease (autosomal dominant myotonia congenita). *Nat Genet* 3: 305-310

10. George AL, Jr., Sloan-Brown K, Fenichel GM, Mitchell GA, Spiegel R, Pascuzzi RM (1994) Nonsense and missense mutations of the muscle chloride channel gene in patients with myotonia congenita. *Hum Mol Genet* 3: 2071-2072

11. Haass A, Ricker K, Hertel G, Heene R (1979) Influence of temperature on isometric contraction and passive muscular tension in paramyotonia congenita (Eulenburg). *J Neurol* 221: 151-162

12. Heene R, Gabriel RR, Manz F, Schimrigk K (1986) Type 2B muscle fibre deficiency in myotonia and paramyotonia congenita. A genetically determined histochemical fibre type pattern? *J Neurol Sci* 73: 23-30

13. Heine R, George AL, Jr., Pika U, Deymeer F, Rudel R, Lehmann-Horn F (1994) Proof of a non-functional muscle chloride channel in recessive myotonia congenita (Becker) by detection of a 4 base pair deletion. *Hum Mol Genet* 3: 1123-1128

14. Heine R, Pika U, Lehmann-Horn F (1993) A novel SCN4A mutation causing myotonia aggravated by cold and potassium. *Hum Mol Genet* 2: 1349-1353

15. Koch MC, Steinmeyer K, Lorenz C, Ricker K, Wolf F, Otto M, Zoll B, Lehmann-Horn F, Grzeschik KH, Jentsch TJ (1992) The skeletal muscle chloride channel in dominant and recessive human myotonia. *Science* 257: 797-800

16. Lehmann-Horn F, Jurkat-Rott K (1999) Voltage-gated ion channels and hereditary disease. *Physiol Rev* 79: 1317-1372

17. Lehmann-Horn F, Küther G, Ricker K, Grafe P, Ballanyi K, Rüdel R (1987) Adynamia episodica hereditaria with myotonia: a non-inactivating sodium current and the effect of extracellular pH. *Muscle Nerve* 10: 363-374

18. Lehmann-Horn F, Mailander V, Heine R, George AL (1995) Myotonia levior is a chloride channel disorder. *Hum Mol Genet* 4: 1397-1402

19. Lehmann-Horn F, Rüdel R, Ricker K (1987b) Membrane defects in paramyotonia congenita (Eulenburg). *Muscle Nerve* 10: 633-641

20. Lerche H, Heine R, Pika U, George AL, Jr., Mitrovic N, Browatzki M, Weiss T, Rivet-Bastide M, Franke C, Lomonaco M, et al. (1993) Human sodium channel myotonia: slowed channel inactivation due to substitutions for a glycine within the III-IV linker. *J Physiol* 470: 13-22

21. Lerche H, Mitrovic N, Dubowitz V, Lehmann-Horn F (1996) Paramyotonia congenita: the R1448P Na+ channel mutation in adult human skeletal muscle. *Ann Neurol* 39: 599-608

22. Lipicky RJ (1979) Myotonic syndromes other than myotonic dystrophy. In *Handbook of Clinical Neurology*, PJ Vinken, GW Bruyn (eds). Elsevier: Amsterdam. pp. 533-571

23. Magee KR, Arbor A (1966) Paramyotonia congenita. Association with cutaneous cold sensitivity and description of peculiar sustained postures after muscle contraction. *Arch Neurol* 14: 590-594

24. McClatchey AI, Van den Bergh P, Pericak-Vance MA, Raskind W, Verellen C, McKenna-Yasek D, Rao K, Haines JL, Bird T, Brown RH, Jr., *et al.* (1992) Temperature-sensitive mutations in the III-IV cytoplasmic loop region of the skeletal muscle sodium channel gene in paramyotonia congenita. *Cell* 68: 769-774

25. Mindell JA, Maduke M, Miller C, Grigorieff N (2001) Projection structure of a ClC-type chloride channel at 6.5 A resolution. *Nature* 409: 219-223

26. Mitrovic N, George AL, Jr., Lerche H, Wagner S, Fahlke C, Lehmann-Horn F (1995) Different effects on gating of three myotonia-causing mutations in the inactivation gate of the human muscle sodium channel. *J Physiol* 487: 107-114

27. Palade PT, Barchi RL (1977) On the inhibition of muscle membrane chloride conductance by aromatic carboxylic acids. *J Gen Physiol* 69: 879-896

28. Ptacek LJ, George AL, Jr., Barchi RL, Griggs RC, Riggs JE, Robertson M, Leppert MF (1992) Mutations in an S4 segment of the adult skeletal muscle sodium channel cause paramyotonia congenita. *Neuron* 8: 891-897

29. Ptacek LJ, Tawil R, Griggs RC, Meola G, McManis P, Barohn RJ, Mendell JR, Harris C, Spitzer R, Santiago F, et al. (1994b) Sodium channel mutations in acetazolamide-responsive myotonia congenita, paramyotonia congenita, and hyperkalemic periodic paralysis. *Neurology* 44: 1500-1503

30. Pusch M, Steinmeyer K, Koch MC, Jentsch TJ (1995) Mutations in dominant human myotonia congenita drastically alter the voltage dependence of the ClC-1 chloride channel. *Neuron* 15: 1455-1463

31. Ricker K, Lehmann-Horn F, Moxley RT (1990) Myotonia fluctuans. *Arch Neurol* 47: 268-272

32. Ricker K, Moxley RT, 3rd, Heine R, Lehmann-Horn F (1994) Myotonia fluctuans. A third type of muscle sodium channel disease. *Arch Neurol* 51: 1095-1102

33. Rüdel R, Ricker K, Lehmann-Horn F (1988) Transient weakness and altered membrane characteristic in recessive generalized myotonia (Becker). *Muscle Nerve* 11: 202-211

34. Saviane C, Conti F, Pusch M (1999) The muscle chloride channel ClC-1 has a double-barreled appearance that is differentially affected in dominant and recessive myotonia. *J Gen Physiol* 113: 457-468

35. Schiffer D, Giordana MT, Monga G, Mollo F (1976) Histochemistry and electron microscopy of muscle fibres in a case of congenital paramyotonia. *J Neurol* 211: 125-133

36. Thomsen J (1876) Tonische Krämpfe in willkürlich beweglichen Muskeln in Folge von ererbter psychischer Disposition. *Arch Psychiatr Nervenkrankh* 6: 702-718

37. Thrush DC, Morris CJ, Salmon MV (1972) Paramyotonia congenita: a clinical, histochemical and pathological study. *Brain* 95: 537-552

38. Vita GM, Olckers A, Jedlicka AE, George AL, Heiman-Patterson T, Rosenberg H, Fletcher JE, Levitt RC (1995) Masseter muscle rigidity associated with glycine1306-to-alanine mutation in the adult muscle sodium channel alpha-subunit gene. *Anesthesiology* 82: 1097-1103

39. Wagner S, Deymeer F, Kurz LL, Benz S, Schleithoff L, Lehmann-Horn F, Serdaroglu P, Ozdemir C, Rudel R (1998) The dominant chloride channel mutant G200R causing fluctuating myotonia: clinical findings, electrophysiology, and channel pathology. *Muscle Nerve* 21: 1122-1128

40. Wegmüller E, Ludin HP, Mumenthaler M (1979) Paramyotonia congenita. A clinical, electrophysiological and histological study of 12 patients. *J Neurol* 220: 251-257

41. Yang N, Ji S, Zhou M, Ptacek LJ, Barchi RL, Horn R, George AL, Jr. (1994) Sodium channel mutations in paramyotonia congenita exhibit similar biophysical phenotypes in vitro. *Proc Natl Acad Sci USA* 91: 12785-12789

Dyskalemic episodic weakness

Karin Jurkat-Rott
Josef Müller-Höcker
Dieter Pongratz
Frank Lehmann-Horn

HyperPP	hyperkalemic periodic paralysis
HypoPP	hypokalemic periodic paralysis
SR	sarcoplasmic reticulum
TTS	T tubular system

Definition of entities

Inexcitability due to lack of action potentials results in muscle weakness. Two dominant episodic types of weakness with or without myotonia are distinguished by the serum K^+ level during the attacks of tetraplegia: hyper- and hypokalemic periodic paralysis (Table 1). In general, the hyperkalemic variant has an earlier onset and more frequent attacks, but these are much shorter and milder than in the hypokalemic form (13). In contrast, the hypokalemic variant more frequently results in degenerative myopathy and permanent disabling weakness of the limbs, and is never associated with myotonia like the hyperkalemic variant (2, 19). Intake of K^+ and glucose have opposite effects in the 2 disorders: while K^+ triggers a hyperkalemic attack and glucose is a remedy, glucose provokes hypokalemic attacks which are ameliorated by K^+ intake.

Molecular pathogenesis

The basis of the myotonia in the hyperkalemic variant is uncontrolled repetitive firing of action potentials, and the underlying defect is a non-inactivating Na^+ inward current (18) through the tetrodotoxin-sensitive Na^+ channel encoded by SCN4A (Table 1) (11). While Na^+ influx at slight depolarization itself generates action potentials and myotonia, stronger depolarizations lead to general inactivation of Na^+ channels both of mutant and wildtype population (in a dominant disorder, both a mutant and a wildtype allele are present) and thus, weakness. The various mutations are situated at several disseminated intracellularly faced positions (28, 32, 42), potentially involved in generating parts of the inactivation apparatus or steric hinderence of its proper function (Figure 2 in chapter 5. 1) (17). The mutations disturb channel inactivation and produce a persistent sodium current (4, 6, 7, 18, 31). Based on the same mechanism of pathogenesis and distribution of mutations, the reader may draw 2 conclusions, both of which are correct: *i)* there could be an overlapping of the phenotypes of hyperkamelic periodic paralysis with paramyotonia congenita and K^+-aggravated myotonia disorders, and *ii)* more severe membrane depolarization found in periodic paralysis may result in more severe morphological findings.

In contrast to the gain of function changes associated to hyperkalemic periodic paralysis, hypokalemic periodic paralysis is associated with a loss-of-function defect of 3 different ion channel types: Na^+, Ca^{2+}, and K^+ (1, 3, 12, 14, 15, 29). In the former 2 channels, the mutations are located solely in special transmembrane voltage-sensing segments (Figure 2 in chapter 5. 1, Figure 1). In the latter, the sole reported mutation is situated in the accessory β subunit not containing the ion-conducting pore, but influencing the gating properties thereof. Functionally, the inactivated state is stabilised in the Na^+ channel mutants (15, 39), while the channel availability is reduced for the Ca^{2+} channel mutants (16, 25). It is still a mystery how the loss-of-function mutations of these 2 cation channels can produce the long lasting depolarisation leading to the weakness (34, 35); however, it does imply that a concomitant myotonia is not to be expected, as is the case. In contrast, for the very rare

Disease entity	Gene name Chromosome	Gene product Functional disturbance	Number of mutations % patients with mutations	Symptoms, prevelance, inheritance
Hyperkalemic periodic paralysis (HyperPP)	SCN4A 17q23	Na^+ channel α subunit gain-of-function	7 missense mutations 55% of patients	~1:200 000; autosomal dominant; childhood onset, episodic attacks of weakness, hyperkalemia during episode, triggering by rest after body exertion or K^+ intake, additional myotonia, no paramyotonia
Hypokalemic periodic paralysis (HypoPP)	CACNA1S 1q32	Ca^{2+} channel α1 subunit loss-of-function	3 missense mutations 35% of patients	~1:100 000; autosomal dominant; teenage onset, episodic attacks of mainly generalised weakness, hypokalemia during episode, triggering by carbohydrate-rich food or exercise, amelioration by K^+ intake, no myotonia
	SCN4A 17q23	Na^+ channel α subunit loss-of-function	4 missense mutations 5% of patients	
	KCNE3 11q13-14	K^+ channel β subunit (MiRP 2) loss-of-function	1 missense mutation 2 families	

Table 1. Voltage-gated channelopathies.

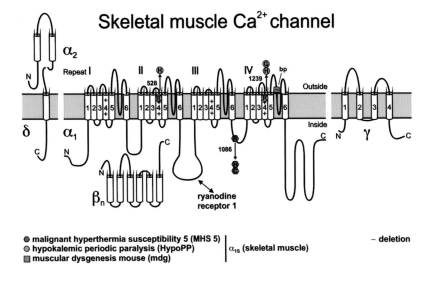

Skeletal muscle Ca²⁺ channel

Figure 1. *Subunits of the voltage-gated L-type calcium channel.* The α1 subunit resembles α of the sodium channel however, the function of the various parts, *e.g.* the III-IV linker, may not be the same. α2/δ, β1 to β4, and γ are auxilliary subunits. Mutations in the here shown α1S subunit of the skeletal muscle L-type calcium channel (= dihydropyridine receptor, DHPR) have been described for man (HypoPP, MHS5) and mice (*mdg*). Conventional 1-letter abbreviations are used for the replaced amino acids. The symbols indicate the diseases as explained at the bottom of the left-hand side.

K⁺ channel variant, a reduced current density has been demonstrated that produces a slight membrane depolarization when heterologously expressed in a muscle cell line (1). This would explain pathogenesis because the K⁺ channel complex is thought to be essential for re-establishing and holding the highly negative resting potential of skeletal muscle fibres after the action potential.

Structural changes

In both types of familial periodic paralysis and in the thyrotoxic hypokalaemic type there is proliferation, regeneration, and dilation of components of the T tubular system (TTS) and the sarcoplasmic reticulum (SR). Changes in the myofibrils and mitochondria and focal increases in muscle glycogen have also been noted, suggesting that the changes in several organelles accounted for the permanent myopathy of the disease (8, 10, 22, 36).

Vacuolation occurs in the following morphologic sequence (9): *i)* abnormal nonvacuolated fibre regions display dilated and proliferating T tubules and TTS networks, and dilated SR profiles (Figure 2); the dilated SR vesicles usually contain amorphous material and are often surrounded by glycogen granules; glycogen deposits, focal decreases in mitochondria, and focal myofibrillar degeneration associated with Z disk streaming are also noted; *ii)* evolving vacuoles appear as areas of rarefaction which react strongly for NADH dehydrogenase and acid phosphatase; these vacuoles lack distinct boundaries and contain amorphous material, cytoplasmic bodies, or myriad vesicles of varying optical density (Figure 3); *iii)* intermediate stage vacuoles are well demarcated spaces with curving or undulating borders and have a clearly defined limiting membrane, contain a variable amount amorphous matrix and relics of structures encountered in the evolving vacuoles; some of the intermediate stage vacuoles contain remnants of calcified SR vesicles (Figure 4); *iv)* mature vacuoles contain only matrix in their interior; T tubules and networks often abut on and communicate with the interior of these spaces (Figure 5); and *v)* remodeled vacuoles are mature vacuoles containing sarcoplasmic invaginations that are dome shaped and usually contain glycogen granules (Figure 5); in some vacuoles, the invaginated membrane is ruptured

and the adjacent myofibrils are highly contracted.

The membranes lining the intermediate stage, mature, and remodelled vacuoles are mechanically stabilized by cytoskeletal proteins. In conclusion, the vacuoles evolve as the result of the proliferation and degeneration of the SR and the TTS. The latter also acts as a membrane source to trap the components of the abnormal fibre regions. Since the evolving and intermediate stage vacuoles react for acid phosphatase, they are autophagic in character. As the intermediate stage and mature vacuoles are limited by and communicate with TTS networks, these spaces are in continuity with the extracellular space indicating that most vacuoles contain extracellular fluid. Furthermore, a rupture of the invaginated sarcoplasmic membranes in remodelled vacuoles exposes the fibre interior to extracellular fluid. This readily explains why the nearby myofibrils are highly contracted and also provides an explanation for the occurrence of fibre necrosis.

In otherwise unaffected fibres, collections of multiple closely packed tubules giving a honeycomb appearance may be viewed in cross sections, mostly on fibre ends (Figure 6). These tubular aggregates are located between longitudinally running myofibrils or beneath the sarcolemma and may contain an internal circular membrane that is not normally seen in the T-tubule or the SR from which they originate (20, 21, 23, 24, 27, 33, 41).

Correlations

Vacuoles evolve as result of the proliferation, dilation and degeneration of components of the T tubular system and the sarcoplasmic reticulum. As early stage may also be present in paramyotonia and K⁺-aggravated myotonia, their pathogenesis is not entirely explainable by the electrical inexcitability. Whether the vacuolar myopathy is conditioned by the abnormal electrolyte milieu within the fibre, electrical inexcitability of the fibre, a still unrecognized factor, or a combination of these, it can result in permanent weakness that may be more disabling than the intermittent paralytic attacks.

At onset of the occurrence of attacks of weakness, the muscle fibres do not show morphologic abnormality even at the ultrastructural level. Morphologic changes follow, or occur independently of the electrical inexcitability of the muscle fibre. The intermittent inexcitability of the muscle fibre might induce proliferation and dilation of the TTS and SR in the same way that denervation causes transient proliferation and dilation of these organelles.

An increased sodium and a decreased potassium content is found in muscle between attacks in both types of familial periodic paralysis (5, 26, 36, 37). This abnormality plus the additional ingress of water and other electrolytes into the fibres during attacks might act as a stimulus for both the proliferation and degeneration of the membranous organelles. Once a membrane-bound vacuole is formed, its lining is indented by sarcoplasmic invaginations. Rupture of these invaginations exposes the muscle fibre interior to the extracellular fluid in the membrane-bound vacuoles and is a likely cause of fibre necrosis. Repeated cycles of vacuole formation and fibre necrosis may contribute to the permanent myopathy.

In some kinships, muscle weakness continues to progress even after the attacks of paralysis have ceased, or a myopathy develops even without attacks of paralysis (38). Attacks of weakness are either not recognized as disease in these families or the myopathy could be caused by a factor unrelated to the paralytic attacks (19). Furthermore, inexcitability of individual muscle fibres may be a more frequent event than the number of clinically recognizable attacks of paralysis. Patients with the permanent myopathy show not only vacuolated muscle fibres, but also focal myofibrillar degeneration, increase in central nuclei, abnormal variation in fibre size, fibre necrosis, and proliferation of connective tissue elements (22),

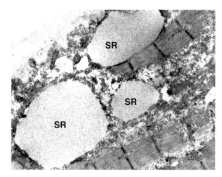

Figure 2. Muscle fibre with regular contractile apparatus and focal dilatations of the sarcoplasmic reticulum (SR). ×10000.

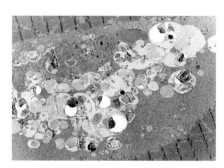

Figure 4. Intermediate stage vacuole containing membraneous material, cell debris, myelin-like figures, and bilaminar membranes ×10000.

Future perspectives and therapy

Local anaesthetics and antiarrhythmic drugs of class I, such as mexiletine and lidocaine derivatives, are antimyotonic agents because they stabilise the inactivated state and lead to the phenomenon called use dependent block. Since the spontaneous attacks of weakness typical for hyperkalemic periodic paralysis are not influenced by mexiletine (30)—because no repetitive action potentials occur that can be attenuated by a use dependent block—diuretics such as hydrochlorothiazide and acetazolamide can be administered. These drugs decrease the frequency and severity of paralytic episodes by lowering serum K^+ and other, so far unexplained, favourable properties, eg, influencing myoplasmic pH and plasmalemmal K^+ channels (40). Therapeutically, long term low dose intake of acetazolamide is also recommended to avoid attacks of weakness in the hypokalemic variant. During acute hypokalemic paralysis phases though, oral K^+ administration has proved to relieve symptoms.

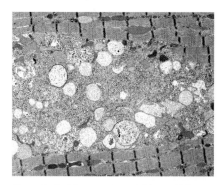

Figure 3. Evolving vacuole containing multiple sarcoplasmic reticulum vesicles filled with granular material. Intermingled are glycogen granules ×10000.

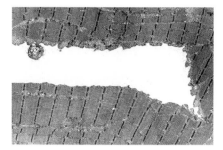

Figure 5. Mature vacuole limited by a membrane and containing fine granular material. The invaginated granular material represents glycogen ×5000.

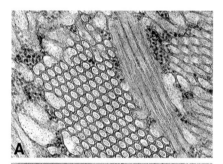

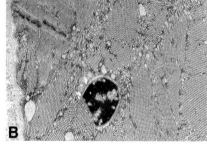

Figure 6. Typical tubular aggregates in a fibre of a hypokalaemic periodic paralysis patient. **A.** ×100000 **B.** ×16500.

From the pathogenetic viewpoint, several clinical phenomena are not yet fully understood, indicating that there could be secondary alterations in muscle of periodic paralysis patients functionally and subsequently morphologically: *i)* why does one frequent hyperkalemic periodic paralysis mutation (T704M) cause severe myopathy with permanent weakness and the others do not, *ii)* what is the pathophysiological mechanism linking a Ca^{2+} mutation to membrane depolarisation and paralysis when the channel does not contribute to the action potential, *iii)* why does the hypokalemia cause depolarisation in patients with hypokalemic periodic paralysis when it hyperpolarises normal muscle, and *iv)* why does the loss-of-function Na^+ channel mutation produce episodic weakness instead of permanent weakness only?

References

1. Abbott GW, Butler MH, Bendahhou S, Dalakas MC, Ptacek LJ, Goldstein SA (2001) MiRP2 forms potassium channels in skeletal muscle with Kv3.4 and is associated with periodic paralysis. *Cell* 104: 217-231

2. Bradley WG, Taylor R, Rice DR, Hausmanowa-Petruzewicz I, Adelman LS, Jenkison M, Jedrzejowska H, Drac H, Pendlebury WW (1990) Progressive myopathy in hyperkalemic periodic paralysis. *Arch Neurol* 47: 1013-1017

3. Bulman DE, Scoggan KA, van Oene MD, Nicolle MW, Hahn AF, Tollar LL, Ebers GC (1999) A novel sodium channel mutation in a family with hypokalemic periodic paralysis. *Neurology* 53: 1932-1936

4. Cannon SC, Strittmatter SM (1993) Functional expression of sodium channel mutations identified in families with periodic paralysis. *Neuron* 10: 317-326

5. Carson MJ, Pearson CM (1964) Familial hyperkalemic periodic paralysis with myotonic features. *J Pediatr* 64: 853-865

6. Cummins TR, Sigworth FJ (1996) Impaired slow inactivation in mutant sodium channels. *Biophys J* 71: 227-236

7. Cummins TR, Zhou J, Sigworth FJ, Ukomadu C, Stephan M, Ptacek LJ, Agnew WS (1993) Functional consequences of a Na+ channel mutation causing hyperkalemic periodic paralysis. *Neuron* 10: 667-678

8. Engel AG (1966) Electron microscopic observations in primary hypokalemic and thyrotoxic periodic paralyses. *Mayo Clin Proc* 41: 797-808

9. Engel AG (1970) Evolution and content of vacuoles in primary hypokalemic periodic paralysis. *Mayo Clin Proc* 45: 774-814

10. Engel AG, Lambert EH, Rosevear JW, Tauxe WN (1965) Clinical and electromyographic studies in a patient with primary hypokalemic periodic paralysis. *Amer J Med* 38: 626-

11. Fontaine B, Khurana TS, Hoffman EP, Bruns GA, Haines JL, Trofatter JA, Hanson MP, Rich J, McFarlane H, Yasek DM, et al. (1990) Hyperkalemic periodic paralysis and the adult muscle sodium channel alpha-subunit gene. *Science* 250: 1000-1002

12. Fontaine B, Vale-Santos J, Jurkat-Rott K, Reboul J, Plassart E, Rime CS, Elbaz A, Heine R, Guimaraes J,

Weissenbach J, *et al.* (1994) Mapping of the hypokalaemic periodic paralysis (HypoPP) locus to chromosome 1q31-32 in three European families. *Nat Genet* 6: 267-272

13. Gamstorp I (1956) Adynamia episodica hereditaria. *Acta Paediat Scand* 45 (suppl 108): 1-126

14. Jurkat-Rott K, Lehmann-Horn F, Elbaz A, Heine R, Gregg RG, Hogan K, Powers PA, Lapie P, Vale-Santos JE, Weissenbach J, et al. (1994) A calcium channel mutation causing hypokalemic periodic paralysis. *Hum Mol Genet* 3: 1415-1419

15. Jurkat-Rott K, Mitrovic N, Hang C, Kouzmenkin A, Iaizzo P, Herzog J, Lerche H, Nicole N, Vale-Santos J, Chauveau D, Fontaine B, Lehmann-Horn F (2000) Voltage sensor sodium channel mutations cause hypokalemic periodic paralysis type 2 by enhanced inactivation and reduced current. *Proc Natl Acad Sci U S A* 97: 9549-9554

16. Jurkat-Rott K, Uetz U, Pika-Hartlaub U, Powell J, Fontaine B, Melzer W, Lehmann-Horn F (1998) Calcium currents and transients of native and heterologously expressed mutant skeletal muscle DHP receptor alpha1 subunits (R528H). *FEBS Lett* 423: 198-204

17. Lehmann-Horn F, Jurkat-Rott K (1999) Voltage-gated ion channels and hereditary disease. *Physiol Rev* 79: 1317-1372

18. Lehmann-Horn F, Küther G, Ricker K, Grafe P, Ballanyi K, Rüdel R (1987a) Adynamia episodica hereditaria with myotonia: a non-inactivating sodium current and the effect of extracellular pH. *Muscle Nerve* 10: 363-374

19. Links TP, Zwarts MJ, Wilmink JT, Molenaar WM, Oosterhuis HJ (1990) Permanent muscle weakness in familial hypokalaemic periodic paralysis. Clinical, radiological and pathological aspects. *Brain* 113: 1873-1889

20. Macdonald RD, Rewcastle NB, Humphrey JG (1968) The myopathy of hyperkalemic periodic paralysis. An electron microscopic study. *Arch Neurol* 19: 274-283

21. Macdonald RD, Rewcastle NB, Humphrey JG (1969) Myopathy of hypokalemic periodic paralysis. An electron microscopic study. *Arch Neurol* 20: 565-585

22. Martin JJ, Ceuterick C, Mercelis R, Amrom D (1984) Familial periodic paralysis with hypokalaemia. Study of a muscle biopsy in the myopathic stage of the disorder. *Acta Neurol Belg* 84: 233-242

23. Meyers KR, Gilden DH, Rinaldi CF, Hansen JL (1972) Periodic muscle weakness, normokalemia, and tubular aggregates. *Neurology* 22: 269-279

24. Morgan-Hughes JA (1998) Tubular aggregates in skeletal muscle: their functional significance and mechanisms of pathogenesis. *Curr Opin Neurol* 11: 439-442

25. Morrill JA, Cannon SC (1999) Effects of mutations causing hypokalaemic periodic paralysis on the skeletal muscle L-type Ca2+ channel expressed in Xenopus laevis oocytes. *J Physiol* 520 Pt 2: 321-336

26. Niall JF, Pak Poy RK (1966) Studies in familial hypokalaemic periodic paralysis. *Aust Ann Med* 15: 352-358

27. Poskanzer DC, Kerr DNS (1961) A third type of periodic paralysis with normokalemia and favorable response to sodium chloride. *American Journal of Medicine* 31: 328-342

28. Ptacek LJ, George AL, Jr., Griggs RC, Tawil R, Kallen RG, Barchi RL, Robertson M, Leppert MF (1991) Identification of a mutation in the gene causing hyperkalemic periodic paralysis. *Cell* 67: 1021-1027

29. Ptacek LJ, Tawil R, Griggs RC, Engel AG, Layzer RB, Kwiecinski H, McManis PG, Santiago L, Moore M, Fouad G, et al. (1994a) Dihydropyridine receptor mutations cause hypokalemic periodic paralysis. *Cell* 77: 863-868

30. Ricker K, Böhlen R, Rohkamm R (1983) Different effectiveness of tocainide and hydrochlorothiazide in paramyotonia congenita with hyperkalemic episodic paralysis. *Neurology* 33: 1615-1618

31. Rojas CV, Neely A, Velasco-Loyden G, Palma V, Kukuljan M (1999) Hyperkalemic periodic paralysis M1592V mutation modifies activation in human skeletal muscle Na+ channel. *Am J Physiol* 276: C259-266

32. Rojas CV, Wang JZ, Schwartz LS, Hoffman EP, Powell BR, Brown RH, Jr. (1991) A Met-to-Val mutation in the skeletal muscle Na+ channel alpha-subunit in hyperkalaemic periodic paralysis. *Nature* 354: 387-389

33. Rosenberg NL, Neville HE, Ringel SP (1985) Tubular aggregates. Their association with neuromuscular diseases, including the syndrome of myalgias/cramps. *Arch Neurol* 42: 973-976

34. Rüdel R, Lehmann-Horn F, Ricker K, Küther G (1984) Hypokalemic periodic paralysis: in vitro investigation of muscle fiber membrane parameters. *Muscle Nerve* 7: 110-120

35. Ruff RL (1999) Insulin acts in hypokalemic periodic paralysis by reducing inward rectifier K+ current. *Neurology* 53: 1556-1563

36. Shy GM, Wanko T, Rowley PT, Engel AG (1961) Studies in familial periodic paralysis. Exp Neurol 3: 53-121

37. Staffurth JS (1964) The total exchangeable potassium in patients with hypokalemia. *Postgrad Med* J 40: 4

38. Stevens JR (1954) Familial periodic paralysis, myotonia, progressive amyotrophy, and pes cavus in members of a single family. *Arch Neurol Psychiat* 72: 726

39. Struyk AF, Scoggan KA, Bulman DE, Cannon SC (2000) The human skeletal muscle Na channel mutation R669H associated with hypokalemic periodic paralysis enhances slow inactivation. *J Neurosci* 20: 8610-8617

40. Tricarico D, Barbieri M, Camerino DC (2000) Acetazolamide opens the muscular KCa2+ channel: a novel mechanism of action that may explain the therapeutic effect of the drug in hypokalemic periodic paralysis. *Ann Neurol* 48: 304-312

41. van Engelen BG, Ter Laak HJ (1999) Images in neurology. Tubular aggregates: their continuity with sarcoplasmic reticulum. *Arch Neurol* 56: 1410-1411

42. Wagner S, Lerche H, Mitrovic N, Heine R, George AL, Lehmann-Horn F (1997) A novel sodium channel mutation causing a hyperkalemic paralytic and paramyotonic syndrome with variable clinical expressivity. *Neurology* 49: 1018-1025

Malignant hyperthermia and central core disease associated with defects in Ca²⁺ channels of the sarcotubular system

David H. MacLennan
Julian C. P. Loke

ARVD2	arrhythmogenic right ventricular cardiomyopathy type 2
bp	base pair
CPVT	catecholaminergic polymorphic ventricular tachycardia
DHPR	dihydropyridine receptor
CCD	central core disease
MH	malignant hyperthermia
MHS	MH susceptible
OMIM	Online Mendelian Inheritance in Man (www.ncbi.nlm.nih.gov/omim)
RYR	ryanodine receptor

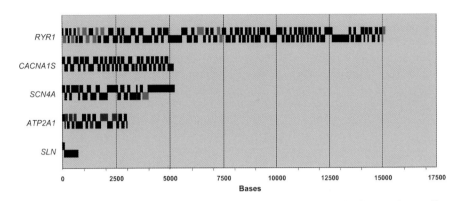

Figure 1. Structure of cDNAs spliced from causal genes for: Malignant hyperthermia (*RYR1*, ryanodine-sensitive Ca²⁺ release channel of skeletal muscle sarcoplasmic reticulum isoform 1; *CACNA1S*, α-subunit of the skeletal muscle slow or L-type, dihydropyridine-sensitive Ca²⁺ channel; *SCN4A*, α-subunit of the skeletal muscle Na⁺ channel); Central core disease (*RYR1*), and Brody disease (*ATP2A1*, thapsigargin-sensitive sarco(endo)plasmic reticulum Ca²⁺ ATPase isoform 1, expressed in fast-twitch skeletal muscle fibres). Segmented bars indicate the exon boundaries within the cDNA for each of the specified genes. Coloured bars show the exons containing disease-causing mutations. MH and CCD mutations (red) are clustered in three regions of the *RYR1* gene, and one segment of the CACNA1S and SCN4A α-subunit genes, while Brody disease-causing stop-codon and point mutations are scattered throughout the *ATP2A1* gene. The SLN gene is included, although it has not been shown to be disease-causing.

Definition of entities

The sarcotubular system, made up of the sarcoplasmic reticulum and transverse tubular membranes, regulates Ca²⁺ concentrations within muscle cells, thereby regulating muscle contraction and relaxation. Key proteins in the regulation of muscle Ca²⁺ are the Ca²⁺ release channels in the junctional terminal cisternae of the sarcoplasmic reticulum (ryanodine receptors or RyRs) and the voltage-dependent, dihydropyridine-sensitive, slow or L-type Ca²⁺ channels located in the transverse tubule (dihydropyridine receptors or DHPRs). These proteins interact functionally and physically to release Ca²⁺ from the lumen of the sarcoplasmic reticulum, elevating sarcoplasmic Ca²⁺ in the process of excitation-contraction coupling (19). This chapter focuses on malignant hyperthermia and central core disease associated with defects in Ca²⁺ channels of the sarcotubular system. In addition, we cover conditions termed "catecholaminergic polymorphic ventricular tachycardia and arrhythmogenic right ventricular cardiomyopathy type 2."

Molecular genetics and pathophysiology

RYR genes. RYR1 (OMIM 180901), located on human chromo-some 19q13.1, is the major ryanodine receptor isoform expressed in both fast- and slow-twitch skeletal muscle, while RYR2, located on human chromosome 1q42.1-43, is expressed highly in cardiac muscle (10). The human RyR1 protein contains 5037 amino acids with a mass of 565 000 Da, but the active Ca²⁺ release channel forms a tetrameric complex with a mass of about 2 300 000 Da. RYR1 cDNA is over 15 000 base pairs (bp) long and the gene from which it is derived is 159 000 bp. The gene contains 106 exons, of which 2 are alternatively spliced into mRNA to create different forms of the protein (17). Transmembrane sequences near the C-terminus of the protein form the Ca²⁺ release channel pore and cytosolic sequences form a huge regulatory domain that interacts with ligands and with sequences in the dihydropyridine receptor. Mutations in the RYR1 gene cause both malignant hyperthermia (MH) and central core disease (CCD)

(3, 20, 28). The codons that give rise to MH and CCD mutations are clustered in 3 regions of the RYR1 gene (Figure 1). MH/CCD region 1 lies between Met1 and Arg614 encoded by exons 2 to 18; MH/CCD region 2 lies between Arg2162 and Arg2458 encoded by exons 39 to 46; and MH/CCD region 3 lies between about Leu4800 and Asp4900 encoded by exons 100 to 104. Less than half of MH families are linked to RYR1 using markers on chromosome 19q, but phenotypic assays (caffeine- and halothane-induced contracture tests carried out in vitro) have high specificity and lower sensitivity, leading to potential phenotypic error (1, 16).

CACNA1S gene. Several genes encode the various subunits and different isoforms of dihydropyridine-sensitive Ca²⁺ channels. The *CACNA1S3* gene (OMIM 114208) encodes the α1-subunit of the human skeletal muscle

DHPR (Figure 1). Some transmembrane sequences in this protein form the voltage sensor of the DHPR and others form the Ca^{2+} channel pore; cytosolic sequences interact with cytosolic sequences in the ryanodine receptor to regulate Ca^{2+} release channel opening. The *CACNA1S* gene represents a second MH locus (14). Mutations are localized in the cytoplasmic III-IV loop of the α1-subunit, which interacts with the ryanodine receptor. MH mutations are encoded in exon 26, distant from exon 5, which houses mutations causal for hypokalemic periodic paralysis (OMIM #170400). These observations highlight the fact that RyR1 and DHPR α1-subunits interact physically and functionally in excitation-contraction coupling, even to the extent that mutations in either protein can give rise to MH.

SCN4A gene. Linkage of MH to the SCN4A Na^+ channel α-subunit gene (OMIM 603967) on human chromosome 17q in several families makes this gene a candidate for MH (Figure 1) (9). However, abnormal responses to succinylcholine, including muscle rigidity, are considered to be secondary to the primary disease, myotonia fluctuans, which arises from demonstrated defects in the sodium channel α-subunit protein (6, 27). The Na^+ channel α-subunit functions upstream of the functions of the DHPR and RyR channels in the cascade of excitation-contraction coupling, providing a potential functional linkage to the defects in Ca^{2+} regulation that characterize MH.

Malignant hyperthermia

Human malignant hyperthermia (OMIM #145600) usually occurs in response to exposure to potent inhalational anesthetics and depolarizing skeletal muscle relaxants (2). In an MH reaction, MH susceptible (MHS) individuals can experience a rising end tidal CO_2, skeletal muscle rigidity, tachycardia, unstable and rising blood pressure, hyperventilation, cyanosis, falling arterial oxygen tension, increasing arterial carbon dioxide tension, lactic acidosis, and eventually, fever. Muscle cell damage brings about electrolyte imbalance, with early elevation of serum K^+ and Ca^{2+} and a later elevation of muscle proteins such as creatine kinase and myoglobin in the serum and urine. If therapy is not initiated immediately, the patient may die within minutes from ventricular fibrillation, within hours from pulmonary oedema or coagulopathy, or within days from post anoxic neurological damage and cerebral oedema or myoglobinuric renal failure, resulting from the release of muscle proteins into the circulation.

Inheritance of MH is autosomal dominant. The incidence of MH reactions is about 1 in 15 000 anesthetics in children and about 1 in 50 000 to 1 in 100 000 anesthetics in adults. Expressivity appears to be age- and gender-dependent with a preponderance of MH reactions occurring in young males. Non-anaesthetic reactions, such as sudden death, have also been described.

When clinical indicators of a MH crisis (8) occur during the course of surgery, the MH-triggering anaesthetic must be stopped and an alternative anaesthetic administered. The patient is hyperventilated with 100% oxygen and treated with dantrolene, a direct-acting skeletal muscle relaxant (5), until muscles relax, fever, heart rate and respiratory rate decline significantly, and blood gases normalize. Death can still occur, especially if dantrolene therapy is not available or administration is delayed. Definitive diagnosis of MH in survivors involves exclusion of different diagnoses and the in vitro contracture testing of muscle biopsies (4, 7). Family members at risk can then be given alternate anaesthetics, which reduce but do not completely prevent MH crises (2).

In the interictal period of MH, muscle fibres show either no or only minor non-specific changes. During an MH crisis massive acute muscle fibre necrosis is present.

Central core disease

Central core disease (CCD) (OMIM #117000), also covered in chapter 4.2.1, is a rare, congenital myopathy, inherited as an autosomal dominant trait, usually with complete penetrance (20, 28). It is characterised by hypotonia and proximal muscle weakness, which presents in infancy and leads to the delay of motor milestones (23). Both clinical and histological variability is observed, but the clinical course is usually slow or non-progressive in adults. Although symptoms may be severe, with significant muscle weakness, up to 40% of patients demonstrating central cores may have normal clinical performance. Additional variable clinical features include pes cavus, kyphoscoliosis, foot deformities, congenital hip dislocation and joint contractures (22).

Diagnosis is made on the basis of histological examination, which has been described and illustrated in chapter 4.2.1. Briefly, a typical biopsy reveals the lack of oxidative or phosphorylase activity in central regions (cores) of both type 1 and type 2 fibres. Electron microscopy shows disintegration of the contractile apparatus, ranging from blurring and streaming of the Z lines to total loss of myofibrillar structure (chapter 4.2.1). The sarcoplasmic reticulum and transverse tubular systems are greatly increased in content and, in general, are less well structured. Mitochondria are depleted in the cores, but may be enriched around the surfaces of the cores. Glycogen granules are decreased. Desmin intermediate fibres are reduced in the core regions and overexpressed in the periphery.

CCD is usually closely associated with MH so that CCD patients are normally considered to be MH susceptible (15, 21). However, an exception has been found in a kindred in which all affected members suffered from a clinically severe and highly penetrant form of CCD (11). In this family, none of the affected individuals had any anaesthetic complications.

There is no proven therapy for central core disease. Exercise is a major benefit, perhaps because it increases

Ca²⁺ fluxes in the muscle, thereby improving myofilament assembly (11).

Differentiation between MH and CCD mutations

A defect in the Ca^{2+} release channel, giving rise to an unregulated elevation of Ca^{2+} in skeletal muscle cells following the administration of anaesthetics and muscle relaxants, can account for all of the signs of MH (12). Abnormalities induced by elevated Ca^{2+} include skeletal muscle contracture and activation of phosphorylase kinase, which increases both glycogenolysis and glycolysis. These hypermetabolic responses lead to depletion of ATP, glycogen and oxygen; the production of excess lactic acid and CO_2; and ultimately, to the disruption of intracellular and extracellular ion balances, with consequent muscle cell damage. A high turnover of ATP could contribute to the elevated temperatures associated with MH episodes.

Mutations in *RYR1*, however, can lead to a spectrum of pathophysiological responses ranging from muscle hypertrophy to muscle atrophy. It has been proposed that muscle hypertrophy might be induced by spontaneous Ca^{2+} leaks and spontaneous contractions, while muscle atrophy might be caused by larger Ca^{2+} leaks, resulting in Ca^{2+}-induced damage to the core of the fibre where homeostasis cannot be maintained through compensatory mechanisms (10, 13). The hypothesis suggests that these different pathophysiological responses result from differences in the properties of different RyR1 mutants; those with less severe defects in Ca^{2+} release leading to disturbances in Ca^{2+} homeostasis that can be compensated for within muscle fibres, and those with more severe defects in Ca^{2+} release leading to disturbances in Ca^{2+} homeostasis that can be compensated for only in the periphery of the muscle cell. It is proposed that the formation of the central core is a protective mechanism to isolate the core of the fibre where Ca^{2+} homeostasis cannot be maintained.

Studies of 15 MH and CCD mutant Ca^{2+} release channels expressed in heterologous cell culture showed each channel mutant in MH regions 1 and 2 to be more sensitive to the triggering action of halothane and caffeine than wild-type, accounting for the ability of halothane to trigger an MH response in susceptible individuals, but not in normal individuals (26). Ca^{2+} release channels with MH or CCD mutations in these two regions were found to be more permeable than wild-type channels (25). CCD mutant channels could be distinguished from MH mutant channels by their higher permeability. A severe CCD mutation in MH region 3 (the pore-forming region) was found to be the most highly permeable with open probability approaching unity (11). Diminished Ca^{2+} stores in severe forms of CCD might lead to skeletal muscle weakness and might even lead to resistance to MH-triggering drugs.

Elevations in resting Ca^{2+} concentrations were found to induce elevated synthesis of the SERCA2b isoform of the sarco(endo)plasmic reticulum Ca^{2+} ATPase, the pump that returns Ca^{2+} released through channels to organellar stores. It is the activity of Ca^{2+} pumps that replenishes Ca^{2+} stores and establishes the resting Ca^{2+} concentration in the cytosol of muscle and non-muscle cells. The induced synthesis of Ca^{2+} pumps represents a compensatory mechanism aimed at the restoration of Ca^{2+} homeostasis. The size of the releasable Ca^{2+} store and the elevation in resting Ca^{2+} concentration appear to be determined by the level of compensation that can be achieved.

Catecholaminergic polymorphic ventricular tachycardia and arrhythmogenic right ventricular cardiomyopathy type 2

Catecholaminergic polymorphic ventricular tachycardia (CPVT) (OMIM #604772) occurs both in response to stress and in the absence of either structural heart disease or prolonged QT interval. Juvenile sudden death or stress-induced syncope is present in one-third of cases. Arrhythmogenic right ventricular cardiomyopathy

type 2 (ARVD2) (OMIM #600996) is characterised by partial degeneration of the myocardium of the right ventricle, electrical instability, and sudden death. Both of these dominantly inherited diseases are linked to mutations in *RYR2* (OMIM #180902) (18, 24). The mutations are located in regions of the gene that correspond to MH regions 1 and 2 in *RYR1* and which affect cytosolic regulatory regions of the two proteins.

Since *RYR2* is not expressed in skeletal muscle, neither MH nor CCD manifest in these diseases. It is probable that CPVT and ARVD2, like MH and CCD, are differentiated on the basis of the severity of the alteration in RyR2 channel function and that the pathological changes in the heart are the result of poorly regulated cytosolic Ca^{2+} arising from defective Ca^{2+} release channels.

Future perspectives

During the past decade, it has been possible to investigate the role of defects in genes encoding Ca^{2+} regulatory proteins in inherited muscle diseases. Genetic linkage analysis, the discovery and analysis of specific causal genes, and the development of hypotheses concerning the pathophysiology of these diseases have advanced our understanding of Ca^{2+} dysregulation. However, much remains to be done. Alternative causal genes for MH and Brody disease (Chapter 5.3) have yet to be discovered. Animal models have not yet been developed for all of these diseases and "chip" technology has not yet been applied to these diseases to understand the compensatory mechanisms that bring about disease.

References

1. Allen GC, Larach MG, Kunselman AR (1998) The sensitivity and specificity of the caffeine-halothane contracture test: a report from the North American Malignant Hyperthermia Registry. The North American Malignant Hyperthermia Registry of MHAUS. *Anesthesiology* 88: 579-588

2. Britt BA (1991) Malignant hyperthermia: a review. In *Thermoregulation: Pathology, Pharmacology and Therapy*, E Schonbaum, P Lomax (eds). Pergamon Press Inc: New York. pp. 179-129

3. Gillard EF, Otsu K, Fujii J, Khanna VK, de Leon S, Derdemezi J, Britt BA, Duff CL, Worton RG, MacLennan DH (1991) A substitution of cysteine for arginine 614 in the ryanodine receptor is potentially causative of human malignant hyperthermia. *Genomics* 11: 751-755

4. Group TEMH (1984) Malignant hyperpyrexia, a protocol for the investigation of malignant hyperthermia (MH) susceptibility. *Br J Anaesth* 56: 1267-1269

5. Harrison GG (1975) Control of the malignant hyperpyrexic syndrome in MHS swine by dantrolene sodium. *Br J Anaesth* 47: 62-65

6. Iaizzo PA, Lehmann-Horn F (1995) Anesthetic complications in muscle disorders. *Anesthesiology* 82: 1093-1096

7. Larach MG (1989) Standardization of the caffeine halothane muscle contracture test. North American Malignant Hyperthermia Group. *Anesth Analg* 69: 511-515

8. Larach MG, Localio AR, Allen GC, Denborough MA, Ellis FR, Gronert GA, Kaplan RF, Muldoon SM, Nelson TE, Ording H, et al. (1994) A clinical grading scale to predict malignant hyperthermia susceptibility. *Anesthesiology* 80: 771-779

9. Levitt RC, Olckers A, Meyers S, Fletcher JE, Rosenberg H, Isaacs H, Meyers DA (1992) Evidence for the localization of a malignant hyperthermia susceptibility locus (MHS2) to human chromosome 17q. *Genomics* 14: 562-566

10. Loke J, MacLennan DH (1998) Malignant hyperthermia and central core disease: disorders of Ca2+ release channels. *Am J Med* 104: 470-486

11. Lynch PJ, Tong J, Lehane M, Mallet A, Giblin L, Heffron JJ, Vaughan P, Zafra G, MacLennan DH, McCarthy TV (1999) A mutation in the transmembrane/luminal domain of the ryanodine receptor is associated with abnormal Ca2+ release channel function and severe central core disease. *Proc Natl Acad Sci USA* 96: 4164-4169

12. MacLennan DH, Phillips MS (1992) Malignant hyperthermia. *Science* 256: 789-794

13. MacLennan DH, Phillips MS, Zhang Y (1996) The Genetic and physiological basis of malignant hyperthermia. In *Molecular Biology of Membrane Transport Disorders*, SG Schultz, T Andreoli, AM Brown, D Fambrough, J Hoffman, MJ Welsh (eds). Plenum Publishing Corp: New York. pp. 81-200

14. Monnier N, Procaccio V, Stieglitz P, Lunardi J (1997) Malignant-hyperthermia susceptibility is associated with a mutation of the alpha 1-subunit of the human dihydropyridine-sensitive L-type voltage-dependent calcium-channel receptor in skeletal muscle. *Am J Hum Genet* 60: 1316-1325.

15. Mulley JC, Kozman HM, Phillips HA, Gedeon AK, McCure JA, Iles DE, Gregg RG, Hogan K, Couch FJ, MacLennan DH, et al. (1993) Refined genetic localization for central core disease. *Am J Hum Genet* 52: 398-405.

16. Ording H, Brancadoro V, Cozzolino S, Ellis FR, Glauber V, Gonano EF, Halsall PJ, Hartung E, Heffron JJ, Heytens L, Kozak-Ribbens G, Kress H, Krivosic-Horber R, Lehmann-Horn F, Mortier W, Nivoche Y, Ranklev-Twetman E, Sigurdsson S, Snoeck M, Stieglitz P, Tegazzin V, Urwyler A, Wappler F (1997) In vitro contracture test for diagnosis of malignant hyperthermia following the protocol of the European MH Group: results of testing patients surviving fulminant MH and unrelated low-risk subjects. The European Malignant Hyperthermia Group. *Acta Anaesthesiol Scand* 41: 955-966.

17. Phillips MS, Fujii J, Khanna VK, DeLeon S, Yokobata K, de Jong PJ, MacLennan DH (1996) The structural organization of the human skeletal muscle ryanodine receptor (RYR1) gene. *Genomics* 34: 24-41.

18. Priori SG, Napolitano C, Tiso N, Memmi M, Vignati G, Bloise R, Sorrentino VV, Danieli GA (2001) Mutations in the cardiac ryanodine receptor gene (hRyR2) Underlie Catecholaminergic Polymorphic Ventricular Tachycardia. *Circulation* 103: 196-200.

19. Protasi F, Franzini-Armstrong C, Allen PD (1998) Role of ryanodine receptors in the assembly of calcium release units in skeletal muscle. *J Cell Biol* 140: 831-842.

20. Quane KA, Healy JM, Keating KE, Manning BM, Couch FJ, Palmucci LM, Doriguzzi C, Fagerlund TH, Berg K, Ording H, et al. (1993) Mutations in the ryanodine receptor gene in central core disease and malignant hyperthermia. *Nat Genet* 5: 51-55.

21. Schwemmle S, Wolff K, Palmucci LM, Grimm T, Lehmann-Horn F, Hubner C, Hauser E, Iles DE, MacLen-nan DH, Muller CR (1993) Multipoint mapping of the central core disease locus. *Genomics* 17: 205-207.

22. Shuaib A, Paasuke RT, Brownell KW (1987) Central core disease. Clinical features in 13 patients. *Medicine (Baltimore)* 66: 389-396.

23. Shy GM, Magee KR (1956) A new congenital nonprogressive myopathy. *Brain* 79: 610-621

24. Tiso N, Stephan DA, Nava A, Bagattin A, Devaney JM, Stanchi F, Larderet G, Brahmbhatt B, Brown K, Bauce B, Muriago M, Basso C, Thiene G, Danieli GA, Rampazzo A (2001) Identification of mutations in the cardiac ryanodine receptor gene in families affected with arrhythmogenic right ventricular cardiomyopathy type 2 (ARVD2). *Hum Mol Genet* 10: 189-194.

25. Tong J, McCarthy TV, MacLennan DH (1999) Measurement of resting cytosolic Ca2+ concentrations and Ca2+ store size in HEK-293 cells transfected with malignant hyperthermia or central core disease mutant Ca2+ release channels. *J Biol Chem* 274: 693-702.

26. Tong J, Oyamada H, Demaurex N, Grinstein S, McCarthy TV, MacLennan DH (1997) Caffeine and halo-thane sensitivity of intracellular Ca2+ release is altered by 15 calcium release channel (ryanodine receptor) mutations associated with malignant hyperthermia and/or central core disease. *J Biol Chem* 272: 26332-26339.

27. Vita GM, Olckers A, Jedlicka AE, George AL, Heiman-Patterson T, Rosenberg H, Fletcher JE, Levitt RC (1995) Masseter muscle rigidity associated with glycine1306-to-alanine mutation in the adult muscle sodium channel alpha-subunit gene. *Anesthesiology* 82: 1097-1103.

28. Zhang Y, Chen HS, Khanna VK, De Leon S, Phillips MS, Schappert K, Britt BA, Browell AK, MacLennan DH (1993) A mutation in the human ryanodine receptor gene associated with central core disease. *Nat Genet* 5: 46-50.

Brody disease associated with defects in a Ca²⁺ pump

David H. MacLennan
Julian C. P. Loke

NCE	Na⁺/Ca²⁺ exchanger
OMIM	Online Mendelian Inheritance in Man (*http://www.ncbi.nlm.nih.gov/omim*)
PMCA	plasma membrane Ca²⁺ ATPase
SERCA	sarco(endo)plasmic reticulum Ca²⁺ ATPase
SLN	sarcolipin

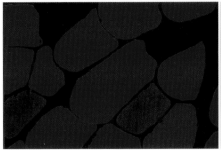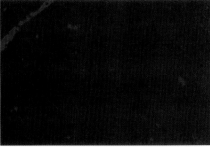

Figure 1. The left panel shows normal immunostaining of type 2 fibres for SERCA1 in a muscle without microscopic pathology. By contrast, in the right panel, a Brody patient's muscle shows complete absence of immunoreactive SERCA 1. Type 1 fibres remain unreactive in either specimen. Primary monoclonal mouse antibody for SERCA 1, and secondary rabbit anti-mouse antibody labelled with Cy3. ×350.

Definition of entities

Ca²⁺ released into muscle cells must be removed quickly to prevent deleterious effects of elevated Ca²⁺. Removal is achieved by the action of sarco-(endo) plasmic reticulum Ca²⁺ ATPases (SERCAs) in skeletal muscle or by a combination of SERCAs, plasma membrane Ca²⁺ ATPases (PMCAs) or Na⁺/Ca²⁺ exchangers (NCEs) in cardiac muscle. Mitochondria can act as a temporary Ca²⁺ buffer, but not as a Ca²⁺ store. This chapter concerns Brody disease and Brody syndrome associated with defects in a Ca²⁺ pump.

Brody disease. Brody myopathy (OMIM 601003) is a disorder of muscle function characterised by painless muscle cramping and exercise-induced impairment of muscle relaxation (4) The term Brody disease is reserved for those cases in which mutations in the *ATP2A1* gene have been identified, while Brody syndrome describes those cases where the molecular aetiology is unknown (8).

Patients with Brody disease experience a lifelong history of difficulty in performing sustained, strenuous muscular activities, such as running upstairs, because the muscles stiffen during exercise, and temporarily, cannot be used (12). The exercise-induced delay in muscle relaxation involves the legs, arms and eyelid and may be worse in cold weather. Distal limb and craniofacial muscles are the major muscles related to the involvement of the bladder sphincter in some cases. Clinical examination demonstrates normal strength with a single effort, but progressive difficulty in relaxing muscles during repeated forceful contraction. Stretch reflexes are not affected and percussion myotonia is absent. To a variable degree, pain develops in the exercised muscle. Muscle relaxation becomes slower as exercise proceeds and the force of contraction declines.

Standard needle electromyography shows normal, spontaneous insertion, voluntary activity, and no electrical activity. In particular, there are no myotonic discharges in the muscles after exercise and during the delayed relaxation. Muscle stiffness and pain subside within minutes after cessation of exercise. Creatine kinase levels may be mildly elevated and exertional rhabdomyolysis has been reported (14). However, fixed muscle weakness or wasting is minimal even years after onset of symptoms. Indeed, many patients appear strongly muscled, perhaps as a result of the demand placed upon slow-twitch fibres, which must both compensate for and counteract the diminished relaxation rates of fast-twitch fibres. Inheritance of Brody disease is autosomal recessive (12), although there is a heavy male preponderance. The incidence of Brody disease is less than 1 in 10 000 000 births, corresponding to a carrier frequency of about 1 in 1600 for autosomal recessive inheritance.

Brody syndrome. Brody syndrome is distinguished from Brody disease by the following features: *i)* Brody disease symptoms are lifelong, while symptoms of Brody syndrome have a later onset, usually appearing in the late teens, *ii)* most muscle groups are involved in Brody disease, but only a subset may be involved in Brody syndrome, *iii)* inheritance of Brody disease is autosomal recessive, while inheritance of Brody syndrome may appear to be either autosomal dominant or autosomal recessive, and *iv)* in Brody disease, inactivating mutations can be detected in the *ATP2A1* gene encoding SERCA1, while no *ATP2A1* mutations are detected in Brody syndrome. In patients being investigated for Brody myopathy, Brody disease can be misdiagnosed if information from genetic testing is not available. Clinical criteria such as exercise-induced contractures in the absence of electrical activity are not sufficient, since more than half of patients with Brody myopathy will be classified as having Brody syndrome.

Molecular genetics

SERCA1 gene. In mammalian skeletal muscles, SERCA1, encoded by the *ATP2A1* gene (OMIM 108730) located on human chromosome 16p12.1-p12.2, is expressed almost exclusively in fast-twitch (type 2) skeletal muscle, while SERCA2a, encoded by *ATP2A2* (OMIM 108740) located on chromosome 12q23-q24.1, is expressed in cardiac and slow twitch (type 1) skeletal muscle (3). The adult human SERCA1a protein contains 994 amino acids with a mass of about 110 000 Da. The coding sequence of the *ATP2A1* cDNA is some 3000 bp long and the *ATP2A1* gene is about 26 000 bp long and contains 23 exons; the last two of which are involved in alternative splicing to create neonatal and adult forms of the protein. Mutations throughout SERCA1 (Figure 1, chapter 5.2) cause Brody disease (12).

Brody disease. Diminished SERCA activity has been reported in all cases of Brody disease studied to date. However, estimates of the remaining fraction of Ca^{2+} ATPase activity vary from near 0% to about 50% (1, 6, 7, 16). Antibodies raised against the Ca^{2+} ATPase from chicken fast-twitch skeletal muscle sarcoplasmic reticulum did not react with histochemical type 2 (fast-twitch) fibres in sections of the skeletal muscle of 4 Brody disease patients (6, 7). However, the antibodies did react with the Ca^{2+} ATPase in type 1 (slow-twitch) fibres, suggesting that the Ca^{2+} ATPase protein was absent from type 2 fibres. These characteristics typify Brody disease.

In a later study of Dutch Brody families (1), an antibody specific for SERCA1, the fast-twitch Ca^{2+} ATPase isoform, was used in muscle homogenates from 10 Brody patients and controls to demonstrate that 83% of the total Ca^{2+} ATPase was SERCA1. Moreover, the content of total SERCA and of SERCA1 protein, measured both by immunoreactivity and by phosphorylation, was identical in a comparison of patients and controls. Nevertheless, Ca^{2+}-stimulated ATPase activity in Brody muscle homogenates was reduced to 50% of normal. The sarcoplasmic Ca^{2+} concentration at rest and the increase in intracellular Ca^{2+} concentration after addition of acetylcholine were found to be the same in muscle cells cultured from patients and controls. However, in cells derived from patients, the time required to reach resting intracellular Ca^{2+} levels after Ca^{2+} release was increased several-fold. Thus the phenotype was consistent with reduced SERCA activity, but not with complete loss of SERCA function. These characteristics typify Brody syndrome.

In patients reported to lack immunoreactive Ca^{2+} ATPase in fast-twitch fibres and in some untested families, premature stop codons were found in the coding sequence for SERCA1 (10, 12). A protein encoded by such mutated genes would be truncated, unstable, and degraded within the muscle cell, consistent with the lack of SERCA1 immunoreactivity. A homozygous point mutation was also detected in the *ATP2A1* gene in a Brody disease family. Analysis of the mutant protein showed that it was expressed in a heterologous system, but was non-functional. Thus, while the absence of immunostaining is often diagnostic of Brody disease, the detection of SERCA1 by immunostaining in muscle biopsies does not rule out Brody disease, since a non-functional protein might be present.

In spite of the absence of SERCA1 in those Brody disease patients who inherited *ATP2A1* gene defects, all are able to relax their fast-twitch skeletal muscles, although at a significantly reduced rate. Thus Ca^{2+} concentrations in Brody disease muscle must be lowered through a combination of other mechanisms resulting in compensatory Ca^{2+} removal—by PMCAs and NCEs in the plasma membrane, by mitochondria (5), or by upregulation of the SERCA2 gene. Of these possible compensatory processes, only the latter would be predicted to result in Ca^{2+} loading of the sarcoplasmic reticulum, a process necessary for subsequent muscle contraction. Ca^{2+} loading of depleted stores may also occur through direct entry into organellar spaces from extracellular spaces by a process known as capacitative Ca^{2+} entry (2).

Brody syndrome. The molecular basis for Brody syndrome is unknown. Since Ca^{2+} ATPase activity is reduced in Brody syndrome, molecules, which might modulate the activity of SERCA1, are candidate causes of Brody syndrome. A prime candidate was sarcolipin (SLN) encoded by the *SLN* gene (13) (Figure 1, chapter 5.2). SLN is a 32 amino acid protein, which is highly and almost exclusively expressed in fast-twitch muscle. It is tightly associated with SERCA1 and inhibits SERCA1 activity at low Ca^{2+} concentrations by decreasing Ca^{2+} affinity. It also activates SERCA1 activity at high Ca^{2+} concentrations by increasing V_{max} (11). A mutation in such a protein might make it highly inhibitory, since specific mutants of a homologous protein, phospholamban, make it a superinhibitor of SERCA2 function in heart (9, 17, 18). Unfortunately, no *SLN* mutations have been found in any of thirteen Brody families studied to date.

Molecular pathogenesis

In Brody disease and Brody syndrome, Ca^{2+} uptake into the sarcoplasmic reticulum is impaired due to an absence or insufficiency of Ca^{2+} pump activity. This results in an elevation in the cytosolic Ca^{2+} concentration in stimulated muscle cells, which increases as exercise progresses, impairing muscle relaxation. Processes known to be Ca^{2+} dependent could then be activated, accounting for any additional deleterious effects on muscle fibres that have been demonstrated in Brody muscle. The activation of phosphorylase kinase by Ca^{2+} leads to the activation of glycogenolysis and glycolysis, resulting in heightened lactate production. The stimulation of Ca^{2+}-dependent proteases, eg, cathepsin, could stimulate protein catabolism and other pathways, possibly leading to apoptosis, which might be responsible for the atrophy of type 2 fibres. The elevation of cytosolic Ca^{2+} increases the risk of fibre necrosis, the probable mechanism by which muscle proteins enter the blood stream in reported cases of myoglobinuria.

The overloading of mitochondria with Ca^{2+} could impair oxidative phosphorylation, leading to diminished energy production.

In some cases, the symptoms of Brody syndrome have been ameliorated by the oral administration of either dantrolene, a direct-acting muscle relaxant that inhibits the Ca^{2+} release channel and is widely used as an antidote to malignant hyperthermia reactions, or L-type Ca^{2+} channel blockers, such as verapamil or nifedipine.

The therapeutic effect of dantrolene sodium may be explained by its ability to inhibit Ca^{2+} release through the Ca^{2+} release channel in the sarcoplasmic reticulum. A reduction in Ca^{2+} release would compensate for impaired reuptake, leading to less deleterious effects on the fibre. The beneficial effect of Ca^{2+} channel blockers, such as verapamil, can also be explained by a similar mechanism, except that they block the activation of the Ca^{2+} release channel indirectly through their effects on the voltage sensor of the DHPR (15).

Structural changes

There are no consistent or discernible myopathological changes. SERCA1 deficiency may be shown by immunocytochemistry as illustrated in Figure 1.

Future perspectives and therapy

As has been pointed out in chapter 5.2, during the past decade, it has been possible to investigate the role of defects in genes encoding Ca^{2+} regulatory proteins in inherited muscle diseases. Genetic linkage analysis, the discovery and analysis of specific causal genes and the development of hypotheses concerning the pathophysiology of these diseases have advanced our understanding of Ca^{2+} dysregulation. However, much remains to be done. Alternative causal genes for MH and Brody disease have yet to be discovered. Animal models have not yet been developed for all of these diseases and "chip" technology has not yet been applied to these diseases to understand the compensatory mechanisms that bring about disease.

References

1. Benders AA, Veerkamps JH, Oosterhof A, Jongen PJ, Bindels RJ, Smit LM, Busch HF, Wevers RA (1994) Ca^{2+} homeostasis in Brody's disease. A study in skeletal muscle and cultured muscle cells and the effects of dantrolene an verapamil. J Clin Invest 94: 741-748

2. Bird GS, Bian X, Putney JW, Jr. (1995) Calcium entry signal? Nature 373: 481-482

3. Brandl CJ, Green NM, Korczak B, MacLennan DH (1986) Two Ca^{2+} ATPase genes: homologies and mechanistic implications of deduced amino acid sequences. Cell 44: 597-607

4. Brody IA (1969) Muscle contracture induced by exercise. A syndrome attributable to decreased relaxing factor. N Engl J Med 281: 187-192

5. Carafoli E (1987) Intracellular calcium homeostasis. Annu Rev Biochem 56: 395-433

6. Danon MJ, Karpati G, Charuk J, Holland P (1988) Sarcoplasmic reticulum adenosine triphosphatase deficiency with probable autosomal dominant inheritance. Neurology 38: 812-815

7. Karpati G, Charuk J, Carpenter S, Jablecki C, Holland P (1986) Myopathy caused by a deficiency of Ca^{2+}-adenosine triphosphatase in sarcoplasmic reticulum (Brody's disease). Ann Neurol 20: 38-49

8. Karpati G, Maclennan DH (1999) In Exercise Intolerance and Muscle Contracture, G Serratrice, J Pouget, J-P Azulay (eds). Springer-Verlag: Berlin. pp. 45-54

9. Kimura Y, Kurzydlowski K, Tada M, MacLennan DH (1997) Phospholamban inhibitory function is activated by depolymerization. J Biol Chem 272: 15061-15064

10. Odermatt A, Barton K, Khanna VK, Mathieu J, Escolar D, Kuntzer T, Karpati G, MacLennan DH (2000) The mutation of Pro789 to Leu reduces the activity of the fast-twitch skeletal muscle sarco(endo)plasmic reticulum Ca2+ ATPase (SERCA1) and is associated with Brody disease. Hum Genet 106: 482-491

11. Odermatt A, Becker S, Khanna VK, Kurzydlowski K, Leisner E, Pette D, MacLennan DH (1998) Sarcolipin regulates the activity of SERCA1, the fast-twitch skeletal muscle sarcoplasmic reticulum Ca2+-ATPase. J Biol Chem 273: 12360-12369

12. Odermatt A, Taschner PE, Khanna VK, Busch HF, Karpati G, Jablecki CK, Breuning MH, MacLennan DH (1996) Mutations in the gene-encoding SERCA1, the fast-twitch skeletal muscle sarcoplasmic reticulum Ca2+ ATPase, are associated with Brody disease. Nat Genet 14: 191-194

13. Odermatt A, Taschner PE, Scherer SW, Beatty B, Khanna VK, Cornblath DR, Chaudhry V, Yee WC, Schrank B, Karpati G, Breuning MH, Knoers N, MacLennan DH (1997) Characterization of the gene encoding human sarcolipin (SLN), a proteolipid associated with SERCA1: absence of structural mutations in five patients with Brody disease. Genomics 45: 541-553

14. Poels PJ, Wevers RA, Braakhekke JP, Benders AA, Veerkamp JH, Joosten EM (1993) Exertional rhabdomyolysis in a patient with calcium adenosine triphosphatase deficiency. J Neurol Neurosurg Psychiatry 56: 823-826

15. Rios E, Pizarro G, Stefani E (1992) Charge movement and the nature of signal transduction in skeletal muscle excitation-contraction coupling. Annu Rev Physiol 54: 109-133

16. Taylor DJ, Brosnan MJ, Arnold DL, Bore PJ, Styles P, Walton J, Radda GK (1988) Ca^{2+}-ATPase deficiency in a patient with an exertional muscle pain syndrome. J Neurol Neurosurg Psychiatry 51: 1425-1433

17. Zhai J, Schmidt AG, Hoit BD, Kimura Y, MacLennan DH, Kranias EG (2000) Cardiac-specific overexpression of a superinhibitory pentameric phospholamban mutant enhances inhibition of cardiac function in vivo. J Biol Chem 275: 10538-10544

18. Zvaritch E, Backx PH, Jirik F, Kimura Y, de Leon S, Schmidt AG, Hoit BD, Lester JW, Kranias EG, MacLennan DH (2000) The transgenic expression of highly inhibitory monomeric forms of phospholamban in mouse heart impairs cardiac contractility. J Biol Chem 275: 14985-14991

CHAPTER 6

Myopathies based on complex molecular defects

6.1 Repeat expansion diseases
    6.1.1 The myotonic dystrophies   108
    6.1.2 PABPN1 dysfunction in oculopharyngeal muscular dystrophy   115
6.2 Large telomeric deletion disease. Facioscapulohumeral dystrophy   119

R ecent studies of several hereditary muscle diseases revealed highly unusual types of pathogenic gene rearrangements. The best example of this is the variable degree of expansion of CTG trinucleotide repeats in the 3′ untranslated region in one allele of the myotonin kinase gene in myotonic dystrophy. It is still uncertain as to how this alteration becomes pathogenic in several cell types. Other forms of trinucleotide repeat expansions also constitute the pathogenic mutation in several CNS diseases as "experiments of nature" that lead to fundamental new clues for the understanding of general molecular mechanisms of the cell.

Another highly unusual molecular defect is the pathogenic mutation in facioscapulo-humeral muscular dystrophy. This consists of a very large deletion in the telomeric region of the long arm of chromosome 4, where there are no genes but many tandemly occurring repeats of identical, long base sequences. This, of course, raises the question as to the mechanism by which such genomic change can become pathogenic for the muscle fibre and perhaps other cells as well. These issues and relevant molecular details are carefully dissected in this chapter.

The myotonic dystrophies

Charles Thornton

CK	creatine kinase
DM	dystrophia myotonica
DM1	myotonic dystrophy 1
DM2	myotonic dystrophy 2
DMPK	DM protein kinase
OMIM	Online Mendelian Inheritance in Man (*www.ncbi.nlm.nih.gov/omim*)
SCA8 gene	spinocerebellar ataxia 8 (SCA8) gene

Definition of entities

Myotonic dystrophy (dystrophia myotonica, DM) is a dominantly-inherited degenerative disease of the skeletal muscles, heart, brain, and lens. The core manifestations of DM in skeletal muscle are weakness, wasting, and myotonia.

Based on genetic locus and disease manifestations, DM is divided into myotonic dystrophy 1 (DM1) and myotonic dystrophy 2 (DM2). DM1 (OMIM 160900) is caused by an expansion of CTG repeats in the *DMPK* gene on chromosome 19q (7). DM1 is divided into congenital, classical, and minimal phenotypes according to the age of symptom onset and disease severity. DM2 (OMIM 602668) is genetically heterogeneous.

The prevalence of DM1, the commonest form of muscular dystrophy in adults, is estimated at 1 in 7400 live births in Europe and North America (21). Evidence suggests a predisposing founder allele that arose after migrations out of Africa, and that the prevalence of DM1 in sub-Saharan Africa is much lower (13). Although the prevalence of DM2 has not been studied, experience suggests that it is 10-fold-less common than DM1.

Classical DM1. Classical DM1 accounts for ~85% of cases that are currently diagnosed. The first symptom is usually grip myotonia that begins in the second, third, or fourth decade. The earliest signs of weakness can be found in the finger flexors, neck flexors, and facial muscles. Muscles of the proximal limb and limb girdle are affected later in the disease. Typical signs at presentation are ptosis, facial weakness, temporalis wasting, and weakness of the neck and distal limb muscles. The extent of contracture and CK elevation is much less than in the sarcolemmal dystrophies (Chapter 2). The most common cause of death is respiratory insufficiency due to involvement of the diaphragm, intercostal, and oropharyngeal muscles (12).

DM1 has important non-myologic manifestations (21). Its main effects in the heart are progressive fibrosis of the conduction system and abnormal excitation. Cardiac arrest due to heart block or ventricular tachyarrhythmia is the second most common cause of death. Effects of DM1 on contractility are much less severe in cardiac than skeletal muscle. The central nervous system manifestations of DM1 can include hypersomnia, hypersensitivity to anaesthetic agents, impaired visuospatial function, abnormal regulation of respiration, apathy, and avoidant behaviour. The cataracts in DM1 are located in the posterior subcapsular zone of the lens and have a distinctive multicolored appearance. Other manifestations include testicular atrophy, balding, insulin resistance, and gastrointestinal disturbance due to involvement of smooth muscle.

Congenital DM1. In 10 to 15% of cases, DM1 presents with neonatal hypotonia, feeding difficulties, and respiratory impairment (20). Failure to develop adequate respiratory function is fatal in 25% of infants with congenital DM1 (44), and more than 75% of affected children have mild or moderate mental retardation. Muscle function often improves in early childhood, but the superimposed signs of classical DM1 begin to emerge in the second or third decade.

Minimal DM1. Small expansions (<100 repeats) of the CTG repeat are associated with a mild phenotype in which cataract may be the only manifestation (43). Signs of muscle wasting and weakness may not appear until after 60 years of age in some individuals. Minimal DM1 is usually undiagnosed unless other members of the family seek medical attention for classical DM1.

Molecular genetics and pathophysiology

DM1. The DM1 mutation is an unstable expansion of CTG repeats in the 3′ untranslated region of the DM protein kinase (*DMPK*) gene (7). Normal *DMPK* alleles have from 4 to 37 CTG repeats, whereas DM1 alleles have from 50 to more than 4000 repeats. Longer expansions correlate with earlier symptom onset and more severe disease. Extensive genetic research has not identified any 19q-linked DM families that do not have an expanded CTG repeat. It appears, therefore, that the pathogenic effect of the expanded CTG repeat cannot be reproduced by point mutations or deletions at the DM1 locus, and that a negative test for the expanded repeat excludes the diagnosis of DM1.

Families with DM1 show marked anticipation. For example, among 61 parent-child pairs the average age of symptom onset was 29 years earlier in offspring than in the affected parent (22). The genetic basis for anticipation is the strong tendency for the expanded repeat to enlarge when transmitted from one generation to the next. The extent of the intergenerational instability depends on repeat length and gender of the transmitting parent. Expansions of less that 100 CTG repeats show greater instability in sperm than ova (9). Consequently, the threshold from minimal to classical DM1 is usually crossed when disease is transmitted through the male germline. By contrast, large expansions that are associated with congenital DM1 are nearly always maternally transmitted, reflecting a bias against very large expansions in sperm (24).

The DM1 mutation also shows dramatic instability in somatic cells. For example, the repeat lengths are 2 to 13-fold larger in skeletal muscle than in peripheral blood cells from the same individual (51, 59). The repeat expansions in skeletal muscle tend to be very large (4-13 kilobase pairs of CTG repeats) in all individuals with symptomatic classical DM1 (51), but the size of these large expansions does not correlate well with the severity of weakness in the sampled muscle (Thornton and Moxley, unpublished data).

DM2. DM2 is linked to chromosome 3q in most (42, 46) but not all (31) kindreds. Inspection of human genome sequence data has not revealed any genes at the *DM2* locus that are highly similar to genes at the DM1 locus. Genetic analysis of DM2 families has not shown evidence for an expanded CTG repeat (42), but repeat sequences with other nucleotide motifs have not been excluded.

Mechanism for repeat instability. Instability of the DM1 mutation is an inherent property of the expanded CTG repeat and its interactions with the normal machinery for DNA replication and repair. Mutations at a second site, such as those that cause genome-wide instability of repetitive sequences in hereditary cancer syndromes, are not required for instability of DM1 alleles, and individuals with DM1 do not have instability at other repeat loci. Both the CTG repeat and its complement, the CAG repeat, are able to form stable intramolecular hairpin loops. The propensity of these sequences to "loop out" from the helix and the susceptibil-

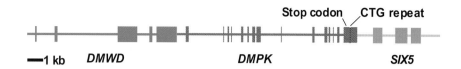

Figure 1. Diagram of *DM1* locus. The *DM1* mutation is in a gene-rich region of chromosome 19q13.3. The CTG repeat is located in the 15th and final exon of *DMPK*, downstream from the translation termination codon. The CTG repeat in DM1 skeletal muscle may expand to a length that is similar to the entire wild-type *DMPK* gene (13 kilobase pairs).

ity of triplet repeats to strand slippage during DNA replication are probably the major factors that lead to instability (36). More than 15 repeat expansion disorders have been identified in humans, whereas none have been found in other species. Furthermore, the marked instability that characterises DM1 is not fully reproduced in any of the transgenic mouse models. These observations suggest that species may differ in there susceptibility to repeat expansion disorders.

The natural history of the somatic instability in DM1 has not been defined. First and second trimester foetuses with DM1 have a fairly uniform population of repeat lengths in different tissues (24), which suggests that rapid growth and cell division in early development are not associated with major somatic instability. Recent evidence suggests that DNA repair rather than mitotic replication is the main process which causes expansion (30), and that enlargement of expanded repeats can continue throughout life (35), even in post-mitotic cells (26). Although the very large expansions in skeletal muscle result mainly from somatic instability, the time course of the enlargement is unknown.

Molecular pathogenesis. The DM1 mutation is in the 3′ untranslated region (Figure 1), a rare position for mutations that have a dominant effect. It is unlikely that the disease mechanism involves a gain-of-function by mutant protein because the coding region of the *DMPK* gene and mRNA remains intact. However, three unconventional effects of the DM1 mutation may contribute to disease pathogenesis. First, the nuclear export of mRNA syn-

thesised from the mutant *DMPK* allele is blocked (11), and levels of DMPK protein in cells are correspondingly reduced. Second, expansion of the CTG repeat silences the expression of flanking genes, such as *SIX5* and *DMWD* (1, 28, 52). Third, the mutant DMPK mRNA is retained in the nucleus in multiple discreet foci, causing nuclear accumulation of expanded CUG repeats (11, 50). To assess their role in pathogenesis, each of these effects has been investigated and reproduced by genetic manipulation in mice.

Altered expression of DMPK. The DM protein kinase is most abundant in skeletal and cardiac muscle (32). This serine/threonine kinase is also expressed at lower levels in other cell types, including neurones and smooth muscle. In muscle fibres, DMPK protein localises to the motor end plate and the terminal cisternae of the sarcoplasmic reticulum (49). Loss of DMPK is associated with abnormalities of calcium homeostasis (4), but its exact role in striated muscle is not understood.

Nuclear retention of the mutant DMPK mRNA would be expected to cause decreased levels of DMPK protein in cells. However, studies of DMPK levels in DM1 have generated conflicting results. Most studies (18, 33), but not all (41), indicate that the levels of DMPK protein in muscle are reduced in classical DM1. To model this result, the *DMPK* gene was disrupted by homologous recombination in mice. One strain of homozygous DMPK knockout mice showed a 40% reduction in force generation and a slight increase in the variability of fibre size in sternomastoid muscle (45). However, muscle histology was normal in a second strain of DMPK knockout mice (23). Although loss of DMPK was associated with changes in gating behaviour of the muscle sodium channel (39), neither strain of DMPK knockout mice showed myotonia. These observations suggest that DMPK is not required for development or maintenance of mammalian skeletal muscle, and that reduced expression of DMPK cannot provide a unitary explanation for the DM1 phenotype. These results may explain why point mutations or deletions in the *DMPK* gene have not been associated with DM. Although absence of DMP*K* may alter excitation-contraction coupling and force generation in murine skeletal muscle, it remains unclear how this finding relates to human DM1 in which DMPK expression is only partially reduced Interestingly, homozygous DMPK knockout mice develop age-related defects in cardiac conduction that are similar to DM (5), although not accompanied by evidence of degeneration or fibrosis in the conduction system.

Altered expression of other genes at the DM1 locus. The intergenic distances that separate the *DMPK*, *DMWD*, and *SIX5* genes at the DM1 locus are small (Figure 1). The CTG repeat is located in the final exon of the *DMPK* gene, only 200 base pairs away from elements that control the expression of *SIX5*. Despite their close physical relationship, these genes are not coordinately regulated (16) or known to have any functional associations. However, CTG repeats are avidly packaged into nucleosomes (58) raising the possibility that an expanded repeat could alter chromatin structure and gene function over the entire region. Studies have confirmed that expression of *SIX5* (28, 52) and *DMWD* (1) is silenced by the expanded repeat in *cis*, but the overall effect (sum of DM-linked and wild type alleles) on expression of either gene is slight (15, 19).

SIX5 (previously known as *DMAHP*) is a member of a small family of transcription factors that share

similar DNA binding motifs, the homeo- and Six-domains (6). The founding member of the family, *sine oculi*, has an essential role in eye development in Drosophila, but the function of SIX5 is unknown. The levels of *SIX5* mRNA in cardiac and skeletal muscle are very low and no effects on striated muscle were observed when the *SIX5* gene was disrupted in mice (27). Although there is no evidence that reduced expression of *SIX5* is involved in the pathogenesis of muscle wasting, the *Six5* knockout mice have an increased frequency of cataract (27, 47) raising the possibility that loss of *SIX5* may contribute to cataract formation in DM1. Less is known about the *DMWD* gene product. A motif in this protein, the WD repeat, is found in some proteins that regulate development. Although the DM-linked *DMWD* allele may also be subject to partial silencing by the expanded CTG repeat (1), the total level of DMWD mRNA levels in DM1 skeletal muscle is not different from controls (15, 19).

Toxicity of expanded CUG repeats. The idea that an expanded CUG repeat could endow mRNA with a toxic property has no biologic precedent and is contrary to the traditional view of mRNA as a labile entity, present in low molar concentration, having no fixed conformation, and whose sole function is to direct the synthesis of protein. Nevertheless, a growing body of evidence suggests that the major pathogenic effect of the DM1 mutation is mediated by the expanded CUG repeat in the mutant DMPK mRNA. The first indication that expanded CUG repeats have biologic effects was the demonstration that the mRNA from the mutant *DMPK* allele, although fully processed and polyadenylated, was retained in the nucleus (11, 50). In a muscle cell line, the expression and nuclear retention of expanded CUG repeats was associated with defects in fusion and myogenic differentiation (2). Direct support for an RNA-mediated disease mechanism comes from studies of transgenic mice that express

expanded CUG repeats in skeletal muscle. These lines of transgenic mice show many DM-related disease phenomena, including multifocal accumulation of expanded CUG repeats in the nucleus, myotonia, and histopathologic changes that resemble DM1, such as ring fibres, atrophic fibres, central nuclei, and increased myonuclei per fibre area (34).

Mechanism of RNA gain-of-function. Expanded CUG repeats have unusual biophysical properties which may underlie their pathogenic effects. Purified expanded CUG repeats adopt a very stable secondary structure in vitro (37, 53). Evidence suggests that this structure is an extended hairpin in which the stem is a duplex with C•G and G•C base pairs separated by U•U mismatch. The stability of this structure is very high, suggesting that it may also form in cells.

Pathogenic effects of expanded CUG repeats may involve interactions with RNA binding proteins. Members in the CELF/ELAV family of RNA binding proteins, CUGBP and Etr3, are able to bind short (8 repeat) CUG oligomers in vitro (54), but they interact with expanded CUG repeats only to a limited extent (37). PKR, the double-stranded-RNA-activated protein kinase, binds preferentially to expanded CUG repeats in vitro, but as yet there is no evidence that it interacts with expanded CUG repeats in vivo (53). A nuclear protein has been isolated that binds expanded CUG hairpins in preference to expanded CAG repeats or non-expanded CUG repeats (38). This protein was identified as the human homologue of *muscleblind*, a protein required for development of striated muscle and photoreceptors in Drosophila (3). Human muscleblind is expressed most highly in cardiac and skeletal muscle (38), and this protein co-localises with expanded CUG repeats in transgenic mice and human DM1 (Mankodi, Swanson, and Thornton, unpublished data). These observations support a model in which muscleblind is sequestered in foci of expanded

CUG repeats and cannot perform its normal, as yet unknown function.

Myotonia results from altered behaviour of ion channels in the muscle fibre membrane. In the non-dystrophic myotonic disorders, myotonia is associated with loss of function for the ClC-1 chloride channel or altered gating properties of the SCN4A sodium channel (chapter 5). Studies of myotonia in DM1 have shown reduced chloride conductance and late re-openings of the sodium channel (17), but neither abnormality was consistently present or clearly sufficient to cause myotonia. However, the myotonia in transgenic mice that express expanded CUG repeats is associated with greater than 80% reduction in chloride conductance (Takahashi and Cannon, unpublished data), an alteration sufficient to cause myotonia. Moreover, the loss of chloride conductance in these transgenic lines can be attributed to aberrant splicing of the ClC-1 mRNA (Mankodi and Thornton, unpublished data). These results support a model in which the accumulation of expanded CUG repeats in the nucleus interferes with processing of particular mRNAs.

Mechanistic interactions. Mice that express expanded CUG repeats in muscle develop myotonia and myopathy. However, these lines of transgenic mice do not develop severe muscle wasting or weakness (34), and thus, do not fully reproduce the muscle phenotype of DM1. Several explanations for this discrepancy are possible. If the disease process in DM1 is multifactorial, as discussed below, some combination of RNA toxicity and partial loss of DMPK or SIX5 may be required to generate the full phenotype. Alternatively, the length of the repeat or the development regulation of its expression may influence its toxicity, or muscle fibres may respond to the toxic mRNA differently in mice than in humans. Species differences have been noted, for example, in the human and murine response to dystrophin deficiency (10).

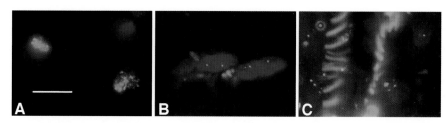

Figure 2. Nuclear foci of expanded CUG repeats. **A.** Fluorescence in situ hybridisation of muscle sections with fluorescein-labeled CAG repeat oligonucleotide shows numerous foci of mutant mRNA (green) in nuclei (blue) of transgenic mice that express expanded CUG repeats. In sections of quadriceps muscle from a patient with DM1, foci are present in nuclei of skeletal (**B**, lipofuscin is brown) and smooth muscle (**C**, an intramuscular vessel, elastic lamina shows green autofluorescence). Bar indicates 10 μm.

Putative disease mechanisms in DM, such as RNA toxicity or partial loss of DMPK or SIX5, are not mutually exclusive. The tools of mouse genetics have been exploited to reproduce each of these mechanisms in isolation, resulting in various phenotypes which resemble aspects of DM. Results from this reductionist approach have been interpreted to suggest that several independent disease mechanisms, such as RNA toxicity for myotonia and myopathy, loss of DMPK for cardiac conduction disease, and loss of SIX5 for cataracts, are required to produce the entire spectrum of disease manifestations in DM1. However, phenotypic similarities suggest that DM1 and DM2 have a shared pathophysiologic mechanism, yet DM2 maps to a locus at which there are no known homologues of *SIX5* or *DMPK*. Therefore, observations on DM2 suggest that a single gene defect can reproduce most aspects of DM1, without invoking a complex, multigenic disease process. Resolution of this paradox awaits the identification of the mutation(s) that causes DM2.

A limitation of the current data is that effects of expanded CUG repeats have not been examined in non-muscle tissues. The discovery of an expanded CTG repeat in the spinocerebellar ataxia 8 (*SCA8*) gene (29) suggests that the deleterious effects of expanded CUG repeats are not restricted to skeletal muscle. *SCA8* may represent a parallel example in which expression of an expanded CUG repeat in neurones causes neurodegeneration. The *SCA8* transcript does not encode a protein, supporting an RNA-mediated disease mechanism.

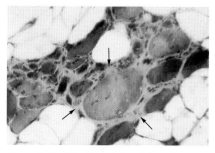

Figure 3. Considerable variation of fibre diameters, endomysial fibrosis (arrows), an increased number of internal nuclei as well as pyknotic nuclear clumps are characteristic findings. Gomori trichrome. Illustration kindly provided by Hans H. Goebel, Mainz, Germany.

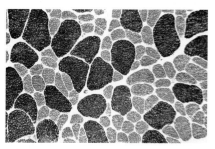

Figure 4. Fibre type disproportion, i.e. predominance and atrophy of type 1 fibres and paucity of normal or enlarged size type 2 fibres characterise early myotonic dystrophy, especially in biceps and deltoid muscles. ATPase pH 9.4. Illustration by Hans H. Goebel.

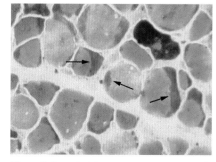

Figure 5. Sarcoplasmic masses can be identified in the Gomori trichrome stain and they react strongly as in this non-specific esterase preparation. Illustration by Hans H. Goebel.

Structural changes

The histopathology of DM1 is characterised by atrophy of muscle fibres and abnormalities of the myonuclei (Figure 3). Although necrosis of muscle fibres is much less conspicuous than in the sarcolemmal dystrophies (chapter 2), the cumulative effect of the disease process is nevertheless severe. At autopsy it is sometimes difficult to find any recognisable skeletal muscle in the limbs. A distinctive feature in many cases is the selective atrophy of type 1 fibres, with or without hypertrophy of type 2 fibres (8, 55) (Figure 4). However, the extent of the muscle fibre atrophy is quite variable and relative smallness of type 1 fibres is not a constant finding. Predominance of type 1 fibres is common and can be pronounced in muscles that are severely affected. Ring fibres and sarcoplasmic masses (Figure 5) are usually present. The increase in endomysial collagen is relatively slight.

Increases in the number of myonuclei and the proportion of central nuclei are among the earliest changes in DM (56, 57) (Figure 3). The central nuclei are found at various depths within the muscle fibre. On longitudinal sections both the subsarcolemmal and central nuclei may be aligned in chains. Pyknotic nuclear clumps are often very abundant. Focal accumulations of CUG repeats in myonuclei can be demonstrated by fluorescence in situ hybridisation with a complementary (CAG repeat) probe. These nuclear foci are very numerous in cultured DM1 myoblasts (50) and muscle sections from transgenic mice that express expanded CUG repeats (34), but in sections from DM1 muscle biopsies there are typically only 1 to 3 foci per nucleus (Figure 2). These foci have not been localised to a particular sub-nuclear structure.

Electron microscopy shows sarcoplasmic masses and dilation of the terminal cisternae of the sarcoplasmic reticulum (14, 40). The myonuclei often have irregular contours and indentations of the nuclear membrane. Although there is one report of intranuclear tubulofilamentous inclusions in DM1 (14), it is unknown whether these structures correspond to the nuclear foci of mutant mRNA.

The muscle histopathology in congenital DM1 shows small fibres with central nuclei and poor fibre type differentiation (48); findings that suggest delayed maturation of muscle fibres. Electron microscopy shows disarray or absence or myofibrils at the periphery of fibres and clusters of tubules with electron dense cores (25).

The pathological features of DM2 are similar to DM1. Pyknotic nuclear clumps and central nuclei are abundant. Selective atrophy of type 1 fibres may favour the diagnosis of DM1 over DM2. However, a detailed comparison of structural findings in these 2 disorders has not yet been reported. Whereas genetic testing has largely supplanted the need for diagnostic muscle biopsy in DM1, histologic examination remains a useful tool in the diagnosis of DM2.

Genotype-phenotype correlations

Repeat lengths above 1000 are associated with congenital or juvenile-onset and severe disease. Repeat lengths of less than 100 repeats are associated with late-onset mild disease. Between these extremes, it appears that the correlation between repeat length and disease severity or age of symptom onset is loose. However, prospective analyses are needed to determine the prognostic value of measuring CTG repeat length in blood leukocytes.

Future perspectives

The intergenerational instability of the expanded CTG repeat has far reaching implications for aspects of DM1 inheritance, such as anticipation. Implications of the somatic instability for disease manifestations and progression may be equally important. The very large repeat expansions in DM1 skeletal muscle result from enlargement of the mutant allele at some time after conception. It will be helpful to determine the mechanism and time course of this process, and to develop strategies by which it can be halted or reversed.

Investigations of DM1 have unexpectedly revealed a new mechanism of genetic dominance, RNA gain-of-function. Exploration of this mechanism is at a very early stage. Currently there is little information about the mechanism for nuclear retention of mature transcripts that have expanded CUG repeats, the structure and protein interactions of expanded CUG repeats in vivo, and the effects that these transcripts may have on genome integrity, nuclear function, and biogenesis of other mRNAs. Model systems are needed to examine the pathogenicity of expanded CUG repeats in other organs. Elucidation of the DM2 mutation may provide insight into this RNA-mediated disease mechanism.

Addendum

DM type 2 is caused by expansion of a CCTG repeat in intron 1 of the *ZNF9* gene (Liquori CL, Ricker K, Moseley ML, Jacobsen JF, Kress W, Naylor SL, Day JW, Ranum LP (2001) Myotonic dystrophy type 2 caused by a CCTG expansion in intron 1 of ZNF9. *Science* 293: 864-867).

References

1. Alwazzan M, Newman E, Hamshere MG, Brook JD (1999) Myotonic dystrophy is associated with a reduced level of RNA from the DMWD allele adjacent to the expanded repeat. *Hum Mol Genet* 8: 1491-1497

2. Amack JD, Paguio AP, Mahadevan MS (1999) Cis and trans effects of the myotonic dystrophy (DM) mutation in a cell culture model. *Hum Mol Genet* 8: 1975-1984

3. Artero R, Prokop A, Paricio N, Begemann G, Pueyo I, Mlodzik M, Perez-Alonso M, Baylies MK (1998) The muscleblind gene participates in the organization of Z-bands and epidermal attachments of Drosophila muscles and is regulated by Dmef2. *Dev Biol* 195: 131-143

4. Benders AA, Groenen PJ, Oerlemans FT, Veerkamp JH, Wieringa B (1997) Myotonic dystrophy protein kinase is involved in the modulation of the Ca2+ homeostasis in skeletal muscle cells. *J Clin Invest* 100: 1440-1447

5. Berul CI, Maguire CT, Aronovitz MJ, Greenwood J, Miller C, Gehrmann J, Housman D, Mendelsohn ME, Reddy S (1999) DMPK dosage alterations result in atrioventricular conduction abnormalities in a mouse myotonic dystrophy model. *J Clin Invest* 103: R1-7

6. Boucher CA, King SK, Carey N, Krahe R, Winchester CL, Rahman S, Creavin T, Meghji P, Bailey ME,

Chartier FL, et al. (1995) A novel homeodomain-encoding gene is associated with a large CpG island interrupted by the myotonic dystrophy unstable (CTG)n repeat. Hum Mol Genet 4: 1919-1925

7. Brook JD, McCurrach ME, Harley HG, Buckler AJ, Church D, Aburatani H, Hunter K, Stanton VP, Thirion JP, Hudson T, et al. (1992) Molecular basis of myotonic dystrophy: expansion of a trinucleotide (CTG) repeat at the 3′ end of a transcript encoding a protein kinase family member. Cell 68: 799-808

8. Brooke MH, Engel WK (1969) The histographic analysis of human muscle biopsies with regard to fiber types. 3. Myotonias, myasthenia gravis, and hypokalemic periodic paralysis. Neurology 19: 469-477

9. Brunner HG, Bruggenwirth HT, Nillesen W, Jansen G, Hamel BC, Hoppe RL, de Die CE, Howeler CJ, van Oost BA, Wieringa B, et al. (1993) Influence of sex of the transmitting parent as well as of parental allele size on the CTG expansion in myotonic dystrophy (DM). Am J Hum Genet 53: 1016-1023

10. Bulfield G, Siller WG, Wight PA, Moore KJ (1984) X chromosome-linked muscular dystrophy (mdx) in the mouse. Proc Natl Acad Sci USA 81: 1189-1192

11. Davis BM, McCurrach ME, Taneja KL, Singer RH, Housman DE (1997) Expansion of a CUG trinucleotide repeat in the 3′ untranslated region of myotonic dystrophy protein kinase transcripts results in nuclear retention of transcripts. Proc Natl Acad Sci USA 94: 7388-7393

12. de Die-Smulders CE, Howeler CJ, Thijs C, Mirandolle JF, Anten HB, Smeets HJ, Chandler KE, Geraedts JP (1998) Age and causes of death in adult-onset myotonic dystrophy. Brain 121: 1557-1563

13. Deka R, Majumder PP, Shriver MD, Stivers DN, Zhong Y, Yu LM, Barrantes R, Yin SJ, Miki T, Hundrieser J, Bunker CH, McGarvey ST, Sakallah S, Ferrell RE, Chakraborty R (1996) Distribution and evolution of CTG repeats at the myotonin protein kinase gene in human populations. Genome Res 6: 142-154

14. Dieler R, Schroder JM (1990) Lacunar dilatations of intrafusal and extrafusal terminal cisternae, annulate lamellae, confronting cisternae and tubulofilamentous inclusions within the spectrum of muscle and nerve fibre changes in myotonic dystrophy. Pathol Res Pract 186: 371-382

15. Eriksson M, Ansved T, Edstrom L, Anvret M, Carey N (1999) Simultaneous analysis of expression of the three myotonic dystrophy locus genes in adult skeletal muscle samples: the CTG expansion correlates inversely with DMPK and 59 expression levels, but not DMAHP levels. Hum Mol Genet 8: 1053-1060

16. Eriksson M, Ansved T, Edstrom L, Wells DJ, Watt DJ, Anvret M, Carey N (2000) Independent regulation of the myotonic dystrophy 1 locus genes postnatally and during adult skeletal muscle regeneration. J Biol Chem 275: 19964-19969

17. Franke C, Hatt H, Iaizzo PA, Lehmann-Horn F (1990) Characteristics of Na+ channels and Cl- conductance in resealed muscle fibre segments from patients with myotonic dystrophy. J Physiol 425: 391-405

18. Fu YH, Friedman DL, Richards S, Pearlman JA, Gibbs RA, Pizzuti A, Ashizawa T, Perryman MB, Scar-lato G, Fenwick RG, Jr., et al. (1993) Decreased expression of myotonin-protein kinase messenger RNA and protein in adult form of myotonic dystrophy. Science 260: 235-238

19. Hamshere MG, Newman EE, Alwazzan M, Athwal BS, Brook JD (1997) Transcriptional abnormality in myotonic dystrophy affects DMPK but not neighboring genes. Proc Natl Acad Sci USA 94: 7394-7399

20. Harper PS (1975) Congenital myotonic dystrophy in Britain. I. Clinical aspects. Arch Dis Child 50: 505-513

21. Harper PS (1989) Myotonic Dystrophy. W.B. Saunders Company: London

22. Howeler CJ, Busch HF, Geraedts JP, Niermeijer MF, Staal A (1989) Anticipation in myotonic dystrophy: fact or fiction? Brain 112: 779-797

23. Jansen G, Groenen PJ, Bachner D, Jap PH, Coerwinkel M, Oerlemans F, van den Broek W, Gohlsch B, Pette D, Plomp JJ, Molenaar PC, Nederhoff MG, van Echteld CJ, Dekker M, Berns A, Hameister H, Wieringa B (1996) Abnormal myotonic dystrophy protein kinase levels produce only mild myopathy in mice. Nat Genet 13: 316-324

24. Jansen G, Willems P, Coerwinkel M, Nillesen W, Smeets H, Vits L, Howeler C, Brunner H, Wieringa B (1994) Gonosomal mosaicism in myotonic dystrophy patients: involvement of mitotic events in (CTG)n repeat variation and selection against extreme expansion in sperm. Am J Hum Genet 54: 575-585

25. Karpati G, Carpenter S, Watters GV, Eisen AA, Andermann F (1973) Infantile myotonic dystrophy. Histochemical and electron microscopic features in skeletal muscle. Neurology 23: 1066-1077

26. Kennedy L, Shelbourne PF (2000) Dramatic mutation instability in HD mouse striatum: does polyglutamine load contribute to cell-specific vulnerability in Huntington's disease? Hum Mol Genet 9: 2539-2544

27. Klesert TR, Cho DH, Clark JI, Maylie J, Adelman J, Snider L, Yuen EC, Soriano P, Tapscott SJ (2000) Mice deficient in Six5 develop cataracts: implications for myotonic dystrophy. Nat Genet 25: 105-109

28. Klesert TR, Otten AD, Bird TD, Tapscott SJ (1997) Trinucleotide repeat expansion at the myotonic dystrophy locus reduces expression of DMAHP. Nat Genet 16: 402-406

29. Koob MD, Moseley ML, Schut LJ, Benzow KA, Bird TD, Day JW, Ranum LP (1999) An untranslated CTG expansion causes a novel form of spinocerebellar ataxia (SCA8). Nat Genet 21: 379-384

30. Kovtun IV, McMurray CT (2001) Trinucleotide expansion in haploid germ cells by gap repair. Nat Genet 27: 407-411

31. Kress W, Mueller-Myhsok B, Ricker K, Schneider C, Koch MC, Toyka KV, Mueller CR, Grimm T (2000) Proof of genetic heterogeneity in the proximal myotonic myopathy syndrome (PROMM) and its relationship to myotonic dystrophy type 2 (DM2). Neuromuscul Disord 10: 478-480

32. Lam LT, Pham YC, Nguyen TM, Morris GE (2000) Characterization of a monoclonal antibody panel shows that the myotonic dystrophy protein kinase, DMPK, is expressed almost exclusively in muscle and heart. Hum Mol Genet 9: 2167-2173

33. Maeda M, Taft CS, Bush EW, Holder E, Bailey WM, Neville H, Perryman MB, Bies RD (1995) Identification, tissue-specific expression, and subcellular localization of the 80- and 71-kDa forms of myotonic dystrophy kinase protein. J Biol Chem 270: 20246-20249

34. Mankodi A, Logigian E, Callahan L, McClain C, White R, Henderson D, Krym M, Thornton CA (2000) Myotonic dystrophy in transgenic mice expressing an expanded CUG repeat. Science 289: 1769-1773

35. Martorell L, Monckton DG, Gamez J, Johnson KJ, Gich I, de Munain AL, Baiget M (1998) Progression of somatic CTG repeat length heterogeneity in the blood cells of myotonic dystrophy patients. Hum Mol Genet 7: 307-312

36. McMurray CT (1999) DNA secondary structure: a common and causative factor for expansion in human disease. Proc Natl Acad Sci USA 96: 1823-1825

37. Michalowski S, Miller JW, Urbinati CR, Paliouras M, Swanson MS, Griffith J (1999) Visualization of double-stranded RNAs from the myotonic dystrophy protein kinase gene and interactions with CUG-binding protein. Nucleic Acids Res 27: 3534-3542

38. Miller JW, Urbinati CR, Teng-Umnuay P, Stenberg MG, Byrne BJ, Thornton CA, Swanson MS (2000) Recruitment of human muscleblind proteins to (CUG)(n) expansions associated with myotonic dystrophy. Embo J 19: 4439-4448

39. Mounsey JP, Mistry DJ, Ai CW, Reddy S, Moorman JR (2000) Skeletal muscle sodium channel gating in mice deficient in myotonic dystrophy protein kinase. Hum Mol Genet 9: 2313-2320

40. Mussini I, Di Mauro S, Angelini C (1970) Early ultrastructural and biochemical changes in muscle in dystrophia myotonica. J Neurol Sci 10: 585-604

41. Narang MA, Waring JD, Sabourin LA, Korneluk R (2000) Myotonic dystrophy (DM) protein kinase levels in congenital and adult DM patients. Eur J Hum Genet 8: 507-512

42. Ranum LP, Rasmussen PF, Benzow KA, Koob MD, Day JW (1998) Genetic mapping of a second myotonic dystrophy locus. Nat Genet 19: 196-198

43. Reardon W, Harley HG, Brook JD, Rundle SA, Crow S, Harper PS, Shaw DJ (1992) Minimal expression of myotonic dystrophy: a clinical and molecular analysis. J Med Genet 29: 770-773

44. Reardon W, Newcombe R, Fenton I, Sibert J, Harper PS (1993) The natural history of congenital myotonic dystrophy: mortality and long term clinical aspects. Arch Dis Child 68: 177-181

45. Reddy S, Smith DB, Rich MM, Leferovich JM, Reilly P, Davis BM, Tran K, Rayburn H, Bronson R, Cros D, Balice-Gordon RJ, Housman D (1996) Mice lacking the myotonic dystrophy protein kinase develop a late onset progressive myopathy. Nat Genet 13: 325-335

46. Ricker K, T. G, Koch MC, Schneider C, Kress W, Reimers C, Schulte-Mattler W, Mueller-Myhsok B, Toyka KV, Mueller CR (1998) Linkage to chromosome 3q in proximal myotonic myopathy (PROMM). Neurology 52: 170-171

47. Sarkar PS, Appukuttan B, Han J, Ito Y, Ai C, Tsai W, Chai Y, Stout JT, Reddy S (2000) Heterozygous loss of Six5 in mice is sufficient to cause ocular cataracts. *Nat Genet* 25: 110-114

48. Sarnat HB, Silbert SW (1976) Maturational arrest of fetal muscle in neonatal myotonic dystrophy. A pathologic study of four cases. *Arch Neurol* 33: 466-474

49. Shimokawa M, Ishiura S, Kameda N, Yamamoto M, Sasagawa N, Saitoh N, Sorimachi H, Ueda H, Ohno S, Suzuki K, Kobayashi T (1997) Novel isoform of myotonin protein kinase: gene product of myotonic dystrophy is localized in the sarcoplasmic reticulum of skeletal muscle. *Am J Pathol* 150: 1285-1295

50. Taneja KL, McCurrach M, Schalling M, Housman D, Singer RH (1995) Foci of trinucleotide repeat transcripts in nuclei of myotonic dystrophy cells and tissues. *J Cell Biol* 128: 995-1002

51. Thornton CA, Johnson K, Moxley RT, 3rd (1994) Myotonic dystrophy patients have larger CTG expansions in skeletal muscle than in leukocytes. *Ann Neurol* 35: 104-107

52. Thornton CA, Wymer JP, Simmons Z, McClain C, Moxley RT, 3rd (1997) Expansion of the myotonic dystrophy CTG repeat reduces expression of the flanking DMAHP gene. *Nat Genet* 16: 407-409

53. Tian B, White RJ, Xia T, Welle S, Turner DH, Mathews MB, Thornton CA (2000) Expanded CUG repeat RNAs form hairpins that activate the double-stranded RNA-dependent protein kinase PKR. *Rna* 6: 79-87

54. Timchenko LT, Miller JW, Timchenko NA, DeVore DR, Datar KV, Lin L, Roberts R, Caskey CT, Swanson MS (1996) Identification of a (CUG)n triplet repeat RNA-binding protein and its expression in myotonic dystrophy. *Nucleic Acids Res* 24: 4407-4414

55. Tohgi H, Kawamorita A, Utsugisawa K, Yamagata M, Sano M (1994) Muscle histopathology in myotonic dystrophy in relation to age and muscular weakness. *Muscle Nerve* 17: 1037-1043

56. Tome FM FM (2000) Nuclear changes in muscle disorders. *Meth Achiev Exp Pathol* 12: 261-296

57. Vassilopoulos D, Lumb EM (1980) Muscle nuclear changes in myotonic dystrophy. *Eur Neurol* 19: 237-240

58. Wang YH, Amirhaeri S, Kang S, Wells RD, Griffith JD (1994) Preferential nucleosome assembly at DNA triplet repeats from the myotonic dystrophy gene. *Science* 265: 669-671

59. Wong LJ, Ashizawa T, Monckton DG, Caskey CT, Richards CS (1995) Somatic heterogeneity of the CTG repeat in myotonic dystrophy is age and size dependent. *Am J Hum Genet* 56: 114-122

PABPN1 dysfunction in oculopharyngeal muscular dystrophy

Bernard Brais

CPSF	cleavage and polyadenylation specificity factor
CTD	c-terminal domains of PolII
INI	intranuclear inclusion
OPMD	oculopharyngeal muscular dystrophy
PABPN	poly(A) binding protein nuclear 1 gene
PAP	poly(A) polymerase
PolII	RNA polymerase II
RV	rimmed vacuole

Definition of entities

Autosomal dominant and recessive oculopharyngeal muscular dystrophy (OPMD) are both caused by short $(GCG)_n$ repeat expansions in the poly(A) binding protein nuclear 1 (*PABPN1*) gene (8). The autosomal dominant form is the most common. It causes a progressive eyelid ptosis and dysphagia, usually after the age of forty-five. Other muscle groups may become weak and develop pathological changes (7). The recessive OPMD clinical phenotype appears similar but with an older age of onset (8).

Dominant OPMD has a worldwide distribution. Cases have been described in more than 30 countries. The regional prevalences appear to be quite variable with higher frequencies in certain populations due to founder effects. The European prevalence may be in the 1 per 100 000 to 200 000 range based on French estimates (11). OPMD is particularly prevalent in the French-Canadian population of Québec (1:1000) and in the Bukhara Jew population living in Israel (1:600) (5, 10). The predicted prevalence of the recessive form is in the order of 1 per 10 000 in Québec, France, and Japan; however, only one confirmed case has been described to date (8).

Molecular genetics and pathophysiology

The OPMD locus maps to chromosome 14q11.1 (8, 10). The dominant form is a genetically homogeneous condition caused by short $(GCG)_{8-13}$

expansions of a $(GCG)_6$ stretch in the first exon of the *PABPN1* gene (previously abbreviated *PABP2*) (Figure 1) (8). The $(GCG)_n$ triplet repeat mutations are mitotically and meiotically stable. The study of 81 non-French-Canadians established the following percentage of families sharing the different six mutation sizes: 5% $(GCG)_8$, 40% $(GCG)_9$, 26% $(GCG)_{10}$, 21% $(GCG)_{11}$, 7% $(GCG)_{12}$, and 1% $(GCG)_{13}$. In the case of severe dominant OPMD cases, approximately 20% carry both a dominant mutation and a $(GCG)_7$ polymorphism in their other copy of the *PABPN1* gene (8). This polymorphism has 1 to 2% prevalence in Japan, North America, and Europe. OPMD compound heterozygotes have been diagnosed in many different countries (8, 17, 19). The molecular basis of autosomal recessive OPMD appears to be, at least in some cases, the double inheritance of the $(GCG)_7$ polymorphism (8). It is still unknown if the observed interfamilial phenotype variability depend on the differences in sizes of the $(GCG)_n$ mutations.

At the protein level, the OPMD mutations cause the lengthening of a predicted N-terminus polyalanine domain (Figure 1). PABPN1 is an abundant, mostly nuclear protein involved in the polyadenylation of all messenger RNAs (Figure 2) (25). The

biphasic polyadenylation process depends on many different proteins (Figure 2). The final rapid elongation of the poly(A) tails is dependent on the adjoining of PABPN1 to the polyadenylation complex. PABPN1 travels with the mRNA to the cytoplasm. The protein falls off when the mRNA is taken over by the translation machinery. PABPN1 is then actively transported back into the nuclei (12).

Polyalanine toxicity gain-of-function pathogenetic models, reminiscent of the ones put forward for CAG/polyQ triplet repeat diseases, have been proposed for OPMD (8, 9, 26). They are all based on the presumed altered physical properties of the expanded polyalanine PABPN1 domain. The abnormal physical characteristics are suggested to cause both PABPN1 accumulation and interfere with normal cellular processes. Different lines of evidence suggest that polyalanine oligomers form resistant macromolecules in vivo and in vitro (3, 15). PABPN1 molecules in OPMD muscle INI are indeed more resistant to salt extraction than the other proteins of the nucleoplasm (13). Various fusion proteins with long polyalanine domains accumulate as INI (16, 20). Lastly, the observation that proteins in the INIs are tagged with ubiquitin without being degraded strongly suggests that the misfolded mutated PABPN1 has acquired new

---

PABPN1 OPMD (GCG)$_n$ dominant mutations

ATG GCG GCG GCG GCG GCG GCG **(GCG)$_{2-7}$** GCA GCA GCA GCG

OPMD dominant expansions in the PABPN1 N terminus polyalanine domain

M A A A A A A A A A A **(A)$_{2-7}$** G A A G G R G S

Figure 1. Genomic *PABPN1* dominant mutations and polyalanine expansions of the homopolymeric polyalanine domain of the PABPN1 protein in OPMD.

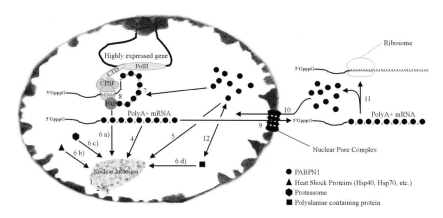

Figure 2. Cellular trafficking of PABPN1 and possible sites of interference of mutated PABPN1 with normal cellular processes. PABPN1 is involved in the polyadenylation of all messenger RNAs (7 and 8). PABPN1 travels with the mRNA to the cytoplasm through nuclear pores (9). It is released from the mRNA on the initiation of translation (11). It is actively transported back to the nucleus to partake in the polyadenylation of other mRNA molecules (10). Based on our understanding of the major role and cellular trafficking and breakdown of PABPN1, mutated forms could interfere with different cellular processes (1-12). Some interferences could be caused by intranuclear inclusion-dependent mechanisms: 1-Physical rupture of the nuclear membrane; 2-Disruption of transcriptional domains; 3-Disruption of chromosomal domains; 4-Sequestering of mRNAs coding for proteins vital for cell survival; 5-Sequestering of PABPN1 in sufficient quantity to interfere with normal mRNA processing; 6-Sequestering of other proteins: a-proteins interacting normally with PABPN1, b-proteins involved in protein folding (eg, chaperones such as Hsp70, Hsp40), c- proteins of the ubiquitin/proteasome pathway or d- other proteins with polyalanine domains. On the other hand, intranuclear inclusion-independent mechanisms could interfere with: 7- normal function of PABPN1 in mRNA polyadenylation; 8- the mRNA processing machinery; 9- PABPN1 and mRNA exit of the nucleus; 10- PABPN1 reimport in the nucleus; 11- the initiation of translation; 12- other soluble polyalanine containing proteins that interact with PABPN1. Abbreviations: PolII (RNA polymerase II); CTD (C-terminal domains of PolII); CPSF (cleavage and polyadenylation specificity factor); PAP (Poly(A) polymerase).

pathogenic physical characteristics (13).

We previously proposed that beyond 10 alanines, the normal number of alanines in PABPN1, the misfolded polyalanine domains polymerise to form stable β-sheets that are resistant to nuclear proteosomal degradation. The polyalanine macromolecules would grow with time to form the OPMD PABPN1-containing intranuclear filaments that are seen on electron microscopy (Figures 3A, B, E, F) (13, 22, 23). When a significant portion of PABPN1 molecules are aggregated in the intranuclear inclusions, this may sufficiently alter normal nuclear or cytoplasmic processes leading to cell death.

Figure 2 summarises in a graphic form the different possible mechanisms that could lead to cellular demise in OPMD. These mechanisms can be either intranuclear inclusion-dependent or inclusion-independent. Numbers on Figure 2 correspond to different mechanisms identified in the legend that could lead to cell death in OPMD.

Many of the suggested means by which mutated PABPN1 could interfere with cell function are dependent on its primary interaction with mRNA. The apparent accumulation of mRNA in the INI, as demonstrated by in situ hybridisation experiments with poly(T) probe, supports this possibility (Figures 3C and D) (13). However, based on the study of mRNA tail sizes in patients homozygotes for (GCG)$_9$ mutations, there does not appear to be any alteration in the PABPN1-dependent final elongation of the poly(A) tails (13). One could speculate that intranuclear mRNA trapping in the inclusions may interfere with the normal cellular traffic of vital poly(A) mRNA, in particular, in the context of an important cellular stress that would ultimately lead to cellular demise (13).

Structural changes

Light microscopy. Different skeletal muscles have been studied in OPMD. Variations in fibre diameter and the presence of atrophic angulated, hyper-

trophic, or segmented muscle fibres are observed (22). Necrotic fibres and ragged red fibres are rarely seen. Predominance of type 1 fibres is often observed, but fibre type grouping does not occur. Rimmed vacuoles (RV) and intranuclear inclusions (INI) are both characteristic of OPMD. Rimmed vacuoles are non-membrane bound and have irregular outlines. Their rimmed borders consist of dark staining material, which extends to the neighbouring cytoplasm. The content of RV is variable. They may contain cytoplasmic debris and myelin bodies. Collection of IBM-like filaments, 15 to 18 nm in diameter, are occasionally observed within the vacuoles and in the neighbouring cytoplasm (1, 18). Acid phosphatase activity is found in many vacuoles. RV are observed in all biopsies, but are usually not numerous. RV mean frequency in muscle fibres is in the order of 0.6% of fibres (range: 0.1-3.5%) (22).

Electron microscopy. The areas containing the INI may be detected on semi-thin sections of material prepared for electron microscopy and embedded in acrylic resins. The INI correspond to clearer zones surrounded by nucleoplasm. Studies of serial semi-thin sections show the presence of clear zones at different levels of most nuclei of the muscle fibres suggesting that all nuclei have inclusions (22, 23). OPMD intranuclear inclusions are formed by tubular filaments (Figure 3E, F).

The INI are about 8.5 nm in outer diameter, 3 nm in inner diameter, and up to 0.25 μm in length. They are often arranged in tangles or palisades. They are found exclusively within the nuclei of muscle fibres, never in the cytoplasm. They are not seen in the nuclei of either satellite cells or other cell types present in the biopsies. The INI replace the normal nuclear structure. They do not contain DNA (Figure 3B). Their size is very variable. In a given ultrathin section, the frequency of nuclei in which filaments inclusions were seen varied from 2% to 5% (mean: 4%) in heterozygote patients.

The percentage of nuclei contaibing INIs appears to be variable between muscles. In the same patient, the INI were found to be present in 8% of nuclei of the more affected cricothyroid pharyngeal compared to 4% in the deltoid muscle (14).

Genotype–phenotype correlations

Gene dosage has a clear influence on the age of onset and severity of the OPMD phenotype (8). The most severe OPMD phenotype is reported for individuals homozygous for a dominant OPMD mutation (4, 6, 8). The study of 4 French-Canadian and 3 Bukhara Jewish OPMD homozygotes documented that on average the onset was 18 years earlier than in $(GCG)_9$ heterozygotes (4). These cases have twice as many muscle nuclei containing intranuclear inclusions than heterozygotes (9.4% vs 4.9%, $p < 0.02$). Severity of the dominant OPMD phenotype is also variable (7). Approximately 20% of these severe cases are compound heterozygotes for the dominant mutation and a $(GCG)_7$ polymorphism in their other copy of the *PABPN1* gene (8). The more severe phenotypes observed in homozygotes and compound heterozygotes for a dominant and a recessive mutation suggest a clear gene dosage effect (4, 8, 9).

At the structural level, the identification of the mutated gene in OPMD has rekindled the efforts to find which proteins are present in the INI. Mutated PABPN1 molecules are an integral part of the OPMD inclusions (2, 13, 24). Using both immunoelectron microscopy and fluorescence confocal microscopy, the OPMD-specific nuclear inclusions are shown in Figure 3A to decorated by anti-PABPN1 antibodies (13). In addition, the inclusions are also recognised by antibodies directed against ubiquitin and proteasomal subunits. This suggests that the polyalanine expansions in PABPN1 induce misfolding and aggregation of ubiquitin-tagged proteins that cells are not able to breakdown through the proteosome machinery. As discussed previously, the nuclear inclusions also

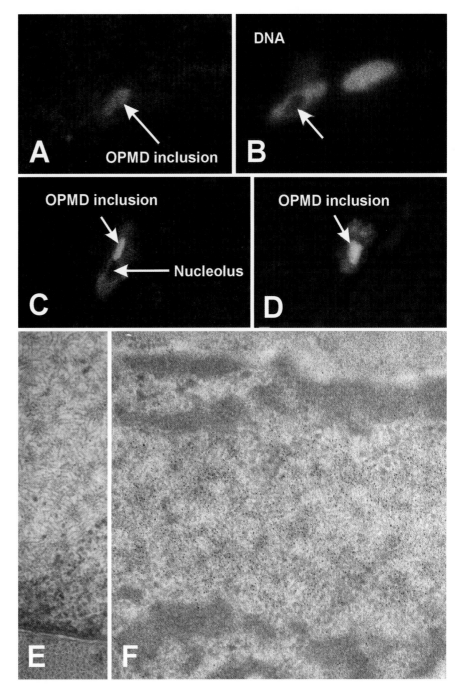

Figure 3. A. The OPMD inclusions contain insoluble PABPN1. Cryostat sections of the deltoid muscle from OPMD patients were treated with 1 M potassium chloride in HPEM buffer for 5 min, at room temperature. Then, the sections were fixed in formaldehyde and immuno-labeled using anti-PABPN1 antibodies. **B**. Nuclei are counterstained with To-Pro, which reveals double-stranded DNA. Note that the PABPN1 protein in the OPMD inclusion resists the salt treatment (arrow), whereas the nucleoplasmic PABPN1 in a nucleus with no detectable inclusion is completely solubilized (arrowhead). **C**. The OPMD inclusions contain poly(A) RNA. Cryostat sections of the deltoid muscle from OPMD patients were hybridized with riboprobes complementary to either the poly(A) tail of mRNA (green staining) or To-Pro (red, C) that shows that DNA is predominantly excluded from the OPMD inclusion and the nucleolus **D**. Shows that the anti-PABPN1 co-localizes with poly(A) RNA in the OPMD inclusions. **E** and **F**. Immunoelectron microscopy of PABPN1 in OPMD nuclei. Biopsy from deltoid muscle from an OPMD patient, aged 60 years. Subsarcolemmal nuclei contain inclusions that consist of unique filaments. These filaments converge to form tangles or palisades, distinctly seen on sections taken from muscle specimens prepared according to standard electron microscopic techniques (**E**). Using anti-PABPN1 antibodies, the filaments are decorated by immuno-gold particles. The labelling is particularly intense at sites of filament convergence (**F**). Theses figures were first published in *Human Molecular Genetics* (13).

sequester poly(A) mRNA (Figure 3C, D) (13).

Future perspectives

The identification of the (GCG)$_n$ *PABPN1* mutations responsible for OPMD has set the stage to the development of cellular and transgenic models of this dystrophy. These will no doubt lead to a greater understanding of its pathophysiology. The demonstration that INI can readily be produced by transfection is very suggestive that overexpression of the mutated protein in different models will produce at least a pathological phenotype reminiscent of OPMD (21). One of the key questions will be to determine if cell death is inclusion-dependent. This issue is not only important in OPMD, but also for CAG/polyQ repeat diseases (26).

The possible role of protein misfolding in OPMD pathogenesis begs the question of finding ways to improve this process in a therapeutic perspective. Considering that PABPN1 is a highly and ubiquitously expressed gene, the perplexing observations of the late onset and relative selectivity of the muscle involvement in OPMD also need to be explained. The importance of studying the pathophysiology of OPMD is further underlined by the fact that at least five other diseases are also caused by the lengthening of polyalanine tracts: synpolydactily, cleidocranial dysplasia, familial holoprosencephaly, hand-foot-genital syndrome and blepharophimosis/ptosis/epicanthus inversus syndrome type II. Lastly, in the field of neuromuscular disorders, the pathological overlap between OPMD and IBM raises the possibility that the latter may also turn out to be a "polyalanine disease."

References

1. Askanas V, Serdaroglu P, Engel WK, Alvarez RB (1991) Immunolocalization of ubiquitin in muscle biopsies of patients with inclusion body myositis and oculopharyngeal muscular dystrophy. *Neurosci Lett* 130: 73-76

2. Becher MW, Kotzuk JA, Davis LE, Bear DG (2000) Intranuclear inclusions in oculopharyngeal muscular dystrophy contain poly(A) binding protein 2. *Ann Neurol* 48: 812-815

3. Blondelle SE, Forood B, Houghten RA, Perez-Paya E (1997) Polyalanine-based peptides as models for self-associated beta-pleated- sheet complexes. *Biochemistry* 36: 8393-8400

4. Blumen SC, Brais B, Korczyn AD, Medinsky S, Chapman J, Asherov A, Nisipeanu P, Codere F, Bouchard JP, Fardeau M, Tome FM, Rouleau GA (1999) Homozygotes for oculopharyngeal muscular dystrophy have a severe form of the disease. *Ann Neurol* 46: 115-118

5. Blumen SC, Nisipeanu P, Sadeh M, Asherov A, Blumen N, Wirguin Y, Khilkevich O, Carasso RL, Korczyn AD (1997) Epidemiology and inheritance of oculopharyngeal muscular dystrophy in Israel. *Neuromuscul Disord* 7 Suppl 1: S38-40

6. Blumen SC, Sadeh M, Korczyn AD, Rouche A, Nisipeanu P, Asherov A, Tome FM (1996) Intranuclear inclusions in oculopharyngeal muscular dystrophy among Bukhara Jews. *Neurology* 46: 1324-1328.

7. Bouchard JP, Brais B, Brunet D, Gould PV, Rouleau GA (1997) Recent studies on oculopharyngeal muscular dystrophy in Quebec. *Neuromuscul Disord* 7 Suppl 1: S22-29

8. Brais B, Bouchard JP, Xie YG, Rochefort DL, Chretien N, Tome FM, Lafreniere RG, Rommens JM, Uyama E, Nohira O, Blumen S, Korczyn AD, Heutink P, Mathieu J, Duranceau A, Codere F, Fardeau M, Rouleau GA, Korcyn AD (1998) Short GCG expansions in the PABP2 gene cause oculopharyngeal muscular dystrophy. *Nat Genet* 18: 164-167

9. Brais B, Rouleau GA, Bouchard JP, Fardeau M, Tome FM (1999) Oculopharyngeal muscular dystrophy. *Semin Neurol* 19: 59-66

10. Brais B, Xie YG, Sanson M, Morgan K, Weissenbach J, Korczyn AD, Blumen SC, Fardeau M, Tome FM, Bouchard JP, et al. (1995) The oculopharyngeal muscular dystrophy locus maps to the region of the cardiac alpha and beta myosin heavy chain genes on chromosome 14q11.2- q13. *Hum Mol Genet* 4: 429-434

11. Brunet G, Tome FM, Eymard B, Robert JM, Fardeau M (1997) Genealogical study of oculopharyngeal muscular dystrophy in France. *Neuromuscul Disord* 7 Suppl 1: S34-37

12. Calado A, Kutay U, Kuhn U, Wahle E, Carmo-Fonseca M (2000a) Deciphering the cellular pathway for transport of poly(A)-binding protein II. *RNA* 6: 245-256

13. Calado A, Tome FM, Brais B, Rouleau GA, Kuhn U, Wahle E, Carmo-Fonseca M (2000b) Nuclear inclusions in oculopharyngeal muscular dystrophy consist of poly(A) binding protein 2 aggregates which sequester poly(A) RNA. *Hum Mol Genet* 9: 2321-2328

14. Coquet M, Vital C, Julien J (1990) Presence of inclusion body myositis-like filaments in oculopharyngeal muscular dystrophy. Ultrastructural study of 10 cases. *Neuropathol Appl Neurobiol* 16: 393-400

15. Forood B, Perez-Paya E, Houghten RA, Blondelle SE (1995) Formation of an extremely stable polyalanine beta-sheet macromolecule. *Biochem Biophys Res Commun* 211: 7-13

16. Gaspar C, Jannatipour M, Dion P, Laganiere J, Sequeiros J, Brais B, Rouleau GA (2000) CAG tract of MJD-1 may be prone to frameshifts causing polyalanine accumulation. *Hum Mol Genet* 9: 1957-1966

17. Hill ME, Creed GA, McMullan TF, Tyers AG, Hilton-Jones D, Robinson DO, Hammans SR (2001) Oculopharyngeal muscular dystrophy: phenotypic and genotypic studies in a UK population. *Brain* 124: 522-526

18. Leclerc A, Tome FM, Fardeau M (1993) Ubiquitin and beta-amyloid-protein in inclusion body myositis (IBM), familial IBM-like disorder and oculopharyngeal muscular dystrophy: an immunocytochemical study. *Neuromuscl Disord* 3: 283-291

19. Mirabella M, Silvestri G, de Rosa G, Di Giovanni S, Di Muzio A, Uncini A, Tonali P, Servidei S (2000) GCG genetic expansions in Italian patients with oculopharyngeal muscular dystrophy. *Neurology* 54: 608-614

20. Rankin J, Wyttenbach A, Rubinsztein DC (2000) Intracellular green fluorescent protein-polyalanine aggregates are associated with cell death. *Biochem J* 348 Pt 1: 15-19

21. Shanmugam V, Dion P, Rochefort D, Laganiere J, Brais B, Rouleau GA (2000) PABP2 polyalanine tract expansion causes intranuclear inclusions in oculopharyngeal muscular dystrophy. *Ann Neurol* 48: 798-802

22. Tomé FM, Chateau D, Helbling-Leclerc A, Fardeau M (1997) Morphological changes in muscle fibers in oculopharyngeal muscular dystrophy. *Neuromuscul Disord* 7 Suppl 1: S63-69

23. Tomé FM, Fardeau M (1980) Nuclear inclusions in oculopharyngeal dystrophy. *Acta Neuropathol* 49: 85-87

24. Uyama E, Tsukahara T, Goto K, Kurano Y, Ogawa M, Kim YJ, Uchino M, Arahata K (2000) Nuclear accumulation of expanded PABP2 gene product in oculopharyngeal muscular dystrophy. *Muscle Nerve* 23: 1549-1554

25. Wahle E, Ruegsegger U (1999) 3'-End processing of pre-mRNA in eukaryotes. *FEMS Microbiol Rev* 23: 277-295

26. Zoghbi HY, Orr HT (2000) Glutamine repeats and neurodegeneration. *Annu Rev Neurosci* 23: 217-247

Large telomeric deletion disease
Facioscapulohumeral dystrophy

George W. Padberg

FRG1	FSHD region gene 1
FSHD	facioscapulohumeral muscular dystrophy

Definition of entities

Recent advances in the molecular analysis of facioscapulohumeral muscular dystrophy (FSHD) have brought to light some unusual mechanisms regarding the pathogenesis of this autosomal dominant myopathy. A high rate of mutation, often somatic in origin, leads to a deletion of an integral number of 3.3 kb D4Z4 repeat units in the subtelomeric region of chromosome 4q. As these repeats do not yield transcripts, the deletion is assumed to cause position effect variegation and a variable, muscle specific dysregulation of transcription.

The prevalence of FSHD is estimated 1 in 20000 (2, 16) and fitness was calculated 0.8 if sporadic cases were included (32).

Neuromuscular features. When Landouzy and Dejerine (12) described the disease for the first time, they emphasized its familial nature and the onset in facial and shoulder girdle muscles in order to discriminate FSHD from Duchenne muscular dystrophy. In subsequent discussions facial muscle involvement has always been considered a classifying requisite, particularly since the mode of inheritance has been uncertain until recently.

Most patients note shoulder girdle weakness as the first symptom of FSHD; a minority presents with foot-extensor weakness. Facial muscle involvement, often mild and asymmetrical, and frequently not recognized by the patients, can be demonstrated in the majority of cases (16, 17).

The disease progresses with varying rates, usually to abdominal and foot-extensor muscles first, and then to upper-arm and pelvic-girdle muscles. In contrast to other neuromuscular diseases, shoulder weakness is often asymmetrical with relative sparing of the deltoid muscles. This clinical pattern is recognized in retrospect by most patients. The descending course of muscle involvement has been related to a diseased replay of ontogeny inspired by the presence of two homeodomains in each deleted repeat unit.

A number of patients have mild cardiac conduction defects, such as a bundle branch block, which are of questionable significance (19). Severe conduction defects at an early age have very rarely been found and related to FSHD (11).

Non-muscular features. When present, scoliosis is often mild. Contractures are unusual with exception of ankle contractures. Pectus excavatum occurs with higher incidence (5%) than in the normal population (16). Occasionally, a subclinical high tone hearing-loss is part of the disease, particularly in infantile onset cases necessitating hearing aids (4). In addition, a subclinical retinal vasculopathy with teleangiectases and capillary microaneurysms demonstrable by fluorescein angiography is frequently present. Directly visible small exudates and haemorrhages are rare and large exudates and haemorrhages resembling Coats' disease occur in less than 1% of the cases (6, 18).

Age at onset and clinical course. Symptoms start on average at age 16 in males and 20 in females, but onset may vary from the first to the sixth decade. In fully examined families, a large number of gene carriers (25-30%) have signs but no complaints of muscle dysfunction. These cases represent the mild end of a clinical spectrum with little or no progression of the disease over years. Within families, the course of the disease may vary considerably. A severe course is most often seen in early onset cases. These cases frequently have large $D_4 Z_4$ deletions. Therefore, a rough correlation exists between size of the deletion, age at onset and rate of progression (18).

Unusual phenotypes. Recently, attention has been drawn to cases with presenting signs of pelvic-girdle weakness and clinical diagnosis as limb-girdle syndromes. Facial weakness and DNA-tests led to the diagnosis of FSHD (23). The rare occurrence of FSHD without facial weakness has also been reported (5).

The infantile form of FSHD was once considered a separate entity because of deafness and retinal vascular disease, but it turned out to be the severe end of the clinical spectrum of FSHD, almost always having large deletions. We found minimally affected parents of many of such cases to be somatic mosaics (24). Epilepsy, mental retardation, and lingual abnormalities have been described in Japanese patients with infantile FSHD (15).

Molecular genetics and pathophysiology

Mode of inheritance. FHSD inherits solely in an autosomal dominant pattern. Sporadic cases, ie, patients without affected first degree relatives, are new mutations and multiple affected sibs of non-affected parents are the result of germ-line mosaicism (10). At least 10% of all living patients are new mutations (18, 32) and more than 45% of these represent somatic mutations (24).

Influence of sex. In completely examined families, more females (40%) than males (20%) tend to be

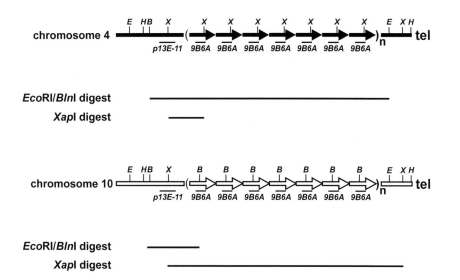

Figure 1. BlnI restriction sites in the chromosome 10 specific repeats and the XapI restriction sites in the chromosome 4 specific repeats in the EcoRI fragments demonstrated by p13E-11, which allow correct indentification of small alleles (<40 kb) in a linear gel.

asymptomatic, and above 30 years a much larger percentage of females (35%) than males (10%) remains asymptomatic. In symptomatic patients, onset of symptoms is later and progression to foot-extensor weakness slower in females than in males (16). Similar observations have been made by others (31). Anecdotal reports of post-menopausal deterioration are in need of a formal study.

Penetrance. Within a family, facial weakness is often the earliest sign with which to make a reliable diagnosis; mild shoulder muscle involvement in FSHD is difficult to detect at an early age. Therefore, penetrance based on clinical examination of persons at risk is age dependent with estimates of 21% for ages 5 to 9, 58% for ages 10 to 14, 86% for ages 15 to 19, and 95% for age 20 years and older (14). Non-penetrance is estimated to be less than 2% after age 50.

Linkage studies. In 1990 linkage was found with markers on 4q35 (29). Probe p13E-11 was subsequently isolated, demonstrating deleted EcoRI fragments causally related to FSHD (30). With probe p13E-11, polymorphic loci on 4q35 and 10q26 can be demonstrated and an invariable locus

(9.5 kb) on the Y- chromosome. In controls the 4q35 fragment varies in size from 35 to 300 kb and contains 11 or more $D_4 Z_4$ repeat units, each of 3.3 kb. In patients this EcoRI fragment is reduced to fewer than 11 repeats by deletion of an integral number of these repeats. The 10q26 locus contains almost identical repeats, and fragment length varies from 15 to more than 200 kb according to the number of repeats. Ten percent of 10q26 fragments are smaller than 35kb, but they do not cause disease; only small fragments on 4q35 are related to FSHD.

Each repeat unit contains hhspm3 and Lsau elements, and two homeodomains. Although the latter reside within a putative open reading frame of 405 bp, no transcript has been obtained in vivo (7). This supported the hypothesis of position effect variegation, and stimulated the search for proximally located genes, as the 25 kb distal to the telomere appeared to be void of genes. Three genes have been identified so far: FRG1 (FSHD-Region-Gene 1) at 100 kb from p13E-11, TUBB4Q at 80 kb, and FRG2 at 37 kb. Based on genetic studies, TUBB4Q is most likely a pseudogene related to the beta-Tubulin gene family (27). Moreover, RT-PCR on patient and control muscles failed to detect TUBB4Q expression.

FRG1 consists of 9 exons, producing a 1042 bp long transcript coding for a protein of 258 amino acids. Allele-specific transcript levels were not altered in FSHD muscles compared to controls (25, 26). The FRG1 protein localizes to the nucleolus and Cajal bodies suggesting a role in RNA processing, but precise functions are not known. Similarly FRG2 function is unknown although its sequence suggests it to be a nuclear protein. FRG2 could be detected in differentiating myoblasts of FSHD patients but not in whole muscle of patients or controls.

RNA subtractive hybridization using normal and FSHD deltoid muscles demonstrated 74 unknown and 34 known, up- or downregulated genes among which genes for structural proteins, regulatory factors, and mitochondrial proteins (22). Similar observations have been made at the protein level. The relationship to the 4q35 repeat deletions is still obscure.

DNA diagnosis. The analysis of the p13E-11 fragments was seriously hampered by the inability to discriminate their chromosomal origins until it was found that the 10q26 repeats harbour BlnI restriction sites. Double digestion of DNA with EcoRI and BlnI leaves chromosome 4 related fragments only (22). We recently demonstrated XapI restriction sites in the 4q35 repeats. XapI digestion shows only chromosome 10 related fragments (13). These findings enable proper identification of the smaller alleles in a standard linear gel in the majority of cases, and identify in the remaining cases the need for pulsed field gel electrophoresis, which allows visualisation of all alleles and also demonstrates the rare occurrence of a p13E-11 deletion (Figure 1). This research has led to the observation of interchromosal exchange of 4q and 10q repeat arrays: in 10% of the normal population BlnI sensitive repeat arrays reside on 10q26 and in another 10% the reverse is present (25, 26). An independent second study confirmed these figures, and in addition, demonstrated that more than 25% of these exchanged repeat arrays are hybrids of 4 and 10 type repeats. These inter- and intra-chromosomal rearrangements make great demands on the quality of DNA-testing (28).

Locus heterogeneity. Worldwide, only a couple of large families have been found not to be linked to 4q35 (8). Small families with a characteristic FSHD phenotype and without an EcoRI/p13E-11 fragment smaller than 38 kb are occasionally observed. Despite an intensive search, no second locus has been found so far.

Mutational mechanism. Studies of the mutations in sporadic cases initially suggested a high frequency of somatic mosaicism in the non-affected mothers of these patients. Full characterization of all alleles in sporadic patients and their parents demonstrated that in males somatic mosaïcism often manifests as a mild or moderate phenotype. Manifestation of FSHD in somatic mosaïcs was found to depend on gender, size of the deletion and percentage of mosaïcism in peripheral blood-leukocytes (24). A number of mosaïcs carried a 4q-type repeat on 10q suggesting this "trisomic state" as a possible premutation. With careful typing of all 4 alleles, a somatic mutational mechanism can be implicated in at least 50% of all de novo FSHD cases. This mechanism might be related to the nuclear chromatid alignement during mitosis (20).

Structural changes

Muscle morphology offers no features characteristic for FSHD. Necrotic and regenerating fibres are present in low frequencies. Small angulated fetal myosin positive fibers and moth-eaten fibres can be found (3). Cellular infiltrates are not rare and are part of the histological picture (1). These infiltrates are HLA-ABC negative and their immunological nature remains obscure. At present we do muscle biopsies only in cases with negative DNA tests to rule in or out the various disorders of the FSH-syndrome.

Future perspectives and therapy

Surgical therapies have so far been applied on a small scale in FSHD for ankle contractures, scoliosis, pectus excavatum, and scapula alata. Prednisone 1.5 mg/kg/dag was tested on 8 patients in a open label study of 12 weeks duration and was found to induce no significant changes in strength or muscle mass (21). Subsequently, albuterol 8 mg/bid was tested in a pilot study of 3 months in 15 patients because of the anabolic effect of beta-2-adrenergic agonists on muscle mass and muscle strength in normal controls (9). A small improvement in strength was found, leading to 2 randomized trials which will be reported soon.

References

1. Arahata K, Ishihara T, Fukunaga H, Orimo S, Lee JH, Goto K, Nonaka I (1995) Inflammatory response in Facioscapulohumeral Muscular Dystrophy (FSHD): immunocytochemical and genetic analyses. *Muscle & Nerve* 2: S56-S66

2. Becker PE (1953) *Dystrophia Musculorum Progressiva. A genetic and clinical investigation muscle dystrophieen.* Georg Thieme Verlag: Stuttgart.

3. Bethlem J, van Wijngaarden GK, de Jong J (1973) The incidence of lobulated fibres in the facioscapulohumeral type of muscular dystrophy and the limb-girdle syndrome. *J Neurol Sci* 18: 351-358

4. Brouwer OF, Padberg GW, Ruys CJ, Brand R, de Laat JA, Grote JJ (1991) Hearing loss in facioscapulohumeral muscular dystrophy. *Neurology* 41: 1878-1881

5. Felice KJ, Moore D, Moore SA (2001) Unusual clinical presentations in patients harboring the facioscapulohumeral dystrophy 4q35 deletion. *Muscle & Nerve* 24: 352-356

6. Fitzsimons RB, Gurwin EB, Bird AC (1987) Retinal vascular abnormalities in facioscapulohumeral muscular dystrophy. A general association with genetic and therapeutic implications. *Brain* 110: 631-648

7. Gabriels J, Beckers MC, Ding H, De Vriese A, Plaisance S, van der Maarel SM, Padberg GW, Frants RR, Hewitt JE, Collen D, Belayew A (1999) Nucleotide sequence of the partially deleted D4Z4 locus in a patient with FSHD identifies a putative gene within each 3.3 kb element. *Gene* 236: 25-32

8. Gilbert JR, Stajich JM, Wall S, Carter SC, Qiu H, Vance JM, Stewart CS, Speer MC, Pufky J, Yamaoka LH, et al. (1993) Evidence for heterogeneity in facioscapulohumeral muscular dystrophy (FSHD). *Am J Hum Genet* 53: 401-408

9. Kissel JT, McDermott MP, Natarajan R, Mendell JR, Pandya S, King WM, Griggs RC, Tawil R (1998) Pilot trial of albuterol in facioscapulohumeral muscular dystrophy. FSH- DY Group. *Neurology* 50: 1402-1406

10. Kohler J, Rupilius B, Otto M, Bathke K, Koch MC (1996) Germline mosaicism in 4q35 facioscapulohumeral muscular dystrophy (FSHD1A) occurring predominantly in oogenesis. *Hum Genet* 98: 485-490

11. Laforet P, de Toma C, Eymard B, Becane HM, Jeanpierre M, Fardeau M, Duboc D (1998) Cardiac involvement in genetically confirmed facioscapulohumeral muscular dystrophy. *Neurology* 51: 1454-1456

12. Landouzy L, Dejerine J (1885) De la myopathie atrophique progressive. *Revue de Médicine* 5: 81-117, 253-366

13. Lemmers RJLF, van Geel M, de Kievit P, van der Wielen MJR, Bakker E, Padberg GW, Frants RR, van der Maarel SM (2001) Complete allele information in diagnosis of facioscapulohumeral muscular dystrophy (FSHD) by triple DNA analysis. in press

14. Lunt PW, Compston DA, Harper PS (1989) Estimation of age dependent penetrance in facioscapulohumeral muscular dystrophy by minimising ascertainment bias. *J Med Genet* 26: 755-760

15. Miura K, Kumagai T, Matsumoto A, Iriyama E, Watanabe K, Goto K, Arahata K (1998) Two cases of chromosome 4q35-linked early onset facioscapulohumeral muscular dystrophy with mental retardation and epilepsy. *Neuropediatrics* 29: 239-241

16. Padberg GW. 1982. *Facioscapulohumeral disease.* Leiden, Leiden

17. Padberg GW (1998) Facioscapulohumeral Muscular Dystrophy. In *Neuromuscular Disorders: clinical and molecular genetics,* E A.E.H. (eds). John Wiley and Sons: Chichester, New York, Weinheim, Brisbane, Singapore. pp. 105-118

18. Padberg GW, Brouwer OF, de Keizer RJ, Dijkman G, Wijmenga C, Grote JJ, Frants RR (1995) On the significance of retinal vascular disease and hearing loss in facioscapulohumeral muscular dystrophy. *Muscle Nerve* 2: S73-80

19. Stevenson WG, Perloff JK, Weiss JN, Anderson TL (1990) Facioscapulohumeral muscular dystrophy: evidence for selective, genetic electrophysiologic cardiac involvement. *J Am Coll Cardiol* 15: 292-299

20. Stout K, van der Maarel S, Frants RR, Padberg GW, Ropers HH, Haaf T (1999) Somatic pairing between subtelomeric chromosome regions: implications for human genetic disease? *Chromosome Res* 7: 323-329

21. Tawil R, McDermott MP, Pandya S, King W, Kissel J, Mendell JR, Griggs RC (1997) A pilot trial of prednisone in facioscapulohumeral muscular dystrophy. FSH-DY Group. *Neurology* 48: 46-49

22. Tupler R, Perini G, Pellegrino MA, Green MR (1999) Profound misregulation of muscle-specific gene expression in facioscapulohumeral muscular dystrophy. *Proc Natl Acad Sci U S A* 96: 12650-12654

23. Van der Kooi AJ, Visser MC, Rosenberg N, van den Berg-Vos R, Wokke JH, Felice KJ, North WA, Moore SA, Mathews KD (2000) FSH dystrophy 4q35 deletion in patients presenting with facial-sparing myopathy. *Neurology* 54: 1927-1931

24. van der Maarel SM, Deidda G, Lemmers RJ, van Overveld PG, van der Wielen M, Hewitt JE, Sandkuijl L, Bakker B, van Ommen GJ, Padberg GW, Frants RR

(2000) De novo facioscapulohumeral muscular dystrophy: frequent somatic mosaicism, sex-dependent phenotype, and the role of mitotic transchromosomal repeat interaction between chromosomes 4 and 10. *Am J Hum Genet* 66: 26-35

25. van Deutekom JC, Bakker E, Lemmers RJ, van der Wielen MJ, Bik E, Hofker MH, Padberg GW, Frants RR (1996) Evidence for subtelomeric exchange of 3.3 kb tandemly repeated units between chromosomes 4q35 and 10q26: implications for genetic counselling and etiology of FSHD1. *Hum Mol Genet* 5: 1997-2003

26. van Deutekom JC, Lemmers RJ, Grewal PK, van Geel M, Romberg S, Dauwerse HG, Wright TJ, Padberg GW, Hofker MH, Hewitt JE, Frants RR (1996) Identification of the first gene (FRG1) from the FSHD region on human chromosome 4q35. *Hum Mol Genet* 5: 581-590

27. van Geel M, van Deutekom JC, van Staalduinen A, Lemmers RJ, Dickson MC, Hofker MH, Padberg GW, Hewitt JE, de Jong PJ, Frants RR (2000) Identification of a novel beta-tubulin subfamily with one member (TUBB4Q) located near the telomere of chromosome region 4q35. *Cytogenet Cell Genet* 88: 316-321

28. van Overveld PG, Lemmers RJ, Deidda G, Sandkuijl L, Padberg GW, Frants RR, van der Maarel SM (2000) Interchromosomal repeat array interactions between chromosomes 4 and 10: a model for subtelomeric plasticity. *Hum Mol Genet* 9: 2879-2884

29. Wijmenga C, Frants RR, Brouwer OF, Moerer P, Weber JL, Padberg GW (1990) Location of facioscapulohumeral muscular dystrophy gene on chromosome 4. *Lancet* 336: 651-653

30. Wijmenga C, Hewitt JE, Sandkuijl LA, Clark LN, Wright TJ, Dauwerse HG, Gruter AM, Hofker MH, Moerer P, Williamson R, et al. (1992) Chromosome 4q DNA rearrangements associated with facioscapulohumeral muscular dystrophy. *Nat Genet* 2: 26-30

31. Zatz M, Marie SK, Cerqueira A, Vainzof M, Pavanello RC, Passos-Bueno MR (1998) The facioscapulohumeral muscular dystrophy (FSHD1) gene affects males more severely and more frequently than females. *Am J Med Genet* 77: 155-161

32. Zatz M, Marie SK, Passos-Bueno MR, Vainzof M, Campiotto S, Cerqueira A, Wijmenga C, Padberg G, Frants R (1995) High proportion of new mutations and possible anticipation in Brazilian facioscapulohumeral muscular dystrophy families. *Am J Hum Genet* 56: 99-105

CHAPTER 7

Developmental disorders of skeletal muscle

7.1 X-linked myotubular myopathy   124
7.2 Congenital fibre type disproportion   130

A great deal of new knowledge has accumulated about the molecular factors and events operating in the embryonic development and growth of skeletal muscle fibres. The most notable of these has been the identification of the nature and activation pattern of muscle specific transcription factors. Experimental perturbations of these molecules in experimental models (simple or combined gene inactivation or overexpression) have produced interesting phenotypes and clarified many aspects of muscle fibre differentiation. However, human skeletal muscle disease has not yet been linked to these molecules.

In this chapter, we have included entities in which a defect of differentiation (general or fibre type specific) or growth of muscle fibres seems to occur.

X-linked myotubular myopathy

Jean-Louis Mandel
Jocelyn Laporte
Anna Buj-Bello
Caroline Sewry
Carina Wallgren-Pettersson

CMT4B	Charcot-Marie-Tooth neuropathy
DM	myotonic dystrophy
PI3P	phosphatidylinositol 3 phosphate
PH	pleckstrin homology
PTP	protein tyrosine phosphatase
SID	SET interacting domain
VPS	vacuolar protein sorting
XLMTM	X-linked myotubular myopathy

Definition of entity

X-linked myotubular myopathy (XLMTM) is a severe congenital myopathy often presenting in the foetal period with polyhydramnios and weak or infrequent movements. Miscarriages and premature birth are common. The floppy male infants have global muscle weakness; many lack spontaneous anti-gravity movements at birth, and some fail to establish spontaneous respiration. Many have feeding difficulties and ophthalmoplegia, and some have contractures of the hips and knees. The disease name was assigned because of the histological resemblance of the patients' muscle fibres to foetal myotubes (34). The causative gene encodes a phosphatase named myo-tubularin (27). The incidence of XLMTM was estimated to be around 1 in 50 000 live-born male infants (Bian-calana and Mandel, unpublished data). For diagnostic criteria see Wallgren-Pettersson and Thomas (45), for a clinical review Wallgren-Pettersson et al (44).

While the cause of death in most affected neonates is from respiratory insufficiency within the first year of life (10), even patients with a very severe neonatal form can survive longer (7, 18, 40, 44). A few mildly affected patients with documented mutations in the *MTM1* gene were alive at ages of 54 (2) and even 65 years (Biancalana et al, unpublished data). The disorder appears non-progressive in long-term survivors (2, 18), and there may even be some improvement

after the neonatal period. Other medical problems may also be associated with XLMTM, such as life-threatening hepatic peliosis (18).

Recent studies indicate that some female carriers of mutations in the myotubularin gene may manifest muscle weakness (14, 35, 43). In at least some of these carriers, the manifestations appear to be caused by skewed X-inactivation (9, 35).

In addition to the X-linked form, a usually less severe autosomal recessive form and a comparatively mild autosomal dominant form have been described, but the corresponding loci have not yet been mapped. An important differential diagnosis is congenital myotonic dystrophy (DM), which can present with similar clinical and morphological features (chapter 6.1.1). This can be excluded by analysis of the CTG repeat at the DM locus.

Molecular genetics and pathophysiology

The MTM1 gene and the myotubularin protein. The gene for XLMTM was assigned to Xq28 by linkage analysis (38, 39). The candidate region was narrowed down by studies of three patients with deletions (9, 19) and the *MTM1* gene was isolated by positional cloning (27). The *MTM1* gene (Figure 1) was found mutated in most of the patients referred for testing (11, 23, 26, 28, 36). An initial claim of genetic heterogeneity in one family with XLMTM was later discounted, as this family was found to have an *MTM1* mutation (13, 29).

The *MTM1* gene is transcribed in all tissues, as indicated by the ubiquitous presence of a 4.0 Kb mRNA. A smaller alternative transcript is also present in muscle, due to the use of a different polyadenylation signal. The functional significance (if any) of this muscle-specific transcript is unknown. The *MTM1*

gene is composed of 15 exons, encompasses 100 Kb at the genomic level, and is located 20 Kb proximal to a homologous gene, *hMTMR1* (20) (Figure 2). Myotubularin defines a new gene/protein family with at least 9 other members in human, which are denominated *hMTM* related (*hMTR1-9*), and which share sequence similarity on a large portion of their length (24, 25) (Figure 3). *hMTR2* has recently been shown to be mutated in a rare recessive form of Charcot-Marie-Tooth neuropathy (CMT4B) (6).

The *MTM1* gene encodes a 603 amino acid protein, myotubularin, which contains the 10 amino acid consensus sequence for the active site of protein tyrosine phosphatases (PTP) or dual specificity protein phosphatases. Myotubularin is highly conserved during evolution and down to the yeasts *Saccharomyces cerevisiae* and *Schizo-saccharomyces pombe*, which at first appeared surprising for a gene implicated in a muscle disorder (Figure 3). A domain that is common to all members of the family is called SID (for SET interacting domain), and was initially defined as mediating interaction of another member of the myotubularin family (*MTMR5/Sbf1*) with some chromatin proteins (8). The function of the SID domain in myotubularin is however unknown.

Initial in vitro studies using phosphorylated peptide substrates suggested that myotubularin is a dual-specificity phosphatase (8). However, in vivo tests in the yeast *S. pombe* and in mammalian cells indicated that myotubularin does not have a broad tyrosine phosphatase activity (5). Expression of human myotubularin in *S. pombe* induced a vacuolar phenotype similar to that of the VPS34 mutant of the vacuolar protein sorting (VPS) pathway, which affects a phosphatidyli-nositol 3-kinase. Indeed, phosphatidylinositol 3 phosphate (PI3P) levels were found decreased in *S. pombe* expressing active human myotubularin, suggesting that myotubularin was a PI3P phosphatase (5). Similar results were obtained by Taylor et al (37) in *S. cerevisae*. In parallel, Taylor et al (37) noted that the catalytic site of myotubularin bears some similarity with that of Sac1p, a yeast phosphoinositide phosphatase implicated in membrane and vesicle trafficking. Finally, myotubularin was shown to dephosphorylate PI3P in vitro (5, 37), even more efficiently than the Sac1p phosphatase, and missense mutations observed in XLMTM patients were shown to abrogate this activity. The presence of phosphoinositide binding domains called FYVE and PH (pleckstrin homology) in several myotubularin homologues is also suggestive of an implication of this protein family in phosphoinositide metabolism (24).

Although preliminary experiments suggested a nuclear localisation for myotubularin (8), this was contradicted by further analyses, as myotubularin is essentially found in the cytoplasm (5, 37) (Laporte, unpublished data). Unfortunately, even though a large panel of specific monoclonal and polyclonal antibodies is now available (22), none of them detect endogenous myotubularin in muscle or other tissue sections. In transfected cells, overexpressed myotubularin appears localised in a dense cytoplasmic network, with occasional staining of the plasma membrane, and does not colocalise with endosomes that contain the major pool of PI3P in the cell (Laporte et al, in preparation). Analysis of a substrate trap mutant suggests that a myotubularin substrate may be present at the plasma membrane (5). Thus, the exact function of myotubularin remains to be deciphered.

Diversity and origin of mutations in the MTM1 gene. One hundred forty-one different disease-associated mutations have been described to date in the *MTM1* gene and account for XLMTM in 213 unrelated families (23) (Bian-

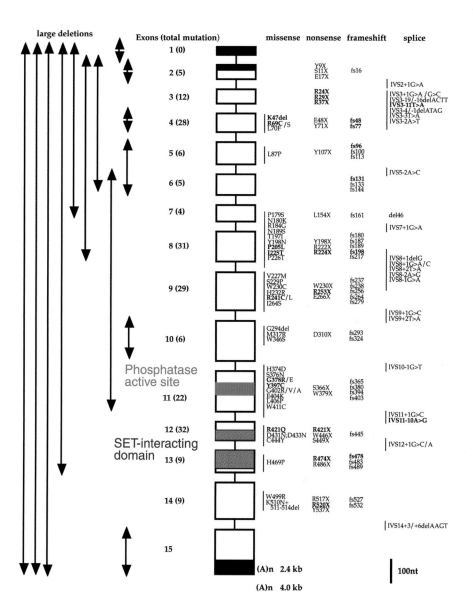

Figure 1. *Schematic representation of the MTM1 gene* showing individual mutations, genomic structure and known protein domains. Updated from Laporte et al. 2000 (22). Exons but not introns are drawn to scale. The start and stop codons are in exon 2 and 15 respectively and the 5′ and 3′ untranslated parts are in black. The 2.4 Kb muscle-specific and testis-specific transcript and the 4.0 ubiquitous transcript differ only by use of an alternative polyadenylation signal in exon 15 (26). The phosphatase consensus active site (PTP) is in exon 11 and the SET interaction domain (SID domain) in exons 12 and 13. On the left: exon deletions, and number of point mutations observed in each exon and flanking splice sites (in parenthesis); on the right : missense, nonsense, frameshift and splice sites mutations. Recurrent mutations in unrelated patients are in bold. The three most frequent mutations are the splice mutation IVS11-10A>G that results in a 3 aminoacid insertion (17 cases), a 4bp deletion in exon 4 (fs48, 11 cases) and the R241C missense (9 cases). Mutations R69C, L70F, L87P, P179S, N180K, I225T, V227M, R241 C, G294del, W346S, E404K, W411C, W499R, R520X and a deletion of exon 15, have been observed in patients with moderate or even mild clinical expression (but severity can vary for patients carrying the same mutation).

calana et al, unpublished data) (Figure 1). A detailed list of the *MTM1* mutations found in the first 198 families has been published (23). See also the Human Gene Mutation Database (I-IGIVID) (*http://www.uwcm.ac.uk/uwcm /mg/search/119439.html*) (21).

Mutations are widespread throughout the gene although 70% of them have been found in 5 exons only (exons 4, 8, 9, 11 and 12) (Figure 1). To date they consist of 60 missense changes (one amino acid replaced by another one), 44 nonsenses, 52 small insertions or deletions, 15 large deletions, and 42

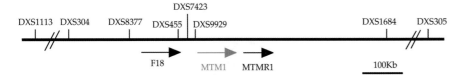

Figure 2. *Map of the MTM1 region* showing the adjacent MTMR1 and F18 genes, and polymorphic markers that can be used for indirect carrier or prenatal diagnosis by linkage analysis.

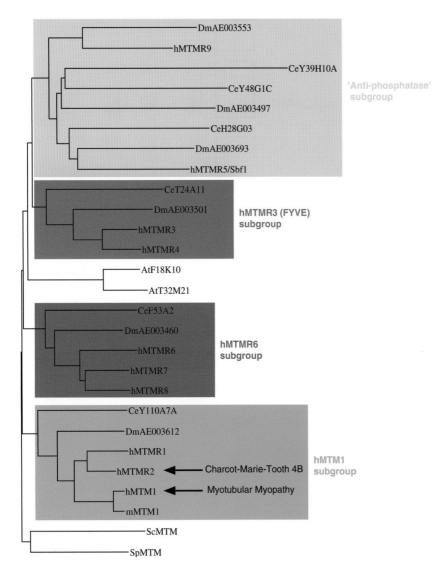

Figure 3. Phylogenetic tree of the myotubularin family. The phylogenetic tree showing the four different myotubularin subgroups was generated using the amino acid alignment from the catalytic aspartate to the end of the SET-interacting domain (amino acids 278 to 486 in hMTM1). The organisms are human (h), *Drosophila melanogaster* (DM), the worm *Caenorhabditis elegans* (Ce), the yeasts *Saccharornyces cerevisiae* (Sc) and *Schizosac-charomyces pombe* (Sp), and the plant *Arabidopsis thaliana* (At). The mouse ortholog of *hMTM1* was included in this analysis (*mMTM1*).

change observed in a patient, it is useful to check whether it affects an amino acid that is conserved at that position during evolution. Indeed, most missense mutations found in patients correspond to positions conserved in the drosophila homologue of the *MTM1* gene (23).

De novo mutations were found in about 21 (17%) of 127 affected boys, suggesting that the ratio of male mutation rate to female mutation rate is about 4. Five instances of mosaicism for a de novo mutation have been documented (2 maternal, 1 grandpaternal, and 2 grandmaternal) (15, 23, 41). In the most extreme case, a de novo mutation was transmitted by a patient's grandfather to 3 of his 4 daughters (41). Germinal mosaicism poses a significant risk of recurrence. Thus, prenatal diagnosis based on mutation analysis should be offered, even when the mother of the index patient has not been found to carry the mutation detected in her son.

Structural changes

Light microscopy. Cross-sections of muscle biopsies show fibre hypotrophy and size variability. The presence of small muscle fibres with large central nuclei, structurally similar to foetal myotubes, is the key diagnostic feature (34) (Figure 4). However, such fibres are also a feature of myotonic dystrophy (chapter 6.1.1). In longitudinal sections, the nuclei are regularly spaced along the length of the fibres; therefore, the plane of section affects the number of central nuclei observed in transverse section. The number of central nuclei can vary between muscles; they can be observed in both type 1 and type 2 fibres (1, 17, 31). Some nuclei are in the normal peripheral position. In some cases, central nuclei may not be apparent at birth. Glycogen and mitochondria often accumulate in the central perinuclear, myofibril-free zone. Thus, histochemically, this central area may be intensely stained for oxidative enzyme activity but lack ATPase staining. Fibres not showing the very dark centres with oxidative enzymes may

splice site mutations. Three recurrent mutations account for the disorder in 17% of the families. Most missense mutations are clustered between exons 8 and 12, around the PTP active site in exon 11 and several change an amino acid in the PTP signature or in the SID domain. The numerous missense mutations in exons 8 and 9 affect regions of unknown function, well conserved in evolution. When assessing the pathogenic significance of a novel missense

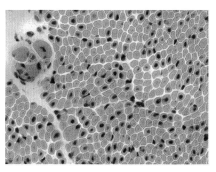

Figure 4. *Muscle biopsy* of a case of myotubular myopathy showing small fibres and the characteristic central nuclei in several fibres. Haematoxyline and eosin.

have a pale peripheral zone that lacks myofibrils and mitochondria. Type 1 fibres are often predominant, a common myopathic feature. Necrosis and fibrosis are not usually features of XLMTM, but it is not known whether the latter may be age-related.

Immunohistochemistry. Immuno-histochemical studies have shown that desmin and vimentin may be abundant in some fibres (30). This has been proposed as evidence of immaturity but is not a universal feature of all fibres with central nuclei. Neonates often have many fibres that express foetal myosin, but again, this is not specific to myotubular myopathy. Older patients have fibres with central nuclei that express mature isoforms of myosin, indicating that they do mature, at least with regard to myosin isoforms (32). Expression of NCAM, utrophin and laminin alpha 5 chain have also been reported (17). Although these relate to immaturity, they are non-specific features. Immunoprecipitation studies identify the absence or very low levels of myotubularin in most patients tested (22), but detection of myotubularin by immunohistochemistry in muscle sections has not yet been achieved.

Electron microscopy. Ultrastructurally, the areas of fibres with the central nuclei are devoid of myofibrils and show accumulations of glycogen and mitochondria (Figure 5). Central nuclei in XLMTM may show condensation of nuclear chromatin (30). Other ultrastructural alterations include disorientation of triads, disorganisation of the

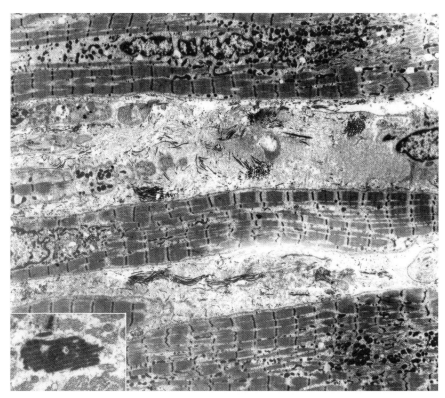

Figure 5. *Low power electron micrograph* showing central nuclei and accumulation of mitochondria in the central area, and some disruption of myofibrils. Inset shows dense tubules that are seen in some cases (origin uncertain, possibly from T tubules).

sarcoplasmic reticulum and dense tubular structures (1, 16). Myofibrils with striations form correctly (30), but zones of disorganised myofibrils may occur (33). Motoneurones and motor endplates appear normal (30), although motor endplate immaturity was suggested in one study of a single case (12).

Genotype-phenotype correlations

Almost all truncating and splice mutations are associated with a severe phenotype. This is also true for the most common mutation that creates a new splice site resulting in an insertion of the three amino acids FIQ after position 420. Two splice site mutations that allowed a low level of correctly spliced RNA were however associated with a severe phenotype (36).

Three male patients with deletions showed, in addition to the XLMTM phenotype, abnormal development of the genitalia (4, 19). These cases present a "contiguous genes syndrome," indicating that a gene located close to the *MTM1* gene (probably on the cen-

tromeric side), is necessary for normal genital development in males (Figure 2).

Only 2 of 14, 1 of 43 and 2 of 39 male patients (5% in total) with respectively large deletions, frameshift and nonsense mutations have a milder phenotype. Among these five patients, two have a R520X and one a deletion of the last exon, suggesting that the C-terminal part of myotubularin after the SID domain does not encompass critically important residues. In apparent contradiction, 2 other very distal mutations—a Y537X nonsense and a splice mutation in intron 14—led to a very severe phenotype; such discrepancy may be linked to the effect of an individual mutation on the stability of the mRNA or protein, which cannot be predicted.

The deletion of exon 1, which is not protein-encoding, was associated with a milder phenotype in one of 2 patients in the same family. Such a mutation might allow synthesis of a partially functional mRNA. Thus, there is only one case where a mutation (frameshift 279) that should not allow synthesis of functional myotubularin was found associated with long survival (deceased, 10 years old). On the other hand, 22 of 57 patients with a missense or a deletion of a single amino acid show a moderate or mild phenotype (missense mutations observed in patients with moderate or mild phenotype are indicated in the legend to Figure 1). The longest survival (patients still alive at the age of 65 or 54) was observed for the mutations N180K and L70F respectively (Biancalana, unpublished) (2). However, missense mutations affecting the phosphatase active site (PTP) or the SID domain appear associated with a severe phenotype, confirming that these domains are essential for the function of myotubularin. Missense mutations in other regions of the protein indicate that other protein domains are important for the stability or function of myotubularin.

Initial results of the detection of myotubularin by immunoprecipitation have shown that the protein is barely detectable in most patient cell lines (21 out of 24) compared with normal controls (22). The only patients showing a normal level of myotubularin have a missense mutation or a small insertion or deletion of amino acids. A missense mutation outside the PTP and SID protein domains, leading to a detectable level of myotubularin, is more likely to be associated with a mild phenotype.

Phenotype variability. In the first reported family, patients survived up to 54 years (2, 40). However, in this family, neonatal deaths of affected males occurred thirty years ago, and might be due to less effective neonatal care at this time. Phenotypic variation was observed for missenses I225T, R241C, R421Q for which both mild and severe forms were observed. Another patient with a mild phenotype carried a deletion of exon 1, but a related male with the same deletion was severely affected.

The occurrence of milder cases with *MTM1* mutations suggests that the classification where severe neonatal hypotonia is thought to indicate XLMTM, while mild adult forms represent autosomal centronuclear myopathy, may not always be valid. However, the age of onset seems a good initial differential parameter (44). Some cases of carrier females with mild to moderate clinical manifestations have been described associated with skewed X inactivation (9, 35). Thus, XLMTM cannot be excluded a priori in a sporadic female patient. Manifesting females should also be examined for the presence of chromosomal abnormalities involving the X chromosome.

In summary, with the exception of some very distal mutations, truncating mutations are nearly always associated with a very poor prognosis. Missense mutations affecting domains other than the PTP or SID are often, but not always, associated with a milder course of the disease.

Future perspectives

The molecular basis of X-linked myotubular myopathy is now well established and we have a good overview of the spectrum of mutations in the *MTM1* gene. Despite the recent advances implicating myotubularin in phosphoinositide metabolism, its physiological role in muscle and other tissues remains elusive. A mouse model of the disease has recently been established by knocking out the mouse *MTM1* homolog. Male mice indeed show a severe muscular phenotype, and histopathology is very reminiscent of the human disease, with presence of small fibres with centrally located nuclei (Buj-Bello et al, unpublished data). This model will be of utmost importance for deciphering the function of myotubularin and the pathophysiology of the muscle defect. It will also allow the testing of the closest related genes (*MTMR1* and *R2*) to see if they have overlapping function and can rescue the muscle phenotype in the mouse model.

The genes responsible for the autosomal cases (or centronuclear myopathy) await mapping and identification. MTM1 related proteins and proteins implicated in PI3P metabolism or function may be good candidates. Unfortunately, only a few informative families with clear autosomal segregation of the specific muscle pathology have been described (44), which impairs positional cloning efforts. A canine model displaying features of autosomal recessive myotubular/centronuclear myopathy is under characterisation, both immunocytochemically and genetically (42).

The most difficult problem will be to get potential therapeutic strategies from knowledge on disease mechanisms, ie, by manipulating PI3P metabolism or by interfering with downstream effects of the absence of myotubularin. At present, this is impaired by the uncertainties on the true cellular functions of myotubularin. However, if studies in the mouse model indicate that *MTMR1* or *MTMR2* can rescue *MTM1* deficiency, one could screen for compounds that would upregulate the expression of these genes in muscle. Similar strategies appear useful for sickle cell anemia or β-thalassemia (upregulation of foetal hemoglobin), and have been proposed for Duchenne muscular dystrophy (upregulation of utrophin). For the 20% of patients who carry a nonsense mutation, one might also consider testing gentamicin, an aminoglycoside that is able to promote low levels of translational readthrough over stop codons (3).

References

1. Ambler MW, Neave C, Singer DB (1984) X-linked recessive myotubular myopathy: II. Muscle morphology and human myogenesis. *Hum Pathol* 15: 1107-1120

2. Barth PG, Dubowitz V (1998) X-linked myotubular myopathy—a long-term follow-up study. *Europ J Paediatr Neurol* 2: 49-56

3. Barton-Davis ER, Cordier L, Shoturma DI, Leland SE, Sweeney HL (1999) Aminoglycoside antibiotics restore dystrophin function to skeletal muscles of mdx mice. *J Clin Invest* 104: 375-381

4. Bartsch O, Kress W, Wagner A, Seemanova E (1999) The novel contiguous gene syndrome of myotubular myopathy (MTM1), male hypogenitalism and deletion in Xq28:report of the first familial case. *Cytogenet Cell Genet* 85: 310-314

5. Blondeau F, Laporte J, Bodin S, Superti-Furga G, Payrastre B, Mandel JL (2000) Myotubularin, a phosphatase deficient in myotubular myopathy, acts on phosphatidylinositol 3-kinase and phosphatidylinositol 3-phosphate pathway. *Hum Mol Genet* 9: 2223-2229

6. Bolino A, Muglia M, Conforti FL, LeGuern E, Salih MA, Georgiou DM, Christodoulou K, Hausmanowa-Petrusewicz I, Mandich P, Schenone A, Gambardella A, Bono F, Quattrone A, Devoto M, Monaco AP (2000) Charcot-Marie-Tooth type 4B is caused by mutations in the gene encoding myotubularin-related protein-2. *Nat Genet* 25: 17-19

7. Buj-Bello A, Biancalana V, Moutou C, Laporte J, Mandel JL (1999) Identification of novel mutations in the MTM1 gene causing severe and mild forms of X-linked myotubular myopathy. *Hum Mutat* 14: 320-325

8. Cui X, De Vivo I, Slany R, Miyamoto A, Firestein R, Cleary ML (1998) Association of SET domain and myotubularin-related proteins modulates growth control. *Nat Genet* 18: 331-337

9. Dahl N, Hu LJ, Chery M, Fardeau M, Gilgenkrantz S, Nivelon-Chevallier A, Sidaner-Noisette I, Mugneret F, Gouyon JB, Gal A, et al. (1995) Myotubular myopathy in a girl with a deletion at Xq27-q28 and unbalanced X inactivation assigns the MTM1 gene to a 600-kb region. *Am J Hum Genet* 56: 1108-1115

10. De Angelis MS, Palmucci L, Leone M, Doriguzzi C (1991) Centronuclear myopathy: clinical, morphological and genetic characters. A review of 288 cases. *J Neurol Sci* 103: 2-9

11. de Gouyon BM, Zhao W, Laporte J, Mandel JL, Metzenberg A, Herman GE (1997) Characterization of mutations in the myotubularin gene in twenty-six patients with X-linked myotubular myopathy. *Hum Mol Genet* 6: 1499-1504

12. Fidzianska A, Goebel HH (1994) Aberrant arrested in maturation neuromuscular junctions in centronuclear myopathy. *J Neurol Sci* 124: 83-88

13. Guiraud-Chaumeil C, Vincent MC, Laporte J, Fardeau M, Samson F, Mandel JL (1997) A mutation in the MTM1 gene invalidates a previous suggestion of nonallelic heterogeneity in X-linked myotubular myopathy. *Am J Hum Genet* 60: 1542-1544

14. Hamman SR, Robinson DO, Moutou C, Kennedy CR, Dennis NR, Hughes PJ, Ellison DW (2000) A clinical and genetic study of a manifesting heterozygote with X-linked myotubular myopathy. *Neuromuscul Disord* 10: 133-137

15. Hane BG, Rogers RC, Schwartz CE (1999) Germline mosaicism in X-linked myotubular myopathy. *Clin Genet* 56: 77-81

16. Heckmatt JZ, Sewry CA, Hodes D, Dubowitz V (1985) Congenital centronuclear (myotubular) myopathy. A clinical, pathological and genetic study in eight children. *Brain* 108: 941-964

17. Helliwell TR, Ellis IH, Appleton RE (1998) Myotubular myopathy: morphological, immunohistochemical and clinical variation. *Neuromuscul Disord* 8: 152-161

18. Herman GE, Finegold M, Zhao W, de Gouyon B, Metzenberg A (1999) Medical complications in long-term survivors with X-linked myotubular myopathy. *J Pediatr* 134: 206-214

19. Hu LJ, Laporte J, Kress W, Kioschis P, Siebenhaar R, Poustka A, Fardeau M, Metzenberg A, Janssen EA, Thomas N, Mandel JL, Dahl N (1996b) Deletions in Xq28 in two boys with myotubular myopathy and abnormal genital development define a new contigu-ous gene syndrome in a 430 kb region. *Hum Mol Genet* 5: 139-143

20. Kioschis P, Wiemann S, Heiss NS, Francis F, Gotz C, Poustka A, Taudien S, Platzer M, Wiehe T, Beckmann G, Weber J, Nordsiek G, Rosenthal A (1998) Genomic organization of a 225-kb region in Xq28 containing the gene for X-linked myotubular myopathy (MTM1) and a related gene (MTMR1). *Genomics* 54: 256-266

21. Krawczak M, Cooper DN (1997) The human gene mutation database. *Trends Genet* 13: 121-122

22. Laporte J, Kress, W., Mandel, I-L (2001) Diagnosis of X-linked Myotubular Myopathy by detection of myotubularin. *Annals of Neurology* in press.

23. Laporte J, Biancalana V, Tanner SM, Kress W, Schneider V, Wallgren-Pettersson C, Herger F, Buj-Bello A, Blondeau F, Liechti-Gallati S, Mandel JL (2000) MTM1 mutations in X-linked myotubular myopathy. *Hum Mutat* 15: 393-409

24. Laporte J, Blondeau F, Buj-Bello A, Mandel J (2001) The myotubularin family: from genetic disease to phosphoinositide metabolism. *Trends Genet* 17: 221-228

25. Laporte J, Blondeau F, Buj-Bello A, Tentler D, Kretz C, Dahl N, Mandel JL (1998) Characterization of the myotubularin dual specificity phosphatase gene family from yeast to human. *Hum Mol Genet* 7: 1703-1712

26. Laporte J, Guiraud-Chaumeil C, Vincent MC, Mandel JL, Tanner SM, Liechti-Gallati S, Wallgren-Pettersson C, Dahl N, Kress W, Bolhuis PA, Fardeau M, Samson F, Bertini E (1997) Mutations in the MTM1 gene implicated in X-linked myotubular myopathy. ENMC International Consortium on Myotubular Myopathy. European Neuro-Muscular Center. *Hum Mol Genet* 6: 1505-1511

27. Laporte J, Hu LJ, Kretz C, Mandel JL, Kioschis P, Coy JF, Klauck SM, Poustka A, Dahl N (1996) A gene mutated in X-linked myotubular myopathy defines a new putative tyrosine phosphatase family conserved in yeast. *Nat Genet* 13: 175-182

28. Nishino I, Minami N, Kobayashi O, Ikezawa M, Goto Y, Arahata K, Nonaka I (1998) MTM1 gene mutations in Japanese patients with the severe infantile form of myotubular myopathy. *Neuromuscul Disord* 8: 453-458

29. Samson F, Mesnard L, Heimburger M, Hanauer A, Chevallay M, Mercadier JJ, Pelissier JF, Feingold N, Junien C, Mandel JL, et al. (1995) Genetic linkage heterogeneity in myotubular myopathy. *Am J Hum Genet* 57: 120-126

30. Sarnat HB (1990) Myotubular myopathy: arrest of morphogenesis of myofibres associated with persistence of fetal vimentin and desmin. Four cases compared with fetal and neonatal muscle. *Can J Neurol Sci* 17: 109-123

31. Sasaki T, Shikura K, Sugai K, Nonaka I, Kumagai K (1989) Muscle histochemistry in myotubular (centronuclear) myopathy. *Brain Dev* 11: 26-32

32. Sewry CA (1998) The role of immunocytochemistry in congenital myopathies. *Neuromuscul Disord* 8: 394-400

33. Silver MM, Gilbert JJ, Stewart S, Brabyn D, Jung J (1986) Morphologic and morphometric analysis of muscle in X-linked myotubular myopathy. *Hum Pathol* 17: 1167-1178

34. Spiro AJ, Shy GM, Gonatas NK (1966) Myotubular myopathy. Persistence of fetal muscle in an adolescent boy. *Arch Neurol* 14: 1-14

35. Tanner SM, Orstavik KH, Kristiansen M, Lev D, Lerman-Sagie T, Sadeh M, Liechti-Gallati S (1999b) Skewed X-inactivation in a manifesting carrier of X-linked myotubular myopathy and in her non-manifesting carrier mother. *Hum Genet* 104: 249-253

36. Tanner SM, Schneider V, Thomas NS, Clarke A, Lazarou L, Liechti-Gallati S (1999a) Characterization of 34 novel and six known MTM1 gene mutations in 47 unrelated X-linked myotubular myopathy patients. *Neuromuscul Disord* 9: 41-49

37. Taylor GS, Maehama T, Dixon JE (2000) Inaugural article: myotubularin, a protein tyrosine phosphatase mutated in myotubular myopathy, dephosphorylates the lipid second messenger, phosphatidylinositol 3-phosphate. *Proc Natl Acad Sci USA* 97: 8910-8915

38. Thomas NS, Sarfarazi M, Roberts K, William H, Cole G, Liechti-Gallati S, Harper PS (1987) X-linkage in myotubular myopathy (XLMTM): evidence for linkage to Xq28 DNA markers. *Cytogenet Cell Genet* 46: 704 (abstract)

39. Thomas NS, Williams H, Cole G, Roberts K, Clarke A, Liechti-Gallati S, Braga S, Gerber A, Meier C, Moser H, *et al.* (1990) X-linked neonatal centronuclear/myotubular myopathy: evidence for linkage to Xq28 DNA marker loci. *J Med Genet* 27: 284-287

40. van Wijngaarden GK, Fleury P, Bethlem J, Meijer AE (1969) Familial "myotubular" myopathy. *Neurology* 19: 901-908

41. Vincent MC, Guiraud-Chaumeil C, Laporte J, Manouvrier-Hanu S, Mandel JL (1998) Extensive germinal mosaicism in a family with X-linked myotubular myopathy simulates genetic heterogeneity. *J Med Genet* 35: 241-243

42. Wallgren-Pettersson C (1998) 58th ENMC workshop: myotubular myopathy 20-22 March, 1998, Naarden, The Netherlands. *Neuromuscul Disord* 8: 521-525

43. Wallgren-Pettersson C (2000) 72nd ENMC International Workshop: myotubular myopathy 1-3 October 1999, Hilversum, The Netherlands. *Neuromuscul Disord* 10: 525-529

44. Wallgren-Pettersson C, Clarke A, Samson F, Fardeau M, Dubowitz V, Moser H, Grimm T, Barohn RJ, Barth PG (1995) The myotubular myopathies: differential diagnosis of the X linked recessive, autosomal dominant, and autosomal recessive forms and present state of DNA studies. *J Med Genet* 32: 673-679

45. Wallgren-Pettersson C, Thomas NS (1994) Report on the 20th ENMC sponsored international workshop: myotubular/centronuclear myopathy. *Neuromuscul Disord* 4: 71-74

Congenital fibre type disproportion

Hans H. Goebel

CFTD	congenital fibre type disproportion
FTD	fibre type disproportion

Definition of entities

Congenital fibre type disproportion (CFTD) (3) is a non-progressive childhood neuromuscular disorder marked by the morphological pattern of fibre type disproportion (FTD), ie, predominance and hypotrophy of type 1 fibres. Clinically, patients show marked variations of their symptoms and signs (6). Respiratory insufficiency is often an important sign (14), which may either improve (23), or result in early death (5). Generalized muscle hypotonia and muscle weakness are non-specific clinical features. Other rare clinical signs are rigid spine (15, 21) and ophthalmoplegia (19).

A large number of other unrelated neuromuscular diseases show myopathological FTD (20). This association with well-defined conditions, especially those affecting the central nervous system (8, 13, 16) casts doubt on CFTD as a separate entity (17).

Molecular background and pathogenesis

Possibly owing to the nosological uncertainty of CFTD, mutated genes have not yet been reported. A single observation (9) concerned a young girl with CFTD showing a balanced chromosomal translocation t(10;17) (p 11.2;q25). This suggested candidate genes located in the breakpoint region of either chromosome 11 or 17 or both (9). CFTD in this family suggested an autosomal dominant transmission (9), but autosomal recessive inheritance has also been proposed (12). CFTD has been described in identical twins (7). Compound heterozygosity in the insulin receptor gene was associated with CFTD in two brothers (13).

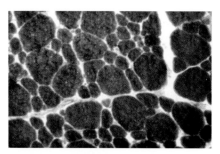

Figure 1. *Congenital fibre type disproportion.* Two populations of muscle fibres: numerous small ones and fewer large ones. Modified trichrome stain.

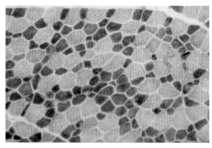

Figure 2. Innumerable small dark type 1 fibres and few large light type 2 fibres, NADH tetrazolium reductase.

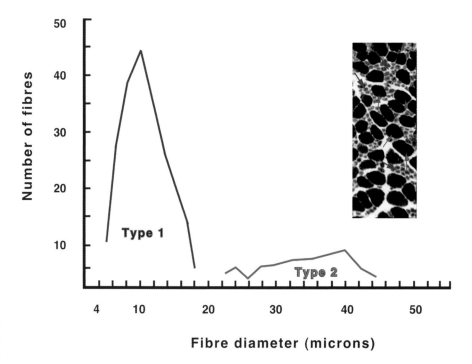

Figure 3. Histogram of a section stained for ATPase pH 9.4 from a muscle biopsy of a child, 4 years and 7 months of age. There are many small type 1 fibres (light, blue arrows and blue line in the graph). The few (25%) large dark type 2 fibres are indicated by red arrows and red line in the graph. Mean diameter of type 1 fibres 9.5 µm and of type 2 fibres 34.9 µm.

The pathogenesis of CFTD is obscure. Dysmaturation, largely based on high numbers of immature, type 2C muscle fibres has been suggested (2, 18). Extramedullary haematopoiesis, usually only seen during fetal life, has been detected in such CFTD muscle specimens (2).

Structural changes

Smallness of type 1 fibres is the cardinal feature which often uniformly affects the muscle specimen (Figures 1-4). It may persist over years (18), change (1), and be detected only in adulthood if the evolution of the disorder is mild. The main difference between the fibre types should be at least 45% (4).

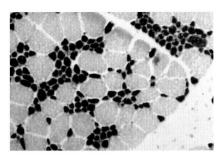

Figure 4. Section stained for ATPase pH 4.2. Numerous small dark type 1 fibres and few large light type 2 fibres are present.

Type 1 fibre smallness also occurs in other neuromuscular diseases (eg, myotonic dystrophy, infantile spinal muscular atrophy, nemaline myopathy) from which fibre type smallness needs to be differentiated.

The other feature is predominance of type 1 fibres, which obviously requires knowledge of the normal distribution pattern of type 1 and type 2 fibres in biopsied skeletal muscle. According to the literature the predominance may vary considerably between 32% (5) and 89% (3). FTD has been seen in peripheral lysosomal neuropathies (8, 13, 16). Decreased intramuscular terminal innervation (22) suggested the possibility of primary neurogenic factors. Expression of the growth-associated protein 43 in small fibres in CFTD has also been considered a sign of developmental delay whereas expression of N-CAM suggested chronic partial denervation of small fibres (10).

Ultrastructural lesions may encompass streaming of the Z band and small minicore-like abnormalities may occur.

Future perspectives

Several lines of investigation ought to be carried out. We should determine *i)* whether CFTD is an entity or not, even a heterogeneous one, *ii)* identify one or several genes responsible for CFTD and their respective gene products, and *iii)* employ markers of muscle fibre development in studies on maturation and maturity of small fibres in CFTD.

References

1. Bartholomeus MG, Gabreels FJ, ter Laak HJ, van Engelen BG (2000) Congenital fibre type disproportion a time-locked diagnosis: a clinical and morphological follow-up study. *Clin Neurol Neurosurg* 102: 97-101.

2. Bove KE, Iannaccone ST, Vogler C (1986) Intramuscular hematopoiesis in hypotonic infants with type 1 muscle fiber dysmaturation. *Arch Pathol Lab Med* 110: 207-211

3. Brooke MH. 1973. *Congenital fiber dysproportion.* Presented at 2nd International Congress on Muscle Diseases, Part 2, Kakulas BA, Editor, Excerpta Medica, Amsterdam, pp. 147-159

4. Brooke MH (1990) Congenital fibre type disproportion. *J Neurol Sci* 98: 100 [abstract 4.1.4]

5. Cavanagh NP, Lake BD, McMeniman P (1979) Congenital fibre type disproportion myopathy. A histological diagnosis with an uncertain clinical outlook. *Arch Dis Child* 54: 735-743.

6. Clancy RR, Kelts KA, Oehlert JW (1980) Clinical variability in congenital fiber type disproportion. *J Neurol Sci* 46: 257-266.

7. Curless RG, Nelson MB (1977) Congenital fiber type disproportion in identical twins. *Ann Neurol* 2: 455-459.

8. Dehkharghani F, Sarnat HB, Brewster MA, Roth SI (1981) Congenital muscle fiber-type disproportion in Krabbe's leukodystrophy. *Arch Neurol* 38: 585-587.

9. Gerdes AM, Petersen MB, Schroder HD, Wulff K, Brondum-Nielsen K (1994) Congenital myopathy with fiber type disproportion: a family with a chromosomal translocation t(10;17) may indicate candidate gene regions. *Clin Genet* 45: 11-16.

10. Heuss D, Engelhardt A, Lochmuller H, Gobel H, Neundorfer B (1994) Expression of growth associated protein 43 and neural cell adhesion molecule in congenital fibre type disproportion with interstitial myositis. *Virchows Arch* 425: 101-105

11. Jaffe M, Shapira J, Borochowitz Z (1988) Familial congenital fiber type disproportion (CFTD) with an autosomal recessive inheritance. *Clin Genet* 33: 33-37.

12. Klein HH, Muller R, Vestergaard H, Pedersen O (1999) Implications of compound heterozygous insulin receptor mutations in congenital muscle fibre type disproportion myopathy for the receptor kinase activation. *Diabetologia* 42: 245-249.

13. Krendel DA, Shutter LA, Holt PJ (1994) Fiber type disproportion in metachromatic leukodystrophy. *Muscle Nerve* 17: 1352-1353.

14. Lenard HG, Goebel HH (1975) Congenital fibre type disproportion. *Neuropädiatrie* 6: 220-231

15. Lössner J, Ziegan J, Oertel G (1979) [An unusual myopathy: the so-called congenital fiber-type disproportion]. *Z Gesamte Inn Med* 34: 685-687.

16. Marjanovic B, Cvetkovic D, Dozic S, Todorovic S, Djuric M (1996) Association of Krabbe leukodystrophy and congenital fiber type disproportion. *Pediatr Neurol* 15: 79-82.

17. Martin JJ, Clara R, Ceuterick C, Joris C (1976) Is congenital fibre type disproportion a true myopathy? *Acta Neurol Belg* 76: 335-344

18. Mizuno Y, Komiya K (1990) A serial muscle biopsy study in a case of congenital fiber-type disproportion associated with progressive respiratory failure. *Brain Dev* 12: 431-436

19. Owen JS, Kline LB, Oh SJ, Miles NE, Benton JW (1981) Ophthalmoplegia and ptosis in congenital fiber type disproportion. *J Pediatr Ophthalmol Strabismus* 18: 55-60.

20. Schröder JM (1996) Congenital fiber type disproportion. In *Handbook of Muscle Disease*, RJM Lane (eds). Marcel Dekker: New York. pp. Chapter 16, 195-200

21. Sulaiman AR, Swick HM, Kinder DS (1983) Congenital fibre type disproportion with unusual clinicopathologic manifestations. *J Neurol Neurosurg Psychiatry* 46: 175-182.

22. ter Laak HJ, Jaspar HH, Gabreels FJ, Breuer TJ, Sengers RC, Joosten EM, Stadhouders AM, Gabreels-Festen AA (1981) Congenital fibre type disproportion. *Clin Neurol Neurosurg* 83: 67-79

23. Tsuji M, Higuchi Y, Shiraishi K, Mitsuyoshi I, Hattori H (1999) Congenital fiber type disproportion: severe form with marked improvement. *Pediatr Neurol* 21: 658-660.

CHAPTER 8

Disorders of catabolic mechanisms

8.1 Lysosomal disorders
    8.1.1 Alpha glucosidase deficiency syndromes   134
    8.1.2 LAMP-2 deficiency   142
    8.1.3 X-linked myopathy with excessive autophagy   145
8.2 Proteolytic disturbances
    8.2.1 Defects of non-lysosomal proteolysis: Calpain3 deficiency   148

Catabolic processes in skeletal muscle fibres take place in lysosomes, proteosomes, and the cytosol. These processes do not generate energy, and in some instances, they may even consume some. The substrates of lysosomal catabolism include proteins, glycogen, complex carbohydrates, triglycerides, complex lipids, nucleic acids, etc. By contrast, in proteosomes and in the cytosol, only proteins are degraded.

Known human skeletal muscle diseases can be related to disordered lysosomal catabolism of glycogen (various forms of alpha glucosidase or acid maltase deficiency) that result in massive accumulation of lysosomal glycogen. Lysosomal excess of glycogen may be secondarily related to a deficiency of a lysosomal membrane protein (LAMP2), as is the case in Danon's disease. Another probable defect of lysosomal biology is called Kalimo's disease (X-linked myopathy with excessive autophagy) in which there is a marked excess of autophagic vacuoles in muscle fibres without apparent storage of a particular substrate. Although in this disease there is no clear evidence of even a secondary catabolic defect, we have included this entity in this chapter.

No human muscle diseases have been attributed to a primary disturbance of proteosomal proteolysis although secondary activation of proteosomes (as evidenced by ubiquitinated masses) seems to occur in sporadic inclusion body myositis. A genetic deficiency of a cytosolic proteolytic enzyme, calpain 3, is the cause of a form of limb girdle dystrophy.

Alpha glucosidase deficiency syndromes

Frank T. Martiniuk

AMD	acid maltase deficiency
GAA	acid α-glucosidase
GSDII	glycogen storage disease

Definition of entities

Lysosomal acid maltase or acid α-glucosidase (GAA) primarily hydrolyses linear α1-4 glucosidic linkage ranging from large polymers (glycogen) to maltose and the artificial substrate 4-methylumbelliferyl-α-D-glucoside (4-MU-Glyc) (38, 49). Genetic deficiency of GAA or glycogen storage disease type II (AMD or GSDII) results in a spectrum of phenotypes including an infantile disorder (Pompe's disease) (27, 28), non-classical infantile, childhood, juvenile, and a late onset adult myopathy (18, 56).

The infantile onset form presents as severe hypotonia in skeletal and heart muscle. In the first few months, respiratory and cardiac difficulties are found with feeding problems. Progressive cardiomegaly, and to a lesser extent hepatomegaly can be observed. Glycogen accumulation is intra-lysosomal and cytoplasmic, primarily in skeletal muscle, liver, and heart; a thickening of the walls of both ventricles and decrease in size of ventricular cavity. Eventually an obstruction in ventricular flow is seen. On EKG, a shortened PR interval and large QRS complexes with inverted T wave can be shown. Mental development is normal. Death is due to cardiorespiratory failure in the first year.

The non-classical infantile form presents with less severe cardiomyopathy and absence of left ventricular flow. Longer survival can be achieved with assisted ventilation and supplemental nutrition (68). The childhood form is the most severe form of late onset AMD and closely mimics Duchenne muscular dystrophy. Patients present at 2 to 3 years of age with difficulty walk-ing, frequently falls and usually become wheelchair bound and respirator-dependent by late childhood and succumb to respiratory failure during adolescence. The juvenile form presents during late childhood or early adolescence with progressive muscle weakness, frequently associated with respiratory failure during late adolescence or early adulthood. Patients with the slowly progressive adult onset form can exhibit varying degrees of enzyme deficiency, even overlapping with that of infantile onset patients. In all cases, pathology is limited to skeletal muscle (17).

Adult onset patients usually develop progressive muscle weakness and wasting during their 20s and 30s with respiratory insufficiency occurring in more than 50% of patients (18, 56). Weakness of respiratory muscles, particularly the diaphragm, with no cardiomegaly is found. There may be a disproportionate atrophy of the paraspinal muscles with a greater involvement of lower than upper limbs. Vital capacity is reduced. Adult patients die due to respiratory failure with pre-terminal signs of pulmonary hypertension and cardiac failure. The later onset forms—childhood, juvenile, and adult—have residual enzyme activity in most tissues with varying amounts of glycogen accumulation, primarily in skeletal muscle. Patients have been studied as to residual enzyme activity, GAA protein detected by antibody and abnormalities in intracellular and posttranslational processing including phosphorylation (9, 10, 46, 49, 63, 64). These studies indicate extensive genetic heterogeneity. Analysis of cells from patients by Reuser et al and others (63, 64, 70) using pulse labelling and immunologic techniques have identified at least 9 different types in 20 patients that included defects in phosphorylation, stability, and processing-degradation.

Molecular genetics

Naturally occurring animal models for GSDII have been identified for

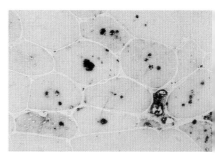

Figure 1. Acid phosphatase positive sites mark lysosomes that are massively distended with glycogen in a case of adult-onset alpha glucosidase deficiency. ×300. Illustration kindly provided by George Karpati, Montreal.

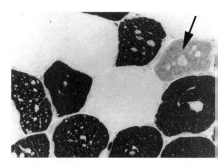

Figure 2. Optically clear spaces represent lysosomal pockets of glycogen mainly in histochemical type 1(dark) fibres. A single, intermediately reacting type 2C fibre indicated by an arrow also contains vacuoles. Myofibrillar ATP-ase, pH 4.6. ×560. Illustration: George Karpati, Montreal.

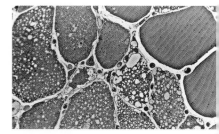

Figure 3. Myriads of variably-sized vacuoles mark lysosomal storage of glycogen in muscle fibres. Sparing of some (presumably type 1) fibres is striking. Infantile alpha glucosidase deficiency (Pompe's disease). Resin section. ×550 Illustration: George Karpati, Montreal.

Lapland dog, Japanese quail, Australian cattle, cat and sheep (19, 31, 39, 48, 59, 60, 65, 76). Two mouse models have been developed (21, 44, 45). Raben et al (62) have developed 2 GAA -/- mice on the 129 background strain, one with an exon 6[neo] disruption that lacks GAA activity in tissues, and accumulates glycogen in cardiac and skeletal muscle by 3 to 4 weeks of age. By 4 weeks, muscle weakness and lack of strength appears. By 8 to 9 months, muscle wasting occurs. This mouse probably represents the childhood-juvenile forms of the human disease. Their second mouse has a deletion of exon 6, and is identical to the exon 6[neo] disrupted mouse with respect to biochemical and pathologic parameters; however, it has unimpaired muscle weakness. This mouse is similar to the GAA -/- mouse by Bijovet et al (6, 11) that was generated by disruption of exon 13. They interpret the differences in the clinical presentation of the -/- mice to genetic background of the strains.

The gene has been localised to the long arm of human chromosome 17 (57, 69) and regionally to 17q21-23 (30, 53). Three allelic forms (GAA 1, 2, and 4) segregate in the general population, reflecting a genetic polymorphism. GAA is a "house-keeping" enzyme with all tissues and cell types exhibiting some activity (55).

The frequency and total number affected by GSDII in the general population was not known until recently. Studies in the United States and the Netherlands using molecular biology techniques to estimate carrier frequencies and live birth records showed that 1 in 40 000 to 50 000 births presented with GSDII (1, 51, 61). Carrier frequency ranged from 1 in 85 to 100. Thus, depending upon country to country variation in birth rates, there could be 3 400 to 4 300 births yearly worldwide with GSDII. The cumulative burden of surviving GSDII cases (later onset forms) worldwide may be 42 900 to 74 580.

Exon(s)	Location	Nucleotide and amino acid
2	-13 bp 5' from exon 2	T→G; exon 2 deleted in mRNA
2	118	C→T; Arg^{40} to stop
2	172	C→T; Gln^{58} to stop
2		Pro^{161}→shift stop codon
2	insertion C^{258}	
2	271	del G^{271}
2	379-380	TG deleted
2	482-483	CC deleted
2	525	T deleted
3	623	T→C; Leu^{208} to Pro
4	del 766-785 (TATATCACAGGCCTCGCCGA), insertion C	
5	875	A→G; Tyr^{292} to Cys
5	896	T→G; Leu^{299} to Arg
5	923	C→T; His^{308} to Leu
5	925	G→A; Gly^{309} to Arg
5	953	T→C; Met^{318} to Thr
6	t→g -22 bp IVS 6	inserts 22 bp & del exon 6 in mRNA
6	971	C→T; Pro^{324} to Leu
9	1411-1414	GAGA deleted
9	1432	G→A; Gly^{478} to Arg
10	1456-1468	13 bp deleted
10	+1 bp 5' in IVS10	GT→CT; deleted1438-1551
11	1555	A→G; Met^{519} to Val
11	1561	G→A; Glu^{521} to Lys
11	1585-1586	TC→GT; Ser^{529} to Val
11	1634	C→G; Pro^{545} to Arg
12	1696	T→C; Ser^{566} to Pro
13	1754	G→T; Arg^{585} to Met
13	1798	C→T; Arg^{600} to Cys
13	del 1821-1836	del 6 aa 607-612
14	1912	G→T; Gly^{638} to Trp
14	1927	G→A; Gly^{643} to Arg
14	1933	G→A; Asp^{645} to Asn
14	1935	C→A; Asp^{645} to Glu
14	1941	C→G; Cys^{647} to Trp
14	1942	G→A; Gly^{648} to Ser
14	2014	C→T; Arg^{672} to Trp
14	2015	G→A; Arg^{672} to Gln
15	2173	C→T; Arg^{725} to Trp
16		IVS16 (+2 T→C); del 16 bp (2315-2330)
16	2303	C→G; Pro^{768} to Arg
16	2237	G→A; Trp^{746} to stop
16	insertion G^{2242}	
16	insertion G^{2243}	
17	insertion C^{2432}	Leu^{811}→shift
18		536 bp deleted; IVS 17-18;exon 18
18	2560	C→T; Arg^{854} to stop
19	2707-2709 del	del Lys^{903}
19	2741	AG→CAGG; Pro^{913} to shift
19	2776	duplication of 18 bp & 6 amino acids (GlyValProValSerAsn) inserted after Asn^{925}
20	2846	T→A: Val^{949} to Asp
16-20		deletion of exons 16-20

Table 1. Salient characteristics of 52 GSDII disease specific mutations.

Structural changes

Morphological alterations are illustrated in Figures 1, 2, and 3 and the microscopic pathology and pathogenesis are summarized by Dr George Karpati: in the *infantile form*, most muscle fibres contain massive, PAS-positive glycogen storage. In many areas of the fibres from where glycogen

	Genotype	Number of patients	References
1.	del exon 18 + ?	17	(13, 16, 52, 74)
2.	del T^{525}-homozygous	12	(41, 42)
3.	del exon 18 + del T525	9	(41, 42)
4.	C^{2560}→TArg^{854} to stop-homozygous	6	(7, 52)
5.	del exon 18-homozygous	6	(3, 16, 35, 42)
6.	C^{2560}→T; Arg^{854} to stop + ?	5	(7, 52)
7.	del exon 18 G^{925}→A; Gly^{309} to Arg	3	(43)
8.	T^{953}→C; Met^{318} to Thr + ?	3	(52, 78)
9.	AG$^{2741-2}$→CAGG; Pro^{913} to shift homozygous	3	(24)
10.	C^{1798}→T; Arg^{600} to Cys + ?	3	(71)
11.	del T^{525} + ?	3	(29, 40)
12.	C^{1935}→A; Asp^{645} to Glu-homozygous (common Chinese mutation)	3	(67, 71)
13.	del T^{525} G^{925}→A; Gly^{309} to Arg	2	(43)
14.	exon 16 insertion G^{2242} + ?	2	(8)
15.	A^{1555}→G; Met^{519} to Val+ ?	2	(34, 52)
16.	del 1411-1414 (GAGA) in exon 8 C^{1935}→A; Asp^{645} to Glu	2	(66)
17.	C^{1941}→G; Cys^{647} to Trp + ?	2	(52)
18.	G1933→A; Asp645 to Asn insertion G^{2243}	1	(37)
19.	C^{1941}→G; Cys^{647} to Trp- homozygous	1	(37)
20.	insertion C^{258}exon 2 + ?	1	(8)
21.	G^{2237}→A:Trp^{746} to stop + ?	1	(8)
22.	@ bp 2776-duplication-18 bp - 6 a.a. after Asn^{925} (GlyValProValSerAsn) G^{2237}→A:Trp^{746} to stop	1	(8)
23.	del 16-20 exons-homozygous	1	(36)
24.	C^{2560}→T ; Arg^{854} to stop T^{2846}→A; Val^{949} to Asp	1	(7)
25.	del exon 18 del TG^{379}	1	(43)
26.	IVS16 (+2T→C), del 16 bp (2315-2330) in exon 16-homozygous	1	(26)
27.	exon 2-C^{118}→T; Arg^{40} to stop-homozygous	1	(41)
28.	G^{1933}→A; Asp^{645} to Asn- homozygous	1	(16)
29.	G^{1561}→A; Glu^{521} to Lys-homozygous	1	(21)
30.	del exon 18 2707-2709 del; del Lys^{903}	1	(14)
31.	del exon 18 T^{896}→G; Leu^{299} to Arg	1	(14)
32.	del exon 18 C^{1941}→G; Cys^{647} to Trp	1	(32)
33.	C^{1941}→G; Cys^{647} to Trp del 1456-1468 in exon 10	1	(32)
34.	C^{2303}→G; Pro^{768} to Arg-homozygous	1	(24)
35.	T^{1696}→C; Ser^{566} to Pro-homozygous	1	(24)
36.	AG$^{2741-2}$→CAGG; Pro^{913} to shift + ?	1	(24)
37.	C^{172}→T; Gln^{58} to stop del T^{525}	1	(35)
38.	C^{1798}→T; Arg^{600} to Cys-homozygous	1	(71)
39.	T^{896}→G; Leu^{299} to Arg + ?	1	(52)
40.	del 1456-68 in exon 10 + ?	1	(52)
41.	C^{1935}→A; Asp^{645} to Glu + ?	1	(52)
42.	2706-2708 del; del Lys^{903} + ?	1	(52)

Table 2. Genotypes Identified in 108 infantile onset patients (Pompe's disease).

has been dissolved during processing, optically empty vacuolar spaces are present (Figure 3). These are positive for acid phosphatase activity indicating their lysosomal nature. The perimeter of the vacuoles tends to show immunostaining for dystrophin, spectrin, and laminin.This feature is not specific for alpha glucosidase deficiency because a similar pattern is present in other forms of abnormal lysosomal storage in muscle fibers.

In addition to the PAS positive glycogen, alcian positive and metachromatically staining material also accumulates in muscle fibres. It has been postulated that this material corresponds to abnormally phosphated derivatives of glycogen.

Electron microscopy shows large lakes of normal appearing glycogen surrounded by a single membrane, consistent with the lysosomal nature of glycogen storage. Many vacuoles contain heterogeneous cell debris including whorls of cytomembranes, implying that the membrane-bound spaces are formed as a result of autophagy. Histochemical techniques to show absent alpha glucosidase activity, or immunoctochemistry demonstrating absent alpha glucosidase protein, are theoretically feasible, but the exceedingly low levels in normal muscle fibers practically precludes the use of these techniques for a precise molecular diagnosis on tissue sections.

In the adult form, the histochemical and electron microscopic features are similar, but the glycogen pockets are smaller and muscle fibres tend to show a "peppering" with numerous vacuoles, mainly in type 1 muscle fibres. This fibres' type predilection is not explained.

Pathogenesis

It is presumed that in normal muscle fibers there is a low grade but constant autophagy of random small cellular regions, perhaps as one mechanism to achieve homeostasis of cell volume and size. Normally, the autophagic vacuoles formed by this process are inconspicuous because the autophagic vacuoles posses all catabolic enzymes required to break down diverse molecules, including glycogen. This would explain the slow emergence of conspicuous lysosomes or autophagic vacuoles filled with undegraded glycogen in the acid maltase deficiency syndromes.

It is further presumed that the main deleterious effect of the massive lysosomal glycogen storage is related to the "space-occupying" effect of the storage masses. An additional deleterious consequence of the lysosomal storage was believed to be focal cellular damage related to "bursting" of the maximally distended lysosomes. However, there is no convincing proof for this mechanism operating.

Genotype-phenotype correlations

We cloned the first authentic cDNA for human GAA in 1986, which is 3.4 kb (54). The structural gene (25 kb) contains 20 exons of various sizes from 100 to 600 bp (50, 73). Barnes and Wynn (5) have shown homology between GAA and sucrase-isomaltase and predicted a catalytic site, a site governing posttranslational modification (phosphorylation of mannose), and a binding site for the high molecular weight substrate, glycogen. Acid maltase deficiency, as other genetic disorders, can be expected to represent an allelic series at the GAA locus, ie, different patients will have various mutations with differing effects, depending upon where they occur in the molecule. There is evidence for extensive heterogeneity responsible for infantile and adult onset forms, not only between, but also among different clinical forms. Mutations can potentially give rise to defects at the level of RNA (in synthesis, stability or nonsense) or at the level of the protein (abnormalities in stability, processing, trafficking, binding of substrate or catalytic sites).

Earlier studies have revealed, not surprisingly, an absence of mRNA in a high proportion of infantile onset patients (25, 45) and a large percentage of adult onset patients containing the exon 2 deletion (12). We hypothesise that many early onset adult patients will be genetic compounds for a mutation also found in infantile onset patients and an "adult onset" mutation. It is well recognised that patients with the adult onset form do not have

	Genotype	Number of patients	Refs.
1.	$C^{2014} \rightarrow T$; Arg^{672} to Trp- homozygous	1	(37)
2.	del T^{525} + IVS1 (-13 T$\rightarrow$G)	1	(42)
3.	$C^{2560} \rightarrow T$; Arg^{854} to stop	1	(2)
	t$\rightarrow$g -22 bp in IVS6-inserts 21 bp in mRNA & del exon 6		
4.	del T^{525} + $C^{1634} \rightarrow G$; Pro^{545} to Arg	1	(20)
5.	del T^{525} + ?	1	(20)
6.	$C^{1634} \rightarrow G$; Pro^{545} to Arg + ?	2	(20, 75)
7.	del exon 18 + ?	1	(16)
8.	$C^{2560} \rightarrow T$; Arg^{854} to stop	1	(15)
	$A^{875} \rightarrow G$; Tyr^{292} to Cys		
9.	$G^{2015} \rightarrow A$; Arg^{672} to Gln-homozygous	2	(71)
10.	$G^{2015} \rightarrow A$; Arg^{672} to Gln + ?	2	(71)
11.	$C^{1798} \rightarrow T$; Arg^{600} to Cys + ?	3	(71)
12.	IVS1 (-13 T$\rightarrow$G) + ?	1	(47)
13.	$C^{971} \rightarrow T$; Pro^{324} to Leu + ?	1	(47)

Table 3. Genotypes identified in 18 in juvenile onset patients.

involvement of the heart, while infantile onset patients have a striking involvement, which is a prominent site of glycogen deposition. This difference cannot be totally explained by differences in residual enzyme activity, since some adult onset patients have essentially no detectable activity and are not distinguishable by enzyme assay from infantile onset patients.

In an attempt to try to correlate clinical phenotype with genotype, we reviewed the literature for confirmed disease specific mutations, which totalled 52 (Table 1). These genetic alterations range from single base substitutions in coding regions that alter significant amino acids or stop codons, deletion of single or multiple base pairs as large as exon(s), insertions of varying lengths, and combinations of the above. Tables 2, 3, and 4 list all the mutations or combinations of mutations found in the infantile, juvenile, or adult onset cases. All of these studies except one, which screened 43 patients for 15 known mutations (52), were directed at identifying a new mutation in an informative patient and then screening other patients for that particular mutation(s). Thus, the percentage of patients carrying unknown mutations remains unclear. Shortly, we will be publishing an extensive study of 113 patients for 30 GSDII mutations, which will address these questions.

There have been at least 28 articles identifying the mutation(s) in infantile onset patients (Table 2). From these studies, 42 different combinations of alleles was found in 108 patients. One hundred-thirteen patients did not contain the mutation studied. Thirty-nine patients were homozygous, 25 were heterozygous with both mutations identified, and 44 were heterozygous with only 1 mutation determined. One hundred seventy-two (80%) of 216 alleles contained a mutation. Forty-five (21%) of 216 alleles contained the del exon 18, while 39 (18%) of 216 alleles contained the del T^{525}.

For later onset patients, there were 10 reports identifying 13 different genotypes in 18 juvenile onset cases (Table 3), and 23 manuscripts describing 40 allelic combinations in 138 adult onset patients (Table 4). Seventeen juvenile and 133 to 162 adult patients did not contain the mutation(s) screened for in that study. In juvenile onset patients, 7 were homozygous, 4 were heterozygous with both alleles found, and 8 were heterozygous with only one allele identified. 25 (69%) of 36 alleles contained mutations. For adult cases, 7 were homozygous, 54 were heterozygous with both alleles found, and 77 were compound heterozygotes with only one allele identified. 104 (38%) of 276 alleles contained the IVS1 (-13T$\rightarrow$G) mutation, 26 (12%) of 276 alleles contained the

	Genotype	Number of patients	References
1.	IVS1 (-13 T→G) + ?	53	(4, 16, 33, 47, 52)
2.	IVS1 (-13 T→G) + del T[525]	21	(4, 42, 44, 77)
3.	IVS1 (-13 T→G) + del exon 18	10	(14, 33, 42, 75)
4.	del exon 18 + ?	8	(13, 29, 33, 47, 52, 77)
5.	del T[525] + ?	5	(20, 29),P
6.	IVS1 (-13 T→G) + del CC[482-483]	2	(58)
7.	TC[1585-6]→GT; Ser[529] to Val-homozygous	2	(71)
8.	TC[1585-6]→GT; Ser[529] to Val + ?	2	(71, 72)
9.	insertion C[258] + ?	2	(8)
10.	IVS1 (-13 T→G) + del TG[370-80]	2	(4)*
11.	IVS6 (-22 T→G) homozygous	2	(75)
12.	C[1634]→G; Pro[545] to Arg + ?	1	(20)
13.	G[1942]→A; Gly[648] to Ser IVS1 (-13 T→G)	1	(37)
14.	C[2014]→T; Arg[672] to Trp deletion 766-785/ insertion C	1	(37)
15.	C[1634]→G; Pro[545] to Arg-homozygous	1	(20)
16.	IVS1 (-13 T→G) + G[925]→A; Gly[309] to Arg	1	(43)
17.	G[1927]→A; Gly[643] to Arg C[2173]→T; Arg[725] to Trp	1	(23)
18.	C[1935]→A; Asp[645] to Glu C[2560]→T; Arg[854] to stop	1	(22)
19.	IVS1 (-13 T→G) IVS10; + 1-GT→CT; deleted 1438-1551	1	(33)
20.	del CC[482-483] + ?	1	(58)
21.	TC[1585-6]→GT; Ser[529] to Val C[1935]→A; Asp[645] to Glu	1	(71)
22.	C[1798]→T; Arg[600] to Cys + ?	1	(71)
23.	IVS1 (-13 T→G) + C[172]→T; Gln[58] to stop	1	(4)
24.	IVS10; + 1-GT→CT; deleted 1438-1551 + ?	1	(52)
25.	C[1935]→A; Asp[645] to Glu + ?	1	(52)
26.	C[2560]→T; Arg[854] to stop + ?	1	(52)
27.	IVS1 (-13 T→G) homozygous	1	(47)
28.	IVS1 (-13 T→G) + T[623]→C; Leu[208] to Pro	1	(47)
29.	IVS1 (-13 T→G) + G[1927]→C; Gly[643] to Arg	1	(47)
30.	IVS1 (-13 T→G) + Pro[161]→shift stop	1	(47)
31.	IVS1 (-13 T→G) + G[1754]→T; Arg[585] to Met	1	(47)
32.	IVS1 (-13 T→G) + C[2560]→T; Arg[854] to stop	1	(47)
33.	IVS1 (-13 T→G) del 1821-1836; del 6 aa 607-612	1	(47)
34.	IVS1 (-13 T→G) + C[118]→T; Arg[40] to stop	1	(47)
35.	G[1927]→C; Gly[643] to Arg + ?	1	(47)
36.	C[923]→T; His[308] to Leu C[2014]→A; Arg[672] to Thr	1	(47)
37.	IVS1 (-13 T→G) + del G[271]	1	(75)
38.	IVS1 (1 13 T→G) + G[1912]→T; Gly[638] to Trp	1	(75)
39.	del exon 18 homozygous	1	(75)
40.	IVS1 (-13 T→G) + insertion C[2432]	1	(75)

Table 4. Genotypes identified in 138 adult onset patients.

del T[525] mutation and 15 (7%) of 276 alleles had the del exon 18 mutation. 130 (72%) of 276 alleles contained mutations.

From this summary, we can predict some genotypes that are clearly phenotype associated. Any genotype underlined in Tables 2, 3, and 4 is probably specific for that subtype and we chose not to include any genotype where the second mutation was not identified. All compound heterozygotes were exclusive to the subtype. For 108 infantile onset patients, 26 (62%) of 42 genotypes were specific for this subtype. For 18 juvenile onset patients, 7 (54%) of 13 genotypes were only found in this subgroup. For 138 adult onset cases, 27 (68%) of 40 genotypes were specific for this phenotype. The most common mutations were: IVS1 (-13 T→G), del exon 18, del T[525] and C[2560]→T; Arg[854] to stop. The IVS1 (-13 T→G) mutation was found in 104 (37%) of 276 adult alleles, 2 (6%) of 36 juvenile alleles, and not in infantile cases. The del exon 18 mutation was found in 20 (7%) of 276 adult, 1 (3%) of 36 juvenile, and 43 (20%) of 216 infantile alleles. The del T[525] mutation was found in 26 (9%) of 276 adult alleles, 3 (8%) of 36 juvenile alleles, and 39 (18%) of 216 infantile alleles. The C2560→T; Arg[854] to stop mutation was identified in 2 (1%) of 276 adult, 1 (3%) of 36 juvenile, and 18 (8%) of 216 infantile alleles. Some general trends can be noted. The del exon 18, del T[525] and C[2560]→T; Arg[854] to stop mutations must be alleles that result in very low residual GAA activity since they homozygous or in combination with each other in the infantile cases. They do occur in later onset cases, but only with the IVS1 (-13 T→G) or an unknown mutation whose residual GAA activity must be much higher. Patients homozygous for a mutation were subtype exclusive, except for the del exon 18 mutation where it was found homozygous in six infantile, no juvenile and one adult patient. We suspect that there are more adult onset patients that are not recognised due to the age of onset and milder clinical presentation (possibly homozygous for the IVS1 (-13 T→G) mutation.

Future perspectives

Currently, there is no cure for GSDII. Future studies that determine the remaining mutations will complete the correlation between genotype and clinical presentation. These data may reveal some clues as to prediction of clinical outcome. However, the influence of other genetic loci and their respective proteins cannot be overlooked. The metabolism, and in particular, glucose pools and energy of the cell, are influenced by the combined expression of all the enzymes and proteins responsible for their production and use. In GSDII, the residual GAA enzyme level, the consequence of the *GAA* genotype, is the most important limiting factor in determining which major subtype the patient presents.

The combination of disease-specific mutations determines the residual GAA activity. In general, the less GAA residual activity, the more severe the subtype. The heterogeneity between and within subtypes may result from a combination of residual GAA activity, the natural decline of GAA activity with age, and the overall expression of genes at other loci, ultimately affecting cellular energy and glucose pools. Newer recombinant DNA technology (microarrays) and availability of the human genome sequence will provide the resources to identify the other loci that influence the clinical presentation of GSDII.

References

1. Abbott GW, Butler MH, Bendahhou S, Dalakas MC, Ptacek LJ, Goldstein SA (2001) MiRP2 forms potassium channels in skeletal muscle with Kv3.4 and is associated with periodic paralysis. Cell 104: 217-231

2. Adams EM, Becker JA, Griffith L, Segal A, Plotz PH, Raben N (1997) Glycogenosis type II: a juvenile-specific mutation with an unusual splicing pattern and a shared mutation in African Americans. Hum Mutat 10: 128-134

3. Ausems MG, Kroos MA, Van der Kraan M, Smeitink JA, Kleijer WJ, Ploos van Amstel HK, Reuser AJ (1996) Homozygous deletion of exon 18 leads to degradation of the lysosomal alpha-glucosidase precursor and to the infantile form of glycogen storage disease type II. Clin Genet 49: 325-328

4. Ausems MG, ten Berg K, Beemer FA, Wokke JH (2000) Phenotypic expression of late-onset glycogen storage disease type II: identification of asymptomatic adults through family studies and review of reported families. Neuromuscul Disord 10: 467-471

5. Barnes AK, Wynn CH (1988) Homology of lysosomal enzymes and related proteins: prediction of posttranslational modification sites including phosphorylation of mannose and potential epitopic and substrate binding sites in the alpha- and beta-subunits of hexosaminidases, alpha-glucosidase, and rabbit and human isomaltase. Proteins 4: 182-189

6. Baudhuim PHG, Hers HG, Loeb H (1964) An electronmicroscopic and biochemical study of type II glycogenosis. Lab Invest 13: 1139-1152

7. Becker JA, Vlach J, Raben N, Nagaraju K, Adams EM, Hermans MM, Reuser AJ, Brooks SS, Tifft CJ, Hirschhorn R, Huie ML, Nicolino M, Plotz PH (1998) The African origin of the common mutation in African American patients with glycogen-storage disease type II. Am J Hum Genet 62: 991-994

8. Beesley CE, Child AH, Yacoub MH (1998) The identification of five novel mutations in the lysosomal acid a-(1- 4) glucosidase gene from patients with glycogen storage disease type II. Mutations in brief no. 134. Online. Hum Mutat 11: 413

9. Beratis NG, LaBadie GU, Hirschhorn K (1978) Characterization of the molecular defect in infantile and adult acid alpha-glucosidase deficiency fibroblasts. J Clin Invest 62: 1264-1274

10. Beratis NG, LaBadie GU, Hirschhorn K (1983) Genetic heterogeneity in acid alpha-glucosidase deficiency. Am J Hum Genet 35: 21-33

11. Bijvoet AG, van de Kamp EH, Kroos MA, Ding JH, Yang BZ, Visser P, Bakker CE, Verbeet MP, Oostra BA, Reuser AJ, van der Ploeg AT (1998) Generalized glycogen storage and cardiomegaly in a knockout mouse model of Pompe disease. Hum Mol Genet 7: 53-62

12. Bijvoet AGA, Kroos MA, van der Kamp EHM, Oostra BA, Verbeet MP, van der Ploeg AT, Reuser AJJ (1995) Transgenic expression of human lysosomal a-glucosidase in the mammary gland: a feasibly study for treatment of glycogen storage disease type II. Am J Hum Genetics 57: A1004

13. Boerkoel C, Raben N, Martiniuk F, Miller F, Plotz P (1992) Identification of a deletion common to adult and infantile onset acid alpha glucosidase deficiency. Am J Hum Gen 51: A347

14. Boerkoel CF, Exelbert R, Nicastri C, Nichols RC, Miller FW, Plotz PH, Raben N (1995) Leaky splicing mutation in the acid maltase gene is associated with delayed onset of glycogenosis type II. Am J Hum Genet 56: 887-897

15. Castro-Gago M, Eiris-Punal J, Rodriguez-Nunez A, Pintos-Martinez E, Benlloch-Marin T, Barros-Angueira F (1999) Severe form of juvenile type II glycogenosis in a compound- heterozygous boy (Tyr-292→Cys/Arg-854→Stop). Rev Neurol 29: 46-49

16. Dagnino F, Stroppiano M, Regis S, Bonuccelli G, Filocamo M (2000) Evidence for a founder effect in Sicilian patients with glycogen storage disease type II. Hum Hered 50: 331-333

17. Engel AG (1970) Acid maltase deficiency in adults: studies in four cases of a syndrome which may mimic muscular dystrophy or other myopathies. Brain 93: 599-616

18. Engel AG, Gomez MR, Seybold ME, Lambert EH (1973) The spectrum and diagnosis of acid maltase deficiency. Neurology 23: 95-106

19. Healy PJ, Sewell CA, Nieper RE, Whittle RJ, Reichmann KG (1987) Control of generalised glycogenosis in a Brahman herd. Aust Vet J 64: 278-280

20. Hermans MM, De Graaff E, Kroos MA, Mohkamsing S, Eussen BJ, Joosse M, Willemsen R, Kleijer WJ, Oostra BA, Reuser AJ (1994) The effect of a single base pair deletion (delta T525) and a C1634T missense mutation (pro545leu) on the expression of lysosomal alpha- glucosidase in patients with glycogen storage disease type II. Hum Mol Genet 3: 2213-2218

21. Hermans MM, de Graaff E, Kroos MA, Wisselaar HA, Oostra BA, Reuser AJ (1991) Identification of a point mutation in the human lysosomal alpha- glucosidase gene causing infantile glycogenosis type II. Biochem Biophys Res Commun 179: 919-926

22. Hermans MM, de Graaff E, Kroos MA, Wisselaar HA, Willemsen R, Oostra BA, Reuser AJ (1993) The conservative substitution Asp-645→Glu in lysosomal alpha- glucosidase affects transport and phosphorylation of the enzyme in an adult patient with glycogen-storage disease type II. Biochem J 289: 687-693

23. Hermans MM, Kroos MA, de Graaff E, Oostra BA, Reuser AJ (1993) Two mutations affecting the transport and maturation of lysosomal alpha- glucosidase in an adult case of glycogen storage disease type II. Hum Mutat 2: 268-273

24. Hermans MM, Kroos MA, Smeitink JA, van der Ploeg AT, Kleijer WJ, Reuser AJ (1998) Glycogen Storage Disease type II: genetic and biochemical analysis of novel mutations in infantile patients from Turkish ancestry. Hum Mutat 11: 209-215

25. Hermans MM, Kroos MA, van Beeumen J, Oostra BA, Reuser AJ (1991) Human lysosomal alpha-glucosidase. Characterization of the catalytic site. J Biol Chem 266: 13507-13512

26. Hermans MM, van Leenen D, Kroos MA, Reuser AJ (1997) Mutation detection in glycogen storage-disease type II by RT-PCR and automated sequencing. Biochem Biophys Res Commun 241: 414-418

27. Hers H, vanHoof F, deBarsy T (1989) Glycogen storage diseases. In The metabolic basis of inherited disease, CR Scriver, AL Beaudet, W Sly, D Valle (eds). McGraw-Hill: New York. pp. 425-452

28. Hers HG (1983) Alpha glucosidase in generalized glycogen storage disease (Pompe's disease). Biochem J 86: 11-16

29. Hirschhorn R, Huie ML (1999) Frequency of mutations for glycogen storage disease type II in different populations: the delta525T and deltaexon 18 mutations are not generally "common" in white populations. J Med Genet 36: 85-86

30. Honig J, Martiniuk F, D'Eustachio P, Zamfirescu C, Desnick R, Hirschhorn K, Hirschhorn LR, Hirschhorn R (1984) Confirmation of the regional localization of the genes for human acid alpha-glucosidase (GAA) and adenosine deaminase (ADA) by somatic cell hybridization. Ann Hum Genet 48: 49-56

31. Howell JM, Dorling PR, Cook RD, Robinson WF, Bradley S, Gawthorne JM (1981) Infantile and late onset form of generalised glycogenosis type II in cattle. J Pathol 134: 267-277

32. Huie ML, Chen AS, Brooks SS, Grix A, Hirschhorn R (1994) A de novo 13 nt deletion, a newly identified C647W missense mutation and a deletion of exon 18 in infantile onset glycogen storage disease type II (GSDII). Hum Mol Genet 3: 1081-1087

33. Huie ML, Chen AS, Tsujino S, Shanske S, DiMauro S, Engel AG, Hirschhorn R (1994) Aberrant splicing in adult onset glycogen storage disease type II (GSDII): molecular identification of an IVS1 (-13T→G) mutation in a majority of patients and a novel IVS10 (+1GT→CT) mutation. Hum Mol Genet 3: 2231-2236

34. Huie ML, Hirschhorn R, Chen AS, Martiniuk F, Zhong N (1994) Mutation at the catalytic site (M519V) in glycogen storage disease type II (Pompe disease). Hum Mutat 4: 291-293

35. Huie ML, Kasper JS, Arn PH, Greenberg CR, Hirschhorn R (1999) Increased occurrence of cleft lip in glycogen storage disease type II (GSDII): exclusion of a contiguous gene syndrome in two patients by presence of intragenic mutations including a novel nonsense mutation Gln58Stop. *Am J Med Genet* 85: 5-8

36. Huie ML, Shanske AL, Kasper JS, Marion RW, Hirschhorn R (1999) A large Alu-mediated deletion, identified by PCR, as the molecular basis for glycogen storage disease type II (GSDII). *Hum Genet* 104: 94-98

37. Huie ML, Tsujino S, Sklower Brooks S, Engel A, Elias E, Bonthron DT, Bessley C, Shanske S, DiMauro S, Goto YI, Hirschhorn R (1998) Glycogen storage disease type II: identification of four novel missense mutations (D645N, G648S, R672W, R672Q) and two insertions/deletions in the acid alpha-glucosidase locus of patients of differing phenotype. *Biochem Biophys Res Commun* 244: 921-927

38. Jeffrey PL, Brown DH, Brown BI (1970) Studies of lysosomal alpha-glucosidase. II. Kinetics of action of the rat liver enzyme. *Biochemistry* 9: 1416-1422

39. Jolly RD, Van-de-Water NS, Richards RB, Dorling PR (1977) Generalized glycogenosis in beef shorthorn cattle--heterozygote detection. *Aust J Exp Biol Med Sci* 55: 14U-50

40. Kleijer WJ, van der Kraan M, Kroos MA, Groener JE, van Diggelen OP, Reuser AJ, van der Ploeg AT (1995) Prenatal diagnosis of glycogen storage disease type II: enzyme assay or mutation analysis? *Pediatr Res* 38: 103-106

41. Kroos MA, Van der Kraan M, Van Diggelen OP, Kleijer WJ, Reuser AJ (1997) Two extremes of the clinical spectrum of glycogen storage disease type II in one family: a matter of genotype. *Hum Mutat* 9: 17-22

42. Kroos MA, Van der Kraan M, Van Diggelen OP, Kleijer WJ, Reuser AJ, Van den Boogaard MJ, Ausems MG, Ploos van Amstel HK, Poenaru L, Nicolino M, et al. (1995) Glycogen storage disease type II: frequency of three common mutant alleles and their associated clinical phenotypes studied in 121 patients. *J Med Genet* 32: 836-837

43. Kroos MA, van Leenen D, Verbiest J, Reuser AJ, Hermans MM (1998) Glycogen storage disease type II: identification of a dinucleotide deletion and a common missense mutation in the lysosomal alpha- glucosidase gene. *Clin Genet* 53: 379-382

44. Kroos MA, Waitfield AE, Joosse M, Winchester B, Reuser AJ, MacDermot KD (1997) A novel acid alpha-glucosidase mutation identified in a Pakistani family with glycogen storage disease type II. *J Inherit Metab Dis* 20: 556-558

45. La Badie GU (1986) *Biochemical and immunologic studies of acid alpha glucosidase deficiency, a genetically heterogeneous, inherited neuromuscular disease.* City University of New York, Mt. Sinai Hospital

46. LaBadie GU, Harris H, Beratis NG, Hirschhorn K (1985) Monoclonal antibodies to acid alpha glucosidase; further evidence for genetic heterogeneity. *Am J Hum Genet* 37: A12 (abstract)

47. Laforet P, Nicolino M, Eymard PB, Puech JP, Caillaud C, Poenaru L, Fardeau M (2000) Juvenile and adult-onset acid maltase deficiency in France: genotype- phenotype correlation. *Neurology* 55: 1122-1128

48. Manktelow BW, Hartley WJ (1975) Generalized glycogen storage disease in sheep. *J Comp Pathol* 85: 139-145

49. Martiniuk F, Bodkin M, Tzall S, Hirschhorn R (1990) Identification of the base-pair substitution responsible for a human acid alpha glucosidase allele with lower "affinity" for glycogen (GAA 2) and transient gene expression in deficient cells. *Am J Hum Genet* 47: 440-445

50. Martiniuk F, Bodkin M, Tzall S, Hirschhorn R (1991) Isolation and partial characterization of the structural gene for human acid alpha glucosidase. *DNA Cell Biol* 10: 283-292

51. Martiniuk F, Chen A, Mack A, Codd W, Hanna B, Arvanitopoulos E, Rom WN (1998) Determination of the frequency of carriers for glycogen storage disease type II or acid maltase deficiency in New York City and estimates of affected individuals born with the disease. *Am J Medical Genetics* 79: 69-72

52. Martiniuk F, Chen A, Mack A, Slonim A, Rom WN (1997) Analysis of 43 patients with glycogen storage disease type II or acid maltase deficiency for fifteen disease specific mutations; prediction of mutations associated with clinical presentation. *Am J Resp Crit Care Med* 155: A462

53. Martiniuk F, Ellenbogen A, Hirschhorn K, Hirschhorn R (1985) Further regional localization of the genes for human acid alpha glucosidase (GAA), peptidase D (PEPD), and alpha mannosidase B (MANB) by somatic cell hybridization. *Hum Genet* 69: 109-111

54. Martiniuk F, Mehler M, Pellicer A, Tzall S, La Badie G, Hobart C, Ellenbogen A, Hirschhorn R (1986) Isolation of a cDNA for human acid alpha-glucosidase and detection of genetic heterogeneity for mRNA in three alpha-glucosidase-deficient patients. *Proc Natl Acad Sci U S A* 83: 9641-9644

55. Martiniuk F, Mehler M, Tzall S, Meredith G, Hirschhorn R (1990) Extensive genetic heterogeneity in patients with acid alpha glucosidase deficiency as detected by abnormalities of DNA and mRNA. *Am J Hum Genet* 47: 73-78

56. Mehler M, DiMauro S (1977) Residual acid maltase activity in late-onset acid maltase deficiency. *Neurology* 27: 178-184

57. Nickel BE, McAlpine PJ (1982) Extension of human acid alpha-glucosidase polymorphism by isoelectric focusing in polyacrylamide gel. *Ann Hum Genet* 46: 97-103

58. Nicolino M, Puech JP, Letourneur F, Fardeau M, Kahn A, Poenaru L (1997) Glycogen-storage disease type II (acid maltase deficiency): identification of a novel small deletion (delCC482+483) in French patients. *Biochem Biophys Res Commun* 235: 138-141

59. Nunoya T, Tajima M, Mizutani M (1983) A new mutant of Japanese quail (Coturnix coturnix japonica) characterized by generalized glycogenosis. *Lab Anim* 17: 138-142

60. O'Sullivan BM, Healy PJ, Fraser IR, Nieper RE, Whittle RJ, Sewell CA (1981) Generalised glycogenosis in Brahman cattle. *Aust Vet J* 57: 227-229

61. Poorthuis BJ, Wevers RA, Kleijer WJ, Groener JE, de Jong JG, van Weely S, Niezen-Koning KE, van Diggelen OP (1999) The frequency of lysosomal storage diseases in The Netherlands. *Hum Genet* 105: 151-156

62. Raben N, Nagaraju K, Lee E, Kessler P, Byrne B, Lee L, LaMarca M, King C, Ward J, Sauer B, Plotz P (1998) Targeted disruption of the acid alpha-glucosidase gene in mice causes an illness with critical features of both infantile and adult human glycogen storage disease type II. *J Biol Chem* 273: 19086-19092

63. Reuser AJ, Kroos M, Oude Elferink RP, Tager JM (1985) Defects in synthesis, phosphorylation, and maturation of acid alpha- glucosidase in glycogenosis type II. *J Biol Chem* 260: 8336-8341

64. Reuser AJ, Kroos M, Willemsen R, Swallow D, Tager JM, Galjaard H (1987) Clinical diversity in glycogenosis type II. Biosynthesis and in situ localization of acid alpha-glucosidase in mutant fibroblasts. *J Clin Invest* 79: 1689-1699

65. Sandstrom B, Westrum I, Ockerman PA (1965) Glycogenosis of the central nervous system of the cat. *Acta Neuropathol* 14: 194-200

66. Shieh JJ, Lin CY (1996) Identification of a small deletion in one allele of patients with infantile form of glycogen storage disease type II. *Biochem Biophys Res Commun* 219: 322-326

67. Shieh JJ, Wang LY, Lin CY (1994) Point mutation in Pompe disease in Chinese. *J Inherit Metab Dis* 17: 145-148

68. Slonim AE, Bulone L, Ritz S, Goldberg T, Chen A, Martiniuk F (2000) Identification of two subtypes of infantile acid maltase deficiency. *J Pediatr* 137: 283-285

69. Solomon E, Swallow D, Burgess S, Evans L (1981) Assignment of the human acid alpha glucosidase gene to chromosome 17 using somatic cell hybrids. *Ann Hum Genet* 42: 273-281

70. Tager JM, Oude Elferink RP, Reuser A, Kroos M, Ginsel LA, Fransen JA, Klumperman J (1987) alpha-Glucosidase deficiency (Pompe's disease). *Enzyme* 38: 280-285

71. Tsujino S, Huie M, Kanazawa N, Sugie H, Goto Y, Kawai M, Nonaka I, Hirschhorn R, Sakuragawa N (2000) Frequent mutations in Japanese patients with acid maltase deficiency. *Neuromuscul Disord* 10: 599-603

72. Tsunoda H, Ohshima T, Tohyama J, Martiniuk F, Sasaki M, Sakuragawa N (1995) Acid alpha glucosidase: Identification of a missense mutation (S529V) in a Japanese adult phenotype. *Human Genetics* 97: 496-499

73. Tzall S, Martiniuk F (1991) Identification of the promoter region and gene expression for human acid alpha glucosidase. Biochem Biophys Res Commun 176: 1509-1515

74. Van der Kraan M, Kroos MA, Joosse M, Bijvoet AG, Verbeet MP, Kleijer WJ, Reuser AJ (1994) Deletion of exon 18 is a frequent mutation in glycogen storage dis-

ease type II. *Biochem Biophys Res Commun* 203: 1535-1541

75. Vorgerd M, Burwinkel B, Reichmann H, Malin JP, Kilimann MW (1998) Adult-onset glycogen storage disease type II: phenotypic and allelic heterogeneity in German patients. *Neurogenetics* 1: 205-211

76. Walvoort HC, Slee RG, Koster JF (1982) Canine glycogen storage disease type II. A biochemical study of an acid alpha-glucosidase-deficient Lapland dog. *Biochim Biophys Acta* 715: 63-69

77. Wokke JH, Ausems MG, van den Boogaard MJ, Ippel EF, van Diggelene O, Kroos MA, Boer M, Jennekens FG, Reuser AJ, Ploos van Amstel HK (1995) Genotype-phenotype correlation in adult-onset acid maltase deficiency. *Ann Neurol* 38: 450-454

78. Zhong N, Martiniuk F, Tzall S, Hirschhorn R (1991) Identification of a missense mutation in one allele of a patient with Pompe disease, and use of endonuclease digestion of PCR-amplified RNA to demonstrate lack of mRNA expression from the second allele. *Am J Hum Genet* 49: 635-645

LAMP-2 deficiency

Ichizo Nishino
Michio Hirano
Salvatore DiMauro

LAMP-2	lysosome-associated membrane-2
Limp-I	lysosome integral membrane protein-I
XMEA	X-linked myopathy with excessive autophagy

Definition of entities

LAMP-2. Lysosome-associated membrane-2 (LAMP-2) is a major lysosomal membrane glycoprotein that coats the inner side of the lysosomal membrane together with its paralogous counterpart, LAMP-1 (5). The *LAMP-2* gene is located on Xq24, while the gene for LAMP-1 is on 13q34. Two functions have been proposed for LAMP-2: *i)* protecting the lysosomal membrane, and thus cytoplasm, from being attacked by proteolytic enzymes in the lysosomal lumen, and *ii)* acting as a receptor for proteins to be imported into and degraded within lysosomes.

Lysosomal glycogen storage disease with normal acid maltase. LAMP-2 deficiency causes X-linked vacuolar cardiomyopathy and myopathy (Danon's disease) (12). This disease was originally reported by Danon et al in 1981, and labelled "lysosomal glycogen storage disease with normal acid maltase"; both clinical manifestations and muscle biopsy findings in their two patients resembled those seen in acid maltase deficiency, although acid maltase activity was normal (3).

There have been 16 case reports of "lysosomal glycogen storage disease with normal acid maltase" in the English literature, but the disorder is probably genetically heterogeneous: in particular, two infantile patients most likely had a distinct disease (9, 14). Despite being part of the original description, glycogen is not always increased in skeletal muscle; therefore, we prefer to call the disease "X-linked vacuolar cardiomyopathy and myopathy" or "Danon's disease."

Clinical manifestations. Typically, the disease is characterised by hypertrophic cardiomyopathy, myopathy, and mental retardation. All probands have been male, but most mothers have had milder later-onset cardiomyopathy, suggesting X-linked dominant inheritance (2, 14).

In probands, cardiac symptoms, such as exertional dyspnoea, start in teenage years. The association of hypertrophic cardiomyopathy and cardiac arrhythmia is common, and patients typically die of cardiac failure or cardiac arrest in their fourth decade.

The myopathy is usually mild and all patients have been ambulant throughout their lives. Even in preclinical subjects, serum creatine kinase levels are 5 to 10-fold above upper normal values. Weakness and atrophy affect predominantly shoulder girdle and neck muscles, but distal muscles can also be involved. Although both original patients reported by Danon et al (3) had mental retardation, this manifestation is mild, or absent in about 40% of the genetically confirmed patients. Liver was primarily affected in some patients (8). In fact, in *LAMP-2* knockout mice, a wider variety of organs is affected, including liver, kidney, pancreas, small intestine, thymus, and spleen, in addition to heart and skeletal muscle (13). Therefore, other organs can potentially be involved in this disease.

Molecular genetics and pathogenesis

Structure of LAMP-2 gene. The open reading frame of the *LAMP-2* gene consists of 9 exons. Human exon 9 exists in 2 forms, exon 9a and 9b, that are alternatively spliced and produce 2 isoforms, LAMP-2a and LAMP-2b (7). LAMP-2a is distributed rather ubiquitously, while LAMP-2b is expressed predominantly in heart and skeletal muscles. LAMP-2 is a type 1 membrane protein, with three domains: luminal, transmembrane, and cytoplasmic. Exons 1 through 8, and part of exon 9, encode the luminal domain, while the remainder of exon 9 encodes both the transmembrane and the cytoplasmic domains.

Primary LAMP-2 deficiency. We have analysed samples from 11 patients, including one of the 2 patients of Danon et al (3), and we have identified *LAMP-2* gene mutations in ten patients (12). Nine of them had stop-codon or frame-shift mutations that are predicted to truncate the protein before the transmembrane domain. One patient had an exon-skipping mutation which deletes one of the 4 loop structures, and therefore, probably produces severe structural changes.

In immunohistochemical and western blot analyses, LAMP-2 protein was virtually absent in all patients, including the one with an exon-skipping mutation. However, in a patient harbouring a mutation in exon 9b, western blot revealed a trace amount of the LAMP-2 protein. This signal most likely represents LAMP-2a because the mutation in exon 9b should affect only the LAMP-2b isoform. These data not only buttress the idea that LAMP-2b is the major isoform in cardiac and skeletal muscles, but also suggest that a deficiency of LAMP-2b by itself is sufficient to cause the disease.

Secondary LAMP-2 deficiency? In one patient with typical clinical manifestations of Danon's disease, we failed to identify a mutation in the *LAMP-2* gene (12). Either a mutation was present, but in a region that we did not

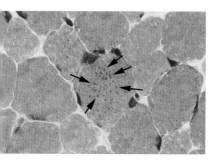

Figure 1. *Light microscopic findings.* Multiple autophagic vacuoles are visible as basophilic granules (arrows) and small intracytoplasmic vacuoles. Haematoxyline and eosin.

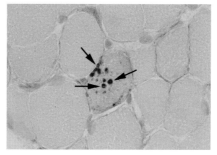

Figure 2. Acetylcholine esterase activity (dark brown staining) is present along the vacuolar membrane (arrows).

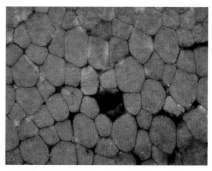

Figure 3. LAMP-2 immunoreactivity is absent.

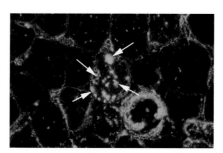

Figure 4. However, limp-l, another lysosomal membrane protein, is abundant in the vacuolar membrane (arrows). Immunohistochemistry for limp-l.

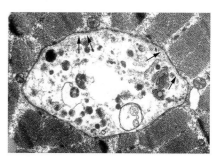

Figure 5. *Electron micrograph* showing an autophagic vacuole in a muscle biopsy of a Danon disease patient. There are various autophagic materials, including myelin figures, electron dense components, and glycogen granules. In addition, basal lamina (arrows) is seen along the inner side of the vacuolar membrane.

sequence (an untranslated region), or this patient had a secondary deficiency of LAMP-2.

Structural changes

Skeletal muscle. Muscle biopsy (Figure 1-4) shows many intracytoplasmic vacuoles which on haematoxylin and eosin staining, often appear like solid basophilic granules, and can be easily overlooked. In fact, these are autophagic vacuoles that typically contain myelin figures, electron-dense bodies, and various cytoplasmic debris. Interestingly, the vacuolar membrane shares properties with the plasma membrane, including such sarcolemma-specific proteins as dystrophin, merosin, and α-sarcoglycan (10, 11) Furthermore, the vacuolar membrane has acetylcholinesterase activity, which can be revealed by histochemical staining for acetylcholine as well as non-specific esterases (11). Electron microscopy (Figure 5) sometimes reveals the presence of basal lamina along the inner surface of autophagic vacuoles.

Heart. Cardiac muscle shows fibrosis and intracytoplasmic vacuoles (4, 10). Electron microscopic examination reveals autophagic vacuoles containing cytoplasmic debris. In *LAMP-2* knockout mice, heart is enlarged and cardiac contractile force is reduced. In the animals, similar autophagic vacuoles are seen not only in skeletal and cardiac muscles, but also in other organs, such as liver and pancreas (13).

Other organs. Although mental retardation is frequent in this disease, brain MRI and EEG are usually normal. Brain histology has not been reported. Liver biopsy in one patient showed mild fatty changes and nuclear vacuolization, although glycogen was not increased (8).

Future perspectives

Despite our knowledge of the defective gene, the pathomechanism leading to the formation of the characteristic vacuoles in this disease still eludes us. Similar pathology can be seen in another vacuolar myopathy, X-linked myopathy with excessive autophagy (XMEA) (6). The locus for XMEA is on Xq28 (1, 15). Hopefully, the genetic cause of this disorder will be identified in the near future; indeed, this may reveal a common pathomechanism for Danon's disease and XMEA.

Future research will include gene therapy, which may require only the expression of LAMP-2b isoform. As indicated by the patient with an exon 9b mutation, expression of LAMP-2b may be sufficient to treat most of the symptoms (12). Presently, cardiomyopathy is the central and life-threatening manifestation, frequently associated with sudden death; treatment should be focused on the prevention of sudden death and cardiac failure. At present, the only effective treatment is cardiac transplantation. This was performed in one patient, who was reportedly well four years after the operation (4).

References

1. Auranen M, Villanova M, Muntoni F, Fardeau M, Scherer SW, Kalino H, Minassian BA (2000) X-linked vacuolar myopathies: two separate loci and refined genetic mapping. *Ann Neurol* 47: 666-669

2. Byrne E, Dennett X, Crotty B, Trounce I, Sands JM, Hawkins R, Hammond J, Anderson S, Haan EA, Pollard A (1986) Dominantly inherited cardioskeletal myopathy with lysosomal glycogen storage and normal acid maltase levels. *Brain* 109: 523-536

3. Danon MJ, Oh SJ, DiMauro S, Manaligod JR, Eastwood A, Naidu S, Schliselfeld LH (1981) Lysosomal glycogen storage disease with normal acid maltase. *Neurology* 31: 51-57

4. Dworzak F, Casazza F, Mora M, De Maria R, Gronda E, Baroldi G, Rimoldi M, Morandi L, Cornelio F (1994) Lysosomal glycogen storage with normal acid maltase: a familial study with successful heart transplant. *Neuromuscul Disord* 4: 243-247

5. Fukuda M (1994) Biogenesis of the lysosomal membrane. *Subcell Biochem* 22: 199-230

6. Kalimo H, Savontaus ML, Lang H, Paljarvi L, Sonninen V, Dean PB, Katevuo K, Salminen A (1988) X-linked myopathy with excessive autophagy: a new hereditary muscle disease. *Ann Neurol* 23: 258-265

7. Konecki DS, Foetisch K, Zimmer KP, Schlotter M, Lichter-Konecki U (1995) An alternatively spliced form of the human lysosome-associated membrane protein-2 gene is expressed in a tissue-specific manner. *Biochem Biophys Res Commun* 215: 757-767

8. Matsumoto S, Yamada T, Tanaka K, Hara H, Nonaka I, Uchida T, Miyagi Y, Fukutomi T, Kira J (1999) [Hepatic involvement in a case of lysosomal glycogen storage disease with normal acid maltase]. *Rinsho Shinkeigaku* 39: 717-721

9. Morisawa Y, Fujieda M, Murakami N, Naruse K, Okada T, Morita H, Sawada K, Miyazaki J, Kurashige T, Nonaka I (1998) Lysosomal glycogen storage disease with normal acid maltase with early fatal outcome. *J Neurol Sci* 160: 175-179

10. Muntoni F, Catani G, Mateddu A, Rimoldi M, Congiu T, Faa G, Marrosu MG, Cianchetti C, Porcu M (1994) Familial cardiomyopathy, mental retardation and myopathy associated with desmin-type intermediate filaments. *Neuromuscul Disord* 4: 233-241

11. Murakami N, Goto Y, Itoh M, Katsumi Y, Wada T, Ozawa E, Nonaka I (1995) Sarcolemmal indentation in cardiomyopathy with mental retardation and vacuolar myopathy. *Neuromuscul Disord* 5: 149-155

12. Nishino I, Fu J, Tanji K, Yamada T, Shimojo S, Koori T, Mora M, Riggs JE, Oh SJ, Koga Y, Sue CM, Yamamoto A, Murakami N, Shanske S, Byrne E, Bonilla E, Nonaka I, DiMauro S, Hirano M (2000) Primary LAMP-2 deficiency causes X-linked vacuolar cardiomyopathy and myopathy (Danon disease). *Nature* 406: 906-910

13. Tanaka Y, Guhde G, Suter A, Eskelinen EL, Hartmann D, Lullmann-Rauch R, Janssen PM, Blanz J, von Figura K, Saftig P (2000) Accumulation of autophagic vacuoles and cardiomyopathy in LAMP-2- deficient mice. *Nature* 406: 902-906

14. Verloes A, Massin M, Lombet J, Grattagliano B, Soyeur D, Rigo J, Koulischer L, Van Hoof F (1997) Nosology of lysosomal glycogen storage diseases without in vitro acid maltase deficiency. Delineation of a neonatal form. *Am J Med Genet* 72: 135-142

15. Villard L, des Portes V, Levy N, Louboutin JP, Recan D, Coquet M, Chabrol B, Figarella-Branger D, Chelly J, Pellissier JF, Fontes M (2000) Linkage of X-linked myopathy with excessive autophagy (XMEA) to Xq28. *Eur J Hum Genet* 8: 125-129

X-linked myopathy with excessive autophagy

Berge Minassian
Nicolas Levy
Hannu Kalimo

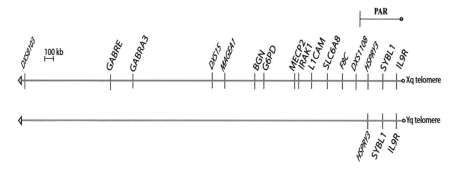

Figure 1. Map sketch of the XMEA gene locus in Xq28 (to scale). Pink, the X chromosome; Blue, the Y chromosome; PAR, the Xq pseudoautosomal region (the X and Y chromosomes have the same sequence and contain the same genes in this region). Some genes in the PAR (e.g. IL9R) are expressed from both the X and Y chromosomes and are therefore not candidates for this X-linked disease. Others (HSPRY3 and SYBL1), are expressed only from the X chromosome and remain therefore positional candidates (2).

Definition of entity

The first family with *X-linked myopathy with excessive autophagy* (XMEA) was described in 1988 by Kalimo et al (5) (OMIM 310440). It is a slowly progressive inherited myopathy characterised by membrane bound sarcoplasmic vacuoles. Therefore, it has been also reported as X-linked vacuolated myopathy, XVM (10). So far, 16 families have been identified in Europe and North America (4).

XMEA patients are males with onset in early childhood. The affected boy is unable to keep up with his companions in running and climbing. Serum creatine kinase values are elevated already during the first years of life by 2.5 to 3 times and may, during adolescence, rise to 10 to 15 times normal. Proximal muscles of the lower limbs are mainly affected, but shoulder girdle muscles are also involved. No other organs appear to be diseased, and the patients have no cardiomyopathy or cognitive deficits. XMEA is slowly progressive and ambulation is usually preserved until later age, but some patients become wheelchair bound around 50 to 60 years of age. XMEA patients have a normal life expectancy. Female carriers are usually without symptoms or only very mildly affected.

EMG findings are characteristic with abundant myotonic and high frequency discharges, without clinical myotonia. This is observed even in clinically unaffected muscles. MRI discloses fatty degeneration with typical distribution. (Jääskeläinen et al, unpublished data).

Molecular genetics and pathophysiology

Genetic linkage was recently established between XMEA and markers in a 10 cM span of the most telomeric band of the long arm of chromosome X (Xq28) (1, 11). A recent unpublished observation of a recombination event in a new family defines marker DXS8103 as the centromeric limit of the XMEA region. The telomeric limit is in the extreme tip of the chromosome within the Xq pseudoautosomal region (PAR) (Figure 1). Based on the completed human genome sequence (*http://www.celera.com*), the segment between DXS8103 and PAR contains 5 million base-pairs of DNA coding for at least 100 genes.

Two main pathogentic mechanisms have been suggested. As the name implies, Kalimo et al (5) suggested that the vacuoles are autophagosomes clearing sarcoplasm of debris after a sublethal injury to the myofibre, and the debris is further extruded from the fibres between the multiple layers of basal lamina. This view is supported by the presence of lysosomal enzymes in both the vacuoles and around the fibres and by the immunopositivity of XMEA

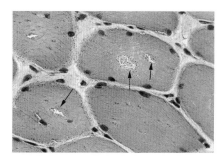

Figure 2. The vacuoles of XMEA (arrows) contain delicate basophilic granules, which are also present around the affected fibres between the multiplied layers of basal lamina, cf. Figure 6. H & E. ×80

vacuoles for LAMP-2, a protein in lysosomal membranes considered to be important in autophagy (8, 9). Even if autophagy appears to have a key role in XMEA, it maybe only secondary to a still unknown primary injury. Villanova et al (10) suggested a "reverse" pathogenesis, ie, the injury is induced by deposition of MAC on myofibres with secondary invagination and/or endocytosis, one of the arguments being that immunopositivity for dystrophin and laminin should not exist on lysosomal membranes. On the other hand, basal lamina is also present in the vacuoles of LAMP-2 deficiency (8), and MAC and calcium deposition may be only secondary to the debris around the affected myofibres (Meri, personal communication).

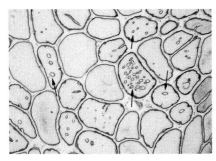

Figure 3. The size variation of myofibres is increased and fibre splitting occurs. Numerous dystrophin-positive vacuoles (arrows) are present in the sarcoplasm of most fibres. Anti-dystrophin 2. ×52

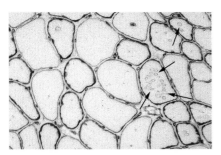

Figure 4. In an adjacent section, many (examples indicated by arrows) but not all vacuoles are weakly positive for muscle specific laminin 2 (merosin), which identifies basal lamina. Note that the affected fibres are surrounded by thickened basal lamina (cf. Figure 6). Anti-laminin 2. ×52

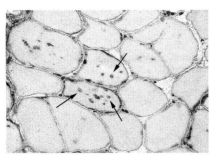

Figure 5. (D) α1-antirypsin-positivity is seen within the vacuoles (arrows) and surrounding the affected fibres. α1-antirypsin.

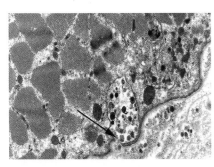

Figure 6. Electron micrograph of affected fibres. Granular debris is present both within a small subsarcolemmal vacuole opening to the surface of the fibre (arrow) and between the multiple layers of basal lamina around the fibre. ×2640

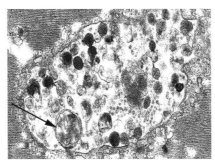

Figure 7. Another vacuole deep in the sarcoplasm contains a degenerating mitochondrion (arrow), small vesicles and granular debris. The vacuole is surrounded by a single membrane without a definite basal lamina. ×8000

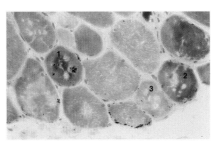

Figure 8. Black deposits of calcium are seen both around some affected fibres and within the vacuoles of one fibre (fibre 1), while in other fibres (fibres 2-3) the vacuoles are negative. ×80

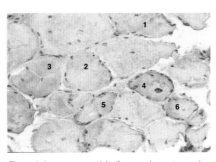

Figure 9. Immmunoreactivity for complement complex 5b-9 (membrane attack complex, MAC) is present on the sarcolemma of fibres 1-6 and within one vacuole in fibre 4. 80x.

Structural changes

Fibre size variation of both fibre types is markedly increased. Definite necrosis, phagocytosis, inflammation, or fibrosis are not observed at younger ages, but later, fibrosis and fat accumulation occur. The key feature is vacuolation of sarcoplasm (Figure 2). In contrast to common rimmed vacuoles, these are bound by a dystrophin positive membrane (Figure 3). Many of the vacuoles are also immunopositive for laminin, and the affected fibres are surrounded by multiple layers of basal lamina (Figure 4); both features being

discernible in detail by electron microscopy (Figures 6, 7). The vacuoles contain cell debris (degenerating organelles, granular material, and membrane whorls), which is also present between the layers of the multiplied basal lamina, and both compartments stain positively for acid phosphatase and other lysosomal enzymes (Figure 5). The surface of the affected fibres is also decorated by deposited calcium (Figure 8) and complement C5b-9 membrane attack complex (MAC; Figure 9) (5, 6, 10).

Of the numerous forms of inherited muscular dystrophies only one, Danon's disease (3), exhibits the principal pathological feature seen in XMEA, namely vacuoles decorated by antibodies to dystrophin and laminin and containing lysosomal enzymes (chapter 8.1.2). Moreover, all Danon patients have cardiomyopathy and many have mental retardation (7, 8). Like XMEA, Danon's disease is X-linked, but the 2 conditions are not allelic, the latter resulting from defects in LAMP-2, the gene of which maps to Xq24 (8). The possibility that Emery-Dreifuss muscular dystrophy, the gene of which is also located in the Xq28 region, were allelic with XMEA despite its clearly different clinical picture has been excluded by direct sequencing of the emerin gene (11).

Future perspectives

Establishing the definite pathogenesis of this peculiar inherited myopathy must await identification of the gene defect. The Xq28 locus contains a vast number of genes, and an international collaborative effort is underway to study candidate genes for mutations. This work would however be greatly advanced through the identification of recombination events in new families.

References

1. Auranen M, Villanova M, Muntoni F, Fardeau M Scherer SW, Kalimo H, Minassian BA (2000) X-linked vacuolar myopathies: two separate loci and refined genetic mapping. *Ann Neurol* 47: 666-669

2. Ciccodicola A, D'Esposito M, Esposito T, Gianfrancesco F, Migliaccio C, Miano MG, Matarazzo MR Vacca M, Franze A, Cuccurese M, Cocchia M, Curci A

Terracciano A, Torino A, Cocchia S, Mercadante G, Pannone E, Archidiacono N, Rocchi M, Schlessinger D, D'Urso M (2000) Differentially regulated and evolved genes in the fully sequenced Xq/Yq pseudoautosomal region. *Hum Mol Genet* 9: 395-401

3. Danon MJ, Oh SJ, DiMauro S, Manaligod JR, Eastwood A, Naidu S, Schliselfeld LH (1981) Lysosomal glycogen storage disease with normal acid maltase. *Neurology* 31: 51-57

4. ENMC (2000) European Neuromuscular Centre, Workshop 77, *http://www.enmc.org/workshops/reports.html*

5. Kalimo H, Savontaus ML, Lang H, Paljärvi L, Sonninen V, Dean PB, Katevuo K, Salminen A (1988) X-linked myopathy with excessive autophagy: a new hereditary muscle disease. *Ann Neurol* 23: 258-265

6. Louboutin JP, Villanova M, Lucas-Heron B, Fardeau M (1997) X-linked vacuolated myopathy: membrane attack complex deposition on muscle fiber membranes with calcium accumulation on sarcolemma. *Ann Neurol* 41: 117-120

7. Muntoni F, Catani G, Mateddu A, Rimoldi M, Congiu T, Faa G, Marrosu MG, Cianchetti C, Porcu M (1994) Familial cardiomyopathy, mental retardation and myopathy associated with desmin-type intermediate filaments. *Neuromuscul Disord* 4: 233-241

8. Nishino I, Fu J, Tanji K, Yamada T, Shimojo S, Koori T, Mora M, Riggs JE, Oh SJ, Koga Y, Sue CM, Yamamoto A, Murakami N, Shanske S, Byrne E, Bonilla E, Nonaka I, DiMauro S, Hirano M (2000) Primary LAMP-2 deficiency causes X-linked vacuolar cardiomyopathy and myopathy (Danon disease). *Nature* 406: 906-910

9. Tanaka Y, Guhde G, Suter A, Eskelinen EL, Hartmann D, Lullmann-Rauch R, Janssen PM, Blanz J, von Figura K, Saftig P (2000) Accumulation of autophagic vacuoles and cardiomyopathy in LAMP-2-deficient mice. *Nature* 406: 902-906

10. Villanova M, Louboutin JP, Chateau D, Eymard B, Sagniez M, Tome FM, Fardeau M (1995) X-linked vacuolated myopathy: complement membrane attack complex on surface membrane of injured muscle fibers. *Ann Neurol* 37: 637-645

11. Villard L, des Portes V, Levy N, Louboutin JP, Recan D, Coquet M, Chabrol B, Figarella-Branger D, Chelly J, Pellissier JF, Fontes M (2000) Linkage of X-linked myopathy with excessive autophagy (XMEA) to Xq28. *Eur J Hum Genet* 8: 125-129

Defects of non-lysosomal proteolysis: Calpain3 deficiency

Hiroyuki Sorimachi
Jacques S. Beckmann

CAPN3	calpain3 or p94 gene
LGMD	limb girdle muscular dystrophy
μCL	mu-calpain
mCL	m-calpain
TMD	Tibial muscular dystrophy

Definition

Although in this chapter, the calpains relationship with nuclear molecules is discussed, it is important to note that calpains also occur in the cytoplasm. Calpainopathy belongs to the limb girdle muscular dystrophy (LGMD) group of diseases. They include conditions with autosomal dominant (type 1, LGMD1A-1E) and recessive (AR) inheritance (type 2, LGMD2A- 2H) (5, 35). In the past, the limb girdle dystrophies were grouped together due to the lack of clear-cut diagnostic criteria for the individual entities. Fortunately, recent discoveries regarding the etiology of many LGMD types have made it possible to define specific discriminating features (18). Thus, calpainopathy corresponds to the juvenile form of progressive muscular dystrophy, described by Erb (10) some two centuries ago.

The discovery in the late 80s of a cluster of LGMD patients on the isle of La Réunion prompted genetic studies of this disease (11) and the overall symptoms fulfilled the proposed criteria for LGMD (41). Pectoral and pelvic girdle muscles are preferentially affected, presenting a histopathological pattern of muscle dystrophy, while facial and cardiac muscles are spared. The mean age of onset is between 8 and 12 years with a range from 3 to 30 years (12). The disease is slowly progressive; about 50% of the cases lead to severe disability with loss of ambulation in the early twenties. Serum creatine kinase level is moderately to markedly increased. The study by Fardeau et al (12) served as a basis for the mapping of the *LGMD2A* locus to chromosome 15 (13). The calpain3 or p94 gene (*CAPN3*) was eventually identified at the *LGMD2A* locus, and the disease classified as "calpainopathy" (27). Interestingly, some patients have 2 null mutations, indicating that loss of calpain3 has a pathogenetic significance.

Ten years ago, the prevalence of the LGMDs was estimated to be around 10^{-5} (9); calpain3-deficiency being probably the most frequent type accounting for 30 to 60% of the reported AR-LGMDs. Richard et al (28) estimated that calpain3-deficient families constitute nearly 40% of the families with LGMD. Similar high incidences have been reported from Brazil (25), Turkey (8) and Japan (19). Recently, Chou et al (6) identified 9 (8 unrelated) calpainopathy patients out of 107 heterogeneous dystrophin-positive muscular dystrophy patients, and Minami et al (22) found mutations in 5 of 14 patients with sporadic LGMD. Therefore, the incidence of calpainopathy among the LGMDs is probably high in most ethnic groups.

Molecular genetics and pathogenesis

To date, more than 100 pathogenic independent mutations in the calpain3 gene (Figure 1) have been identified (22, 29), (Leiden Database at *http://www.dmd.nl/capn3_home.html*) These mutations are relatively evenly distributed over all exons of the calpain3 gene, which spans over 45 Kb of genomic DNA. Most mutations represent private variants, except for particular calpain3 alleles prevailing in specific populations due to founder effects. With more than half of the mutations being of a missense type, their localisation in the determined 3D-backbone structure of calpain (Figure 2) may point to possible relationships between molecular mechanisms of calpainopathy and functions of calpain3 (16, 17, 35, 37).

Understanding the LGMD pathophysiology is still in its infancy. Six of the identified gene defects involve membrane proteins pointing to a sarcolemmal "structuropathy." However, calpain3 is a proteolytic enzyme of the calpain superfamily, and its role is not known. As a matter of fact, little is known about the physiological roles or even substrates of each calpain. The first member of this family was discovered in 1964 and purified in 1978 (34). It is a non-lysosomal, soluble Ca^{2+}-requiring cysteine protease characterised by ubiquitous and intracellular expression. Various intracellular kinases, phosphatases, phospholipases, transcription factors, and cytoskeletal proteins are processed by calpain, resulting in modification of their structures and activities. This strongly suggests that calpain plays significant roles in intracellular signal transduction systems.

So far, 2 isozymes, the ubiquitous μ- and m-calpains have been extensively studied in mammals. They consist of a distinct large subunit of about 80 kDa, abbreviated "μCL" and "mCL" respectively, and a common small subunit of approximately 28 kDa, abbreviated as "30K," forming a heterodimer. In humans, μCL, mCL, and 30K are encoded by distinct genes: *CAPN1*, *CAPN2*, and *CAPN4*, respectively. μCL and mCL can be divided into 4 domains: a pro domain, which is autolyzed upon activation (I); a cysteine protease domain (II); a C2-like Ca2+-binding domain (III); and a calmodulin-like Ca2+-binding domain that contains 5 EF-hand motifs (IV) (Figure 1). The 2 subunits associate at their C-terminus. A specific calpain inhibitor protein, calpastatin, is expressed ubiquitously and regulates calpain activity.

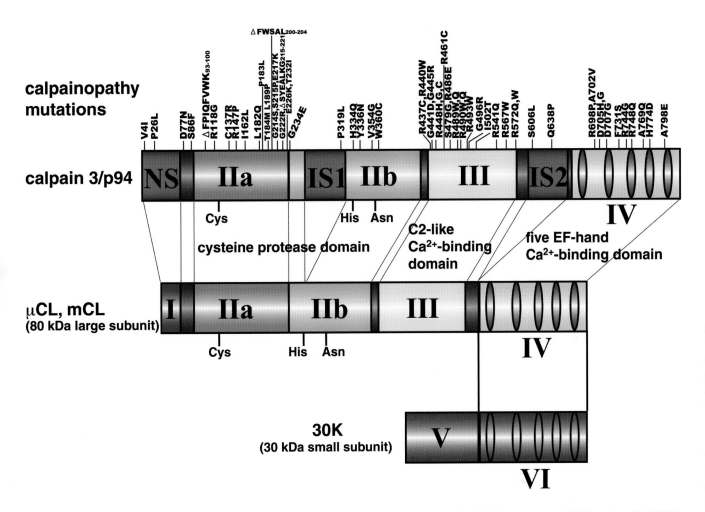

Figure 1. *Schematic primary structure of conventional calpains and calpain3.* Positions of pathogenic missense and small deletion mutations of *CAPN3* gene found in LGMD2A patients are shown on calpain 3. Both calpain 3 and conventional calpain large subunits (μCL and mCL, standing for μ and m-calpain large subunit, respectively) have 3 functional domains: protease (IIa (red) and IIb (orange), C2-like Ca²⁺-binding, III (yellow), and 5-EF-hand Ca²⁺-binding IV (blue striated golden yellow) domains, which are joined with short linker regions (black). In the N-terminus, calpain 3 and conventional calpain large subunits have specific region (NS) and autolyzed α-helix, respectively. In addition, calpain 3 has 2 specific insertion sequences, IS1 and IS2. The small subunit of conventional calpains has 2 distinct domains, Gly-rich hydrophobic (V), and 5-EF-hand Ca²⁺-binding (VI) domains. Domains IVs and VI have ca. 50% amino acid sequence identity.

Calpain3 was first identified in 1989 (31). Analyses of the protein were very difficult, since calpain3 undergoes very quick and exhaustive autolysis, resulting in rapid disappearance. Its half-life in vitro is less than 10 minutes. The amino acid sequence of calpain3 is significantly similar to those of μCL and mCL, but it contains 3 specific insertion sequences: NS, IS1, and IS2 (Figure 1). The latter 2 are essential for rapid autolysis (32). IS2 contains a nuclear translocation signal-like sequence, and calpain3 is located both in the cytosol and the nucleus (3, 32). In skeletal muscle cells, calpain3 binds specifically to the N₂-line region (N2A) and the C-terminus of titin, also called connectin (33). Most of the effective

calpain inhibitors, such as calpastatin, leupeptin, and EDTA, cannot inhibit the proteolytic activity of calpain3. Moreover, calpastatin is a good substrate for calpain3 (33). Although calpain3 has Ca²⁺-binding domains highly similar to those of μCL and mCL, it shows no apparent Ca²⁺-dependency.

The mouse and human calpain3 genes have been extensively characterised. The mouse *Capn3* gene, is composed of 25 exons, which are alternatively spliced to generate several variants of calpain3 mRNA(15, 21, 27). For example, a lens-specific alternative splicing product of calpain3, Lp82, lacks exons 6, 15, and 16, and uses exon 1′ instead of exon 1, resulting in exclusion of the three calpain3-

specific regions: NS, IS1, and IS2 (15). This calpain3 isoform is missing in humans (14).

The following recent reports suggest that calpainopathy results from the loss of proper substrate processing activity of calpain3. First, 10 pathogenic mutations of calpain3 commonly showed inactivity in processing its potential substrates such as fodrin and calpastatin (23). Second, transgenic mice expressing a dominant-negative protease-inactive mutant, calpain3: C129S—whose protease active site Cys-129 is substituted by Ser—showed both accumulation of the calpain3: C129S protein and significant myopathy phenotypes similar to calpain3-deficiency. The latter included presence

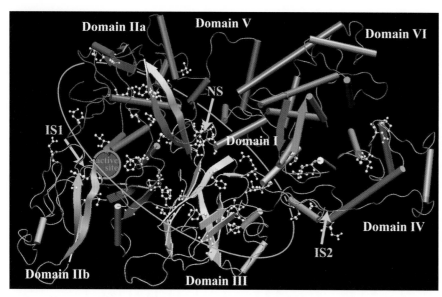

Figure 2. *Schematic 3D structure of human m-calpain and positions of pathogenic mutations leading to calpain3-deficiency.* Cylinders and flat arrows indicate α-helices and β-strands, respectively. Blue arrows show the positions of insertion of the calpain 3-specific regions, NS, IS1, and IS2. The pathogenic missense mutations (see A) are shown by stick and ball structures of the amino acid side chains (white). These mutations generally localised on a plane surrounding the active site (green elliptic line).

of central nuclei, splitting and lobulated fibres (38). Third, mutant mice lacking exons 2 and 3, which encode the proteolytic active site, showed clear calpainopathy-like dystrophy phenotypes (30). Thus, the substrate processing activity of calpain3 is essential for proper functions or maintenance of skeletal muscle.

Which molecular mechanisms may connect a defect of calpain3 protease activity and the final degeneration of muscle proteins? Involvement of apoptosis has been proposed (3). Calpain3 was also shown to proteolyse I-κB, an inhibitor for NF-κB. Preliminary data strongly suggest that calpain3 proteolytically regulates various enzymes, structural proteins, and transcription factors to modulate cellular signal transduction systems (30). Perturbation of several signaling pathways involving calpain3 could lead to calpainopathy. It is noteworthy that calpain3 belongs to a large family of calcium dependent proteases, of which more than 12 members are recognized in mammals, and 7 at least are expressed in skeletal muscle. The latter include calpain3, μ-, and m-calpains. Thus the calpain superfamily could form a proteolytic system network in muscle cells,

as well as in other cell types. Hence, a defect of calpain3 might distort the calpain system, leading to over-activation of other calpains.

Calpainopathy is unique among LGMDs, and also among all muscular dystrophies in that the gene product, calpain3, is a non-membrane-related molecule with proteolytic activity. A membrane hypothesis has also been proposed to explain the processes by which muscle fibres degenerate and undergo necrosis (24). Muscle membrane vulnerability may permit an influx of extracellular Ca^{2+} into the sarcoplasm leading to myofibrillar hypercontraction (opaque fibres). At high Ca^{2+} concentrations, Ca^{2+}-dependent proteases, including calpains (especially m-calpain), are activated and subsequently digest myofibril proteins, resulting in muscle fibre necrosis. The membrane hypothesis, however, cannot be simply applied to calpainopathy since calpain3 is localized primarily in the myofibril and not at the sarcolemma (33). Moreover, sarcoglycan complex at the membrane is normal in calpain3-deficient muscle.

Structural changes

Muscle pathology includes marked variations in fibre size with necrotic

and regenerating processes (Figures 3-6). In the advanced stage, interstitial fibrosis progresses, as in the case of other muscular dystrophies. One of the striking findings in the later stages of calpainopathy is an abnormal lobulation of type 1 fibres (Figures 3, 4) (22). Since the lobulated fibres are also occasionally seen in FSH muscular dystrophy, their presence is not a specific feature of LGMD2A. Nevertheless, the presence of lobulated fibres is highly suggestive of LGMD2A. The pathophysiological significance of the lobulated fibres in LGMD2A remains unknown. Immunocytochemical studies show normal sarcolemmal labeling with anti-dystrophin, anti-utrophin and the different anti-sarcoglycan antibodies.

Molecular diagnosis

As recommended by Kaplan et al (18), muscle sampling is mandatory, as clinical diagnosis must be complemented by a molecular diagnosis, mainly guided by a normal or sub-normal level of dystrophin, and of the other LGMD proteins known to date. Spencer et al (36) reported absence of calpain3 in calpainopathy. Anderson et al (1) showed that most of the calpain3-deficient patients they examined had no or reduced amounts of calpain3 protein in muscle, and that there was no simple relationship between the protein level and clinical severity. Although not completely definitive, western blot detection of calpain3 protein in muscle is nevertheless an easy and useful method for primary screening of calpainopathy. However, functional defect of the encoded calpain3 should be confirmed for the definitive diagnosis of calpainopathy (23) since other myopathies lead to a secondary deficit in calpain3, pointing to shared pathophysiological pathways (2, 40).

Future perspectives and therapy

What kind of strategy for the therapy of calpainopathy can be considered? First, one ought to consider the necessity to compensate for the lack of multiple calpain3 isoforms. Second, since calpain3 is an intracellular protease with strong activity, just over-expression of calpain3 in the cell might be very toxic. Thus, there is a risk that a "simple" gene therapy may not only be ineffective, but also dangerous unless expression of calpain3 is tightly controlled as it is in the normal muscles.

An important alternative involves the utilization of calpain3's in vivo substrate(s), for the latter could also have crucial roles for a therapy of calpain3-deficiency. Such a strategy depends on how many and what kind of molecules they are. For example, if the target for calpain3 is a cytoskeletal protein, which has different functions once processed by calpain3, then controlled expression of the processed form of this protein would be a possibility to alleviate the symptoms. If the target is a protease (eg, a conventional calpain), which is suppressed by processing, then specific inhibitors for this protease could be considered as therapeutic agent. Finally, the identification and utilization of putative modifier genes, or of those genes controlling the fine tissue selectivity, will also open alternative promising avenues for such therapy.

What have we learned from the genetic analyses of the LGMDs? Namely different pathogenic mechanisms may be at hand. Loss of calpain3's proteolytic activity points to an "enzymopathy." Yet, its association with titin, and the demonstrated etiologic role of dystrophin, the sarcoglycans and the other structural proteins suggest a "structuropathy." Evidence supporting a role for calpain3 in signaling pathway indicates a potential "signalopathy." So which one of these mechanisms is involved? Perhaps all three? Whatever the case, the fact that large intrafamilial phenotypic variability occurs (26) suggests that other genetic players, possibly the other LGMD loci, have a role.

Recent reports suggesting the involvement of titin in muscle diseases are noteworthy. Tibial muscular dystrophy (TMD) was mapped to the titin locus (2q31). Thus, it is likely that a partial defect of titin may cause muscu-

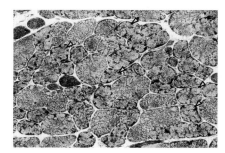

Figure 3. Deltoid muscle biopsy showing a late stage of LGMD with calpainopathy (mutation 946-1 AA to AG). Courtesy of Professor Michel Fardeau, Paris, France for illustrations 3 – 6. In addition to variation in fibre size, many fibres are lobulated fibres. Examples indicated by arrows. NADH-tetrazolium reductase.

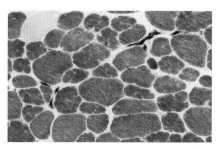

Figure 4. Note the lobulation of fibres and marked type 1 fibre predominance (brown stained fibres). ATPase at 4.35.

lar dystrophy (7). If so, the molecular mechanism of TMD shares common features with calpainopathy. Since the calpain3 binding sites are located near titin's N$_2$-, and M-lines, it is possible that TMD mutations involve either of these regions or regions affecting indirectly this binding. More recently, involvement in cardiomyopathy of a mutation in the N-terminal region of titin has also been suggested (39). Comparative studies of calpainopathy, TMD, and cardiomyopathy may provide us with important clues to solve a novel molecular mechanism of muscular dystrophies distinct from that of DMD, sarcoglycanopathies, and so on.

The recent finding of decreased calpain3 levels in LGMD2B patients is intriguing (2). LGMD2B is caused by a defect in the gene for dysferlin, another membrane-related protein (4, 20). Although there is still no evidence connecting physiologically dysferlin and calpain3, their results strongly suggest a cross-talking mechanism between calpainopathy and other muscular dystrophies caused by a defect of mem-

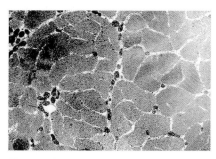

Figure 5. Electron micrograph showing the typical structure of a lobulated fibre and accumulation of mitochondrial profiles. Transverse section.

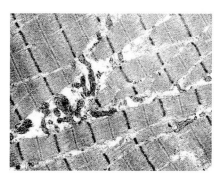

Figure 6. Electron micrograph, longitudinal section.

brane-related proteins. The relationship between dysferlin and calpain3 must be urgently studied. Likewise, the behavior of calpain3 in other muscular dystrophies should be examined more carefully and more broadly.

To sum up, progress achieved towards the elucidation of the molecular etiology of the progressive muscular dystrophies has been stunning. It involved the merging of clinical, molecular, genetic and histological information, with structural information on the horizon. We have all the reasons to be optimistic that this trend will continue for the benefit of the patient's well being and, eventually, for adequate treatments of these disorders.

References

1. Anderson LV, Davison K, Moss JA, Richard I, Fardeau M, Tome FM, Hubner C, Lasa A, Colomer J, Beckmann JS (1998) Characterization of monoclonal antibodies to calpain 3 and protein expression in muscle from patients with limb-girdle muscular dystrophy type 2A. *Am J Pathol* 153: 1169-1179

2. Anderson LV, Harrison RM, Pogue R, Vafiadaki E, Pollitt C, Davison K, Moss JA, Keers S, Pyle A, Shaw PJ, Mahjneh I, Argov Z, Greenberg CR, Wrogemann K, Bertorini T, Goebel HH, Beckmann JS, Bashir R, Bushby KM (2000) Secondary reduction in calpain 3 expression in patients with limb girdle muscular dys-

trophy type 2B and Miyoshi myopathy (primary dysferlinopathies). *Neuromuscul Disord* 10: 553-559

3. Baghdiguian S, Martin M, Richard I, Pons F, Astier C, Bourg N, Hay RT, Chemaly R, Halaby G, Loiselet J, Anderson LV, Lopez de Munain A, Fardeau M, Mangeat P, Beckmann JS, Lefranc G (1999) Calpain 3 deficiency is associated with myonuclear apoptosis and profound perturbation of the IkappaB alpha/NF-kappaB pathway in limb- girdle muscular dystrophy type 2A. *Nat Med* 5: 503-511

4. Bashir R, Britton S, Strachan T, Keers S, Vafiadaki E, Lako M, Richard I, Marchand S, Bourg N, Argov Z, Sadeh M, Mahjneh I, Marconi G, Passos-Bueno MR, Moreira E, Zatz M, Beckmann JS, Bushby K (1998) A gene related to Caenorhabditis elegans spermatogenesis factor fer-1 is mutated in limb-girdle muscular dystrophy type 2B. *Nat Genet* 20: 37-42

5. Beckmann JS, Brown RH, Muntoni F, Urtizberea A, Bonnemann C, Bushby KM (1999) 66th/67th ENMC sponsored international workshop: The limb-girdle muscular dystrophies, 26-28 March 1999, Naarden, The Netherlands. *Neuromuscul Disord* 9: 436-445

6. Chou FL, Angelini C, Daentl D, Garcia C, Greco C, Hausmanowa-Petrusewicz I, Fidzianska A, Wessel H, Hoffman EP (1999) Calpain III mutation analysis of a heterogeneous limb-girdle muscular dystrophy population. *Neurology* 52: 1015-1020

7. de Seze J, Udd B, Haravuori H, Sablonniere B, Maurage CA, Hurtevent JF, Boutry N, Stojkovic T, Schraen S, Petit H, Vermersch P (1998) The first European family with tibial muscular dystrophy outside the Finnish population. *Neurology* 51: 1746-1748

8. Dincer P, Leturcq F, Richard I, Piccolo F, Yalnizoglu D, de Toma C, Akcoren Z, Broux O, Deburgrave N, Brenguier L, Roudaut C, Urtizberea JA, Jung D, Tan E, Jeanpierre M, Campbell KP, Kaplan JC, Beckmann JS, Topaloglu H (1997) A biochemical, genetic, and clinical survey of autosomal recessive limb girdle muscular dystrophies in Turkey. *Ann Neurol* 42: 222-229

9. Emery AE (1991) Population frequencies of inherited neuromuscular diseases — a world survey. *Neuromuscul Disord* 1: 19-29

10. Erb W (1884) Über die juvenile Form der progressiven Muskelatrophie und ihre Beziehungen zur sogennten Psuedohypetrophie der Muskeln. *Dtsch Arch Klin Med* 34: 467-519

11. Fardeau M, Hillaire D, Mignard C, Collin H (1989) Limb-girdle muscular dystrophy frequent in Reunion Island. in *Proceedings of the XIVth World Congress of Neurology*. India: Neurology

12. Fardeau M, Hillaire D, Mignard C, Feingold N, Feingold J, Mignard D, de Ubeda B, Collin H, Tome FM, Richard I, Beckmann J (1996) Juvenile limb-girdle muscular dystrophy. Clinical, histopathological and genetic data from a small community living in the Reunion Island. *Brain* 119: 295-308

13. Fougerousse F, Broux O, Richard I, Allamand V, de Souza AP, Bourg N, Brenguier L, Devaud C, Pasturaud P, Roudaut C, et al. (1994) Mapping of a chromosome 15 region involved in limb girdle muscular dystrophy. *Hum Mol Genet* 3: 285-293

14. Fougerousse F, Bullen P, Herasse M, Lindsay S, Richard I, Wilson D, Suel L, Durand M, Robson S, Abitbol M, Beckmann JS, Strachan T (2000) Human-mouse differences in the embryonic expression patterns of developmental control genes and disease genes. *Hum Mol Genet* 9: 165-173

15. Herasse M, Ono Y, Fougerousse F, Kimura E, Stockholm D, Beley C, Montarras D, Pinset C, Sorimachi H, Suzuki K, Beckmann JS, Richard I (1999) Expression and functional characteristics of calpain 3 isoforms generated through tissue-specific transcriptional and posttranscriptional events. *Mol Cell Biol* 19: 4047-4055

16. Hosfield CM, Elce JS, Davies PL, Jia Z (1999) Crystal structure of calpain reveals the structural basis for Ca(2+)- dependent protease activity and a novel mode of enzyme activation. *Embo J* 18: 6880-6889

17. Jia Z, Petrounevitch V, Wong A, Moldoveanu T, Davies PL, Elce JS, Beckmann JS (2001) Mutations in Calpain 3 associated with Limb Girdle Muscular Dystrophy: Analysis by molecular modelling and by mutation in m-Calpain. *Biophys J* 80: 2590-2596

18. Kaplan JC, Beckmann JS, Fardeau M. Limb girdle muscular dystrophies (2001) In *Disorders of voluntary muscle* G. Karpati, D. Hilton-Jones, R.C. Griggs, eds Cambridge University Press 7th ed, Chapter 19

19. Kawai H, Akaike M, Kunishige M, Inui T, Adachi K, Kimura C, Kawajiri M, Nishida Y, Endo I, Kashiwagi S, Nishino H, Fujiwara T, Okuno S, Roudaut C, Richard I, Beckmann JS, Miyoshi K, Matsumoto T (1998) Clinical, pathological, and genetic features of limb-girdle muscular dystrophy type 2A with new calpain 3 gene mutations in seven patients from three Japanese families. *Muscle Nerve* 21: 1493-1501

20. Liu J, Aoki M, Illa I, Wu C, Fardeau M, Angelini C, Serrano C, Urtizberea JA, Hentati F, Hamida MB, Bohlega S, Culper EJ, Amato AA, Bossie K, Oeltjen J, Bejaoui K, McKenna-Yasek D, Hosler BA, Schurr E, Arahata K, de Jong PJ, Brown RH, Jr (1998) Dysferlin, a novel skeletal muscle gene is mutated in Miyoshi myopathy and limb girdle muscular dystrophy. *Nat Genet* 20: 31-36

21. Ma H, Shih M, Fukiage C, Azuma M, Duncan MK, Reed NA, Richard I, Beckmann JS, Shearer TR (2000) Influence of specific regions in Lp82 calpain on protein stability, activity, and localization within lens. *Invest Ophthalmol Vis Sci* 41: 4232-4239

22. Minami N, Nishino I, Kobayashi O, Ikezoe K, Goto Y, Nonaka I (1999) Mutations of calpain 3 gene in patients with sporadic limb-girdle muscular dystrophy in Japan. *J Neurol Sci* 171: 31-37

23. Ohno K, Brengman J, Tsujino A, Engel AG (1998) Human endplate acetylcholinesterase deficiency caused by mutations in the collagen-like tail subunit (ColQ) of the asymmetric enzyme. *Proc Natl Acad Sci USA* 95: 9654-9659

24. Ozawa E, Noguchi S, Mizuno Y, Hagiwara Y, Yoshida M (1998) From dystrophinopathy to sarcoglycanopathy: evolution of a concept of muscular dystrophy. *Muscle Nerve* 21: 421-438

25. Passos-Bueno MR, Moreira ES, Marie SK, Bashir R, Vasquez L, Love DR, Vainzof M, Iughetti P, Oliveira JR, Bakker E, Strachan T, Bushby K, Zatz M (1996) Main clinical features of the three mapped autosomal recessive limb- girdle muscular dystrophies and estimated proportion of each form in 13 Brazilian families. *J Med Genet* 33: 97-102

26. Penisson-Besnier I, Richard I, Dubas F, Beckmann JS, Fardeau M (1998) Pseudometabolic expression and phenotypic variability of calpain deficiency in two siblings. *Muscle Nerve* 21: 1078-1080

27. Richard I, Broux O, Allamand V, Fougerousse F, Chiannilkulchai N, Bourg N, Brenguier L, Devaud C, Pasturaud P, Roudaut C, et al. (1995) Mutations in the proteolytic enzyme calpain 3 cause limb-girdle muscular dystrophy type 2A. *Cell* 81: 27-40

28. Richard I, Brenguier L, Dincer P, Roudaut C, Bady B, Burgunder JM, Chemaly R, Garcia CA, Halaby G, Jackson CE, Kurnit DM, Lefranc G, Legum C, Loiselet J, Merlini L, Nivelon-Chevallier A, Ollagnon-Roman E, Restagno G, Topaloglu H, Beckmann JS (1997) Multiple independent molecular etiology for limb-girdle muscular dystrophy type 2A patients from various geographical origins. *Am J Hum Genet* 60: 1128-1138

29. Richard I, Roudaut C, Saenz A, Pogue R, Grimbergen JE, Anderson LV, Beley C, Cobo AM, de Diego C, Eymard B, Gallano P, Ginjaar HB, Lasa A, Pollitt C, Topaloglu H, Urtizberea JA, de Visser M, van der Kooi A, Bushby K, Bakker E, Lopez de Munain A, Fardeau M, Beckmann JS (1999) Calpainopathy-a survey of mutations and polymorphisms. *Am J Hum Genet* 64: 1524-1540

30. Richard I, Roudaut C, Marchand S, Baghdiguian S, Herasse M, Stockholm D, Ono Y, Suel L, Bourg N, Sorimachi H, Lefranc G, Fardeau M, Sebille A, Beckmann JS (2000) Loss of calpain 3 proteolytic activity leads to muscular dystrophy and to apoptosis-associated IkappaBalpha/nuclear factor kappaB pathway perturbation in mice. *J Cell Biol* 151: 1583-1590

31. Sorimachi H, Imajoh-Ohmi S, Emori Y, Kawasaki H, Ohno S, Minami Y, Suzuki K (1989) Molecular cloning of a novel mammalian calcium-dependent protease distinct from both m- and mu-types. Specific expression of the mRNA in skeletal muscle. *J Biol Chem* 264: 20106-20111

32. Sorimachi H, Toyama-Sorimachi N, Saido TC, Kawasaki H, Sugita H, Miyasaka M, Arahata K, Ishiura S, Suzuki K (1993) Muscle-specific calpain, p94, is degraded by autolysis immediately after translation, resulting in disappearance from muscle. *J Biol Chem* 268: 10593-10605

33. Sorimachi H, Kinbara K, Kimura S, Takahashi M, Ishiura S, Sasagawa N, Sorimachi N, Shimada H, Tagawa K, Maruyama K, et al. (1995) Muscle-specific calpain, p94, responsible for limb girdle muscular dystrophy type 2A, associates with connectin through IS2, a p94- specific sequence. *J Biol Chem* 270: 31158-31162

34. Sorimachi H, Ishiura S, Suzuki K (1997) Structure and physiological function of calpains. *Biochem J* 328: 721-732

35. Sorimachi H (2000) Structure and function of calpain and its homologues. *Seikagaku* 72: 1297-1315

36. Spencer MJ, Tidball JG, Anderson LV, Bushby KM, Harris JB, Passos-Bueno MR, Somer H, Vainzof M, Zatz M (1997) Absence of calpain 3 in a form of limb-girdle muscular dystrophy (LGMD2A). *J Neurol Sci* 146: 173-178

37. Strobl S, Fernandez-Catalan C, Braun M, Huber R, Masumoto H, Nakagawa K, Irie A, Sorimachi H, Bourenkow G, Bartunik H, Suzuki K, Bode W (2000) The crystal structure of calcium-free human m-calpain suggests an electrostatic switch mechanism for activation by calcium. *Proc Natl Acad Sci USA* 97: 588-592

38. Tagawa K, Taya C, Hayashi Y, Nakagawa M, Ono Y, Fukuda R, Karasuyama H, Toyama-Sorimachi N, Katsui Y, Hata S, Ishiura S, Nonaka I, Seyama Y, Arahata K, Yonekawa H, Sorimachi H, Suzuki K (2000) Myopathy phenotype of transgenic mice expressing active site-mutated inactive p94 skeletal muscle-specific calpain, the gene product responsible for limb girdle muscular dystrophy type 2A. *Hum Mol Genet* 9: 1393-1402

39. Towbin JA (2000) Molecular genetics of hypertrophic cardiomyopathy. *Curr Cardiol Rep* 2: 134-140

40. Udd B (1992) Limb-girdle type muscular dystrophy in a large family with distal myopathy: homozygous manifestation of a dominant gene? *J Med Genet* 29: 383-389

41. Walton JN, Nattrass FJ (1954) On the classification, natural history and treatment of the myopathies. *Brain* 77: 169-231

CHAPTER 9

Neuromuscular transmission defects

9.1 Myasthenia gravis   156
9.2 The Lambert-Eaton myasthenic syndrome   166
9.3 Congenital myasthenic syndromes   170

Autoimmune myasthenia gravis is the best understood and studied autoimmune disease. It has also provided major opportunities for a better understanding of general immunopathological mechanisms and the design of specific immunotherapies. A detailed expose of all that is provided in this chapter.

Mutations affecting the various subunits of the acetylcholine receptor (AchR) are the cause of the congenital myasthenic syndromes. Knowledge in this field has exploded during the last decade due to very resourceful application of microphysiology combined with molecular biology. The AchR subunit mutations either alter channel kinetics or cause a significant reduction of the number of AchRs. This chapter contains an exceptionally detailed but still practical overview of this subject.

Myasthenia gravis

Jon Lindstrom

ACh	acetylcholine
AChR	acetylcholine receptors
EAMG	experimental autoimmune myasthenia gravis
MG	myasthenia gravis
MIR	main immunogenic region

Definition of entities

Recognition that myasthenia gravis (MG) is caused by an antibody-mediated autoimmune response to nicotinic acetylcholine receptors (AChRs) at synapses on skeletal muscle initially resulted from realizing that the muscular weakness caused by immunizing animals with purified AChRs resembled the weakness and fatigability characteristic of MG (51). These immunized animals have provided a model of MG, experimental autoimmune myasthenia gravis (EAMG), which initially permitted elucidation of the pathological mechanisms by which neuromuscular transmission is impaired in both MG and EAMG (40, 44). The availability of genetically modified mice continues to help refine understanding of the regulation of this autoimmune response (9). Both EAMG and idiopathic canine MG provide prehuman systems in which novel specific immunosuppressive therapies for MG could be evaluated (28, 29, 60, 61).

Recognition of the autoimmune nature of MG has permitted immunodiagnostic detection of the autoantibodies to AChRs that define it and has permitted distinction of MG from other diseases resulting from defective neuromuscular transmission, such as: seronegative MG caused by an antibody-mediated autoimmune response to MUSK, the receptor tyrosine kinase that mediates AChR clustering during synapse formation and other components (26), Eaton Lambert syndrome caused by an antibody-mediated autoimmune response to presynaptic voltage-gated calcium channels (49),

and congenital myasthenic syndromes caused by mutations in AChRs, ACh esterase, choline acetyltransferase and other synaptic components (23). Recognition of the autoimmune nature of MG has also resulted in such therapeutic improvements as use of plasmapheresis for acute therapy of severely affected patients, improved use of a range of nonspecific immunosuppressive drugs, treatment with normal IgG, and increased emphasis on immunosuppressive effects of thymectomy in addition to the standard symptomatic therapy with inhibitors of acetylcholine esterase (16).

However, despite the tremendous increase in understanding since the initial development of EAMG of the molecular structure of AChRs, their antigenic structure, and the cellular regulation of the immune response, there has been only limited progress in specific immunotherapy of EAMG and no progress sufficient to permit testing of specific therapies in canine or human MG (44).

The initial mechanisms, which might provoke an autoimmune response to AChRs, remain unknown, but it is possible that the greatest future hope for a cure might lie in discovering what initiates and sustains the autoimmune response. There may well be several parallel mechanisms of initiation reflected in the various recognized patient subgroups leading to a final common pathway of an autoantibody-mediated autoimmune response to AChRs.

Developments in other diseases provide perspective on the specificity and possible origin of autoimmune responses to receptors. Lambert-Eaton myasthenic syndrome is usually a paraneoplastic disease in which an autoimmune response to voltage-gated calcium channels on small cell lung carcinomas of tobacco smokers holds the tumor in

check at the price of impairing neuromuscular transmission (49). The antigen source to initiate and sustain the autoimmune response to muscle AChRs is unknown. Although about 12% of MG patients have a thymoma, few if any of the tumor cells express AChRs (6). An antibody-mediated autoimmune response to the AChRs, which mediate transmission in autonomic ganglia, has been found in certain dysautonomias (70). These autoantibodies to ganglionic AChRs do not cross react with the homologous AChRs of muscle, even though monoclonal antibodies (mAbs) to the main immunogenic region (MIR) recognized by MG patients on muscle AChRs react very well with human ganglionic AChRs (72). Immunization of animals with expressed fragments of cloned glutamate receptors causes fatal epilepsy; autoantibodies to certain subtypes of glutamate receptors have been found in Rasmussen's encephalitis and forms of cerebellar degeneration, and plasmapheresis has been at least transiently beneficial in treatment of Rasmussen's encephalitis (56, 74). Thus, antibody-mediated autoimmune responses to neurotransmitter receptors can also cause central nervous system diseases. Perhaps the most provocative recent discovery about the autoimmune response to glutamate receptors is that infection of mice with the murine leukemia virus LP-BM5 provokes the formation of autoantibodies to glutamate receptors which, like those in Rasmussen's encephalitis, activate the receptors causing excitotoxic brain lesions (35). Anecdotal stories of flu-like diseases occasionally preceding MG have long been around, but no specific association between a virus or bacterial infection and MG has yet been found. Additionally, no microbial infection has yet been found to induce an immune response that cross reacts with AChRs and causes EAMG. Such discoveries might in the future provide whole new approaches to understanding both the cause and cure of MG.

Several recent books on MG provide important facts and references, which are necessarily missing from this brief focused overview (11, 21, 54). Also, recent books on the structure, function and medical aspects of AChRs from muscles and nerves are also available (4, 10).

Molecular background and pathogenesis

AChR structure and function. AChRs are part of a group of homologous neurotransmitter receptors, which also includes receptors for glycine, γ amino butyric acid, and the 5 HT$_3$ type of serotonin receptor (31, 37). All are transmitter-gated ion channels formed from five homologous subunits organized around a central ion channel to which they all contribute part of the structure. cDNAs for 17 types of AChR subunits have been cloned: α subunits numbered 1 to 10, β subunits numbered 1 to 4, γ, δ, and ϵ subunits (41, 44). AChRs at synapses in adult skeletal muscle have the following subunit stoichiometry and subunit arrangement around the central cation channel: $\alpha1\epsilon\alpha1\delta\beta1$. In fetal muscle, or after denervation, a fetal form of the AChR in which γ subunits are substituted for ϵ is expressed all over the muscle surface. Fetal muscle AChRs turn over more rapidly and have longer channel open times than adult muscle AChRs. Other AChR subtypes are expressed in various neurons and some non-neuronal tissues including developing muscle. Figure 1 depicts the structures of AChR subunits and their transmembrane orientation. Figure 2 depicts the organization of subunits within some prominent AChR subtypes.

Low resolution (4.6 Å) electron crystallographic studies of muscle type AChRs have defined the basic size and shape of AChRs and the extent of conformation changes that they make (68). The AChR molecule is about 80 Å in

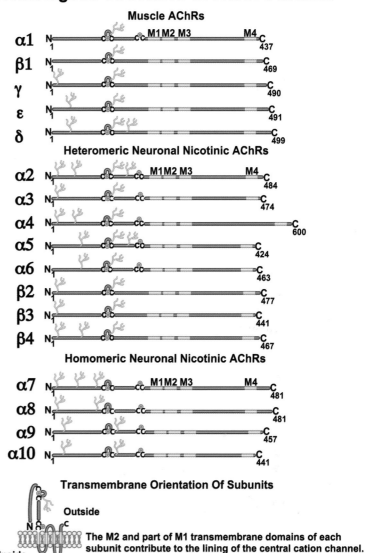

Figure 1. Homologous structures of AChR subunits. Prominent structural features shared by AChR subunits are indicated. These include a disulfide-linked loop in the large extracellular domain, glycosylation sites, and four transmembrane domains number M1-M4. A signal sequence at the N-terminal end of each subunit is cleaved during translation. Only the sequence of the mature subunit is shown. Modified from Lindstrom (44).

diameter and 120 Å long, with 65 Å extending on the extracellular surface, 40 Å crossing the lipid bilayer, and 15 Å extending beneath the bilayer into the cytoplasm (Figure 2). The extracellular vestibule of the channel is about 25 Å in diameter and surrounded by walls about 25 Å thick. The actual lumen of the channel through the lipid bilayer is quite narrow (<10 Å diameter), but wide enough to permit the rapid flow of hydrated ions. The chan-

nel gate is near the cytoplasmic end of the channel (75).

The two acetylcholine binding sites which regulate opening of the channel are in the extracellular domain at specific interfaces between $\alpha1$ and δ, or ϵ, subunits located about 35 Å above the lipid bilayer (13, 24, 31).

The whole AChR molecule is involved in concerted conformation changes between the resting, activated, and desensitized states (13) as reflected both by subtle changes in the accessi-

Prominent AChR Subtypes

Muscle AChRs   Subunits: α1, β1, γ, δ, ε

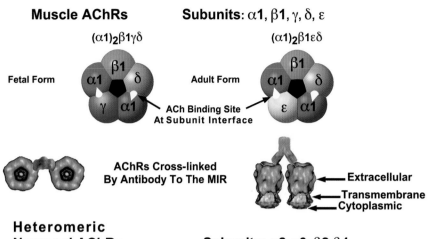

Fetal Form $(\alpha 1)_2\beta 1\gamma\delta$

Adult Form $(\alpha 1)_2\beta 1\varepsilon\delta$

ACh Binding Site At Subunit Interface

AChRs Cross-linked By Antibody To The MIR

← Extracellular
← Transmembrane
← Cytoplasmic

Heteromeric Neuronal AChRs   Subunits: α2-α6, β2-β4

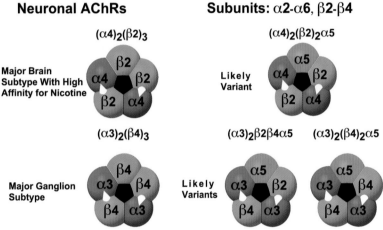

$(\alpha 4)_2(\beta 2)_3$

Major Brain Subtype With High Affinity for Nicotine

$(\alpha 4)_2(\beta 2)_2\alpha 5$

Likely Variant

$(\alpha 3)_2(\beta 4)_3$

Major Ganglion Subtype

$(\alpha 3)_2\beta 2\beta 4\alpha 5$ $(\alpha 3)_2(\beta 4)_2\alpha 5$

Likely Variants

α5 and β3 may occupy only positions camparable to β1 in which they do not participate in forming ACh binding sites.
α6 can participate in forming ACh binding sites, but can also assemble in AChRs with, for example, α3 or α4 subunits.

Homomeric Neuronal AChRs   Subunits: α7-α10

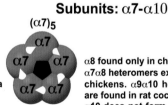

$(\alpha 7)_5$

Major Subtype With High Affinity for αBgt in Both Brain and Ganglia

α8 found only in chickens. α7α8 heteromers exist in chickens. α9α10 heteromers are found in rat cochlea. α10 does not form functional homomers.

Figure 2. AChR subtypes. The arrangements of subunits thought to exist for some prominent AChR subtypes is indicated. Acetylcholine binding sites are depicted at the interface between the "+" side of α subunits and the "-" side of γ, δ, ε, β2, or β4 subunits. Subunits β1, β3, and α5 are depicted as occupying positions that do not participate in forming acetylcholine binding sites, yet these subunits are expected to participate in and influence the concerted conformation changes involved in activation and desensitization as well as contribute to the properties of the cation channel. Modified from Lindstrom (44).

bility to water of various amino acids composing the channel (75) and by small changes in the tilt angles between the rod-like subunits organized like barrel staves around the channel (68).

All AChR subunits have a basically similar structure (13, 41) (Figure 1).

There is an N-terminal extracellular sequence of about 220 amino acids. A disulfide-linked loop homologous to one between cysteines 128 and 142 of α1 subunits is found in all subunits of all receptors in this gene family. All subunits are glycosylated. In most AChR subunits there is an N-glycosylation site at 141, but there may also be other sites. In α subunits, there is a disulfide-linked pair of adjacent cysteines corresponding to 192, 193 of α1. This is one of several parts of the extracellular domain that combine to form the acetylcholine-binding site. Three closely spaced, highly conserved transmembrane domains (M1-M3) extend between the large extracellular domain and the large cytoplasmic domain. A fourth transmembrane domain leads to a short extracellular C-terminal sequence. The large cytoplasmic domain of 110-270 amino acids is the most variable in sequence between subunits.

Neuromuscular transmission. There is normally a substantial safety factor for neuromuscular transmission to ensure that signaling is always effective (20, 47). This results from two features: *i)* cytoarchitecture, which places presynaptic active zones at which acetylcholine is released immediately adjacent to the tips of folds in the postsynaptic membrane where AChRs are concentrated and, *ii)* the magnitude of the junction which ensures an excess of acetylcholine and AChR over the minimum which is required for depolarization of the motor nerve ending to trigger an action potential in the muscle. The net effect of neuromuscular transmission is to act as an impedance-matching device to permit an action potential in a small myelinated axon to trigger an action potential in a large multinucleated muscle fiber.

The development and physiological functional aspects of neuromuscular transmission are known in great detail (59). Despite the robustness of this system, its critical importance for motility and respiration make it a favorite target for toxins in the venoms of many species. Both cobra venom toxin, which competitively inhibits AChR function, and autoantibodies to AChRs in MG patients, which act by several largely noncompetitive mechanisms to reduce the amount of AChR, cause weakness and fatigability by postsynaptically impairing neuromuscular transmission.

Clinical aspects of MG. Clinical features of MG are well known (16). In the United States, MG has a prevalence of about 1 in 25 000. Women 20 to 30 years old are the most frequently affected, but men older than 60 are another prominent group. About 12% of MG patients have thymomas. The frequencies of various HLA markers in these groups differ, as do other features, suggesting that these groups reflect not only the prevalence of young females in several types of autoimmune responses, but perhaps also differences in genetic susceptibilities of immune response genes that might influence different mechanisms by which an immune response to AChRs could be initiated (71). The characteristic weakness and fatigability of skeletal muscles is generalized in 85% of patients and most obvious only in extraocular and eyelid muscles in 15%. MG exhibits spontaneous remissions and exacerbations, and life-long therapy is often required, although now it rarely causes death. Symptomatic therapy with inhibitors of acetylcholinesterase to increase the concentration and prolong the duration of acetylcholine to compensate for the loss of AChRs is beneficial, as are thymectomy and immunosuppressive drug treatments. However, there is a need for improved therapy both to increase efficacy of treatment and reduce side effects.

Pathological mechanisms which impair neuromuscular transmission. The net effect of the autoimmune response in MG and chronic EAMG is to reduce the amount of AChR in muscle and to disrupt the structure of the postsynaptic membrane (16, 39). Most

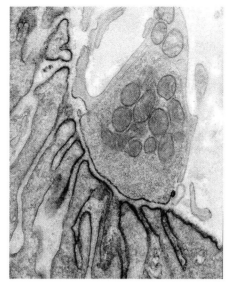
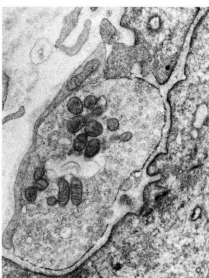

Figure 3. Electronmicroscopic view of control (**A**) and MG patient (**B**) external intercostal muscle endplates. Note the complex folded structure of the postsynaptic membrane in the control and intense labeling for AChRs (with peroxidase-α bungarotoxin) at the tips of the folds. Contrast this with the simplified, lightly labeled postsynaptic membrane in the MG patient Reproduced from Engel et al (22).

of the remaining AChRs have antibodies bound. When more than two-thirds of the AChRs are lost, the safety factor for neurotransmission is exceeded and muscular weakness and fatigability become obvious.

Both MG and chronic EAMG exhibit neuromuscular junctions, in which the postsynaptic membrane is disrupted, resulting in impaired neuromuscular transmission (21, 39). This is revealed by smaller spontaneous miniature endplate potentials, decreased evoked potentials, decreased responses to successive nerve firings, and an increased probability of failure of transmission on successive stimulations or after exercise. These features can be transferred to mice with IgG from MG patients (64), and can be transmitted from one rat to another by mAbs to the extracellular surface of AChRs, but not by their Fab fragments (52).

In both MG and EAMG, both antibody and complement are bound to the postsynaptic membrane and to fragments shed from it (21, 39). Inhibition of complement prevents the passive transfer of EAMG (38). Complement targeted by antibodies bound to AChRs is clearly important for causing focal lysis of the postsynaptic membrane, and thereby also contributing to disrup-

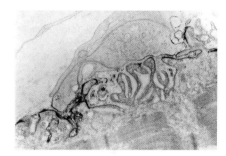

Figure 4. Electronmicroscopic view of an MG patient intercostal muscle endplate labeled for IgG with peroxidase conjugated to protein A. This is a rather mildly affected patient whose postsynaptic membrane is still largely intact. However, the asterisk marks a degenerating fold and the arrow marks bits of lysed membrane in the synaptic cleft. Reproduced from Engel et al (22).

tion of the localization of presynaptic active zones next to the tips of folds in the postsynaptic membrane where AChRs are normally packed in a semicrystalline array. In EAMG, there is an early acute form of muscle weakness 7 to 10 days after immunization with AChR, if suitable adjuvants are used. A similar form occurs within 1 to 2 days of passive transfer of antibodies (42, 43). This acute form of EAMG depends on antibody-dependent complement fixation and release of the chemotactic fragment of the C3 component of complement to attract macrophages to attack the postsynaptic membrane and

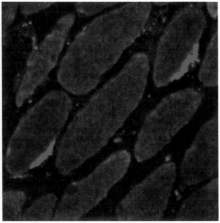

Figure 5. Immunofluorescent localization of acetylcholine esterase (**A**) and the lytic membrane attack complex of complement (**B**) in double labeled muscle sections from an MG patient. The presence of esterase marks the location of two endplates, both of which are heavily labeled for complement. Reproduced from Nakano and Engel (48).

thereby greatly amplify the effects of a small amount of bound antibody (21, 39). This mechanism does not occur in MG, presumably because the deposition of autoantibodies on the postsynaptic membrane occurs much more slowly. In MG, neither macrophages nor cytotoxic T cells are seen at the neuromuscular junction (21).

Antibodies to the extracellular surface of AChRs can cause antigenic modulation, which is an increase in the rate of AChR turnover due to crosslinking of AChRs by antibodies that facilitate their endocytosis and lysosomal destruction (16, 39). This mechanism can quickly and substantially reduce the AChR content of muscle cells in culture. These cells have extrajunctional AChRs which turn over in a few hours. The AChRs at mature rat neuromuscular junctions can be extensively labeled with antibodies without impairing transmission if complement is inhibited (38). This, and other experiments, show that very few antibodies to AChR directly impair AChR function by either competitive or noncompetitive mechanisms (39). This experiment also suggests that at the mature junction, where the AChRs are firmly anchored to the cytoskeleton and their turnover may take many days, antigenic modulation may have a limited effect until complement-mediated focal lysis begins to disrupt the system.

In response to the autoimmune assault, there is a repeated process of focal denervation and reinnervation seen histologically. The abandonment of regions of old complement-labeled postsynaptic membrane as the nerve endings move to adjacent areas results in the larger endplate characteristic of MG.

Specificities of autoantibodies to AChR. The main immunogenic region (MIR) is the part of the extracellular region of muscle AChR α1 subunits at which more than half of the autoantibodies in human or canine MG or rats with EAMG are directed (60, 66, 67). It is a conformation-dependent region at the tips of α1 subunits which is angled outward from the central axis of the AChR (8). Because of this orientation, bound antibodies are well positioned to bind complement and to crosslink adjacent AChRs to induce antigenic modulation. The outward angle of the MIR prevents crosslinking of the two α1 subunits within a single AChR molecular by a single antibody. mAbs bound to the MIR do not inhibit AChR function. The MIR is formed at least in part by amino acids within the sequence 66-76 of α1 subunits. It may owe the conformation dependence of its antigenicity in part to contributions from adjacent sequences as well. The high immunogenicity of the MIR probably depends on its unique conformation and the two MIR in an AChR, which may increase its avidity for B lymphocytes. When AChRs are denatured and the MIR is disrupted, they can be used to provoke the formation of high concentrations of antibody; however, it is very difficult to induce EAMG (40).

The large cytoplasmic domain between M3 and M4 of AChR subunits is the most variable in sequence between subunits (41). When the MIR is destroyed by denaturation, by default these varied sequences become the residual most immunogenic part of the AChR (14). Antibodies to this region are not pathogenic because they cannot bind to AChRs in intact muscle (40).

Sera from MG patients often react better with fetal AChRs than with adult AChRs (5). This may suggest that γ subunit-containing extrajunctional AChRs are often involved in inducing or sustaining the autoimmune response. Rare myoid cells found in thymus express extrajunctional AChRs (71). However, the antibody-producing germinal centers found in MG patient thymus are not centered around myoid cells. Thus, it is unclear whether the beneficial effects of thymectomy in treating MG result from removing this source of immunogen and antibody production. It has been suggested that extraocular muscles express fetal AChRs, which would help explain their selective involvement in MG (27); however, this is controversial (46). Their selective involvement may simply reflect their high average rate of stimulation and the necessity for precise transmission to avoid diplopia. Rare patients have been described who make only autoantibodies against γ subunits, and these antibodies are capable of blocking AChR function (55). They exhibit no signs of MG, but transplacental transfer of such antibodies causes severe fetal weakness resulting in death or the spinal deformities of arthrogryposis multiplex congenita.

Specificities of T lymphocytes to AChRs. T lymphocytes respond to short (≤20 amino acids) peptide fragments of antigens presented bound to antigen presenting proteins on the surfaces of either "professional" antigen presenting cells such as dendritic cells, or "amateurs" such as B lymphocytes. Thus, T lymphocytes usually recognize fundamentally different epitopes on AChRs than do autoantibodies. T lymphocyte epitopes are found throughout the AChR sequence (53, 71). The α1 subunit predominates in the autoimmune response to muscle AChRs not only at the autoantibody level as a result of autoantibodies to the MIR, but also at the T cell level. Some T cell epitopes are especially prominent (6, 12).

Cellular regulation of the autoimmune response to AChRs. The dependence of EAMG and presumably MG on B cells is illustrated by showing that B cell-deficient mice are resistant to developing EAMG (15). These mice remain, of course, fully sensitive to passive EAMG mediated by a mAb to the MIR.

CD4+ helper lymphocytes are necessary for the production of antibodies to AChRs in both MG and EAMG (11). Recently, this was illustrated in a rather elegant way. MG patient blood lymphocytes can passively transfer MG to severe combined immune deficiency (SCID) mice because both B and T cells found in human blood are able to survive in these mice for long periods and produce antibodies which crossreact with mouse AChRs (73). Depletion of CD4+ helper lymphocytes prevented transfer, but depletion of CD8+ killer lymphocytes did not. Reconstitution of CD4+ lymphocytes specific for three prominent epitopes on AChR α1 subunits permitted transfer. Mice genetically deficient in MHC class I antigen presenting molecules and the CD8+ lymphocytes that would recognize antigens presented on this carrier can develop EAMG (62). Conversely, genetic deficiency of MHC class II antigen presenting protein that is involved in activating CD4+ lymphocytes causes resistance to EAMG (32). Mutation of only three amino acids in the class II protein also inhibits EAMG by inhibiting the response to some prominent AChR epitopes while permitting some residual antibody response to AChRs (7). T cells commu-

nicate with B cells and other T cells by lymphokines which are not antigen-specific. Thus, T cells specific for a synthetic AChR peptide can provide help for a heterogeneous anti-AChR antibody response (79).

Structural changes

The microscopic pathological features of MG and EAMG have been determined in detail by a series of studies by Andrew Engel and his colleagues. Some of these features are illustrated here.

Figure 3 contrasts the postsynaptic membrane morphology and the AChR content at an endplate from a control subject with an endplate from an MG patient with moderately severe generalized MG. In the normal endplate, the postsynaptic membrane is expanded into folds, and AChRs labeled with peroxidase conjugated to the snake venom toxin α bungarotoxin are concentrated at the tips of the folds. Diffusion of the peroxidase substrate results in some spurious staining of adjacent presynap-

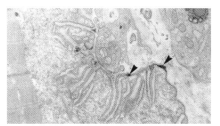
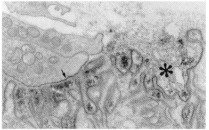

Figure 6. Ultrastructural localization of C9 at MG endplates. Prior to fixation muscle was labeled successively with rabbit antibody to C9 and peroxidase conjugated to goat anti-rabbit IgG. After glutaraldehyde fixation, the sections were reacted for peroxidase. Then, they were fixed with osmium tetroxide and processed without additional staining. In **A**, the synaptic folds are well-preserved. In **B**, the junctional folds are degenerating and labeled debris has accumulated along the right side where the nerve ending is no longer apposed (asterisk). Reproduced from Sahashi et al (58).

tic (arrowhead) and Schwann cell (arrow) membranes. In the MG endplate, the postsynaptic membrane is highly simplified and there is very little labeled AChR.

Figure 4 shows localization of IgG bound to the postsynaptic membrane of an MG patient endplate and to membrane fragments shed into the synaptic cleft from a degenerating synaptic fold. This is a rather mildly affected patient, so the postsynaptic membrane folds are rather well preserved.

Immunocytochemical detection of lytic component (C9) of the membrane attack complex of complement at MG patient endplates is shown at the light microscopic level in Figure 5 and at the electron microscopic level in Figure 6. In Figure 5, the sections are double-labeled with a fluorescently tagged antibody to the membrane attack complex of complement (green in 5A) and a fluorescently tagged antibody to acetylcholinesterase (red in 5B). The acetylcholine esterase marks the two endplates which are present. Both are

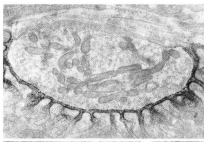
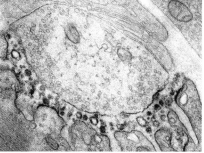

Figure 7. Ultrastructural localization of AChRs in passively transferred EAMG. Rats were injected with IgG from rats with chronic EAMG at time 0. Six hours later, **A** shows an unstained section labeled for AChR with peroxidase conjugated a bungarotoxin. The endplate appears normal with AChRs concentrated at the tips of the postsynaptic folds. After 24 hours, **B** shows a similarly labeled section in which the folds are degenerating and AChRs are found on membrane fragments shed into the synaptic cleft. Reproduced from Engel et al (19).

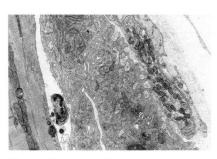

Figure 8. Ultrastructure of a rat neuromuscular junction 48 hours after passive transfer of IgG from a rat with chronic EAMG. The postsynaptic region has disappeared. A macrophage separates the nerve terminal from the muscle fiber to the left. Myeloid scrolls of membrane and smaller fragments lie between the muscle fiber and the macrophage. Z disks of the myofibril near the surface are fragmented. Reproduced from Engel et al (19).

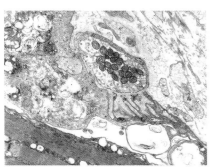

Figure 9. Ultrastructure of acute EAMG. At the peak of the acute response 8-10 days after immunization of rats with *Torpedo* electric organ AChR in complete Freund's adjuvant plus *B. pertussis* as additional adjuvant, there is a massive phagocytic invasion of neuromuscular junctions. The nerve terminal and the muscle fiber are separated by a macrophage which contains phagocytic vacuoles and tentacle-like processes which surround degenerating postsynaptic membrane folds. Reproduced from Engel et al (18).

heavily labeled for complement. Figure 6 shows ultrastructural localization of the C9 component of the membrane attack complex at MG endplates. Intense labeling for complement in unstained sections is seen on the postsynaptic membrane and fragments shed from it into the synaptic cleft and adjacent regions which appear to have been abandoned by the nerve ending.

Although MG and chronic EAMG (seen 30 or more days after immunizing rats) are very similar in their pathological mechanisms, these differ from the early acute phase of EAMG, which is seen 8 to 10 days after immunizing rats using particularly potent adjuvants and from passively transferred EAMG, which is seen 1 to 2 days after transfer

of serum or mAbs from rats with chronic EAMG (39, 44). In acute and passive EAMG the rapid accumulation of antibodies bound to AChRs results in a bolus of complement fixation and release of chemotactic complement fragments. This attracts a phagocytic invasion not seen in MG or chronic EAMG.

Figures 7 and 8 show passive transfer of EAMG by serum from rats with EAMG. Six hours after transfer (Figure 7A), AChRs are ultrastructurally localized at the tips of normal folds of the postsynaptic membrane. After 24 hours (Figure 7B), the synaptic folds are degenerating and AChRs are seen on membrane fragments shed into the synaptic cleft. After 48 hours (Figure 8), the entire postsynaptic region has disappeared leaving the fiber completely denervated, and a macrophage separates the nerve terminal from the muscle fiber. Figure 9 shows an endplate during acute EAMG in which a nerve terminal and muscle fiber are similarly separated by a macrophage.

Potential molecular therapies

Even some "conventional" therapies for MG such as thymectomy remain controversial, and their value has not been established by well-designed therapeutic trials (34). A task force has made recommendations for improving clinical research standards on MG.

Several recent approaches to specific immunotherapies for MG have been investigated using EAMG, but none have yet moved beyond that point. Mucosal tolerance(80) induction by oral or nasal treatment with AChR, bacterially-expressed AChR fragments, or synthetic AChR peptides has proven effective at inhibiting development of EAMG, and in some cases mucosal treatment has been reported to inhibit ongoing EAMG (17, 28-30, 78). Such approaches have been successfully tried on many model autoimmune diseases, but have thus far had very little success in the clinic (36). It is thought that low doses of antigen applied in these regions induce suppressor T cells that release suppressive lymphokines

that inhibit T cells within range of the suppressor cell and antigen. High doses of antigen are thought to produce anergy by causing deletion of reactive lymphocytes. Mechanisms have been studied in some detail using intact *Torpedo* electric organ AChR as antigen (63, 78).

The most promising studies have used only the bacterially-expressed extracellular domain of human α1 subunits (28, 29). We have used a mixture of more nearly complete bacterially-expressed constructs of human α1, β1, γ, δ, ε subunits in hopes of achieving a greater effect than we could with just the extracellular domain of α1 (40) (Kuryatov and Lindstrom, unpublished). However, our success in treating ongoing EAMG has been modest, and rather than suppressing the total autoimmune response, the large amounts of antigen we have used have increased the concentration of total antibodies to AChR but diverted most of these antibodies away to binding to pathologically insignificant epitopes expressed on the cytoplasmic surface of AChRs. The potential for such studies is that large amounts of human AChR subunits can be expressed in bacteria and easily purified. Because they are in a denatured conformation, they stimulate T cells (which only recognize processed peptide fragments) and B cells which produce antibodies that selectively react with denatured AChR or the cytoplasmic surface of native AChRs, but they do not stimulate B cells which produce antibodies to the MIR and other conformation-dependent pathologically significant epitopes. The trick is to selectively stimulate suppressor T cells rather than helper T cells and/or to divert B cells from making antibodies to the MIR. Potentially, genetically modified plants could produce antigen for inducing tolerance (45), or a gene therapy approach could be used to produce the antigen directly in the patient (57). The potential down side to all such antigen therapies is that the antigen could boost the immune response to AChR more than it suppressed or diverted it. Thus, the therapeutic effects would have to be very robust in both EAMG and idiopathic canine MG before trials on human MG would be in order.

Fab fragments of mAbs to the MIR have been expressed in bacteria and investigated for their ability to treat passively transferred EAMG (50, 65). The idea is that the Fab will compete for binding with autoantibodies to the MIR and inhibit both antigenic modulation (because it is monovalent) and complement fixation (because it lacks the Fc region). These effects certainly work in vitro. Unfortunately, Fab is quickly cleared in vivo and large amounts would be required at great expense to get an effect that would not be permanent and might be limited by immune response to the Fab. In a clever variation on the Fab theme, injection of papain was shown to protect against passive transfer of EAMG by a mAb to the MIR by cleaving the mAb into Fab in vivo (52).

A synthetic mimotope of the MIR was able to prevent passively transferred EAMG by competing for the binding of a mAb to the MIR (69). This is very interesting, but much remains to be done. Much higher affinity mimotopes will have to be derived, then tested on chronic EAMG. Even if the mimotopes were not rapidly cleared or did not aggregate and actually stimulate the immune response, prolonged therapy with such mimotopes might prove very expensive. However, if variations on acute therapies targeted by such mimotopes could produce a lasting effect by specifically inhibiting the B cell response to the MIR, such therapies might prove very useful.

Blalock and coworkers have the theory that a peptide with a sequence corresponding to what would be encoded by a nucleotide complementary to the sequence encoding a native peptide would bind to the native peptide and would provoke the formation of antibodies which act as anti-idiotype antibodies to antibodies against the native peptide. They reported that vaccination of rats with a peptide complementary to the *Torpedo* AChR α1 sequence 61-67

(which contributes to the MIR) inhibited development of EAMG (1). This seems amazing both because the theory sounds too simple to be true and because the synthetic α1 61-67 itself has very little structure. Most mAbs to the MIR have little or no affinity for it, and synthetic or denatured α1 peptides do not provoke antibodies to the MIR (44, 66).

Thus, why would a "complementary" peptide efficiently produce anti-idiotype antibodies to the MIR? They also report that a mAb to the complementary peptide prevents EAMG (2). This is surprising because MIR mAbs do not have a single idiotype (33, 66). Further, they report that vaccination of rats with a complementary peptide against a predominant T cell epitope in Lewis rats (α1 100-116) reduced the severity of EAMG subsequently induced in Lewis rats (3).

Different α1 T cell epitopes predominate in other rat strains (Fujii and Lindstrom, 1988) and there is some conflict about which T cell epitopes predominate in MG patients (6, 12) so it would not be expected that the same vaccine would work in other species, even if the proposed mechanism of action were correct. All of these reports concerned inhibition of induction of EAMG rather than therapy of ongoing EAMG.

Work has begun in vitro on specific immunotherapy using genetically engineered antigen presenting cells (76, 77). The idea is to transfect the patient's antigen presenting cells so that they *i)* express both the antigen coupled to a protein that will ensure efficient processing and presentation, *ii)* express Fas L, which induces apoptosis of Fas-expressing activated T cells, and *iii)* express a truncated form of the Fas-associated death domain to inhibit the Fas L from killing the presenting cell. This complex approach works in vitro with either influenza hemagglutinin or AChR as antigen. However, it remains to be determined if this will work on EAMG or other autoimmune diseases in vivo.

Future perspectives

Within a few years some atomic level resolution of the structure of muscle AChR should be available. In addition to enlightening conventional views of the structure and function of the molecule, this should more clearly illuminate the antigenic structure. However, this alone seems unlikely to provide a revolution in concepts about induction or therapy of MG. It may guide the design of better mimotopes of the MIR for potential use in modulating the autoimmune response to the AChR.

Current experimental therapies will be further investigated. Mucosal therapy of EAMG with bacterially-expressed AChR subunits may soon mature to the point where it could face the acid test of treating idiopathic canine MG. Fab therapies, single chain Fv therapies, and MIR mimotope therapies will be tried on chronic EAMG instead of the more straw man model of passive EAMG. Gene therapy using antigen presenting cells and other approaches will be tested in vivo, as well as in vitro, and then it will be easier to evaluate their practicality.

However, a real revolution in our approaches to specific immunosuppressive therapy may await some revolution in our understanding of the pathological mechanisms involved in initiating and sustaining the autoimmune response to AChR in MG. Just as the realization that *H. pylori* causes ulcers rather than stress led to antibiotic therapy (25), understanding what actually sustains the autoimmune response in MG might lead to antimicrobial or other radically different specific immunosuppressive therapies for MG.

References

1. Araga S, LeBoeuf RD, Blalock JE (1993) Prevention of experimental autoimmune myasthenia gravis by manipulation of the immune network with a complementary peptide for the acetylcholine receptor. *Proc Natl Acad Sci USA* 90: 8747-8751

2. Araga S, Galin FS, Kishimoto M, Adachi A, Blalock JB (1996) Prevention of experimental autoimmune myasthenia gravis by a monoclonal antibody to a complementary peptide for the main immunogenic region of the acetylcholine receptors. *J Immunol* 157: 386-392

3. Araga S, Xu L, Nakashima K, Villain M, Blalock JE (2000) A peptide vaccine that prevents experimental autoimmune myasthenia gravis by specifically blocking T cell help. *Faseb J* 14: 185-196

4. Arneric S, Brioni J (1999) *Neuronal Nicotinic Receptors: Pharmacology and Therapeutic Opportunities.* New York: Wiley-Liss.

5. Beeson D, Jacobson L, Newsom-Davis J, Vincent A (1996) A transfected human muscle cell line expressing the adult subtype of the human muscle acetylcholine receptor for diagnostic assays in myasthenia gravis. *Neurology* 47: 1552-1555

6. Beeson D, Bond AP, Corlett L, Curnow SJ, Hill ME, Jacobson LW, MacLennan C, Meager A, Moody AM, Moss P, Nagvekar N, Newsom-Davis J, Pantic N, Roxanis I, Spack EG, Vincent A, Willcox N (1998) Thymus, thymoma, and specific T cells in myasthenia gravis . *Ann N Y Acad Sci* 841: 371-387

7. Bellone M, Ostlie N, Lei SJ, Wu XD, Conti-Tronconi BM (1991) The I-Abm12 mutation, which confers resistance to experimental myasthenia gravis, drastically affects the epitope repertoire of murine CD4+ cells sensitized to nicotinic acetylcholine receptor. *J Immunol* 147: 1484-1491

8. Beroukhim R, Unwin N (1995) Three-dimensional location of the main immunogenic region of the acetylcholine receptor. *Neuron* 15: 323-331

9. Christadoss P, Poussin M, Deng C (2000) Animal models of myasthenia gravis. *Clin Immunol* 94: 75-87

10. Clementi F, Fornasari D, Gotti C (2000) *Handbook of Experimental Pharmacology. Neuronal Nicotinic Receptors.* vol. 144, New York: Springer-Verlag

11. Conti-Fine B, Protti M, Bellone M, Howard J (1997) *Myasthenia Gravis: The Immunobiology of an Autoimmune Disease.* 1997, Texas: RG Landes Company. , Texas: RG Landes Company

12. Conti-Fine BM, Navaneetham D, Karachunski PI, Raju R, Diethelm-Okita B, Okita D, Howard J, Jr., Wang ZY (1998) T cell recognition of the acetylcholine receptor in myasthenia gravis. *Ann N Y Acad Sci* 841: 283-308

13. Corringer PJ, Le Novere N, Changeux JP (2000) Nicotinic receptors at the amino acid level. *Annu Rev Pharmacol Toxicol* 40: 431-458

14. Das MK, Lindstrom J (1991) Epitope mapping of antibodies to acetylcholine receptor alpha subunits using peptides synthesized on polypropylene pegs. *Biochemistry* 30: 2470-2477

15. Dedhia V, Goluszko E, Wu B, Deng C, Christadoss P (1998) The effect of B cell deficiency on the immune response to acetylcholine receptor and the development of experimental autoimmune myasthenia gravis. *Clin Immunol Immunopathol* 87: 266-275

16. Drachman DB. Myasthenia gravis (1994). *N Engl J Med* 330: 1797-1810

17. Drachman DB (1996) Immunotherapy in neuromuscular disorders: current and future strategies. *Muscle Nerve* 19: 1239-1251

18. Engel A, Tsujihata M, Lindstrom J, Lennon V (1976) End-plate fine structure in myasthenia gravis and in experimental autoimmune myasthenia gravis. *Ann N Y Acad Sci* 274: 60-79

19. Engel A, Sakakibara H, Sahashi K, Lindstrom J, Lambert E, Lennon V (1978) Passively transferred experimental autoimmune myasthenia gravis. *Neurology* 29: 179-188

20. Engel A (1994) *Acquired autoimmune myasthenia gravis., in Myology,* Engel A ,Franzini-Armstrong C, Editors. , McGraw-Hill: New York. p. 261-302

21. Engel A (1999) *Myasthenia Gravis and Myasthenic Disorders.* New York: Oxford University Press

22. Engel AG, Lindstrom JM, Lambert EH, Lennon VA (1977) Ultrastructural localization of the acetylcholine receptor in myasthenia gravis and in its experimental autoimmune model. *Neurology* 27: 307-315

23. Engel AG, Ohno K, Sine SM (1999) Congenital myasthenic syndromes: recent advances. *Arch Neurol* 56: 163-167

24. Fairclough RH, Twaddle GM, Gudipati E, Stone RJ, Richman DP, Burkwall DA, Josephs R (1998) Mapping the mAb 383C epitope to alpha 2(187-199) of the Torpedo acetylcholine receptor on the three-dimensional model. *J Mol Biol* 282: 301-315

25. Faller G, Steininger H, Kranzlein J, Maul H, Kerkau T, Hensen J, Hahn EG, Kirchner T (1997) Antigastric autoantibodies in Helicobacter pylori infection: implications of histological and clinical parameters of gastritis. *Gut* 41: 619-23

26. Hoch W, McConville J, Helms S, Newsom-Davis J, Melms A, Vincent A (2001) Auto-antibodies to the receptor tyrosine kinase MuSK in patients with myasthenia gravis without acetylcholine receptor antibodies. *Nat Med* 7: 365-368

27. Horton RM, Manfredi AA, Conti-Tronconi BM (1993) The "embryonic" gamma subunit of the nicotinic acetylcholine receptor is expressed in adult extraocular muscle. *Neurology* 43: 983-986

28. Im S, Barchan D, Fuchs S, Souroujon MC (2000) Mechanism of nasal tolerance induced by a recombinant fragment of acetylcholine receptor for treatment of experimental myasthenia gravis. *J Neuroimmunol* 111: 161-168

29. Im SH, Barchan D, Souroujon MC, Fuchs S (2000) Role of tolerogen conformation in induction of oral tolerance in experimental autoimmune myasthenia gravis. *J Immunol* 165: 3599-3605

30. Karachunski PI, Ostlie NS, Okita DK, Garman R, Conti-Fine BM (1999) Subcutaneous administration of T-epitope sequences of the acetylcholine receptor prevents experimental myasthenia gravis. *J Neuroimmunol* 93: 108-121

31. Karlin A, Akabas MH (1995) Toward a structural basis for the function of nicotinic acetylcholine receptors and their cousins. *Neuron* 15: 1231-1244

32. Kaul R, Shenoy M, Goluszko E, Christadoss P (1994) Major histocompatibility complex class II gene disruption prevents experimental autoimmune myasthenia gravis. *J Immunol* 152: 3152-3157

33. Killen JA, Hochschwender SM, Lindstrom JM (1985) The main immunogenic region of acetylcholine receptors does not provoke the formation of antibodies of a predominant idiotype. *J Neuroimmunol* 9: 229-241

34. Kissel JT, Franklin GM (2000) Treatment of myasthenia gravis: A call to arms. *Neurology* 55: 3-4

35. Koustova E, Sei Y, Fossom L, Wei ML, Usherwood PN, Keele NB, Rogawski MA, Basile AS (2001) LP-BM5 virus-infected mice produce activating autoantibodies to the AMPA receptor. *J Clin Invest* 107: 737-744

36. Krause I, Blank M, Shoenfeld Y (2000) Immunomodulation of experimental autoimmune diseases via oral tolerance. *Crit Rev Immunol* 20: 1-16

37. Le Novere N, Changeux JP (1995) Molecular evolution of the nicotinic acetylcholine receptor: an example of multigene family in excitable cells. *J Mol Evol* 40: 155-172

38. Lennon VA, Seybold ME, Lindstrom JM, Cochrane C, Ulevitch R (1978) Role of complement in the pathogenesis of experimental autoimmune myasthenia gravis. *J Exp Med* 147: 973-983

39. Lindstrom J, Shelton D, Fujii Y (1988) Myasthenia gravis. *Adv Immunol* 42: 233-284

40. Lindstrom J, Peng X, Kuryatov A, Lee E, Anand R, Gerzanich V, Wang F, Wells G, Nelson M (1998) Molecular and antigenic structure of nicotinic acetylcholine receptors. *Ann N Y Acad Sci* 841: 71-86

41. Lindstrom J (2000) The structures of neuronal nicotinic receptors, in: *Handbook of Experimental Pharmacology. Neuronal Nicotinic Receptors,* Clementi F, Gotti C,Fornasari D, Editors. Springer-Verlag: New York. p. 101-162

42. Lindstrom JM, Einarson BL, Lennon VA, Seybold ME (1976) Pathological mechanisms in experimental autoimmune myasthenia gravis. I. Immunogenicity of syngeneic muscle acetylcholine receptor and quantitative extraction of receptor and antibody-receptor complexes from muscles of rats with experimental autoimmune myasthenia gravis. *J Exp Med* 144: 726-738

43. Lindstrom JM, Engel AG, Seybold ME, Lennon VA, Lambert EH (1976) Pathological mechanisms in experimental autoimmune myasthenia gravis. II. Passive transfer of experimental autoimmune myasthenia gravis in rats with anti-acetylcholine receptor antibodies. *J Exp Med* 144: 739-53

44. Lindstrom JM (2000) Acetylcholine receptors and myasthenia. *Muscle Nerve* 23: 453-477

45. Ma SW, Zhao DL, Yin ZQ, Mukherjee R, Singh B, Qin HY, Stiller CR, Jevnikar AM (1997) Transgenic plants expressing autoantigens fed to mice to induce oral immune tolerance. *Nat Med* 3: 793-796

46. MacLennan C, Beeson D, Buijs AM, Vincent A, Newsom-Davis J (1997) Acetylcholine receptor expression in human extraocular muscles and their susceptibility to myasthenia gravis. *Ann Neurol* 41: 423-431

47. Magelby K (1994) Neuromuscular transmission, in: *Myology,* Engel A, Franzini-Armstrong C, Editors. McGraw-Hill: New York. p. 442-463

48. Nakano S, Engel AG (1993) Myasthenia gravis: quantitative immunocytochemical analysis of inflam-

matory cells and detection of complement membrane attack complex at the end-plate in 30 patients. *Neurology* 43: 1167-1172

49. Newsom-Davis J (1998) Autoimmune and genetic disorders at the neuromuscular junction. The 1997 Ronnie Mac Keith lecture. *Dev Med Child Neurol* 40: 199-206

50. Papanastasiou D, Poulas K, Kokla A, Tzartos SJ (2000) Prevention of passively transferred experimental autoimmune myasthenia gravis by Fab fragments of monoclonal antibodies directed against the main immunogenic region of the acetylcholine receptor. *J Neuroimmunol* 104: 124-132

51. Patrick J, Lindstrom J (1973) Autoimmune response to acetylcholine receptor. *Science* 180: 871-872

52. Poulas K, Tsouloufis T, Tzartos SJ. Treatment of passively transferred experimental autoimmune myasthenia gravis using papain. *Clin Exp Immunol* 120: 363-368

53. Protti MP, Manfredi AA, Horton RM, Bellone M, Conti-Tronconi BM (2000) Myasthenia gravis: recognition of a human autoantigen at the molecular level (1993). *Immunol Today* 14: 363-368

54. Richman D (1998) Myasthenia gravis and related diseases. *Ann NY Acad Sci* 841

55. Riemersma S, Vincent A, Beeson D, Newland C, Hawke S, Vernet-der Garabedian B, Eymard B, Newsom-Davis J (1996) Association of arthrogryposis multiplex congenita with maternal antibodies inhibiting fetal acetylcholine receptor function. *J Clin Invest* 98: 2358-2363

56. Rogers SW, Andrews PI, Gahring LC, Whisenand T, Cauley K, Crain B, Hughes TE, Heinemann SF, McNamara JO (1994) Autoantibodies to glutamate receptor GluR3 in Rasmussen's encephalitis. *Science* 265: 648-651

57. Roy K, Mao HQ, Huang SK, Leong KW (1999) Oral gene delivery with chitosan — DNA nanoparticles generates immunologic protection in a murine model of peanut allergy. *Nat Med* 5: 387-391

58. Sahashi K, Engel AG, Lambert EH, Howard FM, Jr. (1980) Ultrastructural localization of the terminal and lytic ninth complement component (C9) at the motor end-plate in myasthenia gravis. *J Neuropathol Exp Neurol* 39: 160-172

59. Sanes JR, Lichtman JW (1999) Development of the vertebrate neuromuscular junction. *Annu Rev Neurosci* 22: 389-442

60. Shelton GD, Cardinet GH, Lindstrom JM (1988) Canine and human myasthenia gravis autoantibodies recognize similar regions on the acetylcholine receptor. *Neurology* 38: 1417-1423

61. Shelton GD, Skeie GO, Kass PH, Aarli JA (2001) Titin and ryanodine receptor autoantibodies in dogs with thymoma and late-onset myasthenia gravis. *Vet Immunol Immunopathol* 78: 97-105

62. Shenoy M, Kaul R, Goluszko E, David C, Christadoss P (1994) Effect of MHC class I and CD8 cell deficiency on experimental autoimmune myasthenia gravis pathogenesis. *J Immunol* 153: 5330-5335

63. Shi FD, Li H, Wang H, Bai X, van der Meide PH, Link H, Ljunggren HG (1999) Mechanisms of nasal tolerance induction in experimental autoimmune myasthenia gravis: identification of regulatory cells. *J Immunol* 162: 5757-5763

64. Toyka KV, Brachman DB, Pestronk A, Kao I (1975) Myasthenia gravis: passive transfer from man to mouse. *Science* 190: 397-399

65. Tsantili P, Tzartos SJ, Mamalaki A (1999) High affinity single-chain Fv antibody fragments protecting the human nicotinic acetylcholine receptor. *J Neuroimmunol* 94: 15-27

66. Tzartos S, Barkas T, Cung M, Mamalaki A, Marraud M, Papanastasiou D, Sakarellos C, Sakarellos-Daitsiotis M, Tsantili P, Tsikaris V (1988) Anatomy of the antigenic structure of a large membrane autoantigen, the muscle-type nicotinic acetylcholine receptor. *Immunol Rev* 163: 89-120

67. Tzartos SJ, Seybold ME, Lindstrom JM (1982) Specificities of antibodies to acetylcholine receptors in sera from myasthenia gravis patients measured by monoclonal antibodies. *Proc Natl Acad Sci USA* 79: 188-192

68. Unwin N (2000) The Croonian Lecture 2000. Nicotinic acetylcholine receptor and the structural basis of fast synaptic transmission. *Philos Trans R Soc Lond B Biol Sci* 355: 1813-1829

69. Venkatesh N, Im S-H, Balass M, Fuchs S, Katchalski-Katzir E (2000) Prevention of passively transferred experimental autoimmune myasthenia gravis by a phage library-derived cyclic peptide. *Proc Natl Acad Sci USA* 97: 761-766

70. Vernino S, Low PA, Fealey RD, Stewart JD, Farrugia G, Lennon VA (2000) Autoantibodies to ganglionic acetylcholine receptors in autoimmune autonomic neuropathies. *N Engl J Med* 343: 847-855

71. Vincent A, Willcox N, Hill M, Curnow J, MacLennan C, Beeson D (1998) Determinant spreading and immune responses to acetylcholine receptors in myasthenia gravis. *Immunol Rev* 164: 157-168

72. Wang F, Nelson ME, Kuryatov A, Olale F, Cooper J, Keyser K, Lindstrom J (1998) Chronic nicotine treatment up-regulates human alpha3 beta2 but not alpha3 beta4 acetylcholine receptors stably transfected in human embryonic kidney cells. *J Biol Chem* 273: 28721-28732

73. Wang ZY, Karachunski PI, Howard JF, Jr. (1999) Conti-Fine BM. Myasthenia in SCID mice grafted with myasthenic patient lymphocytes: role of CD4+ and CD8+ cells. *Neurology* 52: 484-497

74. Whitney KD, McNamara JO (1999) Autoimmunity and neurological disease: antibody modulation of synaptic transmission. *Annu Rev Neurosci* 22: 175-195

75. Wilson G, Karlin A (2001) Acetylcholine receptor channel structure in the resting, open, and desensitized states probed with the substituted-cysteine-accessibility method. *Proc Natl Acad Sci USA* 98: 1241-1248

76. Wu B, Wu JM, Miagkov A, Adams RN, Levitsky HI, Drachman DB (2001) Specific immunotherapy by genetically engineered apcs: the "guided missile" strategy. *J Immunol* 166: 4773-4779

77. Wu B, Wu JM, Miagkov A, Adams R, Drachman D (2001) Specific immunotherapy of experimental masthania gravis *in vitro*: the "guided missile" strategy. *Cell Immunol* 208: 137-147

78. Xiao BG, Link H (1997) Mucosal tolerance: a two-edged sword to prevent and treat autoimmune diseases. *Clin Immunol Immunopathol* 85: 119-128

79. Yeh TM, Krolick KA (1990) T cells reactive with a small synthetic peptide of the acetylcholine receptor can provide help for a clonotypically heterogeneous antibody response and subsequently impaired muscle function. *J Immunol* 144: 1654-1660

80. Zhang GX, Shi FD, Zhu J, Xiao BG, Levi M, Wahren B, Yu LY, Link H (1998) Synthetic peptides fail to induce nasal tolerance to experimental autoimmune myasthenia gravis. *J Neuroimmunol* 85: 96-101

The Lambert-Eaton myasthenic syndrome

Bethan Lang
Angela Vincent

ACh	acetylcholine
AChR	acetylcholine receptor
AZP	active zone particles
CMAP	compound muscle action potential
CSF	cerebrospinal fluid
EMG	electromyography
EPP	endplate potential
LEMS	Lambert-Eaton myasthenic syndrome
MEPP	miniature endplate potential
MG	myasthenia gravis
NCD-LEMS	no cancer detected-LEMS
SCLC	small cell lung cancer
SCLC-LEMS	small cell lung cancer-LEMS
VGCC	voltage-gated calcium channels

Definition of entities

The characteristic features of Lambert-Eaton myasthenic syndrome (LEMS) are weakness and fatigability, which principally affect the proximal limb muscles, but spare the bulbar and ocular muscles. Tendon reflexes are nearly always depressed, in contrast to myasthenia gravis (MG) where they are typically brisk. A diagnostic feature of LEMS is the augmentation in strength following a few seconds of voluntary contraction. This results from presynaptic facilitation and distinguishes LEMS from MG. Many patients also present with varying degrees of autonomic dysfunction, such as dry mouth, constipation, impaired sweating, and in men, impotence (19). The disease can present as a paraneoplastic syndrome, in association with a small cell carcinoma of the lung (SCLC), or in a non-paraneoplastic form. The age of onset of LEMS is lower in the 50% of patients in whom no cancer is detected (NCD-LEMS), but otherwise this subgroup of patients has similar symptoms to those who present with an associated SCLC (SCLC-LEMS). The ratio of males to females is higher in both SCLC-LEMS and NCD-LEMS groups (19). It is now considered that LEMS is an autoimmune disorder, in which autoantibodies are directed against voltage-gated calcium channels situated on the presynaptic nerve terminal.

Physiological abnormalities. The diagnosis of LEMS can be confirmed by electromyographic (EMG) studies. Patients with LEMS show a marked reduction in the compound muscle action potential (CMAP) amplitude following supramaximal nerve stimulation, which decrements further at low stimulation rates (<5 Hz). In contrast to findings in MG, there is an increment in the CMAP amplitude at higher frequency stimulations (eg, 50 Hz) or following voluntary contraction. Intracellular microelectrode recordings from biopsied muscles revealed normal miniature endplate potentials (MEPPs), indicating that the spontaneous release of transmitter and its postsynaptic effect is normal, but the size of the endplate potential (EPP) was markedly reduced and variable in amplitude (5). The ACh content and the choline acetyltransferase activity in biopsied LEMS muscle are within normal limits (16) and the number of acetylcholine receptors (AChR) is also normal. Thus, the main defect in neuromuscular transmission in LEMS patients is a reduction in the number of packets of ACh released (called the quantal content) per nerve impulse. This appears to be caused by a reduced sensitivity of the release mechanism to external calcium, since raising the extracellular calcium ion concentration caused the quantal content to revert towards normal values (4).

Molecular pathology and pathogenesis

An improved understanding of the autoimmune aetiology and pathogenesis of LEMS has arisen from a number of clinical and experimental observations. Firstly, approximately 25% of all LEMS patients have a past history of one or more organ-specific autoimmune diseases, such as hypothyroidism, pernicious anaemia, and coeliac disease (8, 19), with a higher incidence in the NCD patients. Secondly,

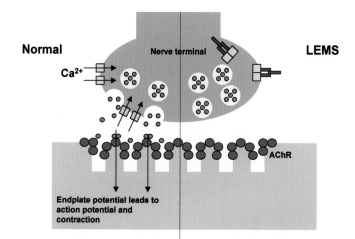

Figure 1. Schematic presentation of essential lesions at the neuromuscular junction in LEMS compared with the normal situation.

there is an increased association with HLA-B8 and IgG heavy chain markers in the non-cancer associated form of the disease (30). Thirdly, there is a strong association with a specific tumour that is known to be of neuroectodermal origin. Finally, the amelioration of the symptoms by immunomodulatory therapy strongly supports the concept that LEMS, in both paraneoplastic and non-paraneoplastic forms, is an autoimmune disorder (Figure 1). This concept has been confirmed by demonstrating the presence of serum antibodies to voltage-gated calcium channels and by achieving passive transfer of disease with injection of immunoglobulins into mice.

Tumour association. The first clinical description of LEMS was by Anderson et al in 1953, who described a patient with a lung neoplasm and a history of proximal weakness (1). Approximately 50% of LEMS patients have a small cell carcinoma of the lung; however, other tumours such as carcinoid and large-cell carcinomas have also been reported (19). Presentation with neurological symptoms will often precede the radiological detection of the lung carcinoma by months or years making follow up screening important. Treatment of the tumour by chemo- or radiotherapy, or resection when possible, will often result in amelioration of the neurological symptoms. The SCLC, which represents approximately 25% of all lung carcinomas, is a very aggressive tumour which mestatasizes rapidly and is strongly associated with smoking. It is thought to be neuroectodermal in origin, being derived from the endocrine Kulchitsky cells of the bronchial epithelium. SCLC cells contain neurosecretory granules, express neurone-specific enolase and have recently been shown to express a number of neuronal proteins that are normally found principally at the mammalian neuromuscular junction (3). The survival time in the SCLC-LEMS is short, especially if untreated. However, in comparison with patients who present with SCLC without neurologi-

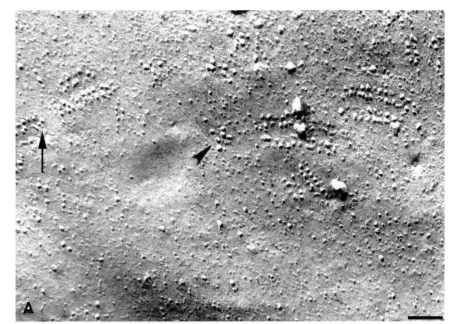

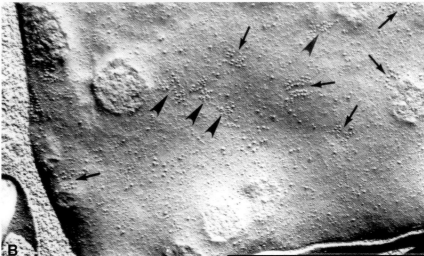

Figure 2. Freeze-fractured presynaptic membranes of the neuromuscular junction display arrays of active zone particles, thought to be the morphological representation of the voltage-gated calcium channels (VGCCs). In LEMS, autoantibodies are directed against the VGCCs, and depletion and disorganisation of these particles is responsible for a reduction in the release of acetylcholine from the presynaptic vesicles and impaired neuromuscular transmission. **A.** Control presynaptic membrane P-faces. The active zones are large (10-12 nm) intramembranous particles arranged in parallel double rows. Some zones display fewer than four rows of particles (arrow). A cluster of large particles occur near the end of an active zone (arrowhead). Magnification: ×98,000, bar = 0.1 μm. **B.** Face-on views of presynaptic membrane P-faces from a LEMS patient. The electronmicrograph displays active zones (arrows) and clusters of large intramembranous particles (arrowheads). The LEMS samples show a marked decrease in active zones and active zone particles per unit area. Magnification:×59,800, bar = 1 μm.

Figures reproduced by kind permission of Professor Andrew Engel, first published in Muscle & Nerve 5:686-697.

cal dysfunction, patients with SCLC-LEMS have an increased survival rate (13) suggesting the presence of an immune response to the tumour that is beneficial.

Immunological basis. The autoimmune nature of LEMS was demonstrat-

ed by the passive transfer to mice of the electrophysiological and morphological changes. Phrenic-nerve diaphragm preparations from mice injected daily with LEMS IgG showed a highly significant reduction in the quantal content of the EPP, compared to preparations from mice injected with control

IgG (11). The effect of IgG on the end-plate quantal content was studied over a range of Ca^{2+} concentrations, which pointed to a direct effect of the IgG on the presynaptic voltage-gated calcium channels (VGCCs) (10). The passive transfer model has also been used to demonstrate a reduction in the number and paucity of the active zone particles (AZPs), similar to those seen at the nerve terminals of LEMS patients (7). Figure 2 (see below).

Similar studies on the bladder and vas deferens of mice with passively transferred LEMS helped to establish an autoimmune aetiology for the autonomic symptoms seen in many patients (29). The results showed a specific down-regulation of one particular subtype of VGCC, namely the P-/Q-type VGCC, which is expressed at the autonomic synapse as well as at the neuromuscular junction.

Autoantibodies against other presynaptic proteins have been found in the sera of a few patients with LEMS, for example synaptotagmin and the intracellular β subunit of the VGCC; however, the pathogenic relevance of these autoantibodies is unknown (25, 27).

Serum antibodies to voltage-gated calcium channels. Voltage-gated calcium channels (VGCC) are a heterogeneous family of oligomeric proteins, the different subtypes distinguished by their individual electrophysiological and pharmacological profiles. The P-/Q-type VGCC subserves neurotransmitter release at the mammalian neuromuscular junction (21) and is the predominant VGCC subtype expressed on the surface of SCLCs (3). Preincubation in LEMS IgG specifically inhibited the influx of $^{45}Ca^{2+}$ into cultured SCLC (9, 22) and down-regulated P-/Q-type calcium currents into another cell line (28). Similar results were seen with both P and Q-type VGCCs on cerebellar Purkinje and granule layer cells (20).

Immunoprecipitation assays to detect antibodies to P/Q type VGCCs were established using a radio-isotopically labelled form of the toxin ω-CmTx MVIIC, derived from the piscivorous marine snail *Conus magus*, to label P-/Q-type VGCC extracted from human brain. VGCC antibodies were detected in the serum of more than 90% of LEMS patients. These antibodies are highly specific for LEMS since positive titres have not been detected in sera from healthy controls (12, 17). Less than 2% of sera from patients with SCLC alone have VGCC antibodies and the levels are generally low. Interestingly, autoantibodies have been found in the serum and CSF of a subset of patients with paraneoplastic cerebellar ataxia with and without concordant LEMS; some of these patients have a small cell lung cancer but others do not (14, 26). Thus, it appears that if VGCC antibodies get into the CNS they can cause cerebellar symptoms.

Structural changes

There are a few reports of mild abnormalities in the muscle fibres of LEMS patients. Squier and colleagues reported a reduction in type 1 fibres leading to a progressive type 2 fibre dominance (23). However, changes at the presynaptic terminal have been more pronounced (Figure 2). Freeze-fracture electron microscopy studies of motor nerve terminals of healthy human muscle biopsies reveal double parallel rows of intramembranous particles, 10 to 12 nm in diameter, which are called active zone particles (AZPs) (6). These structured arrays are associated with the presynaptic active zones, which are known to be close to the transmitter release sites.

The AZPs themselves are considered to be the morphological representation of the voltage-gated calcium channels (VGCCs). These VGCCs respond to depolarisation of the presynaptic nerve terminal by opening, allowing the influx of calcium ions into the terminus. Changes in local Ca^{2+} ion concentrations cause the fusion of synaptic vesicles with the presynaptic terminus and the release of neurotransmitter into the synaptic cleft. Studies of motor nerve terminals taken from patients with LEMS, have shown a highly significant reduction in the number of active zones and in the total number of AZPs. There was also a significant increase in the number of clusters of particles in LEMS patients as compared to controls (6). These clusters lacked the characteristic arrays of the normal terminals. The authors suggest that these changes could be produced by the cross-linking of the AZPs by autoantibodies, causing a functional downregulation of the VGCCs.

Immunological treatment

LEMS can be pharmacologically treated. Historically, guanidine hydrochloride was used to raise the intracellular Ca^{2+} concentration resulting in an increase in ACh release. Currently, aminopyridines, in particular 3,4-diaminopyridine, are used. These compounds inhibit neuronal voltage-gated K^+ ion conductance, which results in lengthening the duration of the action potential. This prolongs the period of Ca^{2+} entry resulting in an increase in neurotransmitter release (15). Acetylcholine esterase inhibitors may also be tried although they are not as helpful as in MG.

Patients with or without an associated carcinoma respond well to immunomodulatory therapy such as plasmapheresis (18) or intravenous immunoglobulin (2). In the latter case, it was shown that a single course of the treatment produced a reduction in the level of specific antibodies against voltage-gated calcium channels. The treatment took effect after a lag period of one to two weeks and lasted for approximately 6 to 8 weeks. Patients without carcinoma have been successfully treated with long-term immunosuppression with drugs such as prednisolone and azathioprine (24).

Future perspectives

LEMS is an autoimmune disorder in which autoantibodies are directed against P-/Q-type VGCC, which are responsible for neurotransmitter release at the mammalian neuromuscular junction and probably also at many central synapses. Although we now understand how these antibodies produce the symptoms present in these patients, we do not yet understand how or why autoantibody production is initiated. In the paraneoplastic form of the disease, it has been demonstrated that the P-/Q-type VGCC are expressed on the surface of SCLC, and it is therefore tempting to speculate that the antibodies are initiated against tumour determinants which can then cross-react with similar VGCCs at the neuromuscular junction. However, the great majority of patients with SCLC do not develop this autoimmune syndrome and patients with LEMS have a better prognosis than those without neurological dysfunction. A better understanding of how and why the immune system responds to the tumour determinants might have important consequences for all SCLC patients.

LEMS patients without an SCLC appear to present with the same clinical phenotype and antibodies of the same specificity as those found in SCLC-LEMS patients. However, the initial antigenic stimulus in this group is unknown. Some patients with NCD-LEMS have been followed for many years without evidence of an underlying occult tumour. Therefore, it is important to identify the exact epitopes on the P-/Q-type VGCC responsible for generation of their immune response and compare them to those identified in the SCLC-LEMS group. This could lead to a much greater understanding of what triggers the immune system in these non-paraneoplastic forms. Moreover, with this information, specific immunotherapies based on the removal of activated T and B cells, using the current tetramer technology might then be possible.

References

1. Anderson HJ, Churchill-Davidson HC, Richardson AT (1953) Bronchial neoplasm with myasthenia. *Lancet* : 1291-1293

2. Bain PG, Motomura M, Newsom-Davis J, Misbah SA, Chapel HM, Lee ML, Vincent A, Lang B (1996) Effects of intravenous immunoglobulin on muscle weakness and calcium- channel autoantibodies in the Lambert-Eaton myasthenic syndrome. *Neurology* 47: 678-683

3. Benatar M, Blaes F, Johnston I, Wilson K, Vincent A, Beeson D, Lang B (2001) Presynaptic neuronal antigens expressed by a small cell lung carcinoma cell line. *J Neuroimmunol* 113: 153-162

4. Cull-Candy SG, Miledi R, Trautmann A, Uchitel OD (1980) On the release of transmitter at normal, myasthenia gravis and myasthenic syndrome affected human end-plates. *J Physiol* 299: 621-638

5. Elmqvist D, Lambert EH (1968) Detailed analysis of neuromuscular transmission in a patient with the myasthenic syndrome sometimes associated with bronchogenic carcinoma. *Mayo Clin Proc* 43: 689-713

6. Fukunaga H, Engel AG, Osame M, Lambert EH (1982) Paucity and disorganisation of presynaptic membrane active zones in the Lambert-Eaton myasthenic syndrome. *Muscle Nerve* 5: 686-697

7. Fukuoka T, Engel AG, Lang B, Newsom-Davis J, Prior C, Wray DW (1987) Lambert-Eaton myasthenic syndrome: I. Early morphological effects of IgG on the presynaptic membrane active zones. *Ann Neurol* 22: 193-199

8. Gutmann L, Crosby TW, Takamori M, Martin JD (1972) The Eaton-Lambert syndrome and autoimmune disorders. *Am J Med* 53: 354-356

9. Johnston I, Lang B, Leys K, Newsom-Davis J (1994) Heterogeneity of calcium channel autoantibodies detected using a small- cell lung cancer line derived from a Lambert-Eaton myasthenic syndrome patient. *Neurology* 44: 334-338

10. Lang B, Newsom-Davis J, Peers C, Prior C, Wray DW (1987) The effect of myasthenic syndrome antibody on presynaptic calcium channels in the mouse. *J Physiol* 390: 257-270

11. Lang B, Newsom-Davis J, Prior C, Wray D (1983) Antibodies to motor nerve terminals: an electrophysiological study of a human myasthenic syndrome transferred to mouse. *J Physiol* 344: 335-345

12. Lennon VA, Kryzer TJ, Griesmann GE, O'Suilleabhain PE, Windebank AJ, Woppmann A, Miljanich GP, Lambert EH (1995) Calcium-channel antibodies in the Lambert-Eaton syndrome and other paraneoplastic syndromes. *N Engl J Med* 332: 1467-1474

13. Maddison P, Newsom-Davis J, Mills KR, Souhami RL (1999) Favourable prognosis in Lambert-Eaton myasthenic syndrome and small- cell lung carcinoma. *Lancet* 353: 117-118

14. Mason WP, Graus F, Lang B, Honnorat J, Delattre JY, Valldeoriola F, Antoine JC, Rosenblum MK, Rosenfeld MR, Newsom-Davis J, Posner JB, Dalmau J (1997) Small-cell lung cancer, paraneoplastic cerebellar degeneration and the Lambert-Eaton myasthenic syndrome. *Brain* 120: 1279-1300

15. McEvoy KM, Windebank AJ, Daube JR, Low PA (1989) 3,4-Diaminopyridine in the treatment of Lambert-Eaton myasthenic syndrome. *N Engl J Med* 321: 1567-1571

16. Molenaar PC, Newsom-Davis J, Polak RL, Vincent A (1982) Eaton-Lambert syndrome: acetylcholine and choline acetyltransferase in skeletal muscle. *Neurology* 32: 1061-1065

17. Motomura M, Johnston I, Lang B, Vincent A, Newsom-Davis J (1995) An improved diagnostic assay for Lambert-Eaton myasthenic syndrome. *J Neurol Neurosurg Psychiatry* 58: 85-87

18. Newsom-Davis J, Murray NM (1984) Plasma exchange and immunosuppressive drug treatment in the Lambert- Eaton myasthenic syndrome. *Neurology* 34: 480-485

19. O'Neill JH, Murray NM, Newsom-Davis J (1988) The Lambert-Eaton myasthenic syndrome. A review of 50 cases. *Brain* 111: 577-596.

20. Pinto A, Gillard S, Moss F, Whyte K, Brust P, Williams M, Stauderman K, Harpold M, Lang B, Newsom-Davis J, Bleakman D, Lodge D, Boot J (1998) Human autoantibodies specific for the alpha1A calcium channel subunit reduce both P-type and Q-type calcium currents in cerebellar neurons. *Proc Natl Acad Sci USA* 95: 8328-8333

21. Protti DA, Reisin R, Mackinley TA, Uchitel OD (1996) Calcium channel blockers and transmitter release at the normal human neuromuscular junction. *Neurology* 46: 1391-1396

22. Roberts A, Perera S, Lang B, Vincent A, Newsom-Davis J (1985) Paraneoplastic myasthenic syndrome IgG inhibits $^{45}Ca^{2+}$ flux in a human small cell carcinoma line. *Nature* 317: 737-739

23. Squier M, Chalk C, Hilton-Jones D, Mills KR, Newsom-Davis J (1991) Type 2 fiber predominance in Lambert-Eaton myasthenic syndrome. *Muscle Nerve* 14: 625-632

24. Streib EW, Rothner AD (1981) Eaton-Lambert myasthenic syndrome: long-term treatment of three patients with prednisone. *Ann Neurol* 10: 448-453

25. Takamori M, Takahashi M, Yasukawa Y, Iwasa K, Nemoto Y, Suenaga A, Nagataki S, Nakamura T (1995) Antibodies to recombinant synaptotagmin and calcium channel subtypes in Lambert-Eaton myasthenic syndrome. *J Neurol Sci* 133: 95-101

26. Trivedi R, Mundanthanam G, Amyes E, Lang B, Vincent A (2000) Autoantibody screening in subacute cerebellar ataxia. *Lancet* 356: 565-566

27. Verschuuren JJ, Dalmau J, Tunkel R, Lang B, Graus F, Schramm L, Posner JB, Newsom-Davis J, Rosenfeld MR (1998) Antibodies against the calcium channel beta-subunit in Lambert-Eaton myasthenic syndrome. *Neurology* 50: 475-479

28. Viglione MP, O'Shaughnessy TJ, Kim YI (1995) Inhibition of calcium currents and exocytosis by Lambert-Eaton syndrome antibodies in human lung cancer cells. *J Physiol* 488: 303-317

29. Waterman SA, Lang B, Newsom-Davis J (1997) Effects of Lambert-Eaton myasthenic syndrome immunoglobulins on autonomic neurones in the mouse. *Ann Neurol* 40: 130-150

30. Willcox N, Demaine AG, Newsom-Davis J, Welsh KI, Robb SA, Spiro SG (1985) Increased frequency of IgG heavy chain marker Glm(2) and of HLA-B8 in Lambert-Eaton myasthenic syndrome with and without associated lung carcinoma. *Hum Immunol* 14: 29-36

Congenital myasthenic syndromes

Andrew G. Engel
Kinji Ohno
Duygu Selcen

AChR	acetyl choline receptor
AChE	acetylcholinesterase
ChAT	choline acetyltransferase
CHAT	gene coding for ChAT
CMAP	compound muscle fibre action potential
ColQ	triple helical collagenic tail subunit of the endplate species of AChE
COLQ	gene coding for the ColQ peptide
EMG	electromyogram or electromyography
EP	endplate
EPP	endplate potential
MEPP	miniature endplate potential
MG	autoimmune myasthenia gravis
m	number of quanta release by nerve impulse
n	number of readily releasable quanta
p	probability of quantal release
TMD	transmernbrane domain

Definition of entities

The congenital myasthenic syndromes (CMS) represent a heterogeneous group of disorders in which the safety margin of neuromuscular transmission is compromised by one or more specific mechanisms. Generic identification of a CMS is often possible on clinical grounds on the basis of myasthenic symptoms since birth or early childhood, a typical pattern of the distribution of weakness with involvement of the cranial muscles and a high arched palate, a history of similarly affected relatives, a decremental electromyographic (EMG) response of the compound muscle fibre action potential (CMAP) on low-frequency (2-3 Hz) stimulation, and negative tests for acetylcholine receptor and calcium channel antibodies.

Some CMS, however, are sporadic or present in later life, a decremental EMG response may not be present in all muscles or at all times, and the weakness may be restricted in distribution and not involve cranial muscles.

In some CMS, a specific diagnosis can be made by simple histologic or EMG studies. In other CMS, in vitro electrophysiologic, ultrastructural, and immunocytochemical investigations

are needed for accurate diagnosis. Table 1 lists tests employed in the investigation of CMS. If these tests point to a defect in a candidate gene or protein, then molecular genetic analysis becomes feasible. If a mutation is discovered in the candidate gene, then expression studies with the genetically engineered mutant molecule can be used to confirm pathogenicity and to analyse the properties of the mutant molecule. However, in some CMS, these investigations provide no clue for genetic analysis, or implicate a gene whose sequence is not yet known, or there are several different proteins or genes that could account for the observed findings.

According to the site of the defect, presently recognised CMS fall into three major categories: presynaptic, synaptic, and postsynaptic. Several different types of presynaptic and postsynaptic CMS exist. Table 2 shows a site-of-defect based classification of 134 CMS kinships investigated at the Mayo Clinic. This classification is useful, but it is still tentative because likely additional types of CMS will be discovered, and because in incompletely studied disorders not listed in Table 1, eg, the limb-girdle CMS or the CMS associated with facial malformation in Iranian Jews, the site of the defect is not known (13, 14).

Choline acetyltransferase deficiency

Clinical background. The distinguishing clinical feature is sudden episodes of severe dyspnoea and bulbar weakness leading to apnea precipitated by infections, fever, or excitement. In some patients, the disease presents at birth with hypotonia and severe bulbar and respiratory weakness requiring ventilatory support that gradually improves, but is followed by apnoeic attacks and bulbar paralysis in later life

(13, 24, 32). Other patients first experience the typical attacks during infancy or early childhood. Variable ptosis and fatigable weakness may persist between the attacks. The clinical features of this disorder were recognised four decades ago (17) and later the disease was dubbed "familial infantile myasthenia," but it was not differentiated from myasthenia gravis (MG) until the autoimmune origin of MG was established and electrophysiological and morphological differences were demonstrated between MG and the congenital syndrome (24). Because all CMS can be familial and because most CMS present in infancy, the term "familial infantile myasthenia" has become a source of confusion and should be avoided (6).

Structural changes and electrophysiology. Morphologic studies reveal no AChR deficiency and the postsynaptic region displays no structural abnormality. The synaptic vesicles are smaller than normal in rested muscle and either increase or do not change in size after stimulation (24). Between attacks, a decremental EMG response is absent in rested muscles, but appears after a conditioning train of 10 Hz stimuli for 5 minutes. The miniature endplate potential (MEPP) is normal in rested muscle, but decreases abnormally during 10 Hz stimulation for 5 minutes (24). Quantal release by nerve impulse is essentially unaltered.

Molecular pathogenesis. The stimulation-dependent decrease of the MEPP amplitude points to a defect in the resynthesis or vesicular packaging of acetylcholine (ACh) and four candidate proteins: the presynaptic high-affinity choline transporter, choline acetyltransferase (ChAT), the vesicular ACh transporter, and the vesicular proton pump. Recent molecular genetic

Clinical Data

- History, examination, response to AChE inhibitor
- EMG: conventional needle EMG, repetitive stimulation, SFEMG
- Serologic tests (AChR antibodies, calcium channel antibodies, tests for botulism)

Morphologic Studies

- Routine histochemical studies
- Cytochemical and immunocytochemical localisation of AChE, AChR, agrin, α2-laminin, utrophin, and rapsyn at the EP
- Estimate of the size shape, and configuration of AChE-reactive EPs or EP regions on teased muscle fibres
- Quantitative electron microscopy; electron cytochemistry

Endplate-Specific ^{125}I-Bungarotoxin Binding Sites

In Vitro Electrophysiology Studies

- Conventional microelectrode studies: MEPP, MEPC, evoked quantal release (m, n, p)
- Single-channel patch-clamp recordings: channel types and kinetics

Molecular Genetic Studies

- Mutation analysis (if candidate gene or protein identified)
- Linkage analysis (if no candidate gene or protein recognised)
- Expression studies (if mutation identified)

*Not all studies need to be performed in all CMS

Additional abbreviations: α-bgt = α-bungarotoxin; MEPC = miniature endplate current; SFEMG = single fibre EMG.

Table 1. Investigation of congenital myasthenic syndromes*.

Presynaptic Defects	
Endplate choline acetyltransferase deficiency (CMS with episodic apnea)	7
Paucity of synaptic vesicles	1
Lambert-Eaton syndrome like CMS	1
Other presynaptic defects	2
Synaptic Defect	
Endplate AChE deficiency	23
Postsynaptic Defects	
Primary kinetic abnormality with or without AChR deficiency	30
Primary AChR deficiency with or without minor kinetic abnormality	65
Myasthenic syndrome with plectin deficiency	1
No identified Defect	4
Total	134

Table 2. Classification of CMS and index patients investigated at the Mayo Clinic.

and biochemical studies established that recessive loss-of-function mutations in CHAT, the gene encoding ChAT, that reduce the expression and/or alter the catalytic efficiency of the mutant enzyme are a cause of this syndrome (32). Pathogenic mutations in other candidate genes have not been observed to date.

Therapeutic approaches. Treatment consists of prophylactic use of pyridostigmine, an AChE inhibitor that increases the lifetime of ACh in the synaptic space and thus the number of AChRs activated by each quantum of ACh. Because apnoeic attacks can occur suddenly, the parents should be provided with an inflatable rescue bag and a fitted mask; be instructed in the IM injection of neostigmine methylsulfate; and advised to install an apnoea monitor in their home. Hypothetically, measures that enhance the concentration of choline and acetyl-CoA in the nerve terminal might be of benefit. Strategies for this approach await development.

Paucity of synaptic vesicles and reduced quantal release

Because only one instance of this disease had been reported (39), it is considered only briefly. The clinical features closely mimic those of autoimmune MG, but EP studies reveal no AChR deficiency. A presynaptic defect is indicated by a severe decrease (to ~20% of normal) in the number of ACh quanta (m) released by nerve impulse. The decrease in m is due to a decrease in the number of readily releasable quanta (n), and this decrease is associated with a comparable decrease (to ~20% of normal) in the numerical density of synaptic vesicles. The putative defect resides in the synthesis or axonal transport of vesicle precursors from the anterior horn cell to the nerve terminal or, less likely, is related to impaired recycling of the synaptic vesicles. Molecular genetic analysis in this disease would be difficult because of the large number of candidate genes and lack of kinships with informative members. This CMS responds partially to AChE inhibitors.

CMS resembling the Lambert-Eaton syndrome

Only two infants with this disorder have been observed (1, 13). EMG studies show a low-amplitude CMAP, a decremental response on low frequency (2 Hz) stimulation, and >100% facilitation of the CMAP on high frequency (20-40 Hz) stimulation. In one patient investigated at the Mayo Clinic, quantal release by nerve impulse was markedly reduced at low frequencies of stimulation due to a decreased probability of quantal release. The pre- and postsynaptic regions were structurally intact and the nerve terminals harboured abundant synaptic vesicles (13). The molecular defect in these patients could reside in a subunit of the presynaptic voltage gated P/Q-type calcium channel or in a component of the synaptic vesicle release complex.

Synaptic acetylcholinesterase deficiency

Clinical background. This CMS is caused by the absence of AChE from the synaptic space (9, 20, 26, 28). In most patients, the disease presents in the neonatal period and is highly disabling, but in one kinship with partial AChE deficiency, it presented after the age of 6 years and became disabling only during the second decade of life (7). The following clinical clues point

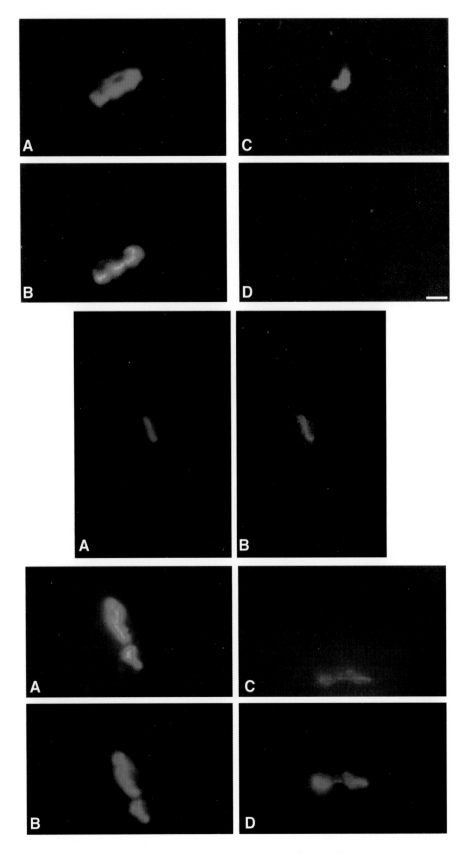

to the diagnosis: *i)* a decremental EMG response; *ii)* a repetitive CMAP elicited from rested muscle by single nerve stimuli; *iii)* no effect of AChE inhibitors on the decremental response, the repetitive CMAP, or the clinical state; and *iv)* a slow pupillary light response. The diagnosis is confirmed by demonstrating absence of AChE from the EP. Presently, there is no satisfactory drug therapy for EP AChE deficiency.

Structural changes and electrophysiology. AChE is absent from the EPs by histochemical, immunocytochemical (Figure 1, upper panels) and electron cytochemical (Figure 2B and C) criteria. Electron microscopy studies of the EP reveal abnormally small nerve terminals (Figure 2A and B), frequently partially or totally isolated from the postsynaptic region by Schwann cell processes extending into the synaptic cleft. Smallness of the nerve terminals and their encasement by Schwann cells restrict the number of quanta that can be released by nerve impulse (*n*), but tend to mitigate postsynaptic injury resulting from overstimulation by unhydrolyzed ACh. Despite this protective mechanism, many EPs display focal degeneration of the junctional folds with loss of AChR (Figure 2A), and the junctional sarcoplasm harbours degenerating organelles, dilated vesicles, and apoptotic nuclei (9, 20).

In vitro electrophysiologic studies demonstrate a prolonged decay of EP potentials and currents reflecting the prolonged lifetime of ACh in the synaptic space; relatively small MEPPs due to loss of AChR from the junctional folds; and reduced quantal release by

Figure 1. Upper panels: Paired fluorescence localisation of AChR (**A** and **C**, red signal) and of AChE (**B** and **D**, green signal) in a control subject (**A** and **B**) and in a patient with endplate AChE deficiency (**C** and **D**). There is no immunostain for AChE at the patient's EP. Bar = 10 μm. Middle panels: Paired fluorescence localisation of AChR with α-bgt (**A**, red signal) and of the γ subunit of the AChR (**B**, green signal) at endplate of a patient with two null mutations in the long cytoplasmic loop of the AChRε subunit. Bottom panels: Paired fluorescence localisation of AChR ε subunit (**A** and **C**, red signal) and of AChE (**B** and **D**, green signal) in a control subject (**A** and **B**) and in a patient homozygous for the ε553del7 null mutation in the AChRε subunit. Note markedly reduced AChR expression at the patient's endplate. Single-channel recordings at the endplate revealed only events generated by AChRs harbouring the γ instead of the ε subunit.

nerve impulse (9, 20). The safety margin of neuromuscular transmission is compromised by reduced quantal release, loss of AChR from the junctional folds, and desensitisation and depolarisation block of AChR at physiologic rates of stimulation.

Molecular pathogenesis. The EP species of AChE is a heteromeric asymmetric enzyme composed of 1, 2, or 3 homotetramers of globular catalytic subunits ($AChE_T$) attached to a triple-stranded collagenic tail (ColQ) (Figure 3B). $AChE_T$ and ColQ are encoded by $ACHE_T$ and *COLQ*, respectively. ColQ has an N-terminal proline-rich region attachment domain (PRAD), a collagenic central domain, and a C-terminal region enriched in charged residues and cysteines (Figure 3A). Each ColQ strand binds an $AChE_T$ tetramer to its PRAD (3). Two groups of charged residues in the collagen domain (heparan sulfate proteoglycan binding domains, or HSPBD) (5) plus other residues in the C-terminal region (7, 28) assure that the asymmetric enzyme is inserted into the synaptic basal lamina. The C-terminal region is also required for initiating the triple helical assembly of ColQ that proceeds from a C- to an N-terminal direction in a zipper-like manner.

In 1998, human *COLQ* cDNA was cloned (7, 25), the genomic structure of *COLQ* determined (25) and the molecular basis of EP AChE deficiency traced to recessive mutations in *COLQ*. Eighteen *COLQ* mutations in 15 kinships have been identified to date (7, 25, 26, 28) (Figure 3A). The mutations are of 3 major types (28): *i)* PRAD mutations prevent attachment of $AChE_T$ to ColQ, *ii)* collagen domain mutations produce a short, single-stranded ColQ that binds a single $AChE_T$ tetramer and is insertion incompetent, and *iii)* C-terminal mutations hinder the triple helical assembly of the collagen domain, or produce an asymmetric species of AChE that is insertion incompetent, or both.

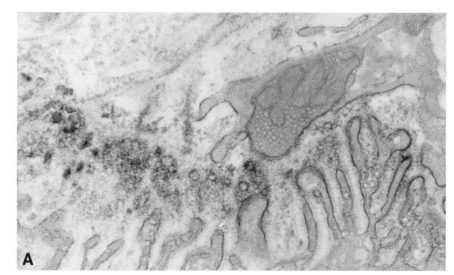

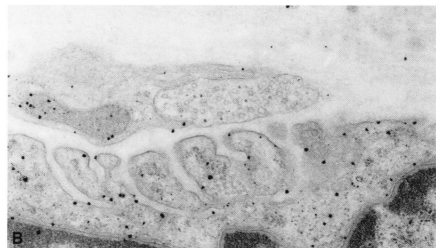

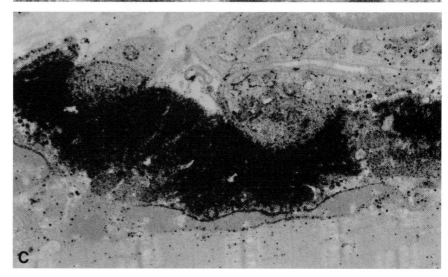

Figure 2. Endplates from an AChE deficient patient (**A**) and (**B**) and from a control subject (**C**). Endplate in (**A**) shows localisation of AChR with peroxidase-labeled α-bungarotoxin and that AChR is lost from degenerating junctional folds. The end-plates imaged in (**B**) and (**C**) were reacted cytochemically for AChE. The nerve terminals are abnormally small (**A** and **B**). In (**B**), there is no reaction for AChE in the synaptic space. In (**C**), dense reaction product fills the entire synaptic space and spreads into adjacent regions. (**A**) and (**B**), ×25, 900; (**C**), ×11,300.

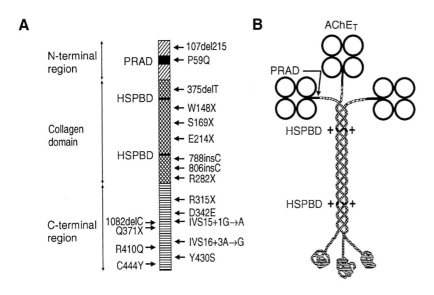

Figure 3. (A) Schematic diagram showing domains of a ColQ strand with 18 identified ColQ mutations and **(B)** components of the A_{12} species of asymmetric AChE. AChE = acetylcholinesterase; HSPBD = heparansulfate proteoglycan binding domain; PRAD = proline rich attachment domain.

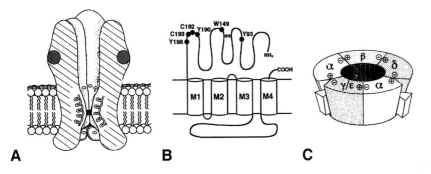

Figure 4. Schematic diagrams: **(A)** AChR in lipid bilayer showing putative site of ACh binding pocket (shaded circles) and the central channel pore. **(B)** Folding pattern of the α subunit; residues indicated on 3 peptide loops are implicated in governing affinity for ACh. **(C)** Cross section of AChR at the level of the ACh binding pocket. Note circular arrangement of AChR subunits and that the ACh binding pockets appear at the interfaces between α and ε/γ subunits, and between the α and δ subunits.

Postsynaptic syndromes

With the exception of the CMS associated with plectin deficiency (2), all postsynaptic CMS identified to date are caused by mutations in AChR subunit genes that either increase or decrease the synaptic response to ACh. We therefore begin with a brief review of the structure and kinetic properties of the muscle species of AChR.

Muscle AChR is a transmembrane macromolecule (Figure 4A) composed of 5 homologous subunits: 2 of α, 1 of β and δ, and 1 of ε in adult AChR (or 1 of γ instead of ε in foetal AChR). The genes coding for α, δ, and γ are at different loci on chromosome 2q, and those coding for β and ε are at different loci on chromosome 17p. The subunits are highly homologous, have similar secondary structures, fold similarly (Figure 4B), and are organised like barrel staves around a central cation channel (Figure 4C). Each subunit has an N-terminal extracellular domain that comprises ~50% of the primary sequence, 4 putative transmembrane domains (TMD1-TMD4), and a small C-terminal extracellular domain. TMD2, which lines the ion channel, forms an α helix interrupted by a short stretch of β sheet. The transmembrane domains are connected by an extracellular TMD2/TMD3 linker and by intracellular TMD1/TMD2 and TMD3/TMD4 linkers.

The TMD3/TMD4 linker forms a long cytoplasmic loop that likely serves as an attachment site for cytoskeletal elements. It also bears phosphorylatable residues that may be important for desensitisation and, in the case of the ε subunit, stabilises the gating mechanism. Each AChR has 2 ACh binding pockets, one at the α/ε (or α/γ), and one at the α/δ interface. Residues contributing to the binding pocket appear on 3 peptide loops on α, and on 4 peptide loops on ε, δ and γ.

Two major kinetic abnormalities of AChR have emerged, resulting in slow channel syndromes and fast-channel syndromes. The 2 kinetic syndromes are physiological and morphological opposites and call for different modalities of therapy (Table 3).

Slow-channel syndromes

Clinical background. The slow channel syndromes are caused by dominant gain-of-function mutations. The clinical phenotypes vary. Some slow channel CMS present in early life and cause severe disability by the end of the first decade (22). Others present later in life and progress slowly, resulting in little disability even in the sixth or seventh decade (10, 14, 38). Most patients show selectively severe involvement of cervical and of wrist and finger extensor muscles. Except for the more severely affected patients, the cranial muscles tend to be spared. Progressive spinal deformities and respiratory embarrassment are common complications during the evolution of the illness.

Structural changes and electrophysiology. The morphologic consequences stem from prolonged activation of the AChR channel that results in cationic overloading of the post-synaptic region. The EP myopathy that develops is like that in EP AChE deficiency but is even more severe, sometimes causing massive destruction of the junctional folds (Figure 5), nuclear apoptosis, and vacuolar degeneration near the EPs (10, 12, 14, 22).

As in EP AChE deficiency, single nerve stimuli evoke a repetitive CMAP, but unlike in AChE deficiency, edrophonium increases the number of repetitive potentials. In vitro microelectrode studies demonstrate very prolonged EP currents that result in staircase summation and a depolarisation block during subtetanic stimulation (12, 29, 38). Single-channel patch-clamp recordings reveal a dual population of AChR channels, one with normal and one with prolonged opening episodes, reflecting the presence of both wild-type and mutant receptors at the EP (12, 22, 29). In addition, the mutant AChR channels are opened, even in the absence of ACh (22, 29) and by choline present in tissue fluids (43) resulting in a continuous cation leak into the postsynaptic region. The safety margin of neuromuscular transmission is compromised by the altered EP geometry, loss of AChR from degenerating junctional folds, depolarisation block during physiologic activity, and an abnormal propensity of some slow-channel mutants to become desensitised on prolonged exposure to ACh.

Molecular pathogenesis. Eleven slow-channel mutations have been reported to date (4, 12, 16, 22, 29, 30, 33, 38, 40). The different mutations occur in different AChR subunits and in different functional domains of the subunits. Patch-clamp studies at the EP, mutation analysis, and expression studies in human embryonic kidney (HEK) cells indicate that the αG153S mutation near an extracellular ACh binding site (38) and the αN217K mutation in the N-terminal part of TMD1 (41) act mainly by enhancing affinity for ACh This slows dissociation of ACh from the binding site and results in repeated channel reopenings during the prolonged receptor occupancy. Another slow-channel mutation near the binding site region, αV156M, probably has the same effect, although its mechanistic consequences have not been investigated (4). Mutations in TMD2 that lines

	Slow-channel syndromes	Fast-channel syndromes
Endplate currents	Slow decay	Fast decay
Channel opening events	Prolonged	Brief
Open states	Stabilised	Destabilised
Closed states	Destabilized	Stabilised
Mechanisms[a]	Increased affinity	Decreased affinity
	Increased β	Decreased β
	Decreased α	Increased α
		Mode-switching kinetics

β =channel opening rate; α = channel closing rate.
[a]Different combinations of mechanisms operate in the individual slow- and fast-channel syndromes.

Table 3. Kinetic abnormalities of AChR.

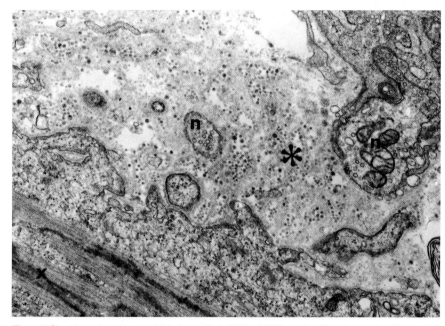

Figure 5. Slow-channel syndrome endplate from patient with the εL269F mutation. There is extensive degeneration of the junctional folds; the synaptic space is widened and contains myriad globular residues of the degenerated folds and remnants of the basal lamina that had invested the preexisting folds (asterisk). Widening of the synaptic space decreases the concentration of ACh reaching the postsynaptic membrane by dilution, and by permitting increased destruction of ACh by AChE. Degeneration of the junctional folds causes loss of AchR. The combination of these factors decreases the efficiency of ACh quanta. Also note focal myofibrillar degeneration beginning at the Z disk (x) in the nearby fibre region. ×17 600. Reproduced by permission from Engel *et al.*, 1999 (13).

the channel pore, (eg, βV266M, εL269F, εT264P and αV249F) promote the open state by affecting channel opening and closing steps (12, 22, 29). Increases in steady-state affinity for ACh are also observed, which are largely accounted for by an increased extent of desensitisation; increased affinity is most marked in the case of αV249F (22) pronounced with εL269F (12), εT264P (29), and not apparent with βV266M (12).

Therapeutic approaches. Following the lead that quinidine is a long-lived open-channel blocker of AChR (37) Fukudome and co-workers (15) showed that clinically attainable levels of quinidine normalise the prolonged opening episodes of mutant slow-channels expressed in HEK cells. On the basis of these findings, Harper and Engel (18) treated slow-channel patients with 200 mg of quinidine sulphate, 3 to 4 times daily, producing serum levels of 0.7 to 2.5 mg/ml (2.1-7.7 mM/L), and found that the patients improved gradually by clinical and EMG criteria.

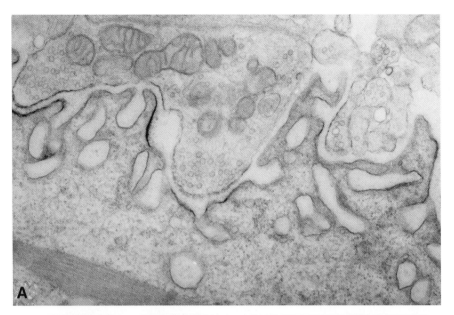

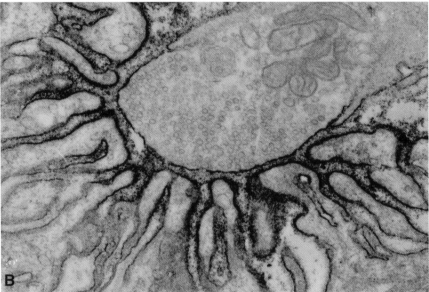

Figure 6. Ultrastructural localisation of AChR with peroxidase-labelled α-bungarotoxin at an EP from a patient homozygous for the ε553del17 mutation (**A**) and at a control EP (**B**). The control EP shows heavy reaction for AChR on the terminal expansions of the junctional folds. At the patient's EP, the junctional folds are simplified and the reaction for AChR is patchy and attenuated. A, ×19700; B, ×25900.

Fast-channel syndromes

Clinical background. The fast-channel mutations derange one or more of the following functions of AChR: affinity for ACh, efficiency of gating, and stabilisation of channel kinetics. The clinical features resemble those of autoimmune myasthenia gravis, but symptoms are mild when the main effect is on gating efficiency (41), moderately severe when channel kinetics are unstable (23, 42), and severe when affinity for ACh, or both affinity and gating efficiency, are impaired (34-36).

Structural changes and electrophysiology. The low-affinity fast-channel syndromes leave no anatomic footprint (34, 36) the structural integrity of the postsynaptic region is maintained, and the density and distribution of AChR on the junctional folds are normal. In the CMS that only affects gating efficiency (41), and in the CMS with unstable channel kinetics (23), the number of AChR per EP is also reduced. In these CMS, multiple small EP regions are dispersed over an extended length of the fibre surface, some postsynaptic regions are simplified, and the expression of AChR on the junctional folds is patchy and attenuated.

The common electrophysiologic features of the fast-channel CMS are rapidly decaying EP currents, abnormally brief channel activation episodes, and a reduced quantal response owing to the reduced probability of channel opening (Table 3).

Molecular pathogenesis. The fast-channel CMS are caused by recessive, loss of function mutations. Five fast-channel mutations have been reported to date. In each instance, the mutated allele causing the kinetic abnormality is accompanied by a null mutation in the second allele. Therefore, the kinetic mutation dominates the clinical phenotype.

Low-affinity fast-channel syndromes. Three identified kinetic mutations fall in this group. Two different substitutions of residue 121 in the extracellular domain of the ε subunit, εP121L (34) and εP121T (35) both result in abnormally brief channel events, reduce the amplitude of the quantal response by decreasing the probability of channel openings, decrease the number of channel reopenings in bursts of openings, and decrease the affinity for ACh in the open channel state. The εP121L mutation also reduces gating efficiency by reducing β, the channel opening rate. In contrast, εP121T mutation does not alter gating efficiency, but reduces closed-state affinity for ACh and thereby stabilises the closed state.

The third mutation in this group occurs in the α subunit, in the most highly conserved domain of the AChR superfamily, the disulfide-bridged β-hairpin formed between cysteine 128 and cysteine 142, or cys-loop. The mutation consists of replacement of a conserved valine at position 132 by a leucine (αV132L). The αV132L mutation markedly reduces closed state affinity for ACh, and impairs gating efficiency by slowing β, the rate of channel opening, and speeding α, the rate of channel closing. The duration of channel opening events is only 15% of normal, and the amplitude of quantal response only 10% of normal (36).

Fast-channel syndrome due to a selective abnormality of gating. Replacement of a valine by an isoleucine at residue 285 in TMD3 of the α subunit (αV285I) selectively reduces gating efficiency by depressing the channel opening rate β and enhancing the channel closing rate α. The αV285I mutation also decreases AChR expression, which further impairs the safety margin of neuromuscular transmission (41)

Fast-channel syndrome due to unstable (mode-switching) kinetics. Two mutations causing unstable channel kinetics have been identified in expression studies, but only one of these, ε1254ins18, was investigated by in vitro microelectrode studies of the EP.

The ε1254ins18 mutation, which is an in-frame duplication of codons 413 to 418 (STRDQE) in the long cytoplasmic loop of ε, also reduces AChR expression at the EP (23). At the EP, ε1254ins18-AChR shows abnormally brief activation episodes during steady-state ACh application. When expressed in HEK cells and exposed to desensitising concentrations of ACh, openings of individual receptors occur in clusters separated by silent periods during which all receptors are desensitised. For the normal receptor, the kinetics of gating within a cluster is essentially uniform and highly efficient. By contrast, the kinetic behaviour of the ε1254ins18-AChR changes abruptly, so that a normal mode activation is replaced by three abnormal and inefficient modes in which the receptor opens slowly and closes more rapidly than normal. In this disorder, the reduced gating efficiency and decreased AChR expression are partially offset by expression of foetal AChR harbouring the γ instead of the ε sub-

unit (γ-AChR); this improves electrical activity at EP and likely rescues the phenotype (23).

The second mutation that destabilises channel kinetics is a nearby missense mutation in the ε subunit, εA411P. When this mutation is expressed in HEK cells, different clusters of channel openings differ widely in their activation kinetics, so that the spread in the distribution of the channel opening and closing rates is greatly expanded (42). Intracellular microelectrode and patch-clamp studies on EPs of patients harbouring this mutation are still unavailable. That both ε1254ins18 and εA411P occur in the amphipathic helix region of the long cytoplasmic loops of the ε subunit implicates this region of ε in stabilisation of channel kinetics.

Therapeutic approaches. The fast-channel syndromes respond well to therapy with 3,4-diaminopyridine, which increases the number of quanta released by nerve impulse, and cholinesterase inhibitors, which increase the number of AChRs activated by each quantum (19). The response is best in those cases in which the level of AChR expression is not reduced.

AChR deficiency with or without minor kinetic abnormality

Clinical background. The clinical phenotypes with these CMS vary from mild to severe. Patients with recessive mutations in the ε subunit are generally less affected than those with mutations in other subunits, but some harbouring ε subunit mutations can also be severely affected. The sickest patients have severe ocular, bulbar, and respiratory muscle weakness from birth, surviving only with respiratory support and gavage feeding. They may be weaned from a respirator and begin to tolerate oral feedings during the first year of life, but have bouts of aspiration pneumonia and may need intermittent respiratory support during childhood and adult life. Motor milestones are severely delayed; they seldom learn to negotiate steps

and can walk for only a short distance. Older patients close their mouth by supporting the jaw with the hand and elevate their eyelids with their fingers. Facial deformities, prognathism, malocclusion, and scoliosis or kyphoscoliosis become noticeable during the second decade. Muscle bulk is reduced. The tendon reflexes are normal or hypoactive.

The least affected patients pass their motor milestones with slight or no delay and only show mild ptosis and limited ocular ductions. They are clumsy in sports, fatigue easily, and cannot run well, climb rope, or do pushups. In some instances, a myasthenic disorder is suspected only when the patient develops prolonged respiratory arrest on exposure to a curariform drug during a surgical procedure.

Patients with intermediate clinical phenotypes experience moderate physical handicaps from early childhood. Ocular palsies and ptosis of the lids become apparent during the first year of life. Patients fatigue easily and cannot keep up with their peers in sports. They have difficulty walking and negotiating stairs, but can perform most activities of daily living.

Structural changes and electrophysiology. Morphologic studies show an increased number of EP regions distributed over an increased span of the muscle fibre. AChR expression at the EP is markedly attenuated (Figure 1, bottom panels). The integrity of the junctional folds is preserved, but some EP regions are simplified and smaller than normal (Figure 6A). The distribution of AChR on the junctional folds is patchy and the density of the reaction for AChR is attenuated (Figure A and B).

The quantal response at the EP, indicated by the amplitude of miniature endplate potentials and currents, is reduced, but quantal release by nerve impulse is frequently higher than normal. In patients with low-expressor or null mutations of the ε subunit, single-channel patch-clamp recordings (21, 31) and immunocytochemical studies

1. Mutations causing premature termination of the translational chain — these mutations are frameshifting, occur at a splice site, or produce a stop codon directly
2. Point mutations in the promoter region of a subunit gene.
3. Missense mutations in a signal peptide region.
4 Mutations involving residues essential for assembly of the pentameric receptor. Mutations of this type were observed at the following sites: in the ε subunit at an N-glycosylation site (εS143L); at cysteine 128 (εC128S), a residue that is an essential part of the C128-Cl42 cysloop in the extracellular domain; in arginine 147 (εR147L) in the extracellular domain, which lies between isoleucine 145 and threonine 150, residues that contribute to subunit assembly; in threonine 51(εT51P); and with a 3 codon deletion in the long cytoplasmic loop of the β subunit (β1276del9).
5. Missense mutations affecting both AChR. expression and kinetics. For example, εR31IW in the long cytoplasmic loop between M3 and M4 decreases, whereas εP245L in the M1 domain increases the open duration of channel events. In the case of εR31IW and εP245L, the kinetic consequences are modest and are likely overshadowed by the reduced expression of the mutant gene. For a complete list of AChR subunit gene mutations and the appropriate references, the reader is referred to a recently published gene table (27).

Table 4. Different types of recessive mutations causing severe EP AChR deficiency.

(11) reveal the presence of fetal γ-AChR at the EP (Figure 1, middle panels).

Molecular pathogenesis. CMS with severe EP AChR deficiency result from different types of homozygous or, more frequently, heterozygous recessive mutations in AChR subunit genes. The mutations are concentrated in the ε subunit. There are two possible reasons for this: *i)* Expression of the foetal type γ subunit, although at a low level, may compensate for absence of the ε subunit (11, 23, 31), whereas patients harbouring null mutations in subunits other than ε might not survive for lack of a substituting subunit, and *ii)* the gene encoding the ε subunit, and especially exons coding for the long cytoplasmic loop, have a high GC content that likely predisposes to DNA rearrangements.

Table 4 lists the different types of recessive mutations causing severe EP AChR deficiency.

Therapeutic approaches. Most patients respond moderately well to anticholinesterase drugs, and some derive additional benefit from 3,4-diaminopyridine (19).

CMS associated with plectin deficiency

We have investigated a single case of this rare disorder (2). Plectin is a highly conserved and ubiquitously expressed intermediate filament-linking protein concentrated at sites of mechanical stress: the postsynaptic membrane of the EP, the sarcolemma, Z-disks in skeletal muscle, hemidesmosomes in skin, and intercalated disks in cardiac muscle. Pathogenic mutations in plectin are associated with a simplex variety of epidermolysis bullosa, a progressive myopathy, and a myasthenic syndrome (2).

Detailed investigation of a patient with epidermolysis bullosa simplex, a progressive myopathy, abnormal fatigability involving of the ocular, facial and limb muscles, a decremental EMG response, and no anti-AChR antibodies, revealed that plectin expression was absent in muscle and severely decreased in skin. Morphologic studies of muscle demonstrated necrotic and regenerating fibres and a wide spectrum of ultrastructural abnormalities. Many EPs had an abnormal configuration with chains of small regions over the fibre surface, and a few EPs displayed focal degeneration of the junctional folds. The EP AChR content was normal. In vitro electrophysiologic studies showed normal quantal release by nerve impulse, small MEPPs, and expression of foetal as well as adult AChR at the EPs. Pyridostigmine failed to improve the patient's symptoms, but 3,4-diarninopyridine (1 mg/kg/day in divided doses) improved her strength and endurance (2).

References

1. Bady B, Chauplannaz G, Carrier H (1987) Congenital Lambert-Eaton myasthenic syndrome. *J Neurol Neurosurg Psychiatry* 50: 476-478

2. Banwell BL, Russel J, Fukudome T, Shen X-M, Stilling G, Engel AG (1999) Myopathy, myasthenic syndrome, and epidermolysis bullosa simplex due to plectin deficiency. *J Neuropathol Exp Neurol* 58: 832-846

3. Bon S, Coussen F, Massoulie J (1997) Quaternary associations of acetylcholinesterase. II. The polyproline attachment domain of the collagen tail. *J Biol Chem* 272: 3016-3021

4. Croxen R, Newland C, Beeson D, Oosterhuis H, Chauplannaz G, Vincent A, Newsom-Davis J (1997) Mutations in different functional domains of the human muscle acetylcholine receptor alpha subunit in patients with the slow-channel congenital myasthenic syndrome. *Hum Mol Genet* 6: 767-774

5. Deprez PN, Inestrosa NC (1995) Two heparin-binding domains are present on the collagenic tail of asymmetric acetylcholinesterase. *J Biol Chem* 270: 11043-11046

6. Deymeer F, Serdaroglu P, Ozdemir C (1999) Familial infantile myasthenia: confusion in terminology. *Neuromuscul Disord* 9: 129-130

7. Donger C, Krejci E, Serradell AP, Eymard B, Bon S, Nicole S, Chateau D, Gary F, Fardeau M, Massoulie J, Guicheney P (1998) Mutation in the human acetylcholinesterase-associated collagen gene, *COLQ*, is responsible for congenital myasthenic syndrome with end-plate acetylcholinesterase deficiency (Type Ic). *Am J Hum Genet* 63: 967-975

8. Engel AG, Lambert EH (1987) Congenital myasthenic syndromes. *Electroencephalogr Clin Neurophysiol Suppl* 39: 91-102

9. Engel AG, Lambert EH, Gomez MR (1977) A new myasthenic syndrome with end-plate acetylcholinesterase deficiency, small nerve terminals, and reduced acetylcholine release. *Ann Neurol* 1: 315-330

10. Engel AG, Lambert EH, Mulder DM, Torres CF, Sahashi K, Bertorini TE, Whitaker JN (1982) A newly recognized congenital myasthenic syndrome attributed to a prolonged open time of the acetylcholine-induced ion channel. *Ann Neurol* 11: 553-569

11. Engel AG, Ohno K, Bouzat C, Sine SM, Griggs RC (1996) End-plate acetylcholine receptor deficiency due to nonsense mutations in the epsilon subunit. *Ann Neurol* 40: 810-817

12. Engel AG, Ohno K, Milone M, Wang H-L, Nakano S, Bouzat C, Pruitt JN, 2nd, Hutchinson DO, Brengman JM, Bren N, Sieb JP, Sine SM (1996) New muta-

tions in acetylcholine receptor subunit genes reveal heterogeneity in the slow-channel congenital myasthenic syndrome. *Hum Mol Genet* 5: 1217-1227

13. Engel AG, Ohno K, Sine SM (1999) Congenital myasthenic syndromes. In *Myasthenia Gravis and Myasthenic Disorders*, AG Engel (eds). Oxford University Press: New York. pp. 251-297

14. Engel AG, Ohno K, Sine SM (1999) Congenital myasthenic syndromes: recent advances. *Arch Neurol* 56: 163-167

15. Fukudome T, Ohno K, Brengman JM, Engel AG (1998) Quinidine normalizes the open duration of slow-channel mutants of the acetylcholine receptor. *Neuroreport* 9: 1907-1911

16. Gomez CM, Maselli R, Gammack J, Lasalde J, Tamamizu S, Cornblath DR, Lehar M, McNamee M, Kuncl RW (1996) A beta-subunit mutation in the acetylcholine receptor channel gate causes severe slow-channel syndrome. *Ann Neurol* 39: 712-723

17. Greer M, Schotland M (1960) Myasthenia gravis in the newborn. *Pediatrics* 26: 101-108

18. Harper CM, Engel AG (1998) Quinidine sulfate therapy for the slow-channel congenital myasthenic syndrome. *Ann Neurol* 43: 480-484

19. Harper CM, Engel AG (2000) Treatment of 31 congenital myasthenic syndrome patients with 3,4-diaminopyridine. *Neurology* 54, supplement 3: A395, abstract

20. Hutchinson DO, Walls TJ, Nakano S, Camp S, Taylor P, Harper CM, Groover RV, Peterson HA, Jamieson DG, Engel AG (1993) Congenital endplate acetylcholinesterase deficiency. *Brain* 116: 633-653

21. Milone M, Ohno K, Pruitt JN, Brengman JM, Sine SM, Engel AG (1996) Congenital myasthenic syndrorne due to frameshifting acetylcholine receptor epsilon subunit mutation. *Soc Neurosci* 22, abstract: 1942

22. Milone M, Wang H-L, Ohno K, Fukudome T, Pruitt JN, Bren N, Sine SM, Engel AG (1997) Slow-channel myasthenic syndrome caused by enhanced activation, desensitization, and agonist binding affinity attributable to mutation in the M2 domain of the acetylcholine receptor alpha subunit. *J Neurosci* 17: 5651-5665

23. Milone M, Wang H-L, Ohno K, Prince R, Fukudome T, Shen XM, Brengman JM, Griggs RC, Sine SM, Engel AG (1998) Mode switching kinetics produced by a naturally occurring mutation in the cytoplasmic loop of the human acetylcholine receptor epsilon subunit. *Neuron* 20: 575-588

24. Mora M, Lambert EH, Engel AG (1987) Synaptic vesicle abnormality in familial infantile myasthenia. *Neurology* 37: 206-214

25. Ohno K, Brengman J, Tsujino A, Engel AG (1998) Human endplate acetylcholinesterase deficiency caused by mutations in the collagen-like tail subunit (ColQ) of the asymmetric enzyme. *Proc Natl Acad Sci USA* 95: 9654-9659

26. Ohno K, Brengman JM, Felice KJ, Cornblath DR, Engel AG (1999) Congenital end-plate acetylcholinesterase deficiency caused by a nonsense mutation and an A→G splice-donor-site mutation at position +3 of the collagenlike-tail-subunit gene (*COLQ*):

how does G at position +3 result in aberrant splicing? *Am J Hum Genet* 65: 635-644

27. Ohno K, Engel AG (2000) Congenital myasthenic syndromes: gene mutations. *Neuromuscul Disord* 10: 534-536

28. Ohno K, Engel AG, Brengman JM, Shen X-M, Heidenreich F, Vincent A, Milone M, Tan E, Demirci M, Walsh P, Nakano S, Akiguchi I (2000) The spectrum of mutations causing end-plate acetylcholinesterase deficiency. *Ann Neurol* 47: 162-170

29. Ohno K, Hutchinson DO, Milone M, Brengman JM, Bouzat C, Sine SM, Engel AG (1995) Congenital myasthenic syndrome caused by prolonged acetylcholine receptor channel openings due to a mutation in the M2 domain of the epsilon subunit. *Proc Natl Acad Sci USA* 92: 758-762

30. Ohno K, Milone M, Brengman JM, Lo Monaco M, Evoli A, Tonali P, Engel AG (1998) Slow-channel congenital myasthenic syndrorne caused by a novel mutation in the acetylcholine receptor ε subunit. *Neurology* 50: A432(abstract)

31. Ohno K, Quiram PA, Milone M, Wang H-L, Harper MC, Pruitt JN, 2nd, Brengman JM, Pao L, Fischbeck KH, Crawford TO, Sine SM, Engel AG (1997) Congenital myasthenic syndromes due to heteroallelic nonsense/missense mutations in the acetylcholine receptor epsilon subunit gene: identification and functional characterization of six new mutations. *Hum Mol Genet* 6: 753-766

32. Ohno K, Tsujino A, Brengman JM, Harper CM, Bajzer Z, Udd B, Beyring R, Robb S, Kirkham FJ, Engel AG (2001) Choline acetyltransferase mutations cause myasthenic syndrome associated with episodic apnea in humans. *Proc Natl Acad Sci USA* 98: 2017-2022

33. Ohno K, Wang H-L, Shen X-M, Milone M, Bernasconi L, Sine SM, Engel AG (2000) Slow-channel mutations in the center of the MI transmembrane domain of the acetylcholine receptor α subunit. *Neurology* 54 supplement 3: AI83(abstract)

34. Ohno K, Wang H-L, Milone M, Bren N, Brengman JM, Nakano S, Quiram P, Pruitt JN, Sine SM, Engel AG (1996) Congenital myasthenic syndrome caused by decreased agonist binding affinity due to a mutation in the acetylcholine receptor epsilon subunit. *Neuron* 17: 157-170

35. Shen X-M, Ohno K, Milone M, Brengman JM, Spilsbury PR, Engel AG (2001) Fast-channel syndrome. *Neurology* 56 supplement 3: A60 (abstract)

36. Shen X-M, Tsujino A, Ohno K, Brengman JM, Gingold M, Engel AG (2000) A novel fast channel congenital myasthenic syndrorne caused by a mutation in the Cys-loop domain of the acetylcholine receptor E subunit. *Neurology* 54,supplement 3: A138, abstract

37. Sieb JP, Milone M, Engel AG (1996) Effects of the quinoline derivatives quinine, quinidine, and chloroquine on neuromuscular transmission. *Brain Res* 712: 179-189

38. Sine SM, Ohno K, Bouzat C, Auerbach A, Milone M, Pruitt JN, Engel AG (1995) Mutation of the acetylcholine receptor alpha subunit causes a slow-channel myasthenic syndrome by enhancing agonist binding affinity. *Neuron* 15: 229-239

39. Walls TJ, Engel AG, Nagel AS, Harper CM, Trastek VF (1993) Congenital myasthenic syndrome associated with paucity of synaptic vesicles and reduced quantal release. *Ann N Y Acad Sci* 681: 461-468

40. Wang H-L, Auerbach A, Bren N, Ohno K, Engel AG, Sine SM (1997) Mutation in the M1 domain of the acetylcholine receptor alpha subunit decreases the rate of agonist dissociation. *J Gen Physiol* 109: 757-766

41. Wang H-L, Milone M, Ohno K, Shen X-M, Tsujino A, Batocchi AP, Tonali P, Brengman JM, Engel AG, Sine SM (1998) Acetylcholine receptor M3 domain: Stereochemical and volume contributions to channel gating. *Nature Neurosci* 2: 226-233

42. Wang H-L, Ohno K, Milone M, Brengman JM, Evoli A, Batocchi AP, Middleton LT, Christodoulou K, Engel AG, Sine SM (2000) Fundamental gating mechanism of nicotinic receptor channel revealed by mutation causing a congenital myasthenic syndrome. *J Gen Physiol* 116: 449-462

43. Zhou M, Engel AG, Auerbach A (1999) Serum choline activates mutant acetylcholine receptors that cause slow channel congenital myasthenic syndromes. *Proc Natl Acad Sci USA* 96: 10466-10471

CHAPTER 10

Myopathies affecting fuel and energy metabolism

10.1 Selected disorders of carbohydrate metabolism   182
10.2 Defects of fatty acid metabolism   189
10.3 Respiratory chain defects   202
10.4 Myoadenylate deaminase deficiency   214

S keletal muscle uses both anaerobic and oxidative metabolism to generate the universal source of chemical energy, ATP. It has also been established that for these processes the principal starting molecules as fuels are fatty acids and glucose, which are derived either from the blood or from catabolism of triglycerides and glycogen respectively. This chapter discusses the genetically determined disorders that affect these processes.

Historically, carbohydrate disorders were the earliest to be recognized as causes of metabolic skeletal and cardiac myopathies. This is partly related to the fact that in many of these myopathies there is excess glycogen accumulation in muscle fibres that is easily recognized in microscopic sections of muscle biopsies. With the advent of molecular science and in vivo magnetic resonance spectroscopy, the diagnostic and pathogenic aspects of these diseases have been greatly advanced. In addition, new entities are continually being discovered.

Even though basic science has taught us that free fatty acids are very important metabolic fuels for skeletal and cardiac muscle fibres, recognition of metabolic muscle diseases related to mismanagement of lipids has been relatively recent. The understanding of the disorders due to disturbed fat metabolism was closely intertwined with the accumulation of new knowledge in mitochondrial biology since the ultimate pathogenic factor in both lipid disorders and mitochondrial myopathies is usually impaired energy supply during exercise, causing either exercise intolerance or massive muscle fibre necrosis.

Mitochondrial diseases are particularly exciting because their discovery as an important type of muscle disease is relatively recent and the field is rapidly growing. Understandably, in many of these diseases, in addition to muscle involvement, other organs with high oxidative metabolism (eg, brain and heart) also show signs and symptoms of disease. While the mitochondrial energy metabolism related to oxidative phosphorylation (OXPHOS) is the cornerstone of many primary mitochondrial diseases, secondary mitochondrial malfunction may have a role in the pathogenesis of such diverse conditions as normal aging and certain CNS diseases such as Parkinson's disease.

Selected disorders of carbohydrate metabolism

Robert J. Beynon
Rosaline C. M. Quinlivan
Caroline A. Sewry

AM	acid maltase
CPT	carnitine palmitoyl transferase
DB	debrancher enzyme
GP	glycogen phosphorylase
LDH	lactate dehydrogenase
MDA	myoadenylate deaminase
OMIM	Online Mendelian Inheritance in Man (*http://www.ncbi.nlm.nih.gov/omim*)
PFK	phosphofructokinase
PGAM	phosphoglycerate mutase
PGM	phosphoglucomutase
PGK	phosphoglycerate kinase
SRCA	sarcoplasmic calcium ATPase

Definitions of entities

The breakdown of glucose (from blood) or intracellular glycogen yields pyruvate that can then enter the TCA cycle (via acetyl CoA in aerobic conditions) or be converted to lactate under ischaemic conditions. Failure in any step in glycogenolysis or glycolysis eliminates or diminishes carbon flux, leading to a rapid decline in high energy phosphates for muscular work, and causing rapid muscle fatigue, cramping, and sometimes rhabdomyolysis. In those conditions where there is a muscle-specific gene product, the symptoms may be restricted to muscle but in other conditions, where there is a single gene encoding the enzyme activity, the effects can be more widespread.

Inherited deficiencies in glyogenolytic/glycolytic enzymes are rare, and are usually autosomal recessive. They generally present as exercise intolerance, elevated serum creatine kinase, with rhabdomyolysis and exertion-induced myoglobinuria (3). One of the less well-understood features of this group of conditions relates to the marked variability in the severity of symptoms, even between individuals carrying the same mutations. This suggests that these enzyme deficiencies must be projected onto additional factors influencing muscle capabilities, whether genetic or environmental. In this respect, the anecdotal evidence of

greater prevalence/severity in males may be relevant (24). In this chapter, we will consider three of the more common of these conditions: McArdle's disease, Tarui's disease, and debrancher deficiency. Some indication of the relative frequencies of these conditions may be gleaned from a survey conducted some years ago as part of the CARMEN programme, (*http://carmen. liv.ac.uk*). Whilst not intended to be exhaustive, these figures (Figure 1) report the total cases from twenty different muscle clinics within the European community, although these data will reflect local interests.

McArdle's disease

McArdle's disease (myophosphorylase deficiency, glycogen storage disease V, OMIM 232600) is a rare autosomal recessive disorder affecting approximately 1 of 100 000 persons (although precise epidemiological data are lacking). The condition was first identified in 1951 by Brian McArdle who reported a patient with myalgia coupled with a failure to produce lactate during ischaemic exercise (21). The condition results from the almost complete absence of functional glycogen phosphorylase in skeletal muscle (4, 8, 9). This enzyme is responsible for the breakdown of glycogen in the sarcoplasm, via phosphorolysis of the substrate, glycogen, and yielding glucose-1-phospate as the product. Of the several metabolic myopathies caused by deficiencies in sarcoplasmic enzymes, McArdle's disease is one of the most common (Figure 1).

McArdle's disease is generally held to be an adult-onset condition although, rarely, cases have been confirmed in childhood. Typically, however, diagnosis is made in the third decade of life and in retrospect, affected individuals are virtually united in their memory, for example, of extreme difficulty in

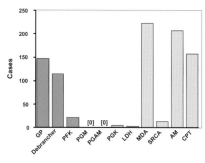

Figure 1. *Analysis of cases in 20 muscle centres.* As part of the background to CARMEN, we surveyed twenty specialist muscle centres throughout Europe and collated their cases for several metabolic myopathies. The conditions shaded in green are considered in this chapter, conditions shaded in pale blue are covered elsewhere in this volume.

school-day physical education. The condition normally presents with exertion-induced fatigue and myalgia, and under extreme exertion, painful muscle cramps and myoglobinuria with the attendant risk of renal failure. However, there is marked heterogeneity in the presentation of this condition, such that some patients maintain a high level of muscle performance whilst others of the same age and with the same genotype are severely disabled with exercise intolerance restricted to a few yards of walking. The disorder is progressive with muscle wasting and weakness occurring from middle age.

McArdle's disease should be suspected by the pattern of symptoms described above. Wasting of the upper body, especially latissimus dorsi, may be seen in contrast with a tendency for bulky lower limb muscles. A raised serum creatine kinase (three to twenty times normal) is common, as in many other conditions where generalised muscle weakness is apparent. An absence of lactate production in an ischaemic forearm test increases suspicion of the diagnosis.

The large number of mutations in this condition, most of them rare, precludes mutation analysis as a uniformly definitive test although the most common mutations in certain ethnic groups, R50X in particular (see below), can provide a conclusive diagnosis in a significant number of cases.

Molecular genetics and pathogenesis. There are three isoenzymic forms of glycogen phosphorylase: *i)* the liver form, encoded on chromosome 14, *ii)* the brain/foetal form, encoded on chromosome 20, and *iii)* the muscle form, encoded on chromosome 11 (proximal part of 11q13). It is only the last of these that is affected in McArdle's disease, and with few exceptions affected patients have virtually no detectable enzyme activity in muscle biopsy. In contrast to other glycogenoses, the restriction to the muscle specific isoform means that there is no liver involvement. In the few patients that have been studied in detail, the lack of enzyme activity is coincident with a lack of immunoreactive protein (Figure 2) or of mRNA (22). Lack of mRNA is a feature of the most common mutation, R50X, which although a nonsense mutation, seems to bring about rapid degradation of mRNA as a consequence of early termination of translation (5). By contrast, a compound het-

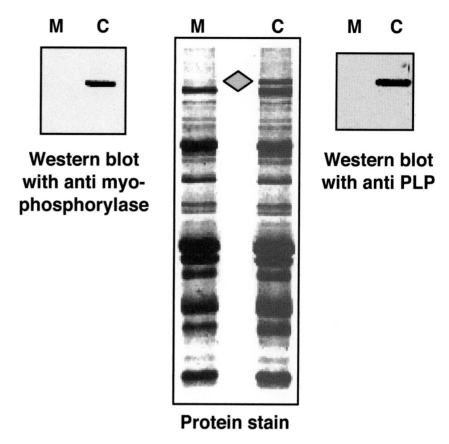

Western blot with anti myophosphorylase

Protein stain

Western blot with anti PLP

Figure 2. *Protein expression in McArdle's disease.* Soluble proteins from muscle biopsies of a normal and a McArdle's patients were separated on linear 12% sodium dodecyl sulphate polyacrylamide gel electrophoresis. The absence of the myophosphorylase band is readily apparent (diamond), as is the lack of immunoreactivity in western blots using an antibody to muscle phosphorylase or to the cofactor, pyridoxal phosphate.

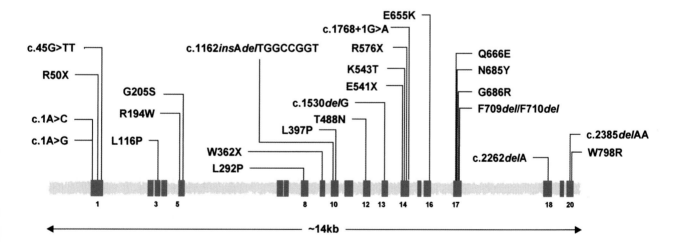

Figure 3. *Mutation map of the myophosphorylase gene.* The figure summarises current information on the known mutations in the myophosphorylase gene. Note that the exact sizes of the two largest introns (5 and 17) are unknown, which precludes a mutation labelling scheme based on the genomic sequence. Accordingly, mutations have been named with reference to the protein sequence, where the initiation methionine residue is numbered 1, or the cDNA sequence, where the first base of the ATG codon for that methionine is numbered 1. Because the protein sequence was previously counted from the second residue (the N-terminal methionine residue is removed from the mature protein), most mutation designations in the literature in the literature are displaced by one residue. Thus, the most common Caucasian mutation, R50X has previously been known as R49X or R49TER. Mutations given with reference to the cDNA sequence are prefaced with "c." In the absence of the full genome sequence, there is no simple way to define a mutation in the first base of intron 14, and the label c.1768+1G>A is used to indicate the mutation that is also known as 1844+1G>A. The detailed bibliography defining these mutations will be presented elsewhere (Quinlivan et al, unpublished).

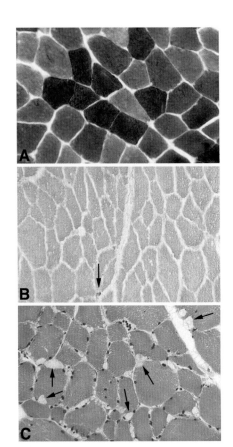

Figure 4. *Histochemical diagnosis of McArdle's disease.* Histochemical demonstration of phosphorylase in **A**. a control and **B**. a case of McArdle's disease. Note the normal fibre typing pattern in the control and absence of the enzyme in most fibres in the McArdle case. Activity is only seen in one very small, regenerating fibre (arrow). The extent of activity staining in regenerating fibres, and the origin of the activity has been discussed recently (20). **C**. In this H & E stain there are subsarcolemmal unstained regions corresponding to deposits of glycogen. Examples indicated by arrows.

erozygote of R50X/G205S revealed a strong mRNA signal on northern blotting (unpublished data). In other groups of patients, a similar heterogeneity in myophosphorylase mRNA levels was observed (13, 30), but these studies predated the discovery of mutations in the gene, and it is not possible to infer anything further about the relationship between genotype and molecular phenotype.

The first report of point mutations in the myophosphorylase gene were made independently by Tsujino et al (38) and Bartram et al (5). These papers reported the identification of the most common mutation R50X (previously known as R49X) in North American and UK patients respectively, The paper by Tsujino et al (38) reported two additional mutations (G205S and K543T), and provided a clear analysis of the apparent pseudodominance of the condition, showing that it was attributable to one parent being a compound heterozygote and the other parent carrying a third mutation. In another early study, the R50X mutation was observed to be the most frequent in a group of German patients (42). However, in southern European countries, the preponderance of R50X is lower and this mutation has never been seen in Japanese patients. In contrast, one common mutation in the last group is F709del/F710del (39), which has never been observed in non-Japanese patients.

Since these early reports, a total of 25 mutations have been identified as of May 2001 (Figure 3). The most common mutation is R50X, but G205S has also been observed in patients from several countries and in different family lines. Many other private mutations are seen in single patients or in isolated family lineages. Of 102 European patients entered in the CARMEN database (*http://carmen.liv.ac.uk*), 46 were homozygous for R50X, and a further 41 were heterozygotes with the same mutation. One patient was homozygous for G205S and a further 5 were heterozygotes that included this mutation.

Structural changes. A definitive diagnosis can only be obtained by skeletal muscle histochemistry (Figure 4). The histochemical method is specific for the isoform present in mature muscle fibres (see below). Thus, regenerating fibres, the immature fibres in spindles, and some smooth muscle fibres will stain but all mature extrafusal fibres will be negative. There is no other known condition where this occurs.

Myophosphorylase is the key enzyme in sarcoplasmic glycogen degradation, but deficiency of this enzyme is not always associated with a marked accumulation of glycogen although there may be some sub-sar-colemmal accumulation of glycogen. The commonly used method relies on activation of nascent enzyme in muscle, and utilises the enzyme in the reverse direction (glycogen synthesis), monitoring the accumulation of glycogen as iodine-reactive material. The colour development is not stable, and it is essential to include a control sample in parallel with the test sample, and observe the outcome as soon as possible in order to avoid a false positive diagnosis.

Future perspectives. Although McArdle's disease is rarely considered to be life threatening, there is a need for treatments that reduce muscle fatiguability and pain, which in turn may diminish the progressive loss of muscle bulk as patients get older. Nutritional and pharmaceutical therapies have not yielded a marked improvement, and no treatment has been universally adopted for this condition (Quinlivan and Beynon, unpublished). The most promising study that has been conducted recently has been a double-blind, placebo-controlled crossover study of oral creatine, which enhanced anaerobic exercise capability although there was no improvement in aerobic exercise ability (41). After a single patient reported improvements with oral vitamin B6 (26), a random, double blind, placebo controlled crossover study failed to confirm a general enhancement of muscle performance (Beynon et al, unpublished).

Gene therapy for McArdle's disease remains a possibility. The availability of animal models, notably in Charolais cattle and Merino sheep, has made future trials feasible. In Charolais cattle, the mutation is R490W, and the resultant molecular phenotype was determined to be zero protein, unknown mRNA (40). In the Merino sheep, the molecular phenotype is unknown, other than for lack of myophosphorylase activity, but the mutation, at the 3′ end of introns 19 invokes a cryptic splice site within exon 20, causing a frame shift and premature termination of translation (35).

Adenoviral-mediated delivery of a myophosphorylase cDNA into myoblasts from McArdle's patients, or myophosphorylase-deficient sheep brought about restoration of activity above normal values. Any toxicity due to over-expression was thought unlikely given the tight controls on the activity of the enzyme (25).

Tarui's disease

Tarui's disease (phosphofructokinase deficiency, glycogen storage disease VII, OMIM 232800) is a deficiency of the enzyme (phosphofructokinase, PFK) that is a key regulator of glycolysis (12, 36). There are three isozymic forms of PFK, the muscle form is encoded at chromosome 12q13 (not on chromosome 1 as originally reported), the liver form at chromosome 21q, and the platelet form at chromosome 10p. The enzyme is tetrameric and in skeletal muscle consists exclusively of M_4 homotetramers. Liver contains exclusively the L_4 homotetramer. The erythrocyte PFK consists of a series of isoenzymic forms: M_4, M_3L, M_2L_2, ML_3, and L_4. The M-type transcript exists in a number of splice variants, but in skeletal muscle the predominant form comprises exons 2 to 24, and intron 2 is retained within the mature transcript. The start codon is located within exon 3 (23).

Deficiency of PFK is a heterogeneous condition, characterised by a myopathy defined by exercise intolerance, muscle cramps, and myoglobinuria. Further, the importance of glycolysis in erythrocytes and the loss of the M-type subunit in these cells means that PFK activity drops to about 50% of normal values, eliciting an associated haemolytic anaemia. There seems to be a particularly high prevalence of the condition among Japanese and those of Ashkenazi Jewish descent (27) although it has been observed in other ethnic groups. A severe fatal infantile form of the condition seems to manifest as a reduction in PFK levels in all tissues examined, which is unlikely to be attributable to single gene mutations

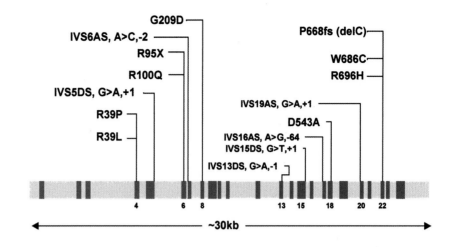

Figure 5. *Pathological mutations in the human PFK gene.* This map is based on that published by Fujii & Miwa (12) but contains additional mutations.

and may reflect some *trans* acting factor (1).

Molecular genetics and pathogenesis. Muscle sections may show some accumulation of glycogen (Figure 5) although this need not be pronounced (6). There is some indication of accumulation of glycogen in abnormal structures in older patients (16, 32). A total of 15 disease-causing mutations in the PFK-M gene have been identified (Figure 6). These range from missense and nonsense mutations to splice variants and single base deletions causing a frameshift and premature termination of translation. In Ashkenazi Jews, the most common mutations are a G to A substitution at the 5′ splice donor site of intron 5, and the deletion of a single base (C) at position 2079 in the mRNA (P688fs in protein-based nomenclature). Together, these 2 mutations account for over 90% of alleles in this group of patients, making feasible a diagnostic strategy based on DNA testing.

The sole reported animal model of PFK deficiency is the dog, specifically, English Springer spaniels (14, 15), which present with classic symptoms of anaemia and exercise intolerance. The PFK-M protein is completely absent by SDS-PAGE or western blotting, and the common causative mutation observed in dogs from the United

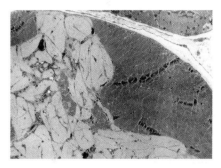

Figure 6. *Section of muscle from GSD VII patient.* Large areas in this muscle fibre are devoid of myofibrils and contain quasi compartments which, on higher power (not shown), contain granular as well as filamentous material and cellular organelles. This picture is from a patient with a metabolic myopathy and hemolytic anemia due to phosphofructokinase defiency. Histochemical reaction for phosphophructokinase activity showed complete negativity (not shown). Electron micrograph. ×2500. Image kindly provided by Dr George Karpati, Montreal.

States and Europe is W742X (33). Some dogs presenting with similar symptoms were heterozygous for this mutation, and it is likely that other mutations exist.

Structural changes. Muscle sections may show some accumulation of glycogen although this need not be pronounced (6). There is some indication of accumulation of glycogen in abnormal structures in older patients (16, 32). Other changes are illustrated in Figure 6.

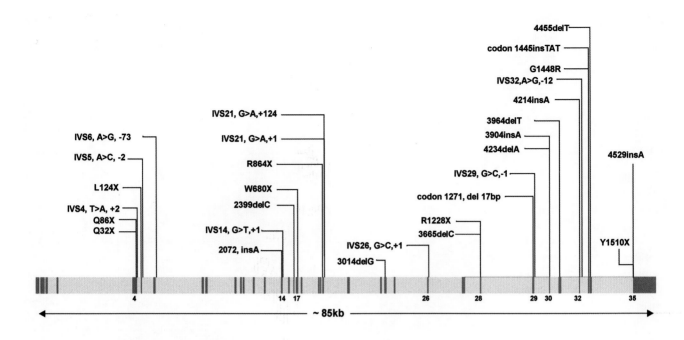

Figure 7. *Pathological mutations in the human debrancher gene (AGL).* The mutations indicated are those that have been specifically associated with GSD IIIa or for which no association may yet be made, as the affected individual was a child. There is some disparity in relation to cDNA base numbering and the mutations have mostly been cited in the same nomenclature as used by the original authors.

Future perspectives. PFK deficiency is rare, and gene-mediated therapies are likely to be consequential to developments in the treatment of other myopathies. At present, a managed lifestyle seems to offer the best option for optimal adjustment to daily life, but there is one report of a ketogenic diet that seemed effective in a severely affected infant (34).

Debrancher deficiency

Debrancher deficiency (Cori-Forbes disease, glycogen storage disease III, OMIM 232400) is a complex set of conditions of variable severity (11, 17). Most patients have liver and muscle involvement (Type IIIa), but approximately 15% of all affected individuals manifest liver involvement without any muscle-specific symptoms (Type IIIb). There may be an associated cardiomyopathy.

The enzyme affected is the product of a single gene (gene name AGL, chromosome 1p21), which encodes a large protein (1,532 amino acids, 175kDa). The enzyme, in concert with glycogen phosphorylase, effects glycogenolysis by removing the 1,6 branch points in the glycogen structure (amylo-1,6-glucosidase activity) and by maintaining the lengths of the 1,4 linked glucose chains for effective phosphorylase action (1,4,glucan-1,4 glycosyl transferase activity). The catalytic sites for these 2 activities are located at different domains of the protein, and in rare cases, either one or the other activity can be selectively disabled (Type IIIc or Type IIId respectively).

Expression of debrancher enzyme is controlled differentially in liver and muscle. There are 6 splice variants involving exons 1 to 3. Variants 1, 5, and 6 are present in liver and muscle, whereas variants 2, 3, and 4 occur in muscle but not liver (2). The start codon is located within exon 3, and variants 1 to 4 encode identical proteins that have an additional 27 amino acids that are absent from variants 5 and 6. In turn, variants 5 and 6 differ at the N-terminal from variant 1 by 10 and 11 amino acids, respectively (2). Tissue specific mRNA or protein variants may explain in part the distinction between Type IIIa and Type IIIb cases—in the latter, enzyme activity is absent in liver but present in muscle, whereas in Type IIIa the enzyme activity is impaired in both tissues. Western blotting of samples from 41 patients with GSD III showed that only patients with defective transferase activity (Type IIId) had cross-reactive material. In all other cases (31 Type IIIa, 4 with type IIIb and three unknown), the cross-reactive material was greatly reduced or absent (10).

In Type IIIa cases, the liver symptoms (hepatomegaly, hypoglycaemia, and hyperlipidaemia) are present in childhood but usually disappear in adulthood. Muscle symptoms may be absent in childhood but appear progressively with age. Because glycogen breakdown is not fully impaired (glycogen phosphorylase activity would be expected to be normal) plasma creatine kinase may be less markedly elevated, and episodes of myoglobinuria are less common than in McArdle's disease or Tarui's disease.

Molecular genetics and pathogenesis. Over 20 mutations have been described for debrancher deficiency Type IIIa (Figure 7). These range from missense and nonsense mutations to splice variations and short deletions within the gene. Whilst the differential-

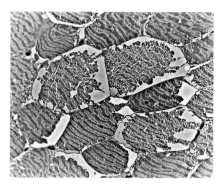

Figure 8. Large sarcolemmal lakes filled with material of groundglass staining appearance (glycogen) are present in many muscle fibres in a case of myopathy caused by glycogen debrancher enzyme deficiency. Semithin resin section. ×550. Image kindly provided by Dr George Karpati, Montreal.

ly expressed mRNA isoforms may explain some differences between Type IIIa and Type IIIb (31), debrancher deficiency, in common with the other myopathies discussed here, demonstrates clinical heterogeneity even within a group of patients homozygous for the same mutation (4455delT). It has been suggested that even in Type IIIa cases, the clinical phenotypes may be further subdivided (18, 19).

Structural changes. Muscle pathology is mild and sections may show glycogen accumulation (Figure 8), often near the periphery of the fibre.

Future perspectives. The explanation for the different clinical phenotypes will undoubtedly extend beyond simple descriptions of the mutations in the gene of interest, and unravelling genetic and environmental factors is a major challenge for debrancher deficiency, just as it is for the other myopathies. There are no specific treatments, although a high-protein diet proved effective in a single case, where failure of respiratory muscles had been precipitated by extreme dieting (18, 19).

A note on "Double Trouble"

The frequency of myoadenylate deaminase deficiency (Chapter 10.4) in the general population is sufficiently high (1-2%) such that is it possible to encounter patients lacking this enzyme and a second enzyme, such as myophosphorylase or phosphofructokinase. This coincidence, often termed "double trouble," has been advanced to explain more severe forms of the conditions (7, 28, 37). However, the pattern of clinical phenotypes again remains elusive, and there are cases where muscle dysfunction seems no worse than others lacking the glycolytic or glycogenolytic enzyme alone (29), or other cases where the conditions are severe. It seems unlikely that "double trouble," where the second component is a deficiency of myoadenylate deaminase, can explain the range of clinical phenotypes observed in these conditions.

References

1. Amit R, Bashan N, Abarbanel JM, Shapira Y, Sofer S, Moses S (1992) Fatal familial infantile glycogen storage disease: multisystem phosphofructokinase deficiency. *Muscle Nerve* 15: 455-458

2. Bao Y, Dawson TL, Jr., Chen YT (1996) Human glycogen debranching enzyme gene (AGL): complete structural organization and characterization of the 5′ flanking region. *Genomics* 38: 155-165

3. Barras BT, Friedmann NR (2000) Metabolic myopathies: A clinical approach II. *Pediatr Neurol* 22: 171-181

4. Bartram C, Edwards RH, Beynon RJ (1995) McArdle's disease-muscle glycogen phosphorylase deficiency. *Biochim Biophys Acta* 1272: 1-13

5. Bartram C, Edwards RH, Clague J, Beynon RJ (1993) McArdle's disease: a nonsense mutation in exon 1 of the muscle glycogen phosphorylase gene explains some but not all cases. *Hum Mol Genet* 2: 1291-1293

6. Bonilla E, Schotland DL (1970) Histochemical diagnosis of muscle phosphofructokinase deficiency. *Arch Neurol* 22: 8-12

7. Bruno C, Minetti C, Shanske S, Morreale G, Bado M, Cordone G, DiMauro S (1998) Combined defects of muscle phosphofructokinase and AMP deaminase in a child with myoglobinuria. *Neurology* 50: 296-298

8. DiMauro S, Haller RG (1999) Metabolic myopathies: substrate utilization defects. In *Muscle Diseases*, RC Griggs, AHV Schapira (eds). Butterworth: Boston. pp. 225-249

9. DiMauro S, Tsujino S (1994) Nonlysosomal glycogenoses. In *Myology*, A Engel, B Banker (eds). McGraw-Hill: New York. pp. 1554-1576

10. Ding JH, de Barsy T, Brown BI, Coleman RA, Chen YT (1990) Immunoblot analyses of glycogen debranching enzyme in different subtypes of glycogen storage disease type III. *J Pediatr* 116: 95-100

11. Forbes GB (1953) Glycogen storage disease. Report of a case with abnormal glycogen structure in liver and skeletal muscle. *J Pediatr* 42: 645-650

12. Fujii H, Miwa S (2000) Other erythrocyte enzyme deficiencies associated with non- haematological symptoms: phosphoglycerate kinase and phosphofructokinase deficiency. *Baillieres Best Pract Res Clin Haematol* 13: 141-148

13. Gautron S, Daegelen D, Mennecier F, Dubocq D, Kahn A, Dreyfus JC (1987) Molecular mechanisms of McArdle's disease (muscle glycogen phosphorylase deficiency). RNA and DNA analysis. *J Clin Invest* 79: 275-281

14. Giger U, Harvey JW (1987) Hemolysis caused by phosphofructokinase deficiency in English springer spaniels: seven cases (1983-1986). *J Am Vet Med Assoc* 191: 453-459

15. Giger U, Reilly MP, Asakura T, Baldwin CJ, Harvey JW (1986) Autosomal recessive inherited phosphofructokinase deficiency in English springer spaniel dogs. *Anim Genet* 17: 15-23

16. Hays AP, Hallett M, Delfs J, Morris J, Sotrel A, Shevchuk MM, DiMauro S (1981) Muscle phosphofructokinase deficiency: abnormal polysaccharide in a case of late-onset myopathy. *Neurology* 31: 1077-1086

17. Illingworth B, Cori GT, Cori CF (1956) Amylo-1,6-glucosidase in muscle tissue in generalized glycogen storage disease. *J Biol Chem* 218: 123

18. Kiechl S, Kohlendorfer U, Thaler C, Skladal D, Jaksch M, Obermaier-Kusser B, Willeit J (1999) Different clinical aspects of debrancher deficiency myopathy. *J Neurol Neurosurg Psychiatry* 67: 364-368

19. Kiechl S, Willeit J, Vogel W, Kohlendorfer U, Poewe W (1999) Reversible severe myopathy of respiratory muscles due to adult-onset type III glycogenosis. *Neuromuscul Disord* 9: 408-410

20. Martinuzzi A, Schievano G, Nascimbeni A, Fanin M (1999) McArdle's disease. The unsolved mystery of the reappearing enzyme. *Am J Pathol* 154: 1893-1897

21. McArdle B (1951) Myopathy due to a defect in muscle glycogen breakdown. *Clin Sci* 10: 13-33

22. McConchie SM, Coakley J, Edwards RH, Beynon RJ (1990) Molecular heterogeneity in McArdle's disease. *Biochim Biophys Acta* 1096: 26-32

23. Nakajima H, Hamaguchi T, Yamasaki T, Tarui S (1995) Phosphofructokinase deficiency: recent advances in molecular biology. *Muscle Nerve* 3: S28-34

24. Nichols RC, Rudolphi O, Ek B, Exelbert R, Plotz PH, Raben N (1996) Glycogenosis type VII (Tarui disease) in a Swedish family: two novel mutations in muscle phosphofructokinase gene (PFK-M) resulting in intron retentions. *Am J Hum Genet* 59: 59-65

25. Pari G, Crerar MM, Nalbantoglu J, Shoubridge E, Jani A, Tsujino S, Shanske S, DiMauro S, Howell JM, Karpati G (1999) Myophosphorylase gene transfer in McArdle's disease myoblasts in vitro. *Neurology* 53: 1352-1354

26. Phoenix J, Hopkins P, Bartram C, Beynon RJ, Quinlivan RC, Edwards RH (1998) Effect of vitamin B6 supplementation in McArdle's disease: a strategic case study. *Neuromuscul Disord* 8: 210-212

27. Rowland LP, DiMauro S, Layzer RB (1986) Phosphofructokinase deficiency. In *Myology*, A Engel, B Banker (eds). McGraw-Hill: New York. pp. 1603-1617

28. Rubio JC, Martin MA, Bautista J, Campos Y, Segura D, Arenas J (1997) Association of genetically proven deficiencies of myophosphorylase and AMP deaminase: a second case of 'double trouble'. *Neuromuscul Disord* 7: 387-389

29. Rubio JC, Martin MA, Del Hoyo P, Bautista J, Campos Y, Segura D, Navarro C, Ricoy JR, Cabello A, Arenas J (2000) Molecular analysis of Spanish patients with AMP deaminase deficiency. *Muscle Nerve* 23: 1175-1178

30. Servidei S, Shanske S, Zeviani M, Lebo R, Fletterick R, DiMauro S (1988) McArdle's disease: biochemical and molecular genetic studies. *Ann Neurol* 24: 774-781

31. Shen J, Bao Y, Liu HM, Lee P, Leonard JV, Chen YT (1996) Mutations in exon 3 of the glycogen debranching enzyme gene are associated with glycogen storage disease type III that is differentially expressed in liver and muscle. *J Clin Invest* 98: 352-357

32. Sivakumar K, Vasconcelos O, Goldfarb L, Dalakas MC (1996) Late-onset muscle weakness in partial phosphofructokinase deficiency: a unique myopathy with vacuoles, abnormal mitochondria, and absence of the common exon 5/intron 5 junction point mutation. *Neurology* 46: 1337-1342

33. Smith BF, Stedman H, Rajpurohit Y, Henthorn PS, Wolfe JH, Patterson DF, Giger U (1996) Molecular basis of canine muscle type phosphofructokinase deficiency. *J Biol Chem* 271: 20070-20074

34. Swoboda KJ, Specht L, Jones HR, Shapiro F, DiMauro S, Korson M (1997) Infantile phosphofructokinase deficiency with arthrogryposis: clinical benefit of a ketogenic diet. *J Pediatr* 131: 932-934

35. Tan P, Allen JG, Wilton SD, Akkari PA, Huxtable CR, Laing NG (1997) A splice-site mutation causing ovine McArdle's disease. *Neuromuscul Disord* 7: 336-342

36. Tarui S, Okuno G, Ikura Y, Tanaka T, Suda M, Nishikawa M (1965) Phosphofructokinase deficiency in skeletal muscle. A new type of glycogenosis. *Biochem Biophys Res Commun* 19: 517-523

37. Tsujino S, Shanske S, Carroll JE, Sabina RL, DiMauro S (1995) Double trouble: combined myophosphorylase and AMP deaminase deficiency in a child homozygous for nonsense mutations at both loci. *Neuromuscul Disord* 5: 263-266

38. Tsujino S, Shanske S, DiMauro S (1993) Molecular genetic heterogeneity of myophosphorylase deficiency (McArdle's disease). *N Engl J Med* 329: 241-245

39. Tsujino S, Shanske S, Goto Y, Nonaka I, DiMauro S (1994) Two mutations, one novel and one frequently observed, in Japanese patients with McArdle's disease. *Hum Mol Genet* 3: 1005-1006

40. Tsujino S, Shanske S, Valberg SJ, Cardinet GH, 3rd, Smith BP, DiMauro S (1996) Cloning of bovine muscle glycogen phosphorylase cDNA and identification of a mutation in cattle with myophosphorylase deficiency, an animal model for McArdle's disease. *Neuromuscul Disord* 6: 19-26

41. Vorgerd M, Grehl T, Jager M, Muller K, Freitag G, Patzold T, Bruns N, Fabian K, Tegenthoff M, Mortier W, Luttmann A, Zange J, Malin JP (2000) Creatine therapy in myophosphorylase deficiency (McArdle disease): a placebo-controlled crossover trial. *Arch Neurol* 57: 956-963

42. Vorgerd M, Kubisch C, Burwinkel B, Reichmann H, Mortier W, Tettenborn B, Pongratz D, Lindemuth R, Tegenthoff M, Malin JP, Kilimann MW (1998) Mutation analysis in myophosphorylase deficiency (McArdle's disease). *Ann Neurol* 43: 326-331

Defects of fatty acid metabolism

Stefano Di Donato
Franco Taroni

ADP	adenosine diphosphate
AFLP	acute fatty liver of pregnancy syndrome
ATP	adenosine triphosphate
CACT	carnitine/acylcarnitine translocase
CoA	acyl-coenzyme A
CPT	carnitine palmitoyltransferase
CT	carnitine transporter
DHA	docosahexaenoic acid
ETF	electron transfer flavoprotein
ETF:QO	ETF:coenzyme Q oxidoreductase
FA	fatty acid
FAD	flavin adenine dinucleotide
FMN	flavin mononucleotide
HELLP	haemolysis, elevated liver enzymes and low platelets
LCAD	long-chain acyl-CoA dehydrogenase
LCEH	long-chain 2-enoyl-CoA hydratase
LCFA	long-chain fatty acids
LCHAD	long-chain L-3-hydroxyacyl-CoA dehydrogenase
LCKT	long-chain 3-ketoacyl-CoA thiolase
MCAD	medium-chain acyl-CoA dehydrogenase
MCKAT	medium-chain 3-ketoacyl-CoA thiolase deficiency
MTP	mitochondrial trifunctional protein
OMIM	Online Mendelian Inheritance in Man (http://www.ncbi.nlm.nih.gov/omim)
PCD	primary carnitine deficiency
RER	respiratory exchange ratio
RR-MADD	riboflavin-responsive multiple acyl-CoA dehydrogenase deficiency
SCAD	short-chain acyl-CoA dehydrogenase
SCHAD	short-chain L-3-hydroxyacyl-CoA dehydrogenase deficiency
SLC22A5	solute carrier family 22 (organic cation transporter), member 5
TCA	tricarboxylic acid
VLCAD	very-long-chain acyl-CoA dehydrogenase deficiency

Definition of entities

Defects of oxidative fatty-acid (FA) metabolism are a heterogeneous group of inherited metabolic disorders caused by abnormalities of any component of the mitochondrial β-oxidation pathway. Mitochondrial oxidative metabolism of lipids is a major source for energy production, particularly at times of stress or fasting. Its contribution to energy homeostasis is especially important in the heart, the liver, and the skeletal muscle (9, 41).

At rest, long-chain fatty acids (LCFA) are the major energy substrate for muscle. Therefore, impairment at any level of mitochondrial β-oxidation pathway can cause skeletal myopathy, possibly associated with other severe metabolic disturbances including cardiomyopathy, hypoketotic hypoglycaemia, and childhood sudden death. Abnormalities of lipid catabolism as possible causes of human disease were first suggested in the late 1960s by morphological observations of excessive accumulation of lipid droplets within muscle fibres of a young woman who had attacks of muscle weakness lasting from a few weeks to several years. In 1970 Engel et al (12) described a lipid storage myopathy in a pair of identical twin sisters who presented with intermittent "cramps" and myoglobinuria induced by exercise, fasting, or a high-fat diet. A possible defect in LCFA utilization, namely a deficiency of carnitine or carnitine palmitoyltransferase (CPT), was hypothesized. CPT deficiency was, in fact, the first enzyme defect of FA oxidation to be discovered. It was identified in 1973 by DiMauro and Melis-DiMauro (11) who described a 29-year-old man who suffered from recurrent episodes of muscle pain and pigmenturia with occasional renal failure. His brother had similar symptoms. The recurrent attacks were triggered by prolonged exercise, especially when the patient fasted. Since this first description in 1973, at least 14 different genetic defects of mitochondrial FA have been reported (Table 1).

Pathophysiology. The immediate source of chemical energy for muscle contraction is the hydrolysis of ATP to ADP. ATP can be regenerated from ADP and the high-energy compound phosphocreatine, but during long-term exercise the rephosphorylation of ADP

to ATP requires the utilization of other fuels, such as carbohydrate mainly glycogen, FA, and ketones, which are degraded in muscle mitochondria. Skeletal muscle can use carbohydrate or lipid as fuel, depending on the degree of activity. The respiratory quotient (RER, respiratory exchange ratio) of resting muscle is close to 0.8, indicating an almost total dependence on the oxidation of FAs (9). During the early phase of exercise (up to approximately 45 minutes), energy is derived mainly from blood glucose and from muscle glycogen metabolism. During prolonged exercise, there is a gradual shift from glucose to FA utilization and, after a few hours, approximately 70% of the skeletal-muscle energy requirements are met by mitochondrial oxidation of LCFA. As with skeletal muscle, the heart is also substantially dependent on LCFA oxidation for its high energy-demanding functional activity (3, 9).

Mitochondrial oxidation of lipids is a complex process that requires a series of enzymatic reactions. Detailed descriptions of the pathway are available (24, 36). Schematically, plasma free FAs delivered into the cytosol are first activated to their corresponding acyl-coenzyme A (CoA) thioesters at the outer mitochondrial membrane by acyl-CoA synthetase(s). Unlike short-chain (C_4–C_6) and medium-chain (C_8–C_{12}) acyl-CoAs, long-chain (C_{14}–C_{20}) acyl-CoAs cannot enter mitochondria directly. The mitochondrial CPT enzyme system, in conjunction with a carnitine/acylcarnitine translocase (CACT), provides the active carnitine-dependent mechanism, whereby long-chain acyl-CoAs are transported from the cytosolic compartment into the mitochondrion where β-oxidation occurs. L-carnitine is supplied for this reaction by a plasma-membrane sodium-dependent carnitine transporter (CT).

Disorder	Myopathic symptoms			Hepatic symptoms		Abnormal Organic Acids	Other features	MIM No.[3]
	Acute[1]	Chronic	Cardiomyopathy	Hypoketotic Hypoglycaemia	Metabolic Encephalopathy[2]			
Long-chain fatty-acid oxidation								
Fatty-acid transport								
CT	–	+	+++	+	+	–	Endocardial fibroelastosis	212140
CPT1	–	–	–	+++	+++	–	Renal tubular acidosis	255120
CACT	?	++	+++[4]	+++	+++	+/–		212138
CPT2, type 1 (muscular)	+++	–	–	–	–	–		255110 600650
CPT2, type 2 (hepatocardiomuscular)	+/–	++	++	++	++	+/–	Recurrent pancreatitis	600649 600650
CPT2, type 3 (lethal neonatal)	–	++	+++	+++	+++	+/–	Brain and kidney dysplasia	600649
β-Oxidation spiral								
VLCAD[5]	+	++	++	++	++	+++		201475
MTP, type 1 (LCHAD)	++	++	++	+++	+++	+++	Retinitis pigmentosa, AFLP, HELLP, lactic acidemia	600890
MTP, type 2 (LCEH/LCHAD/LCKT)	++	++	++	+++	+++	+++	Retinitis pigmentosa, peripheral neuropathy, hypoparathyroidism	143450
Medium- and short-chain fatty-acid oxidation								
β-Oxidation spiral								
MCAD	+/–	+/–	–	+++	+++	+++		201450
SCAD	–	–	–	+/–	+/–	++	Hypotonia, hypertonia mental retardation	201470
MCKAT	++	–	–	++[6,7]	+/–	+++	Vomiting, hyperammonaemia	602199
SCHAD	–	–	–	++[6]	+/–	+++		601609
2,4-Dienoyl-CoA reductase	–	–	–	–	–	–[7]	Microcephaly, dysmorphism	222745
Multiple acyl-CoA dehydrogenation defects								
ETF or ETF:QO, severe				+++	+++	+++[8]	Congenital anomalies, renal dysplasia, dysmorphism	231680 130410 231675
ETF or ETF:QO, mild		+	+/–	+++	+++	+++[9]		231680 130410 231675
Riboflavin responsive	–	+++		+++	+	+++	Leukodystrophy	–

[1] myoglobinuria; [2] Reye-like episodes; [3] Online MIM database (OMIM™): http://www3.ncbi.nlm.nih.gov/omim/; [4] ventricular arrhythmias in most cases; [5] includes cases previously reported as defects of the long-chain acyl-CoA dehydrogenase; [6] ketotic hypoglycaemia; [7] urinary excretion of the unusual carnitine ester decadienoylcarnitine; [8] glutaric acidaemia type II; [9] adipic and ethylmalonic acidaemia.

Table 1. Main clinical features of fatty-acid β-oxidation disorders.

The carnitine-dependent transport of LCFA across the mitochondrial membrane and the intramitochondrial β-oxidation cycle are outlined in Figure 1. Once in the mitochondria, FAs are eventually oxidized by repeated cycles of 4 sequential reactions: acyl-CoA dehydrogenation, 2-enoyl-CoA hydration, L-3-hydroxy-acyl-CoA dehydrogenation, and 3-ketoacyl-CoA thiolysis. The final step of each cycle in the β-oxidation spiral is the release of 2 molecules of acetyl-CoA and a fatty acyl-CoA, which is 2 carbon atoms shorter. Each reaction is catalyzed by multiple enzymes which exhibit partially overlapping chain-length specificity (24). Thus, 4 distinct FAD-dependent acyl-CoA dehydrogenases have been identified with specificity for very-long-, long-, medium-, and short-chain acyl-CoAs. Similarly, there are two 2-enoyl-CoA hydratases, two NAD+-dependent L-3-hydroxy-acyl-CoA dehydrogenases and two 3-ketoa-cyl-CoA thiolases with specificity for long- and short-chain acyl-CoAs. Evidence for the presence of a medium-chain 3-ketoacyl-CoA thiolase has also been reported (23). Therefore, complete catabolism of long-chain acyl-CoAs in mitochondria is accomplished by the action of 2 distinct, albeit coordinated, β-oxidation systems, as outlined in Figure 1 (41).

One system is located on the mitochondrial inner membrane and is specifically involved in the oxidation of LCFA. The other system is composed of soluble enzymes that are located in the mitochondrial matrix and is responsible for the β-oxidation of medium- and short-chain acyl-CoAs. Finally, mitochondrial FA β-oxidation is tightly coupled to both the tricarboxylic acid (TCA) cycle and the respiratory chain. Thus, while acetyl-CoA released can enter the TCA cycle, the electrons are transferred to the respiratory chain. The electrons of the FAD-dependent acyl-CoA dehydrogenases are transferred from FADH$_2$ to coenzyme Q through 2 flavoproteins of the mitochondrial inner membrane, the electron transferring flavoprotein (ETF) and the ETF:coenzyme-Q oxidoreductase (ETF:QO). The NAD+-dependent L-3-hydroxy-acyl-CoA dehydrogenases transfer their electrons from NADH to complex I of the respiratory chain.

Impairment of LCFA transport across the mitochondrial membrane or a defect in the β-oxidation pathway makes FA unavailable for use by the mitochondria. In skeletal muscle, this can result in 2 main phenotypes (9): a chronic myopathy and an acute muscle disorder characterized by rhabdomyolysis with paroxysmal myoglobinuria. In these latter cases, the vulnerability of muscle to the metabolic block may depend on the activity. When affected patients exercise for a prolonged period, glycogen store may be exhausted

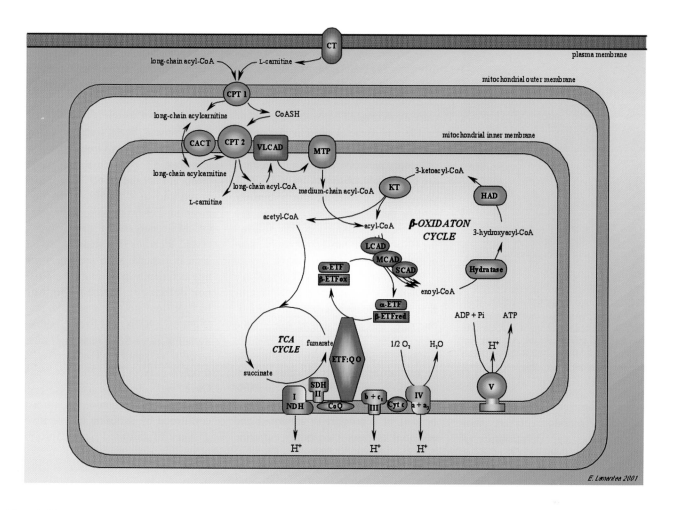

Figure 1. *Schematic representation of the functional and physical organization of FA β-oxidation enzymes in mitochondria. CT,* plasma membrane high-affinity sodium-dependent carnitine transporter (OCTN2); *CPT1,* carnitine palmitoyltransferase 1; *CACT,* carnitine/acylcarnitine translocase; *CPT2,* carnitine palmitoyltransferase 2; *VLCAD, LCAD, MCAD, SCAD,* very-long-, long-, medium-, and short-chain acyl-CoA dehydrogenase, respectively; *MTP,* mitochondrial trifunctional protein; *Hydratase,* 2-enoyl-CoA hydratase; *HAD,* L-3-hydroxyacyl-CoA dehydrogenase; *KT,* 3-ketoacyl-CoA thiolase; *ETF,* electron transfer flavoprotein (*ox,* oxidized; *red,* reduced); *ETF:QO,* ETF:coenzyme Q oxidoreductase; *I,* respiratory chain complex I (*NDH,* NADH:coenzyme Q reductase; *II,* respiratory chain complex II (*SDH,* succinate dehydrogenase); *CoQ,* coenzyme Q; *III,* respiratory chain complex III (*b,* cytochrome *b; c$_1$,* cytochrome *c$_1$*); *Cyt c,* cytochrome *c; IV,* respiratory chain complex IV (cytochrome *c* oxidase) (*a,* cytochrome *a; a$_3$,* cytochrome *a$_3$*); *V,* respiratory chain complex V (ATP synthase). Enzymes which use FAD as a coenzyme are indicated in red colour.

and rhabdomyolysis may occur. Fasting worsens the situation because it reduces the availability of both muscle glycogen and blood glucose, further increasing the dependence of muscle on FA metabolism. In some cases, reduced hepatic production of ketone bodies deprives muscle of another alternative fuel. Diversion of nonoxidized fatty acyl-CoA to triacylglycerol synthesis can explain the formation of lipid vacuoles observed in skeletal muscle of patients presenting with chronic myopathy. The lipid accumulation usually correlates with the oxidative capacity of muscle fibres: it is most marked in type-1 fibres, less marked in

type-2A fibres, and least conspicuous in type-2B fibres (9).

Possible pathogenetic mechanisms for the development of cardiomyopathy in some patients with LCFA oxidation defects include both inadequate energy supply in the heart and myocardial damage and arrhythmogenesis due to the toxic effects of elevated intracellular concentration of acylcarnitines. Long-chain acylcarnitines, which are known to cause myocardial injury and rhythm disturbances during myocardial ischaemia and infarction, are thought to promote arrhythmogenesis via direct activation of Ca^{2+} channels (36).

Clinical phenotypes. The primary presentations of neuromuscular disease in the newborn period are hypotonia and weakness. Although metabolic myopathies are inherited disorders that present from birth and may present with subtle to marked neonatal hypotonia, a number of these defects are diagnosed during childhood, adolescence, or adulthood. Disorders of lipid mitochondrial metabolism may cause 2 main clinical syndromes in muscle, namely, *i*) progressive weakness with hypotonia, eg, carnitine transporter and carnitine/acylcarnitine translocase defects, or *ii*) acute, recurrent, reversible muscle dysfunction with

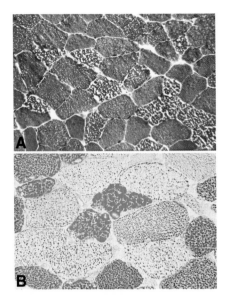

Figure 2. *Lipid storage myopathy in a patient with primary carnitine deficiency* (PCD) *caused by a defect of the high-affinity carnitine transporter (CT).* **A.** *Gomori's modified trichrome staining showing numerous vacuoles mostly in type-1 fibres.* ×160. **B.** *Oil Red O stain showing numerous large (red) lipid droplets within fibres.* ×250.

exercise intolerance and acute muscle breakdown (rhabdomyolysis) with myoglobinuria, eg, deficiencies of CPT2, very-long-chain acyl-CoA dehydrogenase, or trifunctional protein. Notably, some defects may cause both phenotypes, eg, very-long-chain acyl-CoA dehydrogenase, or trifunctional protein deficiencies.

A total of 14 distinct defects, all autosomal recessive, have been identified that involve almost all of the possible enzyme steps in the pathway (Table 1) (8, 36, 41, 51). With the exception of medium-chain acyl-CoA dehydrogenase (MCAD) deficiency, which has a frequency as high as 1 in 10 000 births in Caucasian populations of Northern European origin (36), diagnosis and management of these disorders remain uncommon and the prevalence rate of most of them is unknown.

Overall, the clinical syndromes associated with FA oxidation disorders are the consequence of the failure of FA oxidizing tissues to respond to increased energy demands. The main clinical features of FA oxidation disorders are illustrated in Table 1. Symptomatic hypoglycaemia, characteristically associated with impaired ketogene-sis, is often the earliest clinical manifestation of a defect of FA oxidation and can be observed in nearly all the disorders (41). Because of the dependence of heart and skeletal muscle upon LCFA oxidation, cardiomyopathy, typically hypertrophic but sometimes dilated (3) and skeletal muscle myopathy, either chronic (lipid storage myopathy) or acute (paroxysmal myoglobinuria), are commonly observed in LCFA oxidation defects while they are extremely rare in the disorders of medium- and short-chain FA oxidation. The following disorders are most commonly associated with muscle dysfunction:

Carnitine transporter deficiency (primary carnitine deficiency). L-carnitine (β-hydroxy-g-N-trimethylamino-butyrate) has an essential role in the transport of LCFA into mitochondria for β-oxidation. Although carnitine can be synthesized in liver and kidney, normal adults obtain >75% of carnitine from the diet. Carnitine deficiency can be part of a number of inherited and acquired diseases (secondary carnitine deficiencies) (9, 34, 36).

Primary carnitine deficiency (PCD) is an autosomal recessive disorder characterized by increased losses of carnitine in the urine and decreased concentration (usually less than 5% of normal) in plasma, heart, and skeletal muscle caused by a defect of the high-affinity (K$_m$=5µM) plasma membrane sodium-dependent carnitine transporter (CT, OCTN2) (10, 34).

Two major clinical presentations are associated with CT deficiency (36). The most common phenotype is characterized by slowly progressive hypertrophic or dilated cardiomyopathy with lipid myopathy, which may occur between 1 and 7 years of age. Myopathy is the presenting symptom in a few patients. A second phenotype is characterized by acute recurrent episodes of hypoglycaemic encephalopathy with hypoketonaemia usually with onset between 3 months and 2.5 years of age. These 2 phenotypes cannot be considered mutually exclusive; however, as in some families both an acute metabolic and cardiomuscular presentations have been described.

Differential diagnosis of CT deficiency (PCD) obviously includes secondary carnitine deficiency. In PCD, there is a generalized reduction of carnitine content which is low both in tissues (muscle, heart, liver) and in plasma. Plasma total and free carnitines are less than 5% of normal, but carnitine esters are not increased. Total carnitine is reduced to 1 to 5% of the normal mean in skeletal muscle and heart (15). GC-MS analysis of urine does not reveal dicarboxylic aciduria, which is seen in patients with secondary carnitine deficiency due to fatty-acid oxidation defects (9). Morphologic features include lipid storage in skeletal muscle (Figure 2), heart, and liver. Lipid accumulation in skeletal muscle is characterized by small and numerous lipid droplets in type-1 muscle fibres (9, 10). Once suspected, the defect of plasmalemmal CT should be ultimately confirmed by carnitine uptake investigations in cultured skin fibroblasts (15).

PCD patients respond well to high-dose oral L-carnitine supplementation (usually 100-200 mg/kg per day) (15, 36). Carnitine supplementation restores plasma and liver carnitine levels to normal, whereas muscle carnitine levels remain low (9). Nevertheless, patients gradually recover muscle strength and heart function progressively returns to normal, hence cardiokinetic therapy can be discontinued (36). Also, attacks of hypoglycaemia tend to disappear (15, 36).

Carnitine palmitoyltransferase 2 deficiency. A number of fundamental biochemical and molecular studies have established that the carnitine palmitoyltransferase (CPT) system is composed of 2 distinct acyltransferases, CPT1 located on the inner side of the outer mitochondrial membrane, and CPT2 located on the inner side of the inner mitochondrial membrane (25). Deficiencies of CPT1 and CPT2 have been extensively reviewed (6, 40). Cardiomuscular involvement is extremely rare in CPT1 deficiency, which makes this defect unique among the disorders of LCFA oxidation (Table 1) and can now be explained by the existence of at least 2 tissue-specific isoforms of CPT1 (6, 25) one expressed in liver and fibroblasts (L-CPT1, CPT1A), which would be mutated in patients (21), and another in skeletal muscle and heart (M-CPT1, CPT1B).

Deficiency of CPT2 has been the first FA oxidation defect to be described (11). Three different clinical phenotypes are associated with a defect of CPT2: a myopathic form with juvenile-adult onset, an infantile form with hepatic, muscular, and cardiac involvement, and a lethal neonatal form with developmental abnormalities. In all cases, the enzyme defect can be demonstrated in every tissue examined, eg, skeletal muscle, liver, fibroblasts, platelets and leukocytes.

The most frequent clinical phenotype is commonly referred to as the "muscular" form of CPT deficiency. It is the most frequent disorder of lipid muscle metabolism, one of the most common inherited disorders of mitochondrial FA oxidation (33), and a major cause of hereditary recurrent myoglobinuria in both children and young adults (44). Since the first description in 1973 (11), more than 150 patients suffering from recurrent attacks of aching muscle pain, stiffness, rhabdomyolysis, and myoglobinuria have been reported (6, 54). Muscular CPT2 deficiency can therefore be considered a prototypic disorder for the group of fatty-acid oxidation defects manifesting with paroxysmal myoglobinuria. In approximately 80% of cases, the age of onset is comprised between 6 and 20 years. The first episode usually does not occur until late childhood or adolescence. Among patients with the most typical presentation, ie, exercise-induced myoglobinuria in adults, there is a 5.5:1 predominance of males over females. In general, it seems that affected women or girls have milder symptoms, such as exercise- or fever-induced myalgia with no pigmenturia (40).

The clinical hallmark of the disease is paroxysmal myoglobinuria. Attacks of myoglobinuria are most often precipitated by prolonged exercise, type-1 (exertional) myoglobinuria in the classification by Tein et al (44). Unlike patients with glycolytic defects, patients with CPT2 deficiency do not show reduced tolerance to brief strenuous exercise, do not experience a "second-wind" phenomenon (switch to utilization of fatty acids), and may not feel premonitory symptoms. In a smaller group of patients, mostly children, infection, usually of viral etiology, and/or fever and leucocytosis are the primary precipitating factors, type-2 (toxic) myoglobinuria according to Tein et al (44). Prolonged fasting is also an important precipitant in both exertional and toxic cases. Lesser triggering factors for both groups include cold and emotional stress. In approximately 20% of cases, attacks may occur without any apparent cause. True cramps are not a feature of CPT2 deficiency. Patients describe instead a feeling of "tightness" and pain in exercising limb or trunk muscles before the appearance of myoglobinuria and weakness. Persistent weakness is very uncommon (54). Malignant hyperthermia induced by general anesthesia or postoperative myoglobinuria were the first manifestation of the disease in 3 cases (50).

The "muscular" form of CPT2 deficiency is usually a benign disease with a favourable evolution, provided that acute renal insufficiency, a potential complication of massive myoglobinuria, is adequately managed. There are usually no clinical signs of liver dysfunction. Fasting hypoglycaemia is never observed. Hypertriglyceridemia is noted in approximately 20% of patients. Cardiac involvement is very unusual. In the rare "non-classic" cases, CPT2 deficiency can manifest as a severe life-threatening infantile hepatocardiomuscular form (CPT2 deficiency type 2) or a fatal neonatal-onset form (CPT2 deficiency type 3) (6, 8, 41). The infantile form (approximately ten patients reported) is characterized by hypoketotic hypoglycaemia, liver failure, cardiomyopathy, and mild signs of muscle involvement (7, 41, 43). The disease is often fatal before 1 year of age. In addition to these symptoms, features of brain and kidney dysgenesis are frequently observed in the neonatal-onset variant (41). This form is usually lethal during the first month of life (8).

The striking discrepancy among these different clinical presentations of a single enzymatic defect has not yet received any conclusive explanation. However, Bonnefont et al (7) have shown that a correlation may exist between residual LCFA oxidation rates and phenotypic presentation of CPT2 deficiency and that CPT2 activity has to be reduced below a critical threshold in order for LCFA oxidation to be impaired. In the classic form, outside episodes of myoglobinuria and at rest, serum CK level is normal. During acute episodes of rhabdomyolysis, laboratory findings are dominated by elevated urinary excretion of myoglobin ($\geqslant$200 ng/mL) and a great increase in serum CK (20-400 fold), attributable to the CK-MM isoenzyme. Prolonged fasting or mild exercise may also provoke an increase in serum CK, albeit to a lesser degree (2- to 20-fold above normal). Other serum enzymes may increase during attacks including aldolase, aspartate and alanine aminotransferases, and lactate dehydrogenase. There is no hypoglycaemia, and ketonaemia and ketonuria are appropriate. Serum and muscle carnitine levels are usually normal. Urinary organic acid profile is also normal. Acute tubular necrosis, a life-threatening condition, may develop in patients excreting more than 1000 ng/mL of myoglobin. Following attacks, serum CK levels usually return to normal by 8 to 10 weeks. Between attacks, routine laboratory tests are not contributive to the diagnosis. Prolonged fasting at rest may result in delayed and reduced ketone body production and/or increased serum CK. Challenge with long-chain triglycerides may also demonstrate delayed or mildly insufficient ketogenesis. ECG is normal and EMG is usually described as generical-

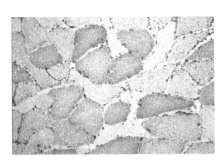

Figure 3. *VLCAD deficiency in a young woman with recurrent paroxysmal myoglobinuria and interictal chronic proximal myopathy. Oil Red O stain shows signs of mild lipid accumulation with numerous fine droplets within most fibres. Lipid droplets exhibit a subsarcolemmal distribution. ×250.*

ly "myopathic." In most cases, muscle biopsies in interictal periods are normal or may show mild signs of muscle involvement with regenerating fibres.

Irrespective of the clinical presentation, diagnosis is ultimately made by demonstrating the enzyme defect in the patients' tissue(s). Widely different results have been obtained on CPT2 levels in normal and diseased tissues, mostly because of the use of different assay conditions for measuring CPT activity. In addition, in most reported cases, the assays used did not discriminate between CPT1 and CPT2 activities. Optimal results are obtained by using the "backward assay" (43) in the presence of 1% octyl glucoside, a strong detergent which fully releases active CP2 but causes complete loss of CPT1 activity (25). Despite the predominant muscular symptomatology, the enzyme defect is expressed in tissues other than skeletal muscle and can thus be detected in fibroblasts, leukocytes, platelets, and liver (54). In a cohort of more than 50 CPT2-deficient patients biochemically evaluated in our laboratory at the Istituto Nazionale Neurologico "C. Besta," Milan, Italy, the magnitude of CPT2 residual activity in peripheral blood leukocytes was found to be similar to that observed in skeletal muscle (approximately 12% and 7%, respectively, when expressed as CPT2-to-citrate-synthase ratio). The enzyme defect was also evident in cultured fibroblasts, albeit with higher residual activity (approximately 25%). Thus, our experience indicates that

muscle biopsy is necessary in virtually none of the cases and the diagnosis can be confidently made by determining CPT2 activity in either fresh or frozen isolated leukocytes.

Effective prevention of attacks may be accomplished by instituting a high-carbohydrate, low-fat diet with frequent and regularly scheduled meals, by avoiding the known precipitating factors (fasting, cold, prolonged exercise), and by increasing slow-release carbohydrate intake during intercurrent illness or sustained exercise (6, 40). Medium-chain triglyceride supplements may be given although their usefulness is questioned (35). Since carnitine is usually normal in this form of the disease, there is no indication for L-carnitine supplementation. Experience in treating the early-onset severe form of CPT2 deficiency is very limited. It seems, however, that restriction of dietary long-chain fat is of primary importance because of the toxic effects of long-chain acylcarnitines, which accumulate in consequence of the metabolic block. As in the classic muscular form, the mainstay of therapy is avoidance of fasting. In general, during period of wellness, patients should be given a diet high in carbohydrate (33, 51).

Very-long-chain acyl-CoA dehydrogenase deficiency. Deficiency of long-chain acyl-CoA dehydrogenation was first described in 1985 and attributed to a defect of the matrical enzyme long-chain acyl-CoA dehydrogenase (LCAD) (41). Following the discovery of VLCAD in 1992, it became clear that the patients originally thought to suffer from LCAD deficiency had, in fact, VLCAD deficiency (51). Since the first reports in 1993, more than 60 VLCAD-deficient patients have been described (1).

The disease is clinically heterogeneous and can be divided into 3 major disease phenotypes: *i)* a form resembling the muscular form of CPT2 deficiency with isolated skeletal muscle involvement, rhabdomyolysis, and myoglobinuria, usually triggered by exercise or fasting; *ii)* a severe child-

hood form, with early onset, dilated or hypertrophic cardiomyopathy, recurrent episodes of hypoketotic hypoglycaemia and a high rate of mortality (50-75%); and *iii)* a milder childhood form, with later onset, usually with hypoketotic hypoglycaemia and dicarboxylic aciduria as the main presenting feature, low mortality and rare cardiomyopathy. Most patients suffer from the severe cardiomyopathic form with early onset and poor outcome. Overall, however, acute metabolic decompensation is the most frequent form of presentation in VLCAD-deficient patients. In several patients, sudden death or severe cardiomyopathy occurred in the first few days of life (1). Isolated recurrent myoglobinuria has been reported in more than 10 patients (1, 26, 30, 37). In these patients the age at onset was older than in patients presenting with acute metabolic decompensation, ranging from 7 to 40 years of age. The episodes were generally precipitated by fasting, exercise, or infections. Except for one case (1), no signs of myopathy were present when the patients overcame the crises. Overall, the leading symptoms resemble the complaints of adult males with CPT2 deficiency, but the myalgia appears to be much more severe and the episodes more numerous and more easily triggered. The diagnosis of VLCAD deficiency in an adult is difficult. Serum CK markedly increases during attacks (20 to >200 fold). However, patients do not exhibit hypoketotic hypoglycaemia nor dicarboxylic aciduria. Elevated $C_{14:1}$ and $C_{14:2}$ plasma acylcarnitines were evident in only one patient, indicating the existence of a defect of LCFA oxidation (37). Available data indicate that the study of plasma LCFA profile by gas chromatograhy-mass spectrometry can be helpful for diagnosis because it may reveal an increase of tetradecenoic ($C_{14:1}$) acid, which persists even after the patient has fully recovered (26, 30). As in CPT2 deficiency, muscle biopsy may not provide any clue to the diagnosis. It may show mild nonspecific morphological alterations with no evidence of lipid accumulation or may demonstrate a diffuse increase of fat droplets mostly in type-1 fibres (26, 30) (Figure 3).

The diagnosis of VLCAD deficiency is ultimately based on the demonstration of reduced palmitoyl-CoA ($C_{16:0}$) dehydrogenation in skeletal muscle or cultured fibroblasts. Residual VLCAD activity in patients with the adult form may range between 15% and 35% of control values. Overall, enzyme studies have not shown any correlation with the different phenotypes while immunoreactive VLCAD protein was barely detectable in all the patients studied (26, 30).

In general, reported patients have been treated with a dietary regimen consisting of avoidance of fasting and a high-carbohydrate, low-fat diet with or without supplementation with medium-chain triglyceride oil, riboflavin, or L-carnitine. This therapy has proved effective in reducing the recurrence of crises and reverting the heart and skeletal muscle involvement in most patients (26, 30).

Mitochondrial trifunctional protein deficiency. MTP deficiency is one of the latest addition to the list of mitochondrial FA oxidation disorders. The enzyme is a heterooctamer of 4 α-subunits, harbouring long-chain 2-enoyl-CoA hydratase (LCEH) and long-chain L-3-hydroxyacyl-CoA de-hydrogenase (LCHAD) activities, and 4 β-subunits harbouring long-chain 3-ketoacyl-CoA thiolase (LCKT) activity. The disease is relatively frequent among FA oxidation disorders, with more than 60 patients reported thus far (47, 51). The clinical manifestations of the disease are characteristically associated with urinary excretion of C_6–C_{14} 3-hydroxydicarboxylic acids. Before the discovery of MTP in 1992, previous cases were reported as LCHAD deficiency (51). Indeed, patients can now be classified into 2 groups (47, 51).

1. Long-chain 3-hydroxyacyl-CoA dehydrogenase deficiency. The vast majority (≥85%) of MTP-deficient patients has an isolated deficiency of LCHAD activity with relative preservation of LCEH and LCKT activities

and nearly normal amounts of both α- and β-subunits (51). The disease is clinically heterogeneous (47). In infancy and early childhood, hypoglycaemic encephalopathy with or without severe hepatic involvement is the most common form of onset. Other manifestations include chronic myopathy, paroxysmal myoglobinuria, and cardiomyopathy. Mortality is high (≈50%), the main cause of death being cardiac decompensation during a metabolic attack. However, cardiomyopathy in patients who survive acute episodes tends to resolve with dietary therapeutic measures (low-fat/high-carbohydrate diet associated with medium-chain triglyceride oil supplementation) (47). Later in childhood, more predominant manifestations are episodes of rhabdomyolysis with muscle pain and weakness. Among the distinctive features of LCHAD deficiency are the occurrence of progressive pigmentary retinopathy, which appears to be related to the duration of the disease (47), and peripheral neuropathy in surviving patients. Also characteristic in this disorder is the occurrence of pregnancy complications such as HELLP (hemolysis, elevated liver enzymes, and low platelets) and AFLP (acute fatty liver of pregnancy) syndromes in pregnant women with an affected fetus (47).

2. MTP deficiency (combined enzyme deficiency). In a smaller group (group 2) of patients, all the activities harboured by MTP are deficient, albeit to different extents, and both α- and β-subunits are hardly detectable by immunoblot (51). In the relatively few patients with verified MTP deficiency, the clinical manifestations of the disease are similar to those observed in patients with isolated LCHAD deficiency, although in general the clinical presentation of MTP-deficient patients is more severe with a higher mortality rate (51). However, in very few cases, a benign late-onset neuromuscular phenotype has been described, characterized by recurrent episodes of exercise-induced rhabdomyolysis (47). The presentation closely resembled the adult form of CPT2 deficiency except

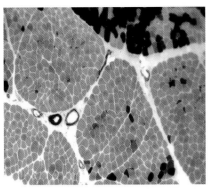

Figure 4. *MTP deficiency.* Muscle biopsy of a 3-year-old child harbouring a mutation in exon 9 of the MTP α-subunit gene *HADHA* (C. Dionisi Vici, E. Bertini, and F. Taroni, submitted manuscript) and presenting with recurrent myoglobinuria and peripheral axonal neuropathy. Staining for ATPase (pH 4.6) shows a clear neurogenic pattern of denervation-reinnervation with type grouping of type-1 (dark) and type-2 (light) fibres. A fascicle with a small group of atrophic type-1 fibres can be observed in the lower part of the figure. ×20 (courtesy of Dr. Enrico Bertini, Rome, Italy)

that the patients had an associated peripheral neuropathy. The occurrence of peripheral sensory-motor polyneuropathy appears to be a distinctive feature of both LCHAD and MTP deficiency, because it has not been reported in patients with any other β-oxidation defect. To date, approximately 10 MTP-deficient patients with sensory-motor polyneuropathy have been reported (47). The neuropathy has been axonal, with sensory predominance in all reported patients. Pathological studies of peripheral nerve have shown signs of both axonal neuropathy and demyelination, with axonal degeneration being predominant on segmental demyelination (5). Unusual among FA oxidation disorders, muscle biopsy may show significant neurogenic features (Figure 4) which correlate with the peripheral nerve involvement. At present, the pathogenesis of MTP-associated neuropathy remains unclarified. A direct nerve toxicity of long-chain 3-hydroxy FA intermediates has been proposed (20). More recently, deficiency of docosahexaenoic acid (DHA), an essential n-3 polyunsaturated FA necessary for nerve myelination, has been documented in MTP-deficient patients, while encouraging response to cod liver oil extract, high in DHA content, has been observed (45).

Riboflavin-responsive multiple acyl-CoA dehydrogenase deficiency. Riboflavin (vitamin B_2) is the water soluble precursor of 2 flavin coenzymes: flavin mononucleotide (FMN) and flavin adenine dinucleotide (FAD). These 2 compounds are essential cofactors in various electron transfer reactions that occur in energy-producing, biosynthetic, detoxifying and electron-scavenging pathways. Riboflavin cannot be synthesized in mammals, which are therefore entirely dependent on the dietary supply. In mitochondria, several flavoproteins play a crucial role in the catabolism of fatty acids, carbohydrates (pyruvate), and amino acids, including the straight-chain acyl-CoA dehydrogenases of the β-oxidation system (SCAD, MCAD, LCAD and VLCAD), the electron transfer flavoprotein (ETF) and its dehydrogenase (ETF:QO), and a number of other dehydrogenases (14).

Riboflavin-responsive multiple acyl-CoA dehydrogenase deficiency, also known as riboflavin-responsive glutaric aciduria type 2, is a genetic metabolic disorder characterized by impaired oxidation of fatty acids due to multiple deficiencies of SCAD, MCAD, LCAD and VLCAD. Two major clinical phenotypes can be observed. An "infantile form" with nonketotic hypoglycaemia, hypotonia, failure to thrive, and acute metabolic episodes reminiscent of Reye's syndrome or MCAD deficiency, and a "juvenile form" characterized by progressive proximal myopathy with lipid storage in type-1 and type-2 muscle fibres (2, 9). There is usually an abnormal urinary excretion of organic acids which is compatible with glutaric aciduria type 2 or ethylmalonic-adipic aciduria (9). Carnitine content in plasma and tissues is variably reduced. Before treatment, all patients show an impairment of muscle fatty-acid oxidation. The reduction is more severe with short- and medium-chain substrates than with long-chain substrates. Culture in riboflavin-depleted medium is necessary to demonstrate the defect in fibroblasts (31). Activities of SCAD, MCAD and (V)LCAD were found to be reduced in isolated muscle mitochondria, with SCAD and MCAD activities being affected to a greater extent (2, 49). Not only are SCAD and MCAD activities severely impaired, but also their protein mass is markedly reduced, as demonstrated by Western blot analysis (2, 49). In 4 adult patients, we have also observed a reduction of VLCAD activity to less than 20% of the control mean (14). ETF and ETF:QO activities appear not to be affected, while reductions of respiratory chain complexes I and II activities have been reported (2, 49).

The clinical, morphological, biochemical, and physiological responses to oral riboflavin supplementation (100-300 mg/day oral riboflavin) are usually dramatic (2, 49), with rapid improvement of muscle weakness and wasting and disappearance of signs of lipid accumulation at muscle biopsy. Riboflavin supplementation also normalizes the activities of SCAD and MCAD, and restores to normal the amount of protein mass.

Other disorders of FA β-oxidation. In addition to CPT1 deficiency, characteristically not associated with myopathy or cardiomyopathy, a number of defects of mitochondrial FA oxidation exist, in which skeletal and cardiac muscle involvement, if any, does not dominate the clinical picture.

1. Carnitine/acylcarnitine translocase deficiency. With carnitine transporter and CPT deficiencies, it belongs to the group of the defects of long-chain fatty-acid transport across the mitochondrial membrane. It seems not to be very rare, as it has been observed in more than 20 patients since the first description in 1992 (36). In most cases, patients present with a life-threatening episode in the neonatal period, characterized by neonatal distress with hyperammonaemia, inconstant hypoglycaemia, heart beat disorders, and early muscle involvement with weakness and high serum CK (8, 36). The disease is often fatal within the first 2 years of life because of the deleterious consequences of long-chain acylcarnitine accumulation, which may cause untreatable episodes of heart beat disorder. The human CACT gene has recently been cloned (19). The transcript is 1.2 kb in length and encodes a 301-amino acid protein composed of 6 transmembrane α-helices. The gene is located on chromosome 3p21.31. The molecular defect has now been identified in several patients (19, 22).

2. Deficiency of medium-chain acyl-CoA dehydrogenase. This is the most common FA oxidation disorder with a prevalent mutation (G^{985}) being found in ≥97% of patients (36). Unlike the defects of LCFA oxidation, skeletal muscle and heart involvement is extremely rare in MCAD deficiency. Ruitenbeek et al described a patient carrying the common mutation who presented late in life with rhabdomyolysis and acute encephalopathy after strenuous exercise (32).

3. Short-chain acyl-CoA dehydrogenase deficiency. This is a rare disorder whose clinical manifestations are uncharacteristic of FA oxidation defects. In fact, the disease presents with neurological abnormalities (hypotonia, hypertonia and seizures) which are not usually found in FA oxidation defects. Furthermore, hypoglycaemia is never observed. A thorough investigation has been reported in few SCAD-deficient patients. Interestingly, a significant association has been observed between a polymorphic SCAD amino acid variant (Gly209Ser) and elevated excretion of ethylmalonic acid (41).

4. Medium-chain 3-ketoacyl-CoA thiolase deficiency. This is one of the latest additions to the list of disorders of mitochondrial FA oxidation. So far, only one case has been described (23), a neonate who presented at 3 days with vomiting, dehydration, metabolic acidosis, and liver dysfunction, and had died after ten days of terminal rhabdomyolysis and myoglobinuria. Biochemical investigations revealed a deficiency of a single enzyme, MCKAT, not previously associated with a metabolic disorder. No lipid accumulation was found in skeletal muscle. No information is yet available on the molecular bases of the disorder.

5. *Short-chain L-3-hydroxyacyl-CoA dehydrogenase deficiency.* Thus far, this has been reported in only 2 patients. There is no muscular involvement and the disease appears to be biochemically and clinically distinct from the other FA oxidation disorders in that it manifests with recurrent episodes of fasting-induced vomiting associated with "ketosis," with or without hypoglycaemia (41).

Molecular genetics and pathogenesis

Almost all of the genes encoding the enzymes involved in mitochondrial FA catabolism have been identified and characterized. In most of the related disorders, the molecular defect has also been delineated.

Carnitine transporter deficiency (primary carnitine deficiency). During the past 2 years, there have been major advances in the molecular characterization of the carnitine transporter. In 1998, the gene encoding OCTN2, a novel organic cation transporter, was identified as a high-affinity sodium-dependent carnitine transporter in humans (39). The OCTN2 cDNA codes for a 557-amino acid protein with 12 transmembrane domains and a predicted molecular mass of approximately 63 kiloDalton (kDa). The corresponding gene, *SLC22A5*, solute carrier family 22 (organic cation transporter), member 5, is composed of 10 exons and is located on chromosome 5q31.1. This locus is syntenic to the murine "*jvs*" (juvenile visceral steatosis) model locus on chromosome 11. OCTN2 is strongly expressed in kidney, skeletal muscle, heart, and placenta (39).

Nezu et al identified 4 mutations in the *SLC22A5* gene in 3 families with the carnitine uptake defect (27). A number of other mutations have been reported since which abolish or severely impair carnitine transport when expressed in heterologous cells (52). Most of the mutations were nonsense mutations associated with no residual

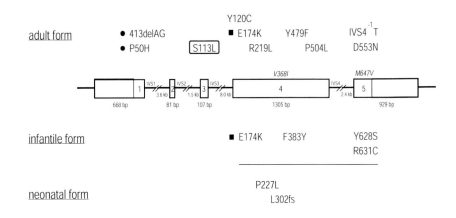

Figure 5. CPT2 gene structure and mutations. The gene is composed of 5 coding exons (48). The dashed boxes in exon 1 and 5 indicate the 5′ and 3′ untranslated regions, respectively. The boxed mutation is the common Ser113Leu substitution which accounts for ≥50% of mutant alleles in the classical adult form of the disease (42). Bullets indicate the two recurrent mutations Pro50His and 413delAG. Squares indicate the Glu174Lys mutation associated with both the adult and the infantile forms of the disease. Two common polymorphisms are indicated in italics.

carnitine transport activity. In a very few cases, "leaky" missense mutations have been identified, which retain residual carnitine transport activity (52). However, there is a clear lack of genotype-phenotype correlation (52). In addition, all types of presentation (metabolic, cardiomyopathic, and myopathic) were observed in the 2 groups. Homozygosity for the same null allele (R282X) was identified in 2 unrelated patients; one presenting with acute metabolic decompensation and one with cardiomyopathy, indicating that the same primary genetic defects may be associated with different phenotypic expression (52).

Carnitine palmitoyltransferase 2 deficiency. Two distinct genes for the liver- and the muscle-type of human CPT1 have been identified. The liver CPT1 gene (L-CPT1, *CPT1A*) is located on chromosome 11q13.1 while the muscle CPT1 gene (M-CPT1, *CPT1B*) is located on chromosome 22q13.33. Mutations in the liver-specific gene *CPT1A* have been reported in 2 patients only (6, 21).

The human CPT2 gene has been identified and characterized (13, 48). It is located on chromosome 1p32 (16) and is composed of 5 exons which encode a transcript of 1.3 kb (Figure 5). Approximately 20 CPT2 gene mutations have been identified (6). Most of

the mutations are "private." However, a prevalent mutation (Ser113Leu) can be identified in ≥50% of mutant alleles of patients of different ethnic origins with the muscular form of CPT2 deficiency (18, 42). Other 2 mutations were found to recur, albeit with a lesser frequency, in myopathic CPT2-deficient patients, the missense mutation Pro50His (38, 48) and the frameshift mutation 413delAG (38). This latter mutation was the second most common mutation identified (20% of mutant alleles) in the group of 59 patients investigated by Taggart et al (38) and all individuals with the mutation were of Ashkenazi Jewish ancestry, suggesting a defined ethnic origin for the mutation. Currently, mutations can be detected in approximately 90% of patients with muscular CPT2 deficiency. With the exception of the 413delAG frameshift mutation, the mutations identified both in myopathic patients (48, 53) and in infants with the hepatocardiomuscular presentation (7, 43, 53) do not completely abolish enzyme activity. By contrast, null mutations have been found in patients with the lethal neonatal-onset form (40). Mutation analysis of CPT2 defects has given some clues for a genotype-phenotype correlation. All mutations reported so far in the homozygous state are strongly associated with a given phenotype, either muscular (Pro50His, Ser113Leu,

Glu174Lys) or generalized (Phe383Tyr, Tyr628Ser, Arg631Cys) (7, 42, 48, 53). Compound heterozygotes between one adult-type mutation and one infantile-type mutation seem at risk for severe episodes: one patient (Glu174Lys/Phe383Tyr) had a severe hepatic presentation ((53), another patient (Ser113Leu/Tyr628Ser) has been reported with a muscular presentation at 6 years who experienced a cardiac arrest (46).

Very-long-chain acyl-CoA dehydrogenase deficiency. VLCAD catalyzes > 90% of palmitoyl-CoA (C_{16}) dehydrogenation in human liver, heart, skeletal muscle, and skin fibroblasts, and is thought to be a rate-limiting enzyme in the LCFA β-oxidation system (51). Unlike the other matrical homotetrameric acyl-CoA dehydrogenases, it is a mitochondrial membrane-bound homodimer with subunit size of approximately 66.5 kDa. The gene (*ACADVL*), which spans ≈ 5.4 kilobases of genomic DNA, has been mapped to chromosome 17p13 (1). More than 60 disease-causing mutation have been identified, but unlike other disorders of FA β-oxidation such as CPT2 and MCAD deficiency, no prevalent mutation was found (1). One splice site mutation seems to be rather common among Italian VLCAD-deficient patients (30). Overall, however, genetic heterogeneity in VLCAD deficiency is large, thus hampering DNA-based diagnosis for this disease. In a molecular survey on 55 unrelated patients, Andresen et al (1) have identified 58 different mutations. They have also shown a clear relationship between the nature of the mutation and the severity of disease. Patients with the severe childhood phenotype have mutations that result in no residual enzyme activity, whereas patients with the milder childhood and adult phenotypes have mutations that may result in residual enzyme activity.

Mitochondrial trifunctional protein deficiency. Both the gene for the α-subunit (*HADHA*) and the gene for the β-subunit (*HADHB*) map to the same region of chromosome 2p23. Since the distance between the 2 loci is quite short, the 2 genes are located side by side, as do the 2 (A and B subunit) genes of the bacterial fatty-acid β-oxidation multienzyme complex. Notably, both *HADHA* and *HADHB* genes share a common bi-directional promoter region which would suggest a tight coupling between the synthesis of the 2 subunits (28).

LCHAD deficiency. LCHAD deficiency appears to be a relatively common β-oxidation defect (47, 51), with an estimated frequency of at least 1 in 50,000 births in Northern Europe (47). Molecular studies have uncovered a prevalent missense mutation (1528G > C) which results in the Glu510Gln amino acid substitution in the LCHAD domain of α-subunit. This mutation fully inactivates the LCHAD component of MTP without affecting the hydratase and thiolase. The mutation can be detected in approximately 90% of LCHAD-deficient alleles (51) thus making molecular screening for the disease quite feasible. However, the relative frequency of this mutation may be lower in Southern Europe (Di Donato and Taroni, unpublished data). No apparent genotype-to-phenotype correlation has been observed, as patients homozygous for this mutation show widely different phenotypes (47, 51). Only very few additional mutations have been reported.

MTP deficiency. Unlike LCHAD deficiency, the molecular basis of MTP deficiency is heterogeneous and mutations have been identified in both α- and β-subunits ((20), which result in severely but more evenly reduced activities of all 3 enzyme components of the MTP (47). Since formation of the $\alpha_4\beta_4$ enzyme complex is essential for MTP function, the α- and β-subunit mutations which underlie the disease in MTP-deficient patients apparently interfere with assembly of the enzyme complex. Overall, genotype-phenotype analysis did not reveal a significant relationship between genetic defect and clinical features. Ibdah et al have suggested that mutations in exon 9 of the α-subunit gene may be associated with a pure neuromuscular phenotype (chronic progressive polyneuropathy and myopathy without hepatic or cardiac involvement) (20) (Figure 4). However, the older sister of a patient harbouring such exon 9 mutation died at 3 years of age of a Reye-like episode with extensive hepatic and cardiac fatty degeneration (Dionisi Vici and Bertini, unpublished data).

Riboflavin-responsive multiple acyl-CoA dehydrogenase deficiency. No information is available on the molecular and genetic bases of this disorder. A reduced availability of intramitochondrial FAD causing an accelerated turnover of apoenzyme proteins seem to be the most likely explanation for RR-MAD. Possible sites of the defect could be alterations in cellular riboflavin uptake, FMN/FAD cellular uptake or synthesis, mitochondrial transport of flavin cofactors and their mitochondrial synthesis. However, cellular riboflavin uptake and FMN/FAD synthesis were found normal in fibroblasts of 2 patients (2, 31). Recently, Pallotta et al demonstrated the existence of a protein involved in flavin transport in isolated mitochondria of *S. cerevisiae* (29). A putative riboflavin/ riboflavin derivative translocator has been also found in rat liver mitochondria (4). Defects in either of these proteins or in recycling of both covalently- and ionically-bound FMN and FAD ("flavinase" deficiency?) might possibly explain intracellular flavin cofactor deficiency observed in RR-MAD patients.

Structural changes

Approximately 40% of patients affected with all kinds of FA oxidation disorders, except CPT1 and MCAD deficiencies, present with significant muscular involvement (33). When a metabolic myopathy involving FA catabolism is suspected, the clinician should only resort to muscle biopsy after obtaining at least preliminary blood tests (carnitine and plasma free fatty acids) and urine tests (organic acid and acylcarnitine profiles), and in some cases an electromyogram. Given the impracticality of testing muscle biopsy tissue for all known FA oxidation defects, the initial clinical and laboratory assessment helps target the biochemical testing of the muscle tissue. However, in many instances, muscle biopsy has provided the initial stimulus for the biochemical studies that eventually uncovered the metabolic basis of the disorder.

Two main clinical syndromes can be observed in muscle: *i)* progressive proximal myopathy (approximately 35% of cases) and *ii)* acute, recurrent muscle dysfunction with myalgia, myolysis, elevated CK, and paroxysmal myoglobinuria (approximately 65% of cases). Chronic progressive myopathy associated with FA oxidation defects is usually characterized by lipid accumulation within muscle fibres (lipid storage myopathy) which represents a prominent or predominant pathological alteration (Figures 2, 3).

The lipid accumulation correlates with the oxidative capacity of the muscle fibres: it is most marked in type-1 fibres, less marked in type-2A fibres, and least conspicuous in type-2B fibres (9). Necrotic or regenerating fibres are absent unless there has been a recent episode of myoglobinuria. Ultrastructurally, the lipid droplets vary from a fraction of a micrometer to several micrometers in diameter, are not membrane-bound, and accumulate in parallel rows between the myofibrils or under the sarcolemma.

Mitochondrial abnormalities consisting of an increase in the number or size of the mitochondria, intramitochondrial inclusions, and indistinct christae can also occur. In the lipid storage myopathies observed to date, the abnormal lipid deposits consisted predominantly of triglycerides. Normal human fibres contain sparse lipid deposits, but the average lipid fraction of the fibre volume is <0.2%. Most muscle pathologists evaluate the lipid content of the biopsy specimen subjectively, ie, by visual inspection.

Although biochemical assay of muscle fibre lipid content would be better than morphological assessment, it would be affected by the varying amount of adipose tissue in the biopsy specimens.

When examining a muscle specimen that shows evidence of lipid accumulation, it is important to bear in mind the following: *i)* some defects of FA oxidation involving skeletal muscle, eg, CPT2 deficiency, do not usually result in a lipid storage myopathy, *ii)* the muscle fibre lipid content can vary markedly in different disorders of lipid metabolism, from patient to patient with the same disorder, or in the same patient during the course of the disease. Furthermore, ischaemia or obesity can also increase the muscle fibre lipid content, *iii)* impaired fatty acid oxidation and lipid accumulation in muscle can be secondary to an error in another metabolic pathway, eg, a defect in the activity of one of the respiratory chain complexes can affect the utilization of LCFA by muscle and *iv)* defects of lipid metabolism are often not restricted to skeletal muscle, and frequently involve liver, heart, and other organs.

The microscopic evaluation of muscle following an episode of metabolic myoglobinuria due to a defect of lipid metabolism is often not contributive. Although the pathologic processes responsible for rhabdomyolysis are diverse, the microscopic features often are similar. There may be some unspecific myopathic changes and isolated necrotic fibres. Typically, a population of muscle fibres shows evidence of injury, with the remainder of the muscle fibres appearing normal. By contrast, muscle specimens obtained several weeks or months after an acute episode are usually normal, reflecting the remarkable regenerative capacity of skeletal muscle. The muscle glycogen content is normal and lipid accumulation, if any, is significantly less than in classical lipid storage myopathy, eg, carnitine transporter deficiency (Figures 2B, 3). The mitochondria are usually ultrastructurally normal.

Future perspectives

Although the incidence of many of the genetic defects of mitochondrial FA β-oxidation is low, altogether they represent important causes of muscle disease. Since most of these defects can be effectively treated, recognition and early diagnosis of the affected patients are of primary importance. During the past decade, our understanding of these diseases has dramatically increased. The emerging clinical significance of FA oxidation disorders has also stimulated the study of mitochondrial β-oxidation. As a result, a number of new defects have been described and new biochemical and molecular tools have been developed which have greatly increased our ability to investigate and categorize patients with suspected FA oxidation disorders. Finally, prevalent mutations have been identified in patients with deficiencies of MCAD, LCHAD, or CPT2, which makes molecular screening for these diseases feasible (17).

References

1. Andresen BS, Olpin S, Poorthuis BJ, Scholte HR, Vianey-Saban C, Wanders R, Ijlst L, Morris A, Pourfarzam M, Bartlett K, Baumgartner ER, deKlerk JB, Schroeder LD, Corydon TJ, Lund H, Winter V, Bross P, Bolund L, Gregersen N (1999) Clear correlation of genotype with disease phenotype in very-long-chain acyl-CoA dehydrogenase deficiency. *Am J Hum Genet* 64: 479-494

2. Antozzi C, Garavaglia B, Mora M, Rimoldi M, Morandi L, Ursino E, Di Donato S (1994) Late-onset riboflavin-responsive myopathy with combined multiple acyl coenzyme A dehydrogenase and respiratory chain deficiency. *Neurology* 44: 2153-2158

3. Antozzi C, Zeviani M (1997) Cardiomyopathies in disorders of oxidative metabolism. *Cardiovasc Res* 35: 184-199

4. Barile M, Brizio C, De Virgilio C, Delfine S, Quagliariello E, Passarella S (1997) Flavin adenine dinucleotide and flavin mononucleotide metabolism in rat liver — the occurrence of FAD pyrophosphatase and FMN phosphohydrolase in isolated mitochondria. *Eur J Biochem* 249: 777-785

5. Bertini E, Dionisi-Vici C, Garavaglia B, Burlina AB, Sabatelli M, Rimoldi M, Bartuli A, Sabetta G, Di Donato S (1992) Peripheral sensory-motor polyneuropathy, pigmentary retinopathy, and fatal cardiomyopathy in long-chain 3-hydroxy-acyl-CoA dehydrogenase deficiency. *Eur J Pediatr* 151: 121-126

6. Bonnefont JP, Demaugre F, Prip-Buus C, Saudubray JM, Brivet M, Abadi N, Thuillier L (1999) Carnitine

palmitoyltransferase deficiencies. *Mol Genet Metab* 68: 424-440

7. Bonnefont JP, Taroni F, Cavadini P, Cepanec C, Brivet M, Saudubray JM, Leroux JP, Demaugre F (1996) Molecular analysis of carnitine palmitoyltransferase II deficiency with hepatocardiomuscular expression. *Am J Hum Genet* 58: 971-978

8. Brivet M, Boutron A, Slama A, Costa C, Thuillier L, Demaugre F, Rabier D, Saudubray JM, Bonnefont JP (1999) Defects in activation and transport of fatty acids. *J Inherit Metab Dis* 22: 428-441

9. Di Donato S (1994) Disorders of lipid metabolism affecting skeletal muscle: carnitine deficiency syndromes, defects in the catabolic pathway, and Chanarin disease. In *Myology*, AG Engel, C Franzini-Armstrong (eds). McGraw-Hill: New York. pp. 1587-1609

10. Di Donato S (1999) Diseases associated with defects of beta-oxidation. In *The Molecular and Genetic Basis of Neurological Diseases*, RN Rosenberg, SB Prusiner, S DiMauro, RL Barchi (eds). Butterworth-Heinemann: Oxford. pp. 939-956

11. DiMauro S, Melis-DiMauro P (1973) Muscle carnitine palmitoyltransferase deficiency and myoglobinuria. *Science* 182: 929-931

12. Engel WK, Vick NA, Glueck CJ, Levy RI (1970) A skeletal muscle disorder associated with intermittent symptoms and a possible defect of lipid metabolism. *N Engl J Med* 282: 697-704

13. Finocchiaro G, Taroni F, Rocchi M, Martin AL, Colombo I, Tarelli GT, Di Donato S (1991) cDNA cloning, sequence analysis, and chromosomal localization of the gene for human carnitine palmitoyltransferase. *Proc Natl Acad Sci U S A* 88: 661-665

14. Garavaglia B (2001) Riboflavin responsive conditions. In *Vitamin Responsive Conditions in Paediatric Neurology*, P Baxter (ed)

15. Garavaglia B, Uziel G, Dworzak F, Carrara F, Di Donato S (1991) Primary carnitine deficiency: heterozygote and intrafamilial phenotypic variation. *Neurology* 41: 1691-1693

16. Gellera C, Verderio E, Floridia G, Finocchiaro G, Montermini L, Cavadini P, Zuffardi O, Taroni F (1994) Assignment of the human carnitine palmitoyltransferase II gene (CPT1) to chromosome 1p32. *Genomics* 24: 195-197

17. Gregersen N, Andresen BS, Bross P (2000) Prevalent mutations in fatty acid oxidation disorders: diagnostic considerations. *Eur J Pediatr* 159 Suppl 3: S213-218

18. Handig I, Dams E, Taroni F, Van Laere S, de Barsy T, Willems PJ (1996) Inheritance of the S113L mutation within an inbred family with carnitine palmitoyltransferase enzyme deficiency. *Hum Genet* 97: 291-293

19. Huizing M, Iacobazzi V, IJlst L, Savelkoul P, Ruitenbeek W, van den Heuvel L, Indiveri C, Smeitink J, Trijbels F, Wanders R, Palmieri F (1997) Cloning of the human carnitine-acylcarnitine carrier cDNA and identification of the molecular defect in a patient. *Am J Hum Genet* 61: 1239-1245

20. Ibdah JA, Tein I, Dionisi-Vici C, Bennett MJ, L IJ, Gibson B, Wanders RJ, Strauss AW (1998) Mild tri-

functional protein deficiency is associated with progressive neuropathy and myopathy and suggests a novel genotype-phenotype correlation. *J Clin Invest* 102: 1193-1199

21. IJlst L, Mandel H, Oostheim W, Ruiter JP, Gutman A, Wanders RJ (1998) Molecular basis of hepatic carnitine palmitoyltransferase I deficiency. *J Clin Invest* 102: 527–531

22. IJlst L, van Roermund CW, Iacobazzi V, Oostheim W, Ruiter JP, Williams JC, Palmieri F, Wanders RJ (2001) Functional analysis of mutant human carnitine acylcarnitine translocases in yeast. *Biochem Biophys Res Commun* 280: 700-706

23. Kamijo T, Indo Y, Souri M, Aoyama T, Hara T, Yamamoto S, Ushikubo S, Rinaldo P, Matsuda I, Komiyama A, Hashimoto T (1997) Medium chain 3-ketoacyl-coenzyme A thiolase deficiency: a new disorder of mitochondrial fatty acid beta-oxidation. *Pediatr Res* 42: 569-576

24. Kunau WH, Dommes V, Schulz H (1995) β-oxidation of fatty acids in mitochondria, peroxisomes, and bacteria: a century of continued progress. Prog Lipid Res 34: 267-342

25. McGarry JD, Brown NF (1997) The mitochondrial carnitine palmitoyltransferase system. From concept to molecular analysis. *Eur J Biochem* 244: 1-14

26. Minetti C, Garavaglia B, Bado M, Invernizzi F, Bruno C, Rimoldi M, Pons R, Taroni F, Cordone G (1998) Very-long-chain acyl-coenzyme A dehydrogenase deficiency in a child with recurrent myoglobinuria. *Neuromuscul Disord* 8: 3-6

27. Nezu J, Tamai I, Oku A, Ohashi R, Yabuuchi H, Hashimoto N, Nikaido H, Sai Y, Koizumi A, Shoji Y, Takada G, Matsuishi T, Yoshino M, Kato H, Ohura T, Tsujimoto G, Hayakawa J, Shimane M, Tsuji A (1999) Primary systemic carnitine deficiency is caused by mutations in a gene encoding sodium ion-dependent carnitine transporter. *Nat Genet* 21: 91-94

28. Orii KE, Orii KO, Souri M, Orii T, Kondo N, Hashimoto T, Aoyama T (1999) Genes for the human mitochondrial trifunctional protein alpha- and beta-subunits are divergently transcribed from a common promoter region. *J Biol Chem* 274: 8077-8084

29. Pallotta ML, Brizio C, Fratianni A, De Virgilio C, Barile M, Passarella S (1998) Saccharomyces cerevisiae mitochondria can synthesise FMN and FAD from externally added riboflavin and export them to the extramitochondrial phase. *FEBS Lett* 428: 245-249

30. Pons R, Cavadini P, Baratta S, Invernizzi F, Lamantea E, Garavaglia B, Taroni F (2000) Clinical and molecular heterogeneity in very-long-chain acyl-coenzyme A dehydrogenase deficiency. *Pediatr Neurol* 22: 98-105

31. Rhead W, Roettger V, Marshall T, Amendt B (1993) Multiple acyl-coenzyme A dehydrogenation disorder responsive to riboflavin: substrate oxidation, flavin metabolism, and flavoenzyme activities in fibroblasts. *Pediatr Res* 33: 129-135

32. Ruitenbeek W, Poels PJ, Turnbull DM, Garavaglia B, Chalmers RA, Taylor RW, Gabreels FJ (1995) Rhabdomyolysis and acute encephalopathy in late onset medium chain acyl- CoA dehydrogenase deficiency. *J Neurol Neurosurg Psychiatry* 58: 209-214

33. Saudubray JM, Martin D, de Lonlay P, Touati G, Poggi-Travert F, Bonnet D, Jouvet P, Boutron M, Slama A, Vianey-Saban C, Bonnefont JP, Rabier D, Kamoun P, Brivet M (1999) Recognition and management of fatty acid oxidation defects: a series of 107 patients. *J Inherit Metab Dis* 22: 488-502

34. Scaglia F, Longo N (1999) Primary and secondary alterations of neonatal carnitine metabolism. *Semin Perinatol* 23: 152-161

35. Schaefer J, Jackson S, Taroni F, Swift P, Turnbull DM (1997) Characterisation of carnitine palmitoyltransferases in patients with a carnitine palmitoyltransferase deficiency: implications for diagnosis and therapy. *J Neurol Neurosurg Psychiatry* 62: 169-176

36. Stanley CA (1995) Carnitine disorders. *Adv Pediatr* 42: 209-242

37. Straussberg R, Harel L, Varsano I, Elpeleg ON, Shamir R, Amir J (1997) Recurrent myoglobinuria as a presenting manifestation of very long chain acyl coenzyme A dehydrogenase deficiency. *Pediatrics* 99: 894-896

38. Taggart RT, Smail D, Apolito C, Vladutiu GD (1999) Novel mutations associated with carnitine palmitoyltransferase II deficiency. *Hum Mutat* 13: 210-220

39. Tamai I, Ohashi R, Nezu J, Yabuuchi H, Oku A, Shimane M, Sai Y, Tsuji A (1998) Molecular and functional identification of sodium ion-dependent, high affinity human carnitine transporter OCTN2. *J Biol Chem* 273: 20378-20382

40. Taroni F (1995) Carnitine palmitoyltransferase deficiency. In *Neurobase*, S Gilman, GW Goldstein, SG Waxman (eds). Arbor Publishing: La Jolla, CA.

41. Taroni F, Uziel G (1996) Fatty acid mitochondrial beta-oxidation and hypoglycaemia in children. *Curr Opin Neurol* 9: 477-485

42. Taroni F, Verderio E, Dworzak F, Willems PJ, Cavadini P, Di Donato S (1993) Identification of a common mutation in the carnitine palmitoyltransferase II gene in familial recurrent myoglobinuria patients. *Nat Genet* 4: 314-320

43. Taroni F, Verderio E, Fiorucci S, Cavadini P, Finocchiaro G, Uziel G, Lamantea E, Gellera C, Di Donato S (1992) Molecular characterization of inherited carnitine palmitoyltransferase II deficiency. *Proc Natl Acad Sci U S A* 89: 8429-8433

44. Tein I, DiMauro S, DeVivo DC (1990) Recurrent childhood myoglobinuria. *Adv Pediatr* 37: 77-117

45. Tein I, Vajsar J, MacMillan L, Sherwood WG (1999) Long-chain L-3-hydroxyacyl-coenzyme A dehydrogenase deficiency neuropathy: response to cod liver oil. *Neurology* 52: 640-643

46. Thuillier L, Sevin C, Demaugre F, Brivet M, Rabier D, Droin V, Aupetit J, Abadi N, Kamoun P, Saudubray JM, Bonnefont JP (2000) Genotype/phenotype correlation in carnitine palmitoyl transferase II deficiency: lessons from a compound heterozygous patient. *Neuromuscul Disord* 10: 200-205

47. Tyni T, Pihko H (1999) Long-chain 3-hydroxyacyl-CoA dehydrogenase deficiency. *Acta Paediatr* 88: 237-245

48. Verderio E, Cavadini P, Montermini L, Wang H, Lamantea E, Finocchiaro G, Di Donato S, Gellera C, Taroni F (1995) Carnitine palmitoyltransferase II deficiency: structure of the gene and characterization of two novel disease-causing mutations. *Hum Mol Genet* 4: 19-29

49. Vergani L, Barile M, Angelini C, Burlina AB, Nijtmans L, Freda MP, Brizio C, Zerbetto E, Dabbeni-Sala F (1999) Riboflavin therapy. Biochemical heterogeneity in two adult lipid storage myopathies. *Brain* 122: 2401-2411

50. Vladutiu GD, Hogan K, Saponara I, Tassini L, Conroy J (1993) Carnitine palmitoyl transferase deficiency in malignant hyperthermia. *Muscle Nerve* 16: 485-491

51. Wanders RJ, Vreken P, den Boer ME, Wijburg FA, van Gennip AH, L IJ (1999) Disorders of mitochondrial fatty acyl-CoA beta-oxidation. *J Inherit Metab Dis* 22: 442-487

52. Wang Y, Taroni F, Garavaglia B, Longo N (2000) Functional analysis of mutations in the OCTN2 transporter causing primary carnitine deficiency: lack of genotype-phenotype correlation. *Hum Mutat* 16: 401-407

53. Wataya K, Akanuma J, Cavadini P, Aoki Y, Kure S, Invernizzi F, Yoshida I, Kira J, Taroni F, Matsubara Y, Narisawa K (1998) Two CPT2 mutations in three Japanese patients with carnitine palmitoyltransferase II deficiency: functional analysis and association with polymorphic haplotypes and two clinical phenotypes. *Hum Mutat* 11: 377-386

54. Zierz S (1994) Carnitine palmitoyltransferase deficiency. In *Myology*, AG Engel, C Franzini-Armstrong (eds). McGraw-Hill: New York. pp. 1577–1586

Oxidative phosphorylation defects

Eric A. Shoubridge
Maria J. Molnar

AdPEO	autosomal dominant PEO
ARCO	autosomal recessive cardiomyopathy, ophthalmoplegia
ATP	adenosine triphosphate
COX	cytochrome c oxidase
CPEO	chronic external ophthalmoplegia syndrome
cytb	cytochrome b
KSS	Kearns-Sayre syndrome
LS	Leigh syndrome
MELAS	mitochondrial encephalopathy, lactic acidosis, stroke-like episodes
MERRF	myoclonic epilepsy, ragged-red fibres
MNGIE	myoneurogastrointestinal encephalopathy
MtDNA	mitochondrial genome DNA
NARP	neuropathy, ataxia, retinitis pigmentosa
PEO	progressive external ophthalmoplegia
PS	Pearson's syndrome
SDH	succinate dehydrogenase

Definition of the entities

The mitochondrial encephalomyopathies are an extremely heterogeneous group of disorders resulting from partial dysfunction of the mitochondrial oxidative phosphorylation. The oxidative phosphorylation system is composed of the 4 enzyme complexes (Complexes I-IV) that make up the mitochondrial respiratory chain, and the ATP synthase complex (Complex V), which uses energy generated by electron transport along the respiratory chain to produce ATP. As most cells in the body rely on ATP generated by oxidative phosphorylation for their normal function, impairment of this system can produce pathology in any organ system. This makes the recognition, diagnosis and classification of these disorders particularly challenging because patients can present with a wide variety of signs and symptoms that often do not fit into neat or convenient categories.

Both the nuclear and mitochondrial genomes are necessary for assembly of the oxidative phosphorylation enzyme complexes. Of the more than 80 structural subunits in the 5 enzyme complexes, 13 are encoded in the mitochon-

drial genome (mtDNA) and are essential for function. In addition to the structural components, a large, but still incompletely characterized set of nuclear-encoded proteins is necessary for the assembly and maintenance of the complexes. Thus, the disorders can exhibit any mode of inheritance: maternal, autosomal dominant or recessive, or sporadic.

This chapter is focused on the principal clinical phenotypes, the molecular pathogenesis, and the characteristic microscopic pathological changes of respiratory chain disorders that involve, at least to some degree, the neuromuscular system. The minimum prevalence of respiratory chain disorders in the adult population has been estimated at approximately 1 in 8500 (15).

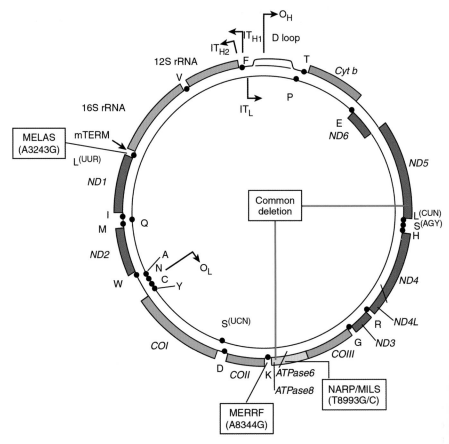

Figure 1. *Structure of human mtDNA.* Human mtDNA is a double-stranded circular molecule of 16 659 base pairs. The two strands are termed heavy (outer circle) and light (inner circle) because of their behaviour in alkaline cesium chloride gradients. The genome codes for 13 polypeptides, 2 rRNAs and 22 tRNAs, which are indicated on the strand containing the coding sequence. The genes coding for polypeptides and rRNAs are depicted as coloured segments on the circle as follows: ND genes of Complex I (blue); Cytb gene of Complex III (purple); CO genes of Complex IV (orange) ATP genes of Complex V (tan); rRNA genes (green). The tRNA genes are shown in the single letter amino acid code. O_H and O_L represent the replication origins of heavy and light strand replication and IT_H and IT_L the transcription initiation sites of each strand. The D-Loop is a triple stranded, non-coding structure that contains several regulatory sequences and a nascent heavy strand. MTERM indicates a binding site for a transcription termination factor that regulates the relative rates of transcription of the rRNA genes and the rest of the genes coded on the H-strand. The sites of the most common mtDNA mutations associated with neuromuscular disease are indicated on the figure.

Mitochondrial genetics

The mitochondrial genome is a double-stranded circular molecule of 16569 base pairs that codes for 13 essential respiratory chain proteins, and the 22 tRNAs and 2 rRNAs that are necessary for their translation within the mitochondrial matrix (Figure 1). Most somatic cells have hundreds to thousands of copies of mtDNA reported to contain, in cultured cells, about 5 copies of mtDNA (range 2-10) per organelle (57, 73). The gametes are exceptional in that the oocyte contains at least 100000 copies (51, 62) and the sperm about 100 (29). MtDNA is thought to exist in a nucleiod structure, complexed with proteins and associated with the matrix face of the inner mitochondrial membrane. There is essentially no information on this point in mammals. However, the structure of the mtDNA nucleoid is beginning to be unraveled in yeast (42).

In mammals, mtDNA is strictly maternally inherited (24). The midpiece of the sperm, which contains the mitochondria and mtDNA, enters the zygote but is actively destroyed in the early embryo by a mechanism that remains obscure, but which may involve ubiquitination of the sperm, targeting it for destruction (83, 84). This apparent surveillance mechanism can be abrogated in interspecific mouse crosses where paternal leakage of mtDNA has been reported (40).

In contrast to nuclear DNA, replication of mtDNA is not linked to the cell cycle (18). This "relaxed" form of replication allows some templates to replicate more than once during the cell cycle, others not at all. Thus, while mtDNA copy number is tightly regulated in a cell- and tissue-specific manner (by unknown mechanisms), sequence variants that arise by germline or somatic mutation can segregate during mitosis due to unequal replication from templates in the parent cell and random sampling of mtDNAs at cytokinesis (5). The presence of more than one sequence variant of mtDNA in a cell or individual is referred to as mtDNA heteroplasmy. In the absence of selection,

the rate of segregation of mtDNA sequence variants depends primarily on two parameters: mtDNA copy number and the number of mitotic divisions. The mtDNA genotype thus varies both temporally and spatially. Because mtDNA is a multicopy genome, the expression of a particular pathogenic mutation depends on the relative proportion of mutant mtDNAs in the cell. Such threshold behaviour is observed for most pathogenic mutations.

Despite the very large copy number ($\sim 10^5$ or more) of mtDNA in the female gamete and the limited number of mitotic divisions in the development of the female germline, mtDNA sequence variants often segregate rapidly between generations. Thus, while most individuals contain a single mtDNA haplotype (mtDNA *homoplasmy*), sequence variation between individuals in human populations is typically of the order of 0.3%, or about 50 nucleotides. New mutations that arise in the female germline produce a transient heteroplasmic state, which usually resolves itself within relatively few generations. These observations were first made in maternal lineages of Holstein cows, where it was observed that a sequence variant in the mtDNA D-loop (the triple stranded, non-coding, hypervariable region of the molecule) could segregate completely in a few generations (27). This led to the hypothesis of an intergenerational bottleneck for the transmission of mtDNA. Rapid segregation of pathogenic mtDNA mutations is also observed in heteroplasmic mice and in human pedigrees, suggesting that the phenomenon is likely to be universal in mammals (38).

Structural changes of skeletal muscle

The most informative feature and the hallmark muscle pathology in many, but not all, patients are ragged-red muscle fibres, which can be demonstrated with the modified Gomori trichrome stain (Figure 2). The modified succinate dehydrogenase (SDH) stain is a more sensitive method to detect these segmental accumulations

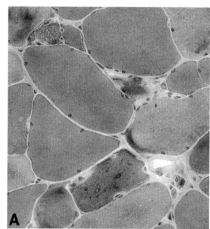

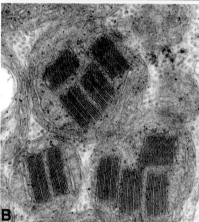

Figure 2. A. Ragged-red fibres demonstrated by the modified Gomori trichrome stain in a transverse section of skeletal muscle from a patient with KSS due to a heteroplasmic large-scale deletion of mtDNA. **B.** Electron micrograph of typical paracrystalline inclusions found in the mitochondria of ragged-red fibres. (magnification ×39,200).

of mitochondria, in which case the fibres appear dark blue. The ragged red and moth eaten appearance of the muscle fibre is due to the accumulation of subsarcolemmal and intermyofibrillar mitochondria, that are genetically, morphologically, and biochemically abnormal.

The percentage of ragged red fibres can range from 2 to 70% and the pathology is segmental; all fibres are affected at multiple locations throughout their length. The boundaries of the affected segments are usually quite sharp (Figure 3). The segmental nature of the biochemical defect generally reflects the underlying distribution of mtDNA mutations, thus from a genetic standpoint the muscle fibres in these patients are linear mosaics.

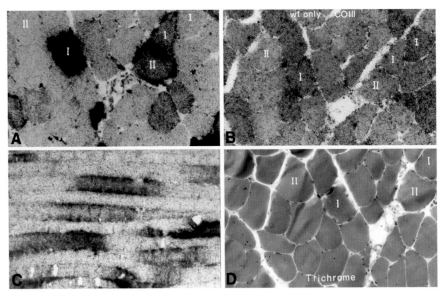

Figure 3. *Molecular pathology of skeletal muscle in a patient with Kearns-Sayre Syndrome due to a large-scale mtDNA deletion.* Panel **A** and **B** are *in situ* hybridization experiments using a probe outside the deletion (**A**), which hybridizes to mtDNA transcripts from both deleted and wild-type mtDNAs, and a probe contained inside the deletion (**B**) which hybridizes to transcripts from wild-type mtDNA only. The probes were labeled with $[\alpha^{35}S]dCTP$ and hybridized to the sections. The slides were then dipped in nuclear track emulsion, developed and counterstained. The large number of silver grains associated with either type 1 (I) or type 2 (II) fibres in **A** represent steady-state levels of ND2 mRNA transcribed off predominantly deleted mtDNAs, as serial sections show much lower numbers of silver grains in the same fibres analyzed with a probe (COIII) that hybridizes to transcripts from wild-type mtD-NAs only (**B**). Similar results are obtained by probing for mtDNA (not shown), demonstrating that transcription from deleted mtDNAs is proportional to the increase in mtDNA copy number. The pathology is segmental as shown in the longitudinal section in panel **C** and those fibres with the largest accumulations of deleted mtDNAs appear as ragged-red with the modified Gomori-trichrome stain (**D**). All fibres with accumulations of deleted mtDNAs would be visible with the modified SDH stain. (**A**), (**B**), and (**D**) are serial sections.

By electron microscopy mitochondria in affected fibre segments appear morphologically abnormal, often with concentric whorls or with abnormal cristae filled with paracrystalline inclusions. These paracrystalline intracristal inclusions contain mitochondrial creatine kinase and possibly other proteins. Ragged-red fibres are usually negative for cytochrome c oxidase (COX) or have much reduced COX activity relative to the increased mitochondrial volume. There is usually a very good correspondence between the proportion of COX-ve fibres and the proportion that are hyper-reactive for SDH. The mitochondrial proliferation that results in ragged-red fibre pathology is presumably an attempt by the cell to compensate for the respiratory chain defect, however, the signals that stimulate increased mitochondrial biogenesis in this circumstance are unknown. Interestingly, ragged-red fibres are nearly always present in patients with mitochondrial translation defects, but only sporadically present in patients with defects in mtDNA protein coding genes.

Molecular genetics and pathogenesis

mtDNA mutations. Mutations in mtDNA can be classified into 3 main categories: large-scale rearrangements, point mutations in tRNAs or rRNAs and point mutations in protein coding genes. The first 2 categories would be expected to affect protein translation, producing multiple deficiencies in the enzymatic activities of the respiratory chain complexes, the latter category produces specific deficiencies in respiratory chain complexes.

Large-scale rearrangements in mtDNA. Large-scale rearrangements in mtDNA generally take one of 2 forms: deletions, which remove multiple tRNA and protein coding genes (32), or duplications, which are dimers of deleted and a wild-type molecules (65, 68). The only real abnormality in a dupli-

cated mtDNA is the sequence around the deletion breakpoint, which is often a truncated or chimeric gene. Most patients with large deletions present as sporadic cases, although there are rare reports of germline transmission. Duplications themselves do not appear to be pathogenic, but can give rise to deletions by mechanisms that remain unknown, but presumably involve resolution of daughter molecules following mtDNA replication (64). Duplications can be maternally transmitted (22).

The mechanism by which deletions in mtDNA are generated is unknown although slip replication and recombination have been suggested (74). Two features of mtDNA deletions lend support to the former mechanism: most deletions are flanked by direct repeat sequences and most occur between the 2 replication origins (O_H and O_L) of mtDNA. A so-called common deletion of approximately 5 kb, present in 30 to 40% of cases, is flanked by a perfect 13 bp repeat sequence, the longest in human mtDNA (53, 74).

All patients with large-scale mtDNA deletions are heteroplasmic (cells homoplasmic for large-scale mtDNA deletions have zero respiratory chain function) and the disease phenotype depends on the load and distribution of mutations inherited at birth. The most common and mildest variant is isolated chronic external ophthalmoplegia syndromes (CPEO) in which clinical signs and symptoms develop during adulthood and are limited to the eyelids and eye muscles (53). CPEO plus refers to a disorder of intermediate severity which has an adolescent or adult onset and variable involvement of tissues other than the eyelids and eye muscles. A more severe variant is Kearns-Sayre Syndrome (KSS) which is characterized by onset of disease manifestations by the second decade and significant multisystem involvement that can include cardiac conduction defects, diabetes mellitus, cerebellar ataxia, retinitis pigmentosa increased CSF protein, and multifocal neurodegeneration. The most severe presentation is called Pearson's syndrome (PS) which is characterized by pancytopenia and dysfunction of the exocrine pancreas dysfunction (70). These patients require frequent transfusions and may have severe systemic manifestations.

In each of these different groups, patients worsen with age. Individuals who are initially classified as isolated CPEO can progress to CPEO plus, patients with Kearns-Sayre syndrome often develop more severe multisystem involvement, and those with Pearsons syndrome progress to KSS in their teenage years (50). The slow progressive nature of these disorders reflects the slow, but apparently inexorable increase in the proportion of deleted mtDNAs with age, especially in post-mitotic tissues like muscle (46) and presumably nerve. Approximately 80% of patients with Kearns-Sayre syndrome, 70% with CPEO plus, and 40% with CPEO harbor mtDNA rearrangements (32, 53).

The deletions in these patients likely arise during oogenesis as in all reported cases, the same molecular species occurs in all tissues where it can be detected. This suggests that the deletion arises early in oogenesis, likely during the generation of primary oocytes, which occurs in fetal life. Deletions arising after this period are likely to be extremely rare (as a proportion of the total mtDNAs in the mature oocyte) and are unlikely to contribute to disease.

How can we explain the very rare transmission of mtDNA deletions and the strikingly different tissue distributions of mtDNA deletions in these patients? A model that can account for these observations is as follows: MtDNA deletions arise at random in the germline and they are for all practical purposes neutral with respect to selection at low levels. Exactly when they appear during oogenesis determines their proportion in any oocyte. In the early embryo, these are randomly distributed in all cells including primordial germ cells. Patients who inherit mtDNA deletions have similar pro-

portions of deleted mtDNA in every tissue at birth, but the percentage varies greatly between individuals. As an example, those who develop CPEO at 40 years of age may have inherited only a few percent of deleted molecules at birth. Even if there is no selection against the presence of these mutant mtDNAs in dividing cells, most will be lost by drift. In fact, if the process is completely stochastic, the proportion of cells predicted to lose the mutation is 1-1/N where N is the initial frequency of the mutant genotype. It is easily seen that in cases where N is small, most cells will have lost the mutation.

Except for those patients with Pearson's syndrome, deletions are not usually found in rapidly dividing tissues like blood. Because of the bottleneck effect, rather few oocytes end up with a high proportion of mutants, so the chance of having a child with detectable mtDNA deletions is low, and probably directly proportional to the frequency of mtDNA deletions received at birth. Patients who develop KSS or PS, both severe phenotypes, would transmit the deletions with a much higher probability than CPEO patients, but they rarely reproduce. This is a rather satisfying model because it can explain why deletions are transmitted in a mouse model of the disease (36) and why pathogenic point mutations in human mitochondrial tRNAs, which produce similar mitochondrial translation defects, are transmitted. In most cases the clinical phenotype of these patients does not preclude reproduction.

The exact size and nature of the deletion has very little effect on the phenotype. Studies on model cell culture systems have demonstrated a mitochondrial translation defect in cells carrying greater than 65% deleted mtDNAs (28). Characteristic of most mtDNA mutations the threshold for the defect is extraordinarily steep as cells carrying 55% deletions have normal respiratory chain function. Thus, below a certain proportion of mtDNA deletions wild-type mtDNAs can complement the mutant molecules, while

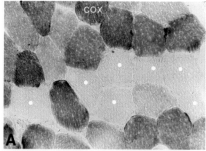

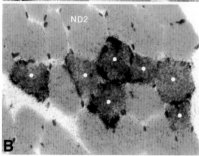

Figure 4. Serial sections of skeletal muscle from a patient with a large-scale deletion and Kearns-Sayre Syndrome showing the correspondence between fibres with large accumulations of deleted mtDNAs, as indicated by *in situ* hybridization with a mtDNA probe outside the deletion (**B**), and those which stain negative for cytochrome c oxidase (**A**).

beyond a certain threshold, this is not possible and in fact the presence of the deleted mtDNAs appears to interfere with the expression from wild-type mtDNAs (28, 76). That the genetic complementation occurs within an organelle was demonstrated by the presence of fusion proteins that could have only be translated from deleted mtDNAs in the presence of wild-type molecules.

The skeletal muscle of patients with large-scale deletions always displays the characteristic ragged-red fibre pathology (Figure 3). In situ hybridization with mtDNA probes contained within or outside of the deletion has demonstrated that these affected fibre segments contain large accumulations of deleted mtDNAs and their transcripts, demonstrating that the mutation does not impair transcription (Figure 3) (76). The relative proportion of wild-type mtDNAs in the affected fibre segments is always reduced, often dramatically and they stain negative for cytochrome c oxidase (Figure 4). Polypeptides encoded in mtDNA are not detectable by immunocytochemistry in these muscle fibres, even those encoded outside the deletion, indicating that translation of mtDNA-encoded genes is virtually zero in these regions.

Mutations in mtDNA protein coding genes. Mutations in the protein coding genes of mtDNA are less common that tRNA mutations or deletions. The first such mutation to be reported was the G11778A mutation in ND4 associated with Leber hereditary optic neuropathy (94). An additional 2 mutations (G3460A and T14484C), also in complex I subunits have been associated with this disorder and can account for the majority of cases (35). In the majority of patients these mutations cause pathology only in the optic nerve. Mutations in several other protein coding genes have been associated with neuromuscular phenotypes.

1. ATP6 mutations: NARP and Leigh syndrome. A mutation in the ATP6 gene (T8993G) was first reported in a complex phenotype that included neuropathy, ataxia, and retinitis pigmentosa (NARP) (33). The result of the T8993G mutation is a leucine to arginine substitution within the proton channel of the F_o segment of complex V. This impairs ATP synthesis (89) and may decrease the stability of the complex (58). A milder mutation at the same position (T8993C) has also been associated with this phenotype, resulting in a leucine to proline substitution (21). The age of onset is during infancy or early childhood. Myopathy is rare, and muscle pathology is not informative, but the liver and heart may be involved. There is a relatively high threshold for expression of the NARP phenotype of about 70% mutant mtDNAs. Patients with heteroplasmy between 70 and 90% show varied disease manifestations. Patients with more than 90% of mutant mtDNAs usually present with Leigh Syndrome (88). This syndrome, also called subacute necrotizing encephalomyelopathy, is characterized by hypotonia, failure to thrive, seizures, respiratory dysfunction, and ataxia. On the T2 weighted MRI images, bilateral hyperintense sig-

nals can be observed in the basal ganglia, cerebellum, or brain stem. The clinical and metabolic status often shows significant worsening during infections.

2. Cytochrome b mutations and Complex I mutations. Several mutations in the cytb gene have recently been reported in patients with exercise intolerance, and myalgia with or without myoglobinuria (1). These patients had either missense mutations or a deletion in the gene coding for cytb. Interestingly, all patients were apparently sporadic, had isolated muscle involvement, and had COX-positive ragged-red muscle fibres. Two sporadic cases of patients with exercise intolerance with mutations in complex I subunits have also been reported (1, 56)

3. Complex IV (COX) subunit mutations. Mutations in all three of the mtDNA-encoded subunits (COI-III) that constitute the catalytic core of COX have been identified. All that have been reported to date are private mutations (associated with single pedigrees) and most were sporadic cases. Three different mutations have been described in COI: a microdeletion associated with motor neuron disease (19); a nonsense mutation in a multisystem disorder (11); and a nonsense mutation in a case of pure myopathy (41). As expected, patients with COX I defects show reductions in COX II, COX III ,and several nuclear-encoded COX subunits due to failure to assemble the holoenzyme complex.

Two different mutations have been reported in COII: an initiation codon mutation producing encephalomyopathy (17) and a missense mutation in a case of myopathy (67). Immunoblot analysis in the latter patient showed the near absence of COX II and COX III with relative preservation of 2 nuclear encoded subunits, COX I and COX Va.

Four mutations have been described in COIII. The first described mutation in this subunit was a 15 bp microdeletion in COIII in a patient with myopathy and myoglobinuria (45). A missense mutation was reported in a patient with MELAS (49) and a non-

sense mutation, predicting truncation of the last 13 amino acids was found in a patient with encephalomyopathy and myopathy (25). Very recently a frameshift mutation was described in the context of a Leigh-like syndrome (90). Patients with COIII mutations show a failure to assemble the holoenzyme complex and instability of the COX I-COX II interaction (31).

All of the mutations described above in COI-III genes are heteroplasmic, and in contrast to the autosomal recessive presentation of isolated COX deficiency, disease onset is generally in late childhood or adulthood. It is not possible to draw any conclusions about genotype-phenotype relationships in these disorders; all are private mutations and the clinical presentations are remarkably different, even among patients with mutations in the same gene. Ragged-red fibres are present in some but not all of these cases.

tRNA and rRNA mutations. Mutations in tRNA genes are the most common class of mtDNA mutations in human disease. More than 50 different mutations in most of the tRNA genes have been reported, the majority showing some neuromuscular or cardiac phenotype. The mutations are always heteroplasmic, nearly always associated with ragged-red fibres, and all display some threshold behaviour in muscle. The majority of mutations are private or semiprivate and we only discuss the most common syndromes associated with myopathy. Thus far, mutations in rRNA genes have been associated with aminoglycoside-induced non-syndromic deafness (66) and cardiomyopathy (2) and are not be discussed further.

1. Mitochondrial encephalomyopathy, lactic acidosis and stroke-like episodes (MELAS). This syndrome, which is one of the most common respiratory chain disorders, is characterized by sudden development of cerebral lesions reminiscent of large or small vessel strokes which cross vascular territories. The onset of the disease is usually under 45 years. In most cases, preexisting migraine headaches and/or seizures are present in the clinical history. Associated symptoms may include myopathy, ataxia, cardiomyopathy, diabetes mellitus, renal tubular dysfunction, retinitis pigmentosa, lactic acidosis, and hyperalaninemia. About 80% of the MELAS cases are due to an A3243G point mutation in the tRNA[leu (UUR)] gene. This mutation significantly increases the risk for diabetes mellitus (39) and it is also an important cause of CPEO (52). Four other mutations in the tRNA[leu (UUR)] gene and 4 in other different tRNA genes have also been found in MELAS cases. Ragged-red fibres are found in muscle biopsy, but in contrast to many other tRNA point mutations and large-scale deletions, they can be positive for COX activity although the activity is usually reduced relative to the mitochondrial proliferation. Blood vessels in these cases also show hyper-reactivity for SDH (26). Although the common MELAS mutation is located in a site in the tRNA[leu] gene that also binds a transcription termination factor responsible for regulating the relative rates of transcription of the two rRNA species and the mRNAs encoded on the same strand, there is no evidence that alteration of transcription termination is part of the pathogenic mechanism of the mutation (16). The A3243G mutation results in a marked decrease in the aminoacylation of tRNA[leu (UUR)]; however, the extent of the defect does not correlate with the leucine content of mitochondrial polypeptides (16). The mechanism has been suggested to be due to a reduced association of mRNA with mitochondrial ribosomes (16).

2. Myoclonic Epilepsy and Ragged-Red Fibres (MERRF). The symptoms may start from the early childhood to the adulthood. The typical clinical symptoms include myoclonic and/or generalized or focal seizures, cerebellar ataxia, and myopathy with ragged-red fibres (Figure 5). The myoclonic jerks occur at rest and worsen during movement (action myoclonus). Associated symptoms may also include corticospinal tract deficits, dementia, optic

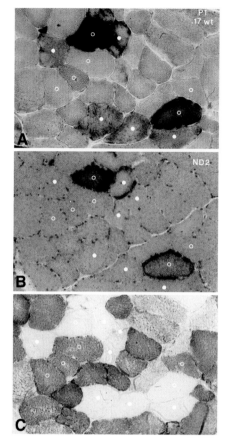

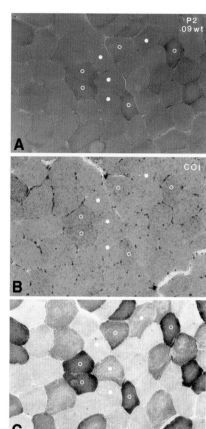

Figure 5. *Molecular pathology of skeletal muscle in two patients carrying the A8344G mutation in tRNA[lys] associated with the MERRF syndrome. The patient on the left, with an overall proportion of 83% mutant mtDNAs in the muscle biopsy, shows abundant ragged-red fibres by SDH staining (**A**). Large accumulations of mtDNA transcripts are seen by in situ hybridization in the same fibres using a probe that detects a mtDNA transcript (**B**). Cytochrome c oxidase activity is undetectable in the affected fibres (**C**). The good correspondence between the SDH staining intensity and the accumulation of mtDNA transcripts shows that the mutation does not interfere with mtDNA transcription. Both type 1 (open circles) and type 2 (closed circles) fibres are affected, and the pathology is segmental (not shown). The patient on the right had 91% of mutant mtDNAs in the biopsy specimen, but no obvious muscle pathology. This is likely due to a more uniform distribution of mutant mtDNAs in the muscle of this patient. Studies of the threshold for expression this mutation in myotubes cultured from patient muscle show that the proportion of mutants must exceed 85% before any biochemical defect is observed.*

atrophy, deafness, peripheral neuropathy, cardiomyopathy, multiple symmetric lipomatosis, and renal tubular dysfunction. Muscle biopsy reveals COX negative ragged red fibres. EEG detects epileptiform discharges, photic hypersensitivity, and large amplitude occipital slow waves. About 80% of the MERRF cases are caused by A8344G mutation in the tRNA[Lysine] gene (75). A smaller percentage of the patients have T8356C mutation in the same gene (77). Unlike the case for large-scale deletions, there is no evidence that the proportion of mtDNAs carrying the A8344G mutation increases substantially in skeletal muscle during life (8). The mutation behaves in a functionally

recessive manner; in cultured myotubes from MERRF patients, no biochemical phenotype is observed until the proportion of mutant mtDNAs exceeds 85% (8). There is a good correlation between the extent of the translation defect and the lysine content of different mtDNA-encoded polypeptides (23). The mutation causes defective aminoacylation of the tRNA[lys], resulting in premature translation termination (23).

3. Mitochondrial myopathy and cardiomyopathy. Hypertrophic cardiomyopathy is a relatively common finding in patients with respiratory chain defects. The congestive heart failure begins in young adulthood. Frequently, bilateral cataracts, insulin dependent diabetes mellitus, and Wolf-Parkinson-White syndrome are associated. The myopathy is of variable severity in these patients. Pathogenic point mutations (A3260G, C3303T) have been reported in tRNA$^{leu\ (UUR)}$ gene (78, 96). The tRNA^{ile} gene appears to be a "hotspot" for mutations associated with cardiomyopathy; at least 5 different point mutations have been reported (2).

Nuclear gene mutations. *Nuclear-mitochondrial communication disorders.* Several different clinical phenotypes have been associated with multiple rearrangements of mtDNA inherited in an autosomal recessive or dominant fashion.

MtDNA depletion syndrome. This is a quantitative error in mtDNA in which the copy number of mtDNA is drastically reduced (below 10%) in a tissue-specific fashion (54). Curiously, different members of the same family may show different tissue involvement. The age of onset is variable but is usually in the first weeks of the life. The infants show failure to thrive, weakness, hypotonia, hepatopathy, proximal renal tubular abnormalities, or encephalopathy depending on which tissues show the depletion. Patients with myopathic symptoms often present later, around 1 year of age (48).

The muscle biopsy may reveal excessive lipid, glycogen accumulation, and excessive numbers of enlarged mitochondria. Muscle fibres show COX deficiency, but ragged-red fibres are not usually present. The genetic basis of the disorder remains a mystery. At least half of the reported cases are sporadic, the rest are compatible with autosomal recessive inheritance. It is not known whether sequence variants in the control region of mtDNA play a role in depletion syndrome, but none have been found. In some cases the mtDNA depletion can be complemented in patient cells with a control nucleus, supporting the notion that the disorder can be caused by a nuclear gene defect (6). A number of nuclear genes thought to play a role in mtDNA replication (eg, single-stranded binding protein, endo G, polymerase gamma, mtTFA and NRF1) have been excluded in one family (79).

Multiple mtDNA deletions. *Progressive external ophthalmoplegia.* PEO can be transmitted in an autosomal dominant (AdPEO) (97), or more rarely autosomal recessive fashion (7). The disease is characterized clinically by ophthalmoparesis and exercise intolerance with onset usually between 18 to 40 years (82). The muscle pathology in these patients is similar to that in patients with sporadic PEO, being characterized by the presence of ragged-red fibres although the proportion is often less than 5% (82). Southern blot analysis of mtDNA shows multiple deletions in postmitotic tissues but not in the mitotically active cells, such as lymphocytes. These may appear as a smear below the wild-type mtDNA or as a series of more or less discrete bands.

Single fibre analysis has demonstrated that affected fibre segments usually contain a single molecular species of deleted mtDNA, suggesting the clonal expansion of a relatively rare somatic mutation event (55). Linkage analysis detected pathogenic loci on chromosome 10q24 (81) and 4q34-35 (44), and there is at least 1 other yet unidentified locus. The gene defect in the chromosome 4 locus has been identified as the adenine nucleotide translocator 1 (ANT1) (43). Although there is no direct evidence to support a role of the carrier in the supply of intramitochondrial dATP, it has been speculated that the molecular genetic basis for the generation of multiple deletions could involve an imbalance in the mitochondrial nucleotide pools (43). The gene defect on chromosome 10 was very recently identified as a mitochondrial DNA helicase related to the phage T7 gene 4 primase/helicase (78a). Mutations in the mitochondrial g DNA polymerase POLG were recently reported in an adPEO family with multiple deletions linked to chromosome 15q22-q26 and in two other families with apparently arPEO (93a).

Myoneurogastrointestinal Encephalopathy (MNGIE). MNGIE is an autosomal recessive disorder characterized by a progressive external ophthalmoplegia, dementia with a progressive leukodystrophy, mitochondrial myopathy, peripheral neuropathy, and prominent involvement of the gastrointestinal tract manifesting as diarrhea, malabsorption, and weight loss with normal pancreatic function. Radiologic investigations may show marked thickening of the small intestines, reflecting the pathological findings of extensive mural thickening and fibrosis of the submucosa and subserosa. This syndrome was linked to chromosome 22q13 (30) and shown to be caused by loss-of-function mutations in the thymidine phosphorylase gene (59). Thymidine phosphorylase converts thymidine to 2-deoxy D-ribose 1-phosphate and may function to regulate thymidine availability for DNA synthesis. Thymidine phosphorylase is widely expressed in human tissues, but paradoxically not in skeletal muscle, in which multiple mtDNA deletions are present in some but not all patients. Although the disease mechanism remains unknown, it may, as with ANT1 mutations, result from an imbalance in the intramitochondrial dNTP pools.

Wolfram syndrome. This disease, also known by the acronym DID-MOAD, is transmitted as an autosomal recessive trait characterized by diabetes insipidus, insulin-dependent diabetes mellitus, optic neuropathy, and deafness. The pathogenic gene was linked to chromosome 4p16 (63) and identified as a transmembrane protein named wolframin (80). This disorder was linked to a respiratory chain abnormality with reports of large-scale mtDNA deletions in some patients (3, 69) and the presence of multiple deletions in a family that linked to the 4p16 locus (3). A recent report has localized the wolframin protein to the endoplasmic reticulum (87). The relationship between mutations in wolframin and the mtDNA abnormalities remains unknown.

Autosomal recessive cardiomyopathy, ophthalmoplegia (ARCO). This childhood disease was described in two families showing severe fatal hypertrophic cardiomyopathy (7). Progressive external ophthalmoplegia and proximal muscle weakness were present in addition to the cardiac symptoms and the muscle biopsy shows raggedred fibres. Multiple mtDNA deletions are present on Southern blot analysis of skeletal muscle, but the gene defect is unknown.

Mutations in nuclear encoded genes associated with isolated respiratory chain complex deficiencies. *Leigh syndrome.* As discussed above, Leigh Syndrome (LS) is an early onset, fatal neurodegenerative disorder characterized pathologically by bilateral lesions in the brainstem, basal ganglia, thalamus, and spinal cord. Occasionally white matter lesions and focal cortical atrophy may present as well. Raggedred fibres are not present in the muscle biopsy. It can be caused by mutations in the ATP6 gene, encoded in mtDNA, or by several different nuclear gene products affecting complexes I, II, or IV of the respiratory chain—all of which are inherited in an autosomal recessive fashion. The first mutations in a respiratory chain subunit in this disorder were found in the Fp subunit of complex II (9, 61). In LS patients with COX deficiency, COX is reduced in all tissues to 10 to 25% of control levels. The majority of patients with this form of LS were assigned to a single genetic complementation group by somatic cell genetics (10). Functional complementation of the defect by microcell-mediated chromosome transfer mapped the gene defect to 9q34 and loss of function mutations were identified in the *SURF1* gene (92, 98). Surf1 appears to be involved in an early step in the assembly of the COX holoenzyme complex (95). All patients so far tested are null for the Surf1 protein by immunoblot analysis (91, 95). A French Canadian form of LS with COX defi-

ciency is biochemically distinct from the classical disorder, and the gene defect in this disease has been mapped by linkage to chromosome 2p16 (47). Several mutations in complex I structural subunits have been reported in cases with complex I deficiency (4, 93).

Infantile hypertrophic cardiomyopathy with encephalopathy. This autosomal recessive disorder, which has an onset in the early postnatal period, manifests with rapidly fatal, severe hypertrophic cardiomyopathy, encephalopathy, respiratory difficulties, and metabolic acidosis. COX activity is severely reduced in the brain, skeletal muscle, and heart, whereas other tissues such as fibroblasts are much less severely affected. Candidate gene analysis identified mutations in the *SCO2* gene, a copper chaperone necessary for the delivery of copper to COX (60). Most cases are compound heterozygotes for an E140K substitution near the putative copper binding site of the protein (37, 60). Recently, patients homozygous for this mutation have been reported to have a comparatively mild phenotype (36a). A minority of patients with a nearly identical severe cardiomyopathic phenotype have *SCO2* mutations (37). Sequencing of 2 other genes in the copper delivery pathway (*SCO1* and *COX17*) have not identified defects in these genes (34). As *SCO2* appears to be a ubiquitously expressed housekeeping gene, the basis for the extreme variability in the extent of the biochemical defect in different tissues of these patients remains unexplained.

Mutations in other mitochondrial protein genes. *Hereditary spastic paraplegia.* This is a genetically heterogeneous group of disorders with autosomal dominant and recesssive and X-linked forms. In one autosomal recessive form which was mapped to chromosome 16q24, patients experience progressive weakness, spasticity, mild decreases in vibratory sensation as their major manifestations, and have raggedred, COX-deficient fibres in their

skeletal muscle. This unique form of hereditary spastic paraplegia, is caused by mutations in the gene called "paraplegin" that is localized to the mitochondria (13). Paraplegin has a high degree of homology to a subclass of ATPases belonging to the AAA family. These ATPases are metalloproteases with both proteolytic and chaperonin functions, suggesting that paraplegin plays a role in the assembly and maintenance of the respiratory chain enzyme complexes.

Friedreich ataxia. This is an autosomal recessive disease with onset in early childhood characterized by severe gait and limb ataxia, pyramidal signs, absent stretch reflexes and an axonal sensory neuropathy. The mutation is in the frataxin gene on the chromosome 9q13. The majority of cases are homozygous for a large expansion of the triplet repeat sequence GAA in the first intron of the frataxin gene (12). Frataxin is targeted to the mitochondrial matrix where it plays a role in the regulation of mitochondrial iron. The intronic mutation results in a severe reduction of the frataxin protein. The lack of frataxin in the mitochondrial matrix results in an increase in mitochondrial iron which appears to increase oxidative stress, resulting in a severe reduction in the activities of enzymes containing Fe-S centers, including Complexes I, II, III, and aconitase (71).

Treatment

Currently there is no specific pharmacological treatment available for respiratory chain disorders. There are a number of mostly anecdotal reports of clinical improvement after administration of a variety of compounds including Coenzyme Q10, menadione, succinate, ascorbate, thiamine, nicotinamide, and riboflavin; however, objective assessment of the efficacy of the metabolic therapies is difficult because of clinical and genetic heterogeneity and uncertainty regarding the natural history of these disorders (review in (14). Idibenone, a Q10 analogue, has been demonstrated to be effective in reversing the cardiomyopathy in patients with Freidrich Ataxia (72). Dichloroacetate (DCA), which stimulates pyruvate dehydrogenase by inhibiting pyruvate dehydrogenase kinase, is used in the treatment of acute lactic acidosis, and there are ongoing trials using this compound in MELAS patients.

A moderate degree of aerobic training has been shown to improve exercise tolerance, the cardiovascular status, and muscle metabolism in a group of patients with mtDNA mutations (85). The effects of strength training have been investigated in one patient with a heteroplasmic tRNA mutation and a CPEO plus syndrome and a very skewed distribution of mutant mtDNAs between the satellite cell population and skeletal muscle (86). In this patient and in nearly all patients with large-scale deletions, mutant mtDNAs are rare or undetectable in the satellite cell population. The muscle hypertrophy that results from strength training requires recruitment of satellite cells. The incorporation of wild-type mtDNAs strength training increased the relative proportion of wild-type genomes in the biceps and decreased the proportion of COX-negative fibres. This approach needs to be tested in a larger patient population to determine if it is generally beneficial.

Prenatal diagnosis

Genetic counseling of women who are carrying mtDNA mutations has been highly problematic (20). If, as the data suggest, segregation of mtDNA sequence variants can be treated as a problem of binomial sampling (38), it ought to be possible to calculate recurrence risks in a future sibling. Whether this will ever be truly useful remains to be seen, as the confidence limits on the estimates of risk might be too large to be of value. While it seems clear that the risk of having an affected child increases with the level of heteroplasmy in the mother, there is no degree of heteroplasmy at which the risk is low enough to be ignored.

The prospects for preimplantation or prenatal diagnosis are considerably brighter. Because the individual's mtDNA genotype is most likely determined by the relative proportions of wild-type and mutant mtDNA in the oocyte, the mtDNA genotype of a blastomere sampled from an 8-cell embryo (or perhaps a polar body) ought to be a random sample of the oocyte's mtDNA complement, and hence a good predictor of the mtDNA genotype of the fetus. The fact that little if any segregation of mtDNA sequence variants occurs during fetal life, even those that have been proven to be pathogenic, suggests that sampling of any fetal tissue after establishment of pregnancy (eg, chorionic villus, amniocytes) ought also to provide a reliable indication of the overall mtDNA mutation load.

Future perspectives

The last decade has seen an explosion in the area of mitochondrial disease research. More than one hundred pathogenic mutations in mtDNA have been described and mutations in nuclear genes coding for structural and assembly/maintenance factors are beginning to be uncovered. The rather surprising outcome of all of this work is the rather close relationship between specific mutations (nuclear or mitochondrial) and particular clinical phenotypes. Equally unexpected is the fact that the same mutation can sometimes produce strikingly different phenotypes. Why mutations that affect the same common biochemical pathway— the ability of the cell to produce ATP by oxidative phosphorylation—should produce such a rich diversity of clinical phenotypes, some with exquisite cellular specificity, is an abiding mystery. The unique genetics of mtDNA goes some way to explaining differential tissue involvement in patients with the same mtDNA mutation, but how tissue-specificity arises from mutations in nuclear housekeeping genes that are ubiquitously expressed remains an unanswered question. In this respect, respiratory chain disorders caused by nuclear gene mutations are similar to the majority of inherited neurodegenerative diseases, in which the culprit gene codes for a ubiquitously expressed protein. For respiratory chain diseases, it seems likely that the cell-specific details of the regulation of assembly of the enzyme complexes, the balance of energy supply and demand, or the relative importance of different enzyme complexes will ultimately provide the answers to specific cellular vulnerability. Sorting out these complexities remains the foremost challenge for the future.

References

1. Andreu AL, Hanna MG, Reichmann H, Bruno C, Penn AS, Tanji K, Pallotti F, Iwata S, Bonilla E, Lach B, Morgan-Hughes J, DiMauro S (1999) Exercise intolerance due to mutations in the cytochrome b gene of mitochondrial DNA. *N Engl J Med* 341: 1037-1044.

2. Arbustini E, Diegoli M, Fasani R, Grasso M, Morbini P, Banchieri N, Bellini O, Dal Bello B, Pilotto A, Magrini G, Campana C, Fortina P, Gavazzi A, Narula J, Vigano M (1998) Mitochondrial DNA mutations and mitochondrial abnormalities in dilated cardiomyopathy. *Am J Pathol* 153: 1501-1510.

3. Barrientos A, Volpini V, Casademont J, Genis D, Manzanares JM, Ferrer I, Corral J, Cardellach F, Urbano-Marquez A, Estivill X, Nunes V (1996b) A nuclear defect in the 4p16 region predisposes to multiple mitochondrial DNA deletions in families with Wolfram syndrome. *J Clin Invest* 97: 1570-1576

4. Benit P, Chretien D, Kadhom N, de Lonlay-Debeney P, Cormier-Daire V, Cabral A, Peudenier S, Rustin P, Munnich A, Rotig A (2001) Large-scale deletion and point mutations of the nuclear NDUFV1 and NDUFS1 genes in mitochondrial complex I deficiency. *Am J Hum Genet* 68: 1344-1352.

5. Birky CW (1995) Uniparental inheritance of mitochondrial and chloroplast genes: mechanisms and evolution. *Proc Natl Acad Sci U S A* 92: 11331-11338

6. Bodnar AG, Cooper JM, Holt IJ, Leonard JV, Schapira AH (1993) Nuclear complementation restores mtDNA levels in cultured cells from a patient with mtDNA depletion. *Am J Hum Genet* 53: 663-669

7. Bohlega S, Tanji K, Santorelli FM, Hirano M, al-Jishi A, DiMauro S (1996) Multiple mitochondrial DNA deletions associated with autosomal recessive ophthalmoplegia and severe cardiomyopathy. *Neurology* 46: 1329-1334.

8. Boulet L, Karpati G, Shoubridge EA (1992) Distribution and threshold expression of the tRNA(Lys) mutation in skeletal muscle of patients with myoclonic epilepsy and ragged-red fibers (MERRF). *Am J Hum Genet* 51: 1187-1200.

9. Bourgeron T, Rustin P, Chretien D, Birch-Machin M, Bourgeois M, Viegas-Pequignot E, Munnich A, Rotig A (1995) Mutation of a nuclear succinate dehydrogenase

gene results in mitochondrial respiratory chain deficiency. *Nat Genet* 11: 144-149.

10. Brown RM, Brown GK (1996) Complementation analysis of systemic cytochrome oxidase deficiency presenting as Leigh syndrome. *J Inherit Metab Dis* 19: 752-760

11. Bruno C, Martinuzzi A, Tang Y, Andreu AL, Pallotti F, Bonilla E, Shanske S, Fu J, Sue CM, Angelini C, DiMauro S, Manfredi G (1999) A stop-codon mutation in the human mtDNA cytochrome c oxidase I gene disrupts the functional structure of complex IV. *Am J Hum Genet* 65: 611-620

12. Campuzano V, Montermini L, Molto MD, Pianese L, Cossee M, Cavalcanti F, Monros E, Rodius F, Duclos F, Monticelli A, et al. (1996) Friedreich's ataxia: autosomal recessive disease caused by an intronic GAA triplet repeat expansion. *Science* 271: 1423-1427

13. Casari G, De Fusco M, Ciarmatori S, Zeviani M, Mora M, Fernandez P, De Michele G, Filla A, Cocozza S, Marconi R, Durr A, Fontaine B, Ballabio A (1998) Spastic paraplegia and OXPHOS impairment caused by mutations in paraplegin, a nuclear-encoded mitochondrial metalloprotease. *Cell* 93: 973-983

14. Chinnery P, Turnbull DM (2001) Epidemiology and treatment of mitochondrial disorders. *Am J Med Genet* 106: 94-101

15. Chinnery PF, Johnson MA, Wardell TM, Singh-Kler R, Hayes C, Brown DT, Taylor RW, Bindoff LA, Turnbull DM (2000) The epidemiology of pathogenic mitochondrial DNA mutations. *Ann Neurol* 48: 188-193

16. Chomyn A, Enriquez JA, Micol V, Fernandez-Silva P, Attardi G (2000) The mitochondrial myopathy, encephalopathy, lactic acidosis, and stroke- like episode syndrome-associated human mitochondrial tRNALeu(UUR) mutation causes aminoacylation deficiency and concomitant reduced association of mRNA with ribosomes. *J Biol Chem* 275: 19198-19209

17. Clark KM, Taylor RW, Johnson MA, Chinnery PF, Chrzanowska-Lightowlers ZM, Andrews RM, Nelson IP, Wood NW, Lamont PJ, Hanna MG, Lightowlers RN, Turnbull DM (1999) An mtDNA mutation in the initiation codon of the cytochrome C oxidase subunit II gene results in lower levels of the protein and a mitochondrial encephalomyopathy. *Am J Hum Genet* 64: 1330-1339

18. Clayton DA (1991) Replication and transcription of vertebrate mitochondrial DNA. *Annu Rev Cell Biol* 7:453-78. *Annu Rev Cell Biol* 7: 453-478

19. Comi GP, Bordoni A, Salani S, Franceschina L, Sciacco M, Prelle A, Fortunato F, Zeviani M, Napoli L, Bresolin N, Moggio M, Ausenda CD, Taanman JW, Scarlato G (1998) Cytochrome c oxidase subunit I microdeletion in a patient with motor neuron disease. *Ann Neurol* 43: 110-116

20. Dahl HH, Thorburn DR, White SL (2000) Towards reliable prenatal diagnosis of mtDNA point mutations: studies of nt8993 mutations in oocytes, fetal tissues, children and adults. *Hum Reprod* 15 Suppl 2: 246-255

21. de Vries DD, van Engelen BG, Gabreels FJ, Ruitenbeek W, van Oost BA (1993) A second missense mutation in the mitochondrial ATPase 6 gene in Leigh's syndrome. *Ann Neurol* 34: 410-412

22. Dunbar DR, Moonie PA, Swingler RJ, Davidson D, Roberts R, Holt IJ (1993) Maternally transmitted partial direct tandem duplication of mitochondrial DNA associated with diabetes mellitus. *Hum Mol Genet* 2: 1619-1624

23. Enriquez JA, Chomyn A, Attardi G (1995) MtDNA mutation in MERRF syndrome causes defective aminoacylation of tRNA(Lys) and premature translation termination. *Nat Genet* 10: 47-55

24. Giles RE, Blanc H, Cann HM, Wallace DC (1980) Maternal inheritance of human mitochondrial DNA. *Proc Natl Acad Sci U S A* 77: 6715-6719

25. Hanna MG, Nelson IP, Rahman S, Lane RJ, Land J, Heales S, Cooper MJ, Schapira AH, Morgan-Hughes JA, Wood NW (1998) Cytochrome c oxidase deficiency associated with the first stop-codon point mutation in human mtDNA. *Am J Hum Genet* 63: 29-36

26. Hasegawa H, Matsuoka T, Goto Y, Nonaka I (1991) Strongly succinate dehydrogenase-reactive blood vessels in muscles from patients with mitochondrial myopathy, encephalopathy, lactic acidosis, and stroke-like episodes. *Ann Neurol* 29: 601-605

27. Hauswirth WW, Laipis PJ (1982) Mitochondrial DNA polymorphism in a maternal lineage of Holstein cows. *Proc Natl Acad Sci U S A* 79: 4686-4690

28. Hayashi J, Ohta S, Kikuchi A, Takemitsu M, Goto Y, Nonaka I (1991) Introduction of disease-related mitochondrial DNA deletions into HeLa cells lacking mitochondrial DNA results in mitochondrial dysfunction. *Proc Natl Acad Sci U S A* 88: 10614-10618

29. Hecht NB, Liem H, Kleene KC, Distel RJ, Ho SM (1984) Maternal inheritance of the mouse mitochondrial genome is not mediated by a loss or gross alteration of the paternal mitochondrial DNA or by methylation of the oocyte mitochondrial DNA. *Dev Biol* 102: 452-461

30. Hirano M, Garcia-de-Yebenes J, Jones AC, Nishino I, DiMauro S, Carlo JR, Bender AN, Hahn AF, Salberg LM, Weeks DE, Nygaard TG (1998) Mitochondrial neurogastrointestinal encephalomyopathy syndrome maps to chromosome 22q13.32-qter. *Am J Hum Genet* 63: 526-533

31. Hoffbuhr KC, Davidson E, Filiano BA, Davidson M, Kennaway NG, King MP (2000) A pathogenic 15-base pair deletion in mitochondrial DNA-encoded cytochrome c oxidase subunit III results in the absence of functional cytochrome c oxidase. *J Biol Chem* 275: 13994-14003

32. Holt IJ, Harding AE, Cooper JM, Schapira AH, Toscano A, Clark JB, Morgan-Hughes JA (1989) Mitochondrial myopathies: clinical and biochemical features of 30 patients with major deletions of muscle mitochondrial DNA. *Ann Neurol* 26: 699-708

33. Holt IJ, Harding AE, Petty RK, Morgan-Hughes JA (1990) A new mitochondrial disease associated with mitochondrial DNA heteroplasmy. *Am J Hum Genet* 46: 428-433

34. Horvath R, Lochmuller H, Stucka R, Yao J, Shoubridge EA, Kim SH, Gerbitz KD, Jaksch M (2000) Characterization of human SCO1 and COX17 genes in mitochondrial cytochrome-c-oxidase deficiency. *Biochem Biophys Res Commun* 276: 530-533

35. Howell N, Bogolin C, Jamieson R, Marenda DR, Mackey DA (1998) mtDNA mutations that cause optic neuropathy: how do we know? *Am J Hum Genet* 62: 196-202

36. Inoue K, Nakada K, Ogura A, Isobe K, Goto Y, Nonaka I, Hayashi JI (2000) Generation of mice with mitochondrial dysfunction by introducing mouse mtDNA carrying a deletion into zygotes. *Nat Genet* 26: 176-181

36a. Jaksch M, Horvath r, Horn N, Auer DP, Macmillan C, Peters J, Gerbitz KD, Kraegeloh-Mann I, Muntau A, Karcagi V, Kalmanchey R, Lochmuller H, Shoubridge EA, Freisinger P (2001) Homozygosity (E140K) in SCO2 causes delayed infantile onset of cardiomyopathy and neuropathy. *Neurology* 57: 1440-1446

37. Jaksch M, Ogilvie I, Yao J, Kortenhaus G, Bresser HG, Gerbitz KD, Shoubridge EA (2000) Mutations in SCO2 are associated with a distinct form of hypertrophic cardiomyopathy and cytochrome c oxidase deficiency. *Hum Mol Genet* 9: 795-801

38. Jenuth JP, Peterson AC, Fu K, Shoubridge EA (1996) Random genetic drift in the female germline explains the rapid segregation of mammalian mitochondrial DNA. *Nat Genet* 14: 146-151

39. Kadowaki H, Tobe K, Mori Y, Sakura H, Sakuta R, Nonaka I, Hagura R, Yazaki Y, Akanuma Y, Kadowaki T (1993) Mitochondrial gene mutation and insulin-deficient type of diabetes mellitus. *Lancet* 341: 893-894

40. Kaneda H, Hayashi J, Takahama S, Taya C, Lindahl KF, Yonekawa H (1995) Elimination of paternal mitochondrial DNA in intraspecific crosses during early mouse embryogenesis. *Proc Natl Acad Sci U S A* 92: 4542-45426

41. Karadimas CL, Greenstein P, Sue CM, Joseph JT, Tanji K, Haller RG, Taivassalo T, Davidson MM, Shanske S, Bonilla E, DiMauro S (20 0) Recurrent myoglobinuria due to a nonsense mutation in the COX I gene of mitochondrial DNA. *Neurology* 55: 644-649

42. Kaufman BA, Newman SM, Hallberg RL, Slaughter CA, Perlman PS, Butow RA (2000) In organello formaldehyde crosslinking of proteins to mtDNA: identification of bifunctional proteins. *Proc Natl Acad Sci U S A* 97: 7772-7777

43. Kaukonen J, Juselius JK, Tiranti V, Kyttala A, Zeviani M, Comi GP, Keranen S, Peltonen L, Suomalainen A (2000) Role of adenine nucleotide translocator 1 in mtDNA maintenance. *Science* 289: 782-785

44. Kaukonen J, Zeviani M, Comi GP, Piscaglia MG, Peltonen L, Suomalainen A (1999) A third locus predisposing to multiple deletions of mtDNA in autosomal dominant progressive external ophthalmoplegia. *Am J Hum Genet* 65: 256-261

45. Keightley JA, Hoffbuhr KC, Burton MD, Salas VM, Johnston WS, Penn AM, Buist NR, Kennaway NG (1996) A microdeletion in cytochrome c oxidase (COX) subunit III associated with COX deficiency and recurrent myoglobinuria. *Nat Genet* 12: 410-416

46. Larsson NG, Holme E, Kristiansson B, Oldfors A, Tulinius M (1990) Progressive increase of the mutated mitochondrial DNA fraction in Kearns-Sayre syndrome. *Pediatr Res* 28: 131-136

47. Lee N, Daly MJ, Delmonte T, Lander ES, Xu F, Hudson TJ, Mitchell GA, Morin CC, Robinson BH, Rioux JD (2001) A genomewide linkage-disequilibrium scan localizes the Saguenay-Lac- Saint-Jean cytochrome oxidase deficiency to 2p16. *Am J Hum Genet* 68: 397-409.

48. Macmillan CJ, Shoubridge EA (1996) Mitochondrial DNA depletion: prevalence in a pediatric population referred for neurologic evaluation. *Pediatr Neurol* 14: 203-210

49. Manfredi G, Schon EA, Moraes CT, Bonilla E, Berry GT, Sladky JT, DiMauro S (1995) A new mutation associated with MELAS is located in a mitochondrial DNA polypeptide-coding gene. *Neuromuscul Disord* 5: 391-398

50. McShane MA, Hammans SR, Sweeney M, Holt IJ, Beattie TJ, Brett EM, Harding AE (1991) Pearson syndrome and mitochondrial encephalomyopathy in a patient with a deletion of mtDNA. *Am J Hum Genet* 48: 39-42

51. Michaels GS, Hauswirth WW, Laipis PJ (1982) Mitochondrial DNA copy number in bovine oocytes and somatic cells. *Dev Biol* 94: 246-251

52. Moraes CT, Ciacci F, Silvestri G, Shanske S, Sciacco M, Hirano M, Schon EA, Bonilla E, DiMauro S (1993) Atypical clinical presentations associated with the MELAS mutation at position 3243 of human mitochondrial DNA. *Neuromuscul Disord* 3: 43-50

53. Moraes CT, DiMauro S, Zeviani M, Lombes A, Shanske S, Miranda AF, Nakase H, Bonilla E, Werneck LC, Servidei S, et al. (1989) Mitochondrial DNA deletions in progressive external ophthalmoplegia and Kearns-Sayre syndrome. *N Engl J Med* 320: 1293-1299

54. Moraes CT, Shanske S, Tritschler HJ, Aprille JR, Andreetta F, Bonilla E, Schon EA, DiMauro S (1991) mtDNA depletion with variable tissue expression: a novel genetic abnormality in mitochondrial diseases. *Am J Hum Genet* 48: 492-501

55. Moslemi AR, Melberg A, Holme E, Oldfors A (1996) Clonal expansion of mitochondrial DNA with multiple deletions in autosomal dominant progressive external ophthalmoplegia. *Ann Neurol* 40: 707-713

56. Musumeci O, Andreu AL, Shanske S, Bresolin N, Comi GP, Rothstein R, Schon EA, DiMauro S (2000) Intragenic inversion of mtDNA: a new type of pathogenic mutation in a patient with mitochondrial myopathy. *Am J Hum Genet* 66: 1900-1904

57. Nass MM (1969) Mitochondrial DNA. I. Intramitochondrial distribution and structural relations of single- and double-length circular DNA. *J Mol Biol* 42: 521-528

58. Nijtmans LG, Henderson NS, Attardi G, Holt IJ (2001) Impaired ATP synthase assembly associated with a mutation in the human ATP synthase subunit 6 gene. *J Biol Chem* 276: 6755-6762

59. Nishino I, Spinazzola A, Hirano M (1999) Thymidine phosphorylase gene mutations in MNGIE, a human mitochondrial disorder. *Science* 283: 689-692

60. Papadopoulou LC, Sue CM, Davidson MM, Tanji K, Nishino I, Sadlock JE, Krishna S, Walker W, Selby J, Glerum DM, Coster RV, Lyon G, Scalais E, Lebel R, Kaplan P, Shanske S, De Vivo DC, Bonilla E, Hirano M,

DiMauro S, Schon EA (1999) Fatal infantile cardioencephalomyopathy with COX deficiency and mutations in SCO2, a COX assembly gene. *Nat Genet* 23: 333-337

61. Parfait B, Chretien D, Rotig A, Marsac C, Munnich A, Rustin P (2000) Compound heterozygous mutations in the flavoprotein gene of the respiratory chain complex II in a patient with Leigh syndrome. *Hum Genet* 106: 236-243

62. Piko L, Taylor KD (1987) Amounts of mitochondrial DNA and abundance of some mitochondrial gene transcripts in early mouse embryos. *Dev Biol* 123: 364-374

63. Polymeropoulos MH, Swift RG, Swift M (1994) Linkage of the gene for Wolfram syndrome to markers on the short arm of chromosome 4. *Nat Genet* 8: 95-97

64. Poulton J, Deadman ME, Bindoff L, Morten K, Land J, Brown G (1993) Families of mtDNA re-arrangements can be detected in patients with mtDNA deletions: duplications may be a transient intermediate form. *Hum Mol Genet* 2: 23-30

65. Poulton J, Deadman ME, Gardiner RM (1989) Tandem direct duplications of mitochondrial DNA in mitochondrial myopathy: analysis of nucleotide sequence and tissue distribution. *Nucleic Acids Res* 17: 10223-10229

66. Prezant TR, Agapian JV, Bohlman MC, Bu X, Oztas S, Qiu WQ, Arnos KS, Cortopassi GA, Jaber L, Rotter JI, et al. (1993) Mitochondrial ribosomal RNA mutation associated with both antibiotic- induced and non-syndromic deafness. *Nat Genet* 4: 289-294

67. Rahman S, Taanman JW, Cooper JM, Nelson I, Hargreaves I, Meunier B, Hanna MG, Garcia JJ, Capaldi RA, Lake BD, Leonard JV, Schapira AH (1999) A missense mutation of cytochrome oxidase subunit II causes defective assembly and myopathy. *Am J Hum Genet* 65: 1030-1039

68. Rotig A, Bourgeron T, Chretien D, Rustin P, Munnich A (1995) Spectrum of mitochondrial DNA rearrangements in the Pearson marrow- pancreas syndrome. *Hum Mol Genet* 4: 1327-1330

69. Rotig A, Cormier V, Chatelain P, Francois R, Saudubray JM, Rustin P, Munnich A (1993) Deletion of mitochondrial DNA in a case of early-onset diabetes mellitus, optic atrophy and deafness (DIDMOAD, Wolfram syndrome). *J Inherit Metab Dis* 16: 527-530

70. Rotig A, Cormier V, Koll F, Mize CE, Saudubray JM, Veerman A, Pearson HA, Munnich A (1991) Site-specific deletions of the mitochondrial genome in the Pearson marrow-pancreas syndrome. *Genomics* 10: 502-504

71. Rotig A, de Lonlay P, Chretien D, Foury F, Koenig M, Sidi D, Munnich A, Rustin P (1997) Aconitase and mitochondrial iron-sulphur protein deficiency in Friedreich ataxia. *Nat Genet* 17: 215-217

72. Rustin P, von Kleist-Retzow JC, Chantrel-Groussard K, Sidi D, Munnich A, Rotig A (1999) Effect of idebenone on cardiomyopathy in Friedreich's ataxia: a preliminary study. *Lancet* 354: 477-479

73. Satoh M, Kuroiwa T (1991) Organization of multiple nucleoids and DNA molecules in mitochondria of a human cell. *Exp Cell Res* 196: 137-140

74. Schon EA, Rizzuto R, Moraes CT, Nakase H, Zeviani M, DiMauro S (1989) A direct repeat is a hotspot for large-scale deletion of human mitochondrial DNA. *Science* 244: 346-349

75. Shoffner JM, Lott MT, Lezza AM, Seibel P, Ballinger SW, Wallace DC (1990) Myoclonic epilepsy and ragged-red fiber disease (MERRF) is associated with a mitochondrial DNA tRNA(Lys) mutation. *Cell* 61: 931-937

76. Shoubridge EA, Karpati G, Hastings KE (1990) Deletion mutants are functionally dominant over wild-type mitochondrial genomes in skeletal muscle fiber segments in mitochondrial disease. *Cell* 62: 43-49

77. Silvestri G, Moraes CT, Shanske S, Oh SJ, DiMauro S (1992) A new mtDNA mutation in the tRNA(Lys) gene associated with myoclonic epilepsy and ragged-red fibers (MERRF). *Am J Hum Genet* 51: 1213-1217

78. Silvestri G, Santorelli FM, Shanske S, Whitley CB, Schimmenti LA, Smith SA, DiMauro S (1994) A new mtDNA mutation in the tRNA(Leu(UUR)) gene associated with maternally inherited cardiomyopathy. *Hum Mutat* 3: 37-43

78a. Spelbrink JN, Li FY, Tiranti V, Nikali K, Yuan QP, Tariq M, Wanrooij S, Garrido N, Comi G, Morandi L, Santoro L, Toscano A, Fabrizi GM, Somer H, Crozen R, Beeson D, Poulton J, Suomalainen A, Jacobs HT, Zeviani M, Larsson C (2001) Human mitochondrial DNA deletions associated with mutations in the gene encoding Twinkle, a phage T7 gene 4-like protein localized in mitochondria. *Nat Genet* 28: 223-231

79. Spelbrink JN, Van Galen MJ, Zwart R, Bakker HD, Rovio A, Jacobs HT, Van den Bogert C (1998) Familial mitochondrial DNA depletion in liver: haplotype analysis of candidate genes. *Hum Genet* 102: 327-331

80. Strom TM, Hortnagel K, Hofmann S, Gekeler F, Scharfe C, Rabl W, Gerbitz KD, Meitinger T (1998) Diabetes insipidus, diabetes mellitus, optic atrophy and deafness (DIDMOAD) caused by mutations in a novel gene (wolframin) coding for a predicted transmembrane protein. *Hum Mol Genet* 7: 2021-2028

81. Suomalainen A, Kaukonen J, Amati P, Timonen R, Haltia M, Weissenbach J, Zeviani M, Somer H, Peltonen L (1995) An autosomal locus predisposing to deletions of mitochondrial DNA. *Nat Genet* 9: 146-151

82. Suomalainen A, Majander A, Wallin M, Setala K, Kontula K, Leinonen H, Salmi T, Paetau A, Haltia M, Valanne L, Lonnqvist J, Peltonen L, Somer H (1997) Autosomal dominant progressive external ophthalmoplegia with multiple deletions of mtDNA: clinical, biochemical, and molecular genetic features of the 10q-linked disease. *Neurology* 48: 1244-1253

83. Sutovsky P, Moreno RD, Ramalho-Santos J, Dominko T, Simerly C, Schatten G (1999) Ubiquitin tag for sperm mitochondria. *Nature* 402: 371-372

84. Sutovsky P, Moreno RD, Ramalho-Santos J, Dominko T, Simerly C, Schatten G (2000) Ubiquitinated sperm mitochondria, selective proteolysis, and the regulation of mitochondrial inheritance in mammalian embryos. *Biol Reprod* 63: 582-590

85. Taivassalo T, De Stefano N, Argov Z, Matthews PM, Chen J, Genge A, Karpati G, Arnold DL (1998) Effects of aerobic training in patients with mitochondrial myopathies. *Neurology* 50: 1055-1060

86. Taivassalo T, Fu K, Johns T, Arnold D, Karpati G, Shoubridge EA (1999) Gene shifting: a novel therapy for mitochondrial myopathy. *Hum Mol Genet* 8: 1047-1052

87. Takeda K, Inoue H, Tanizawa Y, Matsuzaki Y, Oba J, Watanabe Y, Shinoda K, Oka Y (2001) WFS1 (Wolfram syndrome 1) gene product: predominant subcellular localization to endoplasmic reticulum in cultured cells and neuronal expression in rat brain. *Hum Mol Genet* 10: 477-484

88. Tatuch Y, Christodoulou J, Feigenbaum A, Clarke JT, Wherret J, Smith C, Rudd N, Petrova-Benedict R, Robinson BH (1992) Heteroplasmic mtDNA mutation (T----G) at 8993 can cause Leigh disease when the percentage of abnormal mtDNA is high. *Am J Hum Genet* 50: 852-858

89. Tatuch Y, Robinson BH (1993) The mitochondrial DNA mutation at 8993 associated with NARP slows the rate of ATP synthesis in isolated lymphoblast mitochondria. *Biochem Biophys Res Commun* 192: 124-128

90. Tiranti V, Corona P, Greco M, Taanman JW, Carrara F, Lamantea E, Nijtmans L, Uziel G, Zeviani M (2000) A novel frameshift mutation of the mtDNA COIII gene leads to impaired assembly of cytochrome c oxidase in a patient affected by Leigh-like syndrome. *Hum Mol Genet* 9: 2733-2742

91. Tiranti V, Galimberti C, Nijtmans L, Bovolenta S, Perini MP, Zeviani M (1999) Characterization of SURF-1 expression and Surf-1p function in normal and disease conditions. *Hum Mol Genet* 8: 2533-2540

92. Tiranti V, Hoertnagel K, Carrozzo R, Galimberti C, Munaro M, Granatiero M, Zelante L, Gasparini P, Marzella R, Rocchi M, Bayona-Bafaluy MP, Enriquez JA, Uziel G, Bertini E, Dionisi-Vici C, Franco B, Meitinger T, Zeviani M (1998) Mutations of SURF-1 in Leigh disease associated with cytochrome c oxidase deficiency. *Am J Hum Genet* 63: 1609-1621

93. Triepels RH, Van Den Heuvel LP, Trijbels JM, Smeitink JA (2001) Respiratory chain complex I deficiency. *Am J Med Genet* 106: 37-45

93a. Van Goethern G, Dermaut B, Lofgren A, Martin JJ, Van Broeckhoven C (2001) Mutation of POLG is associated with progressive external opthalmoplegia characterized by mtDNA deletions. *Nat Genet* 28: 211-212

94. Wallace DC, Singh G, Lott MT, Hodge JA, Schurr TG, Lezza AM, Elsas LJ, 2nd, Nikoskelainen EK (1988) Mitochondrial DNA mutation associated with Leber's hereditary optic neuropathy. *Science* 242: 1427-1430

95. Yao J, Shoubridge EA (1999) Expression and functional analysis of SURF1 in Leigh syndrome patients with cytochrome c oxidase deficiency. *Hum Mol Genet* 8: 2541-2549

96. Zeviani M, Gellera C, Antozzi C, Rimoldi M, Morandi L, Villani F, Tiranti V, DiDonato S (1991) Maternally inherited myopathy and cardiomyopathy: association with mutation in mitochondrial DNA tRNA(Leu)(UUR). *Lancet* 338: 143-147

97. Zeviani M, Servidei S, Gellera C, Bertini E, DiMauro S, DiDonato S (1989) An autosomal dominant disorder with multiple deletions of mitochondrial DNA starting at the D-loop region. *Nature* 339: 309-311

98. Zhu Z, Yao J, Johns T, Fu K, De Bie I, Macmillan C, Cuthbert AP, Newbold RF, Wang J, Chevrette M, Brown GK, Brown RM, Shoubridge EA (1998) SURF1, encoding a factor involved in the biogenesis of cytochrome c oxidase, is mutated in Leigh syndrome. *Nat Genet* 20: 337-343

Myoadenylate deaminase deficiency

Richard L. Sabina

AMPD	AMP deaminase
mAMPD	myoadenylate deaminase

Definition of entities

Myoadenylate deaminase (mAMPD) deficiency is a common skeletal muscle disorder of purine nucleotide metabolism with a heterogeneous clinical presentation (8). mAMPD deficiency is divided into four groups: symptomatic inherited, asymptotic inherited, coincidental inherited, and acquired (Table 1). Symptomatic inherited deficiency is associated with exercise intolerance accompanied by aches and cramping. Asymptotic inherited deficiency represents the largest cohort of this inborn error of metabolism. It is unclear whether these individuals are at risk of developing exercise-induced myalgia. Coincidental inherited and acquired deficiencies differ in molecular background, yet share the feature of being secondary to a wide array of other disorders that typically dictate clinical presentation. Whether the enzyme deficiency affects clinical outcome in these two classes of individuals is uncertain. However, symptoms more severe than either condition alone have been reported in several cases of coincidental inherited deficiency where the associated disorder is another inborn error of energy metabolism (10).

Molecular genetics and pathogenesis

Human tissues and cells produce AMP deaminase isoforms through the regulated expression of a multigene family (8). As summarized in Table 2, the *AMPD1* gene encodes isoform M (mAMPD) and is expressed predominantly in skeletal muscle. The *AMPD2* and *AMPD3* genes encode isoforms L and E, respectively, and are widely expressed. In skeletal muscle, mAMPD is most abundant in type 2 (glycolytic) fibres; isoform E is found in smooth muscle cells, type 1 (oxidative) fibres, and nerve bundles; and isoform L is present only in nonmyocyte elements of this tissue (4).

AMPD1 gene mutations (Table 2) are solely (all inherited deficiencies) or partially (acquired deficiency) responsible for mAMPD deficiency. Typically, loss of enzyme activity can be attributed to a single mutant allele characterised by double transitions at nucleotides +34 in exon 2 and +143 in exon 3 (6). The upstream mutation introduces a premature stop codon (Q12X) into AMPD1 mRNA. Consequently, a severely truncated and dysfunctional polypeptide is encoded by this mutant allele. The downstream mutation introduces a P48L substitution into the mAMPD polypeptide, but this occurs only when exon 2-encoded sequence is removed by an alternative splicing event in 0.6 to 2% of *AMPD1*

Groups	Presentation	AMPD1 genotype
Symptomatic inherited	Exercise-induced aches and cramping	Mutant homozygote or rare compound heterozygote
Asymptotic inherited	No clinical complaints	Same as "Symptomatic inherited"
Coincidental inherited	Variable, more severe neuromuscular symptoms	Same as "Symptomatic inherited"
Acquired	Variable, more severe neuromuscular symptoms	Heterozygote (pathology due to associated disorder further reduces enzyme activity into the deficient range.

Table 1. Classification of myoadenylate deaminase deficiency.

Gene	Isoform	Inherited defects	Expression
AMPD1 (myoadenylate deaminase)	M	C34T/C143T (Q12X/P48L) (COMMON-Caucasian and African-American) G468T (Q156H (Rare-Caucasian) C1165T (R388W) (Rare-Japanese) C1277T (R425H) (Rare-Japanese)	Restricted Skeletal muscle: Type 2 fibres Type 1 fibres
AMPD2	L	None identified	Widespread Skeletal muscle: Nerve bundles Smooth muscle Endothelial cells
AMPD3	E	C1717T (R573C) (Japanese) G931C (V311L) (Caucasian) Other rare mutations (Japanese)	Widespread Skeletal muscle: Smooth muscle Type 1 fibres Nerve bundles

Table 2. Molecular basis and identified mutations of AMP deaminase expression.

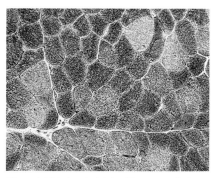

Figure 1. Histochemical stain of frozen muscle tissue for myoadenylate deaminase activity. Control tissue showing the normal intense blue staining of both fibre types. Photographs courtesy of Susan K. Danielson MS, Dept. Neurology, Medical College of Wisconsin, Milwaukee, WI, USA.

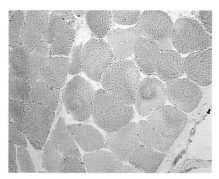

Figure 2. Same staining as in Figure 1 from a patient with deficiency of myoadenylate deaminase. The blue staining seen in the control is lacking. Magnification, ×100.

mRNAs (5). Estimated frequencies of this common mutant allele are 0.10 to 0.14 (3, 6, 7) in Caucasians and 0.19 in African-Americans (6). Consequently, nearly 1 in 4 individuals is a carrier of an inherited deficiency and approximately 2% are mutant homozygotes. The common *AMPD1* mutant allele is not found in the Japanese population, although rare mutations have been identified in one family (1).

Structural changes

An inherited deficiency alone is not associated with structural changes in skeletal muscle. However, coincidental inherited and acquired deficiencies can present with a variety of structural alterations, but these are typical of the associated disorder. Histochemistry can be used to demonstrate absence of myoadenylate deaminase activity compared with that in normal muscle tissue (Figures 1, 2).

Future perspectives

Future studies of mAMPD deficiency should address the following:

i) Molecular distinctions between symptomatic and asymptotic inherited deficiency. Potential determinants include individual variations in alternative splicing of AMPD1 transcripts and AMPD3 gene expression, both of which are dependent on fibre-type composition of muscle. Also, AMPD3 gene mutations responsible for an erythrocyte enzyme deficiency (11, 12) should also be considered in context with the skeletal muscle disorder.

ii) Comparative functional characterizations of *a)* asymptotic and symptomatic inherited mAMPD deficiency, and *b)* combined inherited deficiencies of mAMPD and other inborn errors of energy metabolism ("double trouble") and individuals with either defect alone.

iii) Documentation of an acquired deficiency by complete sequencing of both alleles to rule out a compound heterozygous genotype involving rare mutations (2, 9)

References

1. Abe M, Higuchi I, Morisaki H, Morisaki T, Osame M (2000) Myoadenylate deaminase deficiency with progressive muscle weakness and atrophy caused by new missense mutations in AMPD1 gene: case report in a Japanese patient. *Neuromuscul Disord* 10: 472-477

2. Fishbein WN (1999) Primary, secondary, and coincidental types of myoadenylate deaminase deficiency. *Ann Neurol* 45: 547-548

3. Gross M (1997) Clinical heterogeneity and molecular mechanisms in inborn muscle AMP deaminase deficiency. *J Inherit Metab Dis* 20: 186-192

4. Kuppevelt THV, Veerkamp JH, Fishbein WN, Ogasawara N, Sabina RL (1994) Immunolocalization of AMP-deaminase isozymes in human skeletal muscle and cultured muscle cells: concentration of isoform M at the neuromuscular junction. *J Histochem Cytochem* 42: 861-868

5. Morisaki H, Morisaki T, Newby LK, Holmes EW (1993) Alternative splicing: a mechanism for phenotypic rescue of a common inherited defect. *J Clin Invest* 91: 2275-2280

6. Morisaki T, Gross M, Morisaki H, Pongratz D, Zollner N, Holmes EW (1992) Molecular basis of AMP deaminase deficiency in skeletal muscle. *Proc Natl Acad Sci USA* 89: 6457-6461

7. Norman B, Mahnke-Zizelman DK, Vallis A, Sabina RL (1998) Genetic and other determinants of AMP deaminase activity in healthy adult skeletal muscle. *J Appl Physiol* 85: 1273-1278

8. Sabina RL, Holmes EW (2001) Myoadenylate deaminase deficiency. In *The Metabolic and Molecular Bases of Inherited Disease*, C Scriver, AL Beaudet, WS Sly, D Valle (eds). McGraw-Hill: New York. pp. 2627-2638

9. Verzijl HTFM, Engelen BGM, Luyten JAFM, Steenbergen GCH, Heuvel LPWJ, Laak HJt, Padberg GW, Wevers RA (1999) Primary, secondary, and coincidental types of myoadenylate deaminase deficiency. *Ann Neurol* 45: 548

10. Vladutiu GD (2000) Complex phenotypes in metabolic muscle diseases. *Muscle Nerve* 23: 1157-1159

11. Yamada Y, Goto H, Murase T, Ogasawara N (1994) Molecular basis for human erythrocyte AMP deaminase deficiency: screening for the major point mutation and identification of other mutations. *Hum Mol Genet* 3: 2243-2245

12. Yamada Y, Makarewicz W, Goto H, Nomura N, Kitoh H, Ogasawara N (1998) Gene mutations responsible for human erythrocyte AMP deaminase deficiency in Poles. *Adv Exp Med Biol* 431: 347-350

CHAPTER 11

Dysimmune and infectious myopathies

11.1 Dysimmune myopathies. Definition of entities and experimental models of myositis   218

11.2 Polymyositis and dermatomyositis   221

11.3 Inclusion body myositis   228

11.4 Viral myositis   231

11.5 Bacterial myositis   236

11.6 Fungal, protozoal and other parasitic infections   238

Inflammatory myopathies constitute the largest group of acquired skeletal muscle diseases. To a large extent, the immunopathological basis of these myopathies has been elucidated. This includes the identification of the target cell in muscle (muscle fibres vs vascular endothelium), the predominant dysimmune process (humoral vs cellular or mixed), and the immunocytochemical features, ie, types of inflammatory cells, and the prevalent cytokine or chemokine profile. Detailed knowledge of these items will hopefully permit the development of effective and specific immunotherapies even without identification of the primary offending antigen.

Infectious agents rarely cause skeletal muscle disease. However, they are still important entities in this group. The inflammatory myopathy occurring in AIDS caused by the *human immunodeficiency virus* is one such entity. The acute, potentially fatal necrotizing myopathy caused by a particularly virulent β *hemolytic streptococcus* infection of muscle ("flesh-eating disease") is another important example. More traditional acute inflammatory myopathies, eg, the one caused by *trichinella spiralis*, have diminishing practical importance because of awareness of the preventable source of the infection.

Dysimmune myopathies. Definition of entities and experimental models of myositis

Reinhard Hohlfeld

CTL	cytotoxic T-lymphocyte
DM	dermatomyositis
IBM	inclusion-body myositis
ICAM	intercellular adhesion molecule
LFA	lymphocyte function-associated molecule
MMF	macrophage myofasciitis
N-CAM	neural cell adhesion molecule
NK	natural killer
PM	polymyositis
TNF-α	tumor necrosis factor α

Definition of entities

The dysimmune myopathies are sometimes referred to as "idiopathic inflammatory myopathies," a somewhat misleading term. This heterogeneous group of diseases traditionally includes different forms of polymyositis (PM), dermatomyositis (DM), and inclusion-body myositis (IBM) (1, 8, 11, 18, 21, 22). It is presently thought that in principle, PM is a T-cell mediated disorder, whereas DM is an antibody-mediated vascular disorder. In contrast, the inflammatory changes of IBM are probably secondary to an unknown primary process (degenerative, metabolic, infectious, or other) (1).

The classical triad of PM, DM, and IBM are not the only myopathies that have a conspicuous inflammatory component. For example, inflammation may occur in response to degenerative changes in some of the hereditary myopathies. Notable examples include Duchenne muscular dystrophy, facioscapulohumeral muscular dystrophy (29) and some dysferlinopathies (26).

Muscle inflammation may also occur as a local or generalized response to toxic agents. An interesting example is macrophagic myofasciitis (MMF), a new type of inflammatory myopathy, which was recognized as an unusual reaction to intramuscular injection of aluminium-containing vaccines (5). The main presenting symptom of MMF is diffuse muscle pain and arthralgia. Muscle weakness and fever occur less frequently. MMF is characterised by accumulations of tightly packed macrophages in epi-, peri-, and endomysium. The macrophages contain aluminium inclusions. Aluminium is used as an adjuvant in vaccines against HBV, hepatitis A and tetanus toxoid. Interestingly, MMF may be associated with an inflammatory CNS disease resembling multiple sclerosis, and perhaps with other autoimmune disorders (2)

This chapter concerns in vitro and in vivo models of myositis. The different inflammatory myopathies are presented in chapters 11.2-11.3 with emphasis on their pathophysiology and morphological features.

Experimental models of myositis

Cultured myoblasts and in vitro models. Numerous studies have shown that cultured myoblasts can express a variety of immunologically important molecules (Table 1). Furthermore, myoblasts express a surprising number of cytokines and chemokines (19). For this and other reasons, it seems likely that in myositis, muscle cells play an active immunological role in the affected tissue (18). Myoblasts are extremely useful for functional studies of various aspects of the pathogenesis of myositis. For example, cultured human myoblasts can serve as targets for cytotoxic CD8+ T cells and other cytotoxic effector cells. Perhaps even more interesting, myoblasts can present antigens to CD4+ T cells (14).

Human myoblasts (myogenic stem cells) can be isolated and purified from muscle biopsy specimens and expanded in culture (14). In contrast to fibroblasts, myoblasts express the cytoskeletal protein desmin and the neural cell adhesion molecule N-CAM (CD56/Leu 19/NKH-1) (18). Myoblasts constitutively express HLA class I antigens and a low level of lymphocyte function-associated (LFA-) molecule 3 (LFA-3, CD58). Tumor necrosis factor (TNF)-α, a cytokine secreted by macrophages, T cells, and NK cells

Surface antigen	Constitutive expression	IFN-γ-stimulated expression
Differentiation ag		
NCAM-1 (CD56)	+	+
HLA-molecules		
Classical HLA class I	(+)	+
HLA-DR	-	+
HLA-DP	-	+
HLA-DQ	-	(+)
HLA-G	-	+
Adhesion molecules		
ICAM-1 (CD54)	-	+
LFA-3 (CD58)	(+)	(+)
Costimulatory molecules		
B7.1 (CD80)	-	-
B7.2 (CD86)	-	-
CD40	+	+

Table 1. Immunological properties of human myoblasts. Based on the following reports: (14, 15, 27, 38).

induces myoblasts to express the inter-cellular adhesion molecule-1 (ICAM-1, CD54) (14). Gamma-interferon, a cytokine secreted by T cells and natural killer cells, induces myoblasts to express HLA-DR and ICAM-1 (14, 15, 23). HLA-DP and HLA-DQ are also inducible by gamma-interferon, but the kinetics of induction and the levels of expression vary with the different HLA class II molecules (14).

Cultured myotubes and myoblasts express HLA class I molecules. This qualifies them as potential targets of CD8+ cytotoxic T-lymphocytes (CTL). Lysis of myotubes by CTL was shown in different experimental situations. On the one hand myotubes were lysed by allogeneic CD8+ CTL lines raised against the allogeneic HLA antigens expressed by the myotubes (16). Autologous control myotubes were not lysed. Lysis involved the recognition of allogeneic class I HLA antigens since it was completely blocked by a mono-clonal antibody against a monomorphic determinant of HLA class I (16). Fur-thermore, myotubes were lysed by autologous polyclonal CD8+ T cell lines directly expanded from muscle of patients with different inflammatory myopathies (17). The results obtained in this model system clearly establish that cultured myotubes are fully sus-ceptible to HLA-class I restricted lysis by CD8+ CTL. The autoreactive myocytotoxicity is consistent with the hypothesis that some of the CTL isolat-ed from muscle recognise the same antigen on myotubes in vitro that they recognize on muscle fibres in vivo.

Antigen presentation to CD4+ T cells depends on the constitutive or induced expression of HLA class II on the presenting cell. Myoblasts can be induced to express HLA class II by gamma-interferon (15, 23). Highly purified human myoblasts were tested for their ability to present various pro-tein antigens to autologous CD4+ T cell lines specific for tuberculin, tetanus toxoid or myelin basic protein (14). Non-induced myoblasts, or myoblasts treated with TNF-α alone, could not present any of these antigens

to T cells. However, gamma-interferon-treated myo-blasts induced antigen spe-cific T cell proliferation and were killed by the T cells only in the presence of the relevant antigen (14). Antigen spe-cific lysis was reduced to background level by adding the anti-HLA-DR mon-oclonal antibody L-243. These results suggest that HLA class II-positive human myoblasts can act as facultative local antigen presenting cells in muscle by providing the signals necessary to trigger both antigen specific lysis and T cell proliferation. In addition to presen-tation of exogenous antigens processed in the classical MHC class II-restricted pathway, human myoblasts seem to be capable of presenting endogenous anti-gen to MHC class II restricted CD4+ T cells (6).

It is clear from these studies that myoblasts have more than sufficient immunological "potential" to qualify them for local (re)stimulation of mem-ory and effector T cells. It is not clear, however, to what extent myoblasts can stimulate naive (unprimed T cells). Myoblasts do not express the classical co-stimulatory molecules B7.1 (CD80) and B7.2 (CD86) (3), but they do express CD40, another important co-stimulatory molecule (3, 33). Further-more, a subpopulation of myoblasts express BB-1, a B7-related molecule that has not been molecularly defined (3). The presence of these co-stimulato-ry molecules further emphasizes the important immunological role of myoblasts.

In addition to the classical MHC class I molecules (HLA-A, -B, and -C), myoblasts can be induced to express the non-classical HLA-G (38). HLA-G expression was first observed in cytotrophoblasts of the human placen-ta, and the function of HLA-G is not yet known. Like the classical HLA class I molecules, HLA-G binds anti-genic peptides and CD8. Therefore, it should be capable of presenting anti-genic peptides to T cells in a way simi-lar to the classical HLA class I mole-cules. This raises the possibility that in polymyositis, some of the autoaggres-sive T cells recognize their antigen in

the molecular context of HLA-G. In addition, HLA-G interacts with differ-ent receptors expressed on various types of lymphocytes, monocytes, and dendritic cells. It is thought that the recognition of HLA-G induces immunoregulatory functions in these cells, raising the possibility that HLA-G protects muscle fibres from attack by certain types of immune cells, eg, natu-ral killer cells.

Animal models of myositis. Inflam-matory and necrotising lesions of mus-cle were experimentally induced in var-ious animal species by the injection of Freund's complete adjuvant and homogenates of muscle or muscle pro-tein preparations (7, 9, 10, 12, 13, 28, 34, 36, 37). The majority of these mod-els show only limited resemblance to human polymyositis. The pathological changes in muscle consist of necrotic and regenerating fibres and mononu-clear infiltrates in the perimysium and endomysium, particularly at perivascu-lar sites. In some studies the changes of experimental myositis were transferred with lymphocytes or serum. These early experiments were conducted when little or nothing was known about the mechanisms of antigen recognition and cytotoxicity. Their relevance to the pathogenesis of any human inflamma-tory muscle disease is uncertain.

Several reports described the induc-tion of myositis in the SJL mouse (24, 25, 31, 32). The problem with this "SJL model of myositis" is that SJL/J mice spontaneously develop a necrotising myopathy (20). This myopathy is caused by a deletion in the dysferlin gene, defining a natural model for limb girdle muscular dystrophy (4, 35). Inflammatory changes are not uncom-mon in some human hereditary myopathies and muscular dystrophies, including Duchenne muscular dystro-phy, facioscapulohumoral muscular dystrophy and dysferlinopathies. One important lesson from these observa-tions is that in any myopathy, the pres-ence of inflammatory changes does not necessarily imply an (auto)immune pathogenesis but may be secondary to a metabolic or genetic defect.

A novel transgenic mouse model of myositis was recently described (30). The authors used a controllable muscle-specific promoter system to up-regulate MHC class I expression in skeletal muscles of mice. The transgenic mice developed an inflammatory myopathy accompanied by autoantibodies against histidyl-tRNA synthetase, the most commonly observed antibody specificity in human myositis (30). This model indicates that the sustained upregulation of MHC class I antigen in a tissue that is normally essentially devoid of MHC class I may be sufficient to induce T-cell and antibody responses to antigens expressed in the target tissue.

References

1. Askanas V, Engel WK (2001) Inclusion-body myositis: newest concepts of pathogenesis and relation to aging and Alzheimer disease. *J Neuropathol Exp Neurol* 60: 1-14.

2. Authier FJ, Cherin P, Creange A, Bonnotte B, Ferrer X, Abdelmoumni A, Ranoux D, Pelletier J, Figarella-Branger D, Granel B, Maisonobe T, Coquet M, Degos JD, Gherardi RK (2001) Central nervous system disease in patients with macrophagic myofasciitis. *Brain* 124: 974-983.

3. Behrens L, Kerschensteiner M, Misgeld T, Goebels N, Wekerle H, Hohlfeld R (1998) Human muscle cells express a functional costimulatory molecule distinct from B7.1 (CD80) and B7.2 (CD86) *in vitro* and in inflammatory lesions. *J Immunol* 161: 5943-5951.

4. Bittner RE, Anderson LV, Burkhardt E, Bashir R, Vafiadaki E, Ivanova S, Raffelsberger T, Maerk I, Hoger H, Jung M, Karbasiyan M, Storch M, Lassmann H, Moss JA, Davison K, Harrison R, Bushby KM, Reis A (1999) Dysferlin deletion in SJL mice (SJL-Dysf) defines a natural model for limb girdle muscular dystrophy 2B. *Nat Genet* 23: 141-142.

5. Cherin P, Gherardi RK (2000) Macrophagic myofasciitis. *Curr Rheumatol Rep* 2: 196-200.

6. Curnow J, Corlett L, Willcox N, Vincent A (2001) Presentation by myoblasts of an epitope from endogenous acetylcholine receptor indicates a potential role in the spreading of the immune response. *J Neuroimmunol* 115: 127-134.

7. Currie S (1971) Experimental myositis: the *in vivo* and *in vitro* activity of lymph-node cells. *J Pathol* 105: 169-185.

8. Dalakas MC, Sivakumar K (1996) The immunopathologic and inflammatory differences between dermatomyositis, polymyositis and sporadic inclusion body myositis. *Curr Opin Neurol* 9: 235-239.

9. Dawkins RL (1965) Experimental myositis associated with hypersensitivity to muscle. *J Pathol Bacteriol* 90: 619-625.

10. Dawkins RL (1975) Experimental autoallergic myositis, polymyositis and myasthenia gravis. Autoimmune muscle disease associated with immunodeficiency and neoplasia. *Clin Exp Immunol* 21: 185-201.

11. Engel AG, Hohlfeld R, Banker BQ (1994) The polymyositis and dermatomyositis syndromes. In *Myology*, AG Engel, C Franzini-Armstrong (eds). McGraw Hill: New York. pp. 1335-1383

12. Esiri MM, MacLennan IC (1974) Experimental myositis in rats. I. Histological and creatine phosphokinase changes, and passive transfer to normal syngeneic rats. *Clin Exp Immunol* 17: 139-150.

13. Esiri MM, MacLennan IC (1975) Experimental myositis in rats. II. The sensitivity of spleen cells to syngeneic muscle antigen. *Clin Exp Immunol* 19: 513-520.

14. Goebels N, Michaelis D, Wekerle H, Hohlfeld R (1992) Human myoblasts as antigen-presenting cells. *J Immunol* 149: 661-667.

15. Hohlfeld R, Engel AG (1990a) Induction of HLA-DR expression on human myoblasts with interferon-gamma. *Am J Pathol* 136: 503-508.

16. Hohlfeld R, Engel AG (1990b) Lysis of myotubes by alloreactive cytotoxic T cells and natural killer cells. Relevance to myoblast transplantation. *J Clin Invest* 86: 370-374.

17. Hohlfeld R, Engel AG (1991) Coculture with autologous myotubes of cytotoxic T cells isolated from muscle in inflammatory myopathies. *Ann Neurol* 29: 498-507.

18. Hohlfeld R, Engel AG (1994) The immunobiology of muscle. *Immunol Today* 15: 269-274.

19. Hohlfeld R, Engel AG, Goebels N, Behrens L (1997) Cellular immune mechanisms in inflammatory myopathies. *Curr Opin Rheumatol* 9: 520-526

20. Hohlfeld R, Muller W, Toyka KV (1988) Necrotizing myopathy in SJL mice. *Muscle Nerve* 11: 184-185.

21. Karpati G, Carpenter S (1993) Pathology of the inflammatory myopathies. In *Baillière's Clinical Neurology*, M FL (eds). Baillière Tindal: London, U. pp. 527-556

22. Mantegazza R, Bernasconi P, Confalonieri P, Cornelio F (1997) Inflammatory myopathies and systemic disorders: a review of immunopathogenetic mechanisms and clinical features. *J Neurol* 244: 277-287

23. Mantegazza R, Hughes SM, Mitchell D, Travis M, Blau HM, Steinman L (1991) Modulation of MHC class II antigen expression in human myoblasts after treatment with IFN-gamma. *Neurology* 41: 1128-1132.

24. Matsubara S, Okumura S (1996) Experimental autoimmune myositis in SJL/J mice produced by immunization with syngeneic myosin B fraction. Transfer by both immunoglobulin G and T cells. *J Neurol Sci* 144: 171-175.

25. Matsubara S, Shima T, Takamori M (1993) Experimental allergic myositis in SJL/J mice immunized with rabbit myosin B fraction: immunohistochemical analysis and transfe. *Acta Neuropathol (Berl)* 85: 138-144

26. McNally EM, Ly CT, Rosenmann H, Mitrani Rosenbaum S, Jiang W, Anderson LV, Soffer D, Argov Z (2000) Splicing mutation in dysferlin produces limb-girdle muscular dystrophy with inflammation. *Am J Med Genet* 91: 305-312.

27. Michaelis D, Goebels N, Hohlfeld R (1993) Constitutive and cytokine-induced expression of human leukocyte antigens and cell adhesion molecules by human myotubes. *Am J Pathol* 143: 1142-1149.

28. Morgan G, Peter JB, Newbould BB (1971) Experimental allergic myositis in rats. *Arthritis Rheum* 14: 599-609.

29. Munsat TL, Piper D, Cancilla P, Mednick J (1972) Inflammatory myopathy with facioscapulohumeral distribution. *Neurology* 22: 335-347.

30. Nagaraju K, Raben N, Loeffler L, Parker T, Rochon PJ, Lee E, Danning C, Wada R, Thompson C, Bahtiyar G, Craft J, Hooft Van Huijsduijnen R, Plotz P (2000) Conditional up-regulation of MHC class I in skeletal muscle leads to self-sustaining autoimmune myositis and myositis-specific autoantibodies. *Proc Natl Acad Sci U S A* 97: 9209-9214.

31. Rosenberg NL, Kotzin BL (1989) Aberrant expression of class II MHC antigens by skeletal muscle endothelial cells in experimental autoimmune myositis. *J Immunol* 142: 4289-4294.

32. Rosenberg NL, Ringel SP, Kotzin BL (1987) Experimental autoimmune myositis in SJL/J mice. *Clin Exp Immunol* 68: 117-129.

33. Sugiura T, Kawaguchi Y, Harigai M, Takagi K, Ohta S, Fukasawa C, Hara M, Kamatani N (2000) Increased CD40 expression on muscle cells of polymyositis and dermatomyositis: role of CD40-CD40 ligand interaction in IL-6, IL-8, IL- 15, and monocyte chemoattractant protein-1 production. *J Immunol* 164: 6593-6600.

34. Uemura N (1969) Histological and histochemical studies on experimental allergic myositis and human polymyositis. *Nagoya J Med Sci* 31: 357-377.

35. Vafiadaki E, Reis A, Keers S, Harrison R, Anderson LV, Raffelsberger T, Ivanova S, Hoger H, Bittner RE, Bushby K, Bashir R (2001) Cloning of the mouse dysferlin gene and genomic characterization of the SJL-Dysf mutation. *Neuroreport* 12: 625-629.

36. Webb JN (1970a) Experimental immune myositis in guinea pigs. *J Reticuloendothel Soc* 7: 305-316.

37. Webb JN (1970b) *In vitro* transformation of lymphocytes in experimental immune myositis. *J Reticuloendothel Soc* 7: 445-452.

38. Wiendl H, Behrens L, Maier S, Johnson MA, Weiss EH, Hohlfeld R (2000) Muscle fibers in inflammatory myopathies and cultured myoblasts express the nonclassical major histocompatibility antigen HLA-G. *Ann Neurol* 48: 679-684.

Polymyositis and dermatomyositis

Reinhard Hohlfeld

CK	creatine kinase
DM	dermatomyositis
Hsp	heat shock protein
IBM	inclusion-body myositis
MHC	major histocompatibility complex
MMP	matrix metalloproteinase
NOS	nitric oxide synthase
PM	polymyositis

Definition of entities

In both polymyositis (PM) and dermatomyositis (DM), proximal muscles are usually symmetrically affected. Respiratory, pharyngeal, and neck muscles may be involved during later stages (10, 11, 17, 42). Up to 50% of patients suffer from muscle pain or arthralgia. The history, clinical symptoms and signs, elevated serum levels of muscle enzymes, electrophysiological changes, and histopathological findings together provide the basis for the diagnosis. The main diagnostic criteria and features of the different inflammatory myopathies are compared and summarized in Table 1.

Characteristic skin changes may accompany the muscle weakness in DM. These include heliotropic erythema of the eyelids, cheeks and trunk; chronic skin lesions with de- and hyperpigmentation; painfully dilated capillaries at the base of the fingernails (Keinig's sign); erosions of the knuckles (Gottron's sign); dry and cracked skin of palms and fingers ("mechanic's hands"); subcutaneous calcifications in later stages (mainly juvenile DM); and cutaneous or intestinal ulcerations as a sign of generalised vascular injury (mainly juvenile DM).

In both PM and DM, cardiac involvement with ECG changes, pericarditis, cardiomyopathy, or heart failure can occur during all stages of the disease. Pulmonary complications can be secondary to aspiration or pulmonary restriction if the pharyngeal or respiratory muscles are affected. Further, about 10% of patients with PM or DM develop interstitial lung disease. About 50% of these patients have autoantibodies directed against histidyl transfer RNA (tRNA) synthetase, so-called Jo-1 antibodies. Interstitial lung disease indicates a severe course and poor prognosis.

There are numerous reports on the association of certain HLA haplotypes with subgroups of myositis (17). In Caucasians, PM is associated with HLA-B8 and HLA-DR3. Juvenile DM is associated with HLA-DQA1*0501 in multiple ethnic groups (49). In Japanese patients, HLA-A24 and B52 are significantly decreased in PM as compared to DM, while CW3 is significantly increased in PM versus DM (18). DRB1*08 alleles are significantly increased in PM and DM. DQA1*0501 and DQB1*0301 are significantly decreased (18).

The exact nature of the relation between malignancy and myositis has

	Polymyositis	Dermatomyositis	Inclusion body myositis
Age at manifestation	>18 years	any age, two peaks at 5-15 and 45-65 years	>50 years
Female: male ratio	2:1	2:1	1:3
Muscle involvement	proximal symmetrical	proximal symmetrical	distal to proximal, asymmetrical
Atrophy	+	(+)	++
Muscle pain	(+)	+	(+)
Serum CK	elevated up to 50x	normal, to 50x elevated	normal, to 10x elevated
EMG	myopathic	myopathic	myopathic + mixed large units
Muscle biopsy	peri- and endomysial infiltrate, invasion of MHC I+ fibres	perifascicular atrophy +/- infiltrate (perivascular and perifascicular)	prominent endomysial infiltrate atrophic fibres "rimmed vacuoles" eosinophilic inclusions
Immunohistochemistry	autoinvasive CD8+ T-cells, Mø	B-cells, macrophages CD4+ T-cells	autoinvasive CD8+ T-cells, ß-amyloid, prion-protein
Electron microscopy		tubulovesicular inclusions in capillary endothelium	helical filaments, fibrils

Table 1. Clinical and diagnostic criteria of polymyositis, dermatomyositis, and inclusion body myositis.

ONE DOMINANT ANTIGEN

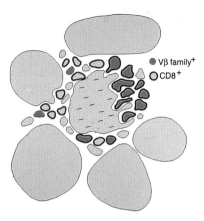

PCR --> MONO- OR OLIGOCLONAL TCRs

Figure 1. Schematic representation of the typical histological changes observed in polymyositis. T cells surround and invade a muscle fibre. The majority of the autoinvasive T cells are CD3+CD8+. All invaded muscle fibres, and some that are noninvaded, show surface reactivity for MHC class I. The autoanvasive T cells are oligoclonal: They express only a few types of T-cell receptor (TCR), as demonstrated by immunohistochemical staining with monoclonal antibodies against TCR Vβ families, in combination with PCR.

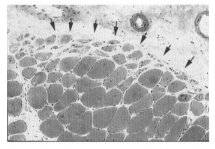

Figure 2. Perifascular atrophy, a typical histological feature of dermatomyositis. Note atrophic fibres at the edge of the fascicle (arrows). H&E.

created continued controversy. Most of the evidence points toward an association between dermatomyositis (DM) with malignancy. The relation with polymyositis is much weaker, if at all present (57). The relative risk of suffering from cancer was calculated to be 4.4 for DM and 2.1 for PM patients. The first 5 years after DM diagnosis is when the risk is greatest for malignancy. Although types of malignancy seen in DM and polymyositis are similar to those in the general population, ovarian cancer seems to be more common in DM. Most experts recommend that otherwise asymptomatic patients with DM

have an age-specific examination for occult malignancy. All suggestive symptoms or clinical clues should be evaluated thoroughly (57).

In the absence of malignancy, 5-year survival rates between 70% and 90% have been reported (17). Indicators for a poor prognosis include increased age, extramuscular organ involvement (heart, lung, pharyngeal muscles), acute onset of the disease, malignancy and late or insufficient treatment. Functional recovery is best if treatment is started within the first six months of the disease.

Of the enzymes released as a consequence of muscle fibre injury, the serum concentration of creatine kinase (CK) provides the best estimate of the extent of muscle damage and clinical activity. Both BB and MM isoenzymes may be elevated in myositis. CK levels can be elevated up to 50 times of normal in active disease phases of PM and adult DM. In contrast, the erythrocyte sedimentation rate is not a reliable parameter for disease activity and is normal in half of the patients.

In a proportion of patients, myositis-specific autoantibodies are detectable in the serum (44, 51). Although the pathogenetic relevance of these autoantibodies has yet to be defined, they are often associated with certain disease characteristics and HLA haplotypes (17, 44). Antibodies specific for aminoacyl tRNA-synthetases (Jo-1 and others) help define the anti-synthetase syndrome (myositis overlapping with polyarthritis, Raynaud's phenomenon, and/or interstitial lung disease).

Pathophysiology

The pathophysiological concepts of PM and DM rest mainly on morphological, especially immunohistochemical studies. In essence, in PM there is a conspicuous endomysial inflammatory exudate containing mainly CD8+ T cells and macrophages that surround and focally invade non-necrotic muscle fibres (Figure 1). Immunelectron microscopy demonstrated that CD8+ T cells and macrophages traverse the basal lamina; focally compress the

fibre; and ultimately replace entire segments of muscle fibre (1). All of the invaded fibres and some noninvaded fibres, express increased amounts of HLA-class I, but not class II molecules (17, 26). By contrast, normal muscle fibres do not express detectable amounts of HLA class I or class II antigens. Taken together, these observations are consistent with an HLA class I-restricted CTL-mediated response against antigen(s) expressed on muscle fibres in PM. Consistent with this hypothesis, CD8+ T cells expanded from muscle of patients with different inflammatory myopathies may show low but significant cytotoxicity against autologous cultured myotubes (24).

In DM, perifascicular atrophy is a highly characteristic microscopic feature (Figure 2) due to the degeneration of muscle fibres at the periphery of muscle fascicles secondary to microvascular damage. Quantitative morphological analyses suggest that the depletion of capillaries is one of the earliest changes in DM. Immunofluorescence studies revealed the deposition of complement in or around microvascular endothelium in a significant proportion of capillaries (43). These observations support the concept that an antibody- or immune-complex-mediated response against a vascular-endothelial component is a primary pathogenetic mechanism in DM.

In juvenile inflammatory myopathies, especially juvenile DM, maternal chimerism has been implicated in the pathogenesis (2, 48a). In one study, the families of 15 boys with DM were investigated for chimerism by PCR. Chimerism was noted in 13 of the 15 affected children with DM, compared with 5 of 35 siblings (48a). Maternal cells among peripheral blood mononuclear cells were detected in 11 of the 15 boys, compared with 5 of 17 unaffected controls, and in muscle tissue of 12 of 15 compared with 2 of 10 unaffected siblings (48a). Very similar results were obtained in another study (2). Microchimerism could induce graft-versus host disease, which could manifest as autoimmune diseases. For example, chimeric cells of fetal origin were identified in skin lesions and peripheral blood of women with systemic sclerosis (3).

Structural changes

General features. A number of studies have investigated the expression of inflammatory molecules such as cytokines, matrix metalloproteases, adhesion molecules, and costimulatory molecules in the different inflammatory myopathies (27). Despite some discrepancies between the different studies, which are probably explained by methodological aspects, it is safe to conclude that inflammatory cells, muscle fibres and endothelial cells express a complex array of different inflammatory mediators, adhesion and costimulatory molecules. The local production of soluble mediators likely induces the expression of cell interaction and adhesion molecules in various cellular components of muscle tissue.

A crucial prerequisite for immunological interaction between muscle fibres and inflammatory T cells is the expression of major histocompatibility complex (MHC, also called HLA) antigens. Muscle fibres normally do not express detectable amounts of MHC class I or II antigens. However, classical studies by the groups of George Karpati (32, 33) and Andrew Engel (14) demonstrated that MHC class I is strongly upregulated in pathological conditions, especially inflammatory myopathies. In principle, muscle fibres also seem to be capable of expressing MHC class II (HLA-DR) antigen, although to a lesser extent (4, 30). Recently, the expression of a "nonclassical" HLA class I molecule (HLA-G) has been demonstrated in muscle of patients with PM, DM, and IBM (56).

In PM, the endomysial inflammatory infiltrate is typically dominated by CD8+ T lymphocytes, which surround, invade and eventually destroy muscle fibres (Figure 1). In a rare subtype of PM, the infiltrate consists of gamma-delta T-lymphocytes (24a). In contrast to noninflamed muscle, the invaded muscle fibres express HLA class I molecules. This is a prerequisite for the immunological interaction with CD8+ T cells. The different stages of CTL-mediated myocytotoxicity were analysed by immunoelectron microscopy (1). Initially, CD8+ cells and macrophages abut on and send spike-like processes into nonnecrotic muscle fibres. Subsequently, an increasing number of CD8+ cells and macrophages traverse the basal lamina and focally replace the fibre.

Approximately one-third of all autoinvasive cells and about one-half of the CD8+ autoinvasive T cells are HLA-DR+, suggesting that they have been activated (16). The vast majority of the inflammatory CD4+ and CD8+ T cells display the phenotype of memory T cells, ie, they express the RO isoform of the leukocyte common antigen CD45 (13). The intensity of the CD45RO signal was similar in all CD8+ T cells regardless of their position relative to the invaded muscle fibre surface. A similar expression pattern was noted for the leukocyte function associated antigen-(LFA-) 1 (12, 28). LFA-1 (CD11a/CD18) is a $\beta2$ integrin that has a key role in mediating leukocyte adhesion to endothelium and T cell adhesion to target cells. ICAM-1, a ligand of LFA-1, was upregulated especially on T cells in the vicinity of invaded muscle fibres, suggesting that the expression of CD45RO and ICAM-1 is differentially regulated (12). Indeed, LFA-1 is mainly constitutively expressed, whereas ICAM-1 is widely inducible on B and T cells. Taken together, these results establish that the autoaggressive (autoinvasive) T cells in the inflammatory lesions of PM and IBM muscle represent activated CD8+ memory T cells.

In contrast to PM, perivascular and perifascicular infiltrates consisting predominantly of B-lymphocytes, macrophages, and CD4+ T lymphocytes prevail in DM. Immunohistochemistry shows immune complexes and C5b9-complement (membrane attack complex) on small blood vessels, suggesting a humoral immune effector mecha-nism (15, 43). The immune processes affecting the muscle microvasculature lead to a reactive proliferation of endothelial cells and a reduction of muscle capillaries. Focal capillary depletion, with marked reduction of the capillary density, can be observed in DM specimens with minimal structural alterations, suggesting that the capillaries are an early and specific target of the disease process (15). Electronmicroscopy demonstrates tubulovesicular inclusions in endothelial cells. Capillary changes are thought to be the cause of the characteristic perifascicular muscle fibre atrophy in DM (Figure 2). Perifascicular atrophy is diagnostic for DM, even in the absence of an inflammatory infiltrate. As in PM, the molecular target of the autoimmune reaction in DM has not yet been defined.

T-cell repertoire studies. The characteristic lesion of PM has several features that make it an ideal paradigm to study CD8+ T cell-mediated immunopathology (Figure 1). First of all, the muscle fibre target cells can be readily distinguished from the effector T cells. Secondly, different populations of inflammatory T cells can be discerned: One population, which deeply invades muscle fibres (the autoaggressive or autoinvasive T cells), and another, which remains in interstitial areas and therefore seems to represent regulatory or bystander cells (the interstitial T cells).

To address the question whether the 2 morphologically defined T-cell populations represent distinct clones, Bender et al (6) combined 2 independent PCR techniques with immunohistochemistry to characterize the T-cell receptor repertoire. The results show that the T-cell repertoire of the autoinvasive T cells is distinct from the repertoire of the interstitial T cells (Figure 1). These findings are consistent with the results of previous studies, although they did not combine sequence with histological analysis of TCR Vβ expression (37, 41, 46). Differences in TCR usage in the different studies presumably reflect differences between

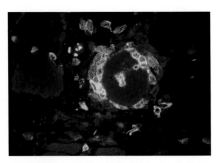

Figure 3. Immunohistological changes in γδ T cell-mediated polymyositis. Localisation of CD3 antigen (a pan-T cell marker) in red, and TiV-δ2 antigen (a marker of the monoclonal γδT cell infiltrate) in green. Note that the autoanvasive T cells appear yellow, because they stain positive for both markers. The noninvasive T cells appear red, because they do not express the γδ T cell receptor. From reference (48).

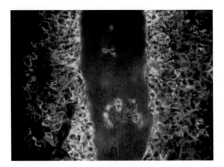

Figure 4. Immunohistological changes in γδ T cell-mediated polymyositis. Paired immunolocalization of CD3 (red) and the unique γδ T cell receptor expressed by the autoinvasive T cells (green). Note that the cells surrounding and invading the muscle fibre appear yellow (positive for both markers). From reference (24a).

individual patients, eg, different HLA types.

A possible clue to the nature of the suspected autoantigen(s) was provided by the discovery of a rare variant of PM. In this variant, CD3+CD4-CD8-TCRγδ+ T cells surrounded and invaded non-necrotic muscle fibres in the same way as CD3+CD8+TCRαβ+ T cells in the more common forms of PM (Figures 3, 4) (24a). The autoaggressive myocytotoxic γδ T cells were essentially monoclonal, and expressed an unusual Vγ3Jγ1Cγ1-Vδ2Jδ3Cδ disulfide-linked TCR (48). In γδ T-cell-mediated PM, all muscle fibres expressed MHC class I antigen and showed intense reactivity with a monoclonal antibody specific for the 65 kDa heat shock protein (hsp) (24a). One possible implication of the striking co-localization of γδ T-cells with the 65

kDa hsp is that the autoinvasive γδ T-cells recognise hsp determinants on muscle fibres. Therefore, hsp may be considered as a candidate autoantigen in some inflammatory myopathies. However, it should be noted that the expression of hsp is not unique to γδ T-cell-mediated PM, but is also observed in other types of inflammatory myopathy (25).

Cytotoxic mechanisms. The precise mechanisms by which muscle fibres are injured in the different inflammatory myopathies remain to be defined. In PM and IBM, there is strong evidence that muscle fibres are directly attacked by cytotoxic T cells. An additional possibility is that locally produced soluble inflammatory mediators and cytokines exert toxic effects on muscle fibres.

Cytotoxic T cells can kill by a variety of different mechanisms (31, 39). A main pathway of cytotoxicty seems to be mediated by the secretion of the pore-forming protein perforin by the cytotoxic T cell. An alternative, nonsecretory pathway relies on the interaction of the Fas ligand that is upregulated during T-cell activation with the apoptosis-inducing Fas receptor on the target cell. In PM, there is evidence that a perforin- and secretion-dependent mechanism contributes to the muscle fibre injury. Perforin has been localised in inflammatory T cells by immunohistochemistry (21, 47) and by in situ hybridisation (8). In PM but not DM, the autoinvasive T cells orient their perforin-containing cytotoxic granules towards the target muscle fibre (Figures 4, 5) (21), providing suggestive evidence that secretion of this cytotoxic effector molecule contributes to muscle fibre injury.

Perforin is not the only potentially cytotoxic molecule expressed in inflammatory myopathies. For example, muscle fibres in myositis display distinct up-regulation both of inducible and neuronal nitric oxide synthase (NOS) (54). It may be speculated that the enhanced expression of NOS with production of nitric oxide contributes to oxidative stress, mediating muscle

fibre damage. Furthermore, different matrix metalloproteinases (MMPs) have been shown to be expressed in PM and DM muscle (9, 34). Matrix metalloproteinases are zinc-dependent endopeptidases capable of degrading extracellular matrix. MMP-1 (interstitial collagenase) is localised around the sarcolemma of injured muscle fibres and to fibroblast-like cells, whereas MMP-9 (gelatinase B) is present mainly in inflammatory T lymphocytes (34). The matrix-degrading action of the MMPs could directly contribute to muscle fibre injury, or it could facilitate the access of cytotoxic factors and cells to muscle fibres.

If perforin is indeed involved in muscle fibre injury, why does the surface membrane of muscle fibres appear intact at the light microscopic (16) and electronmicroscopic (1) level in the early stages of muscle fibre invasion? Pore-like structures could not be detected in the sarcolemma of muscle fibres attacked by T cells in PM (1). One possible explanation is that perforin pores/channels on nucleated cells in vivo are smaller in size than the pores generated in vitro on erythrocytes and other target cells by the addition of purified perforin. Perforin pores containing less than 10 to 20 monomers would escape detection by electron microscopy (38). Another explanation for the lack of morphologically visible muscle cell damage is that the surface membrane of the muscle fibre is rapidly repaired at least during the early stages of muscle fibre invasion. Repair could occur, for example, by shedding or endocytosis of pore-damaged membrane (23).

It is interesting to note that the volume of a 25 mm long and 50 μm wide muscle fibre is nearly 28 000-fold larger than, for example, that of a spherical 15 μm tumor cell (1). Perforin pores would allow the influx of calcium. Consistent with this assumption is the observation that invaded muscle fibres show signs of focal myofibrillar degeneration near invading cells (1). These changes could be a consequence of membrane insertion of perforin and focal protease activation (1). Another indirect sign of muscle fibre damage is the intense focal regenerative activity noted in areas immediately adjacent to autoinvasive T cells (1).

In addition to the perforin-mediated killing mechanism, ocytotoxic T cells can kill by a nonsecretory, ligand-mediated mechanism (31, 39) . This second killing mechanism requires the interaction between Fas (expressed on the target cell) and Fas-ligand (expressed on the T cell). Fas-mediated cytotoxicity is thought to induce programmed cell death ("apoptosis") rather than "necrosis," although it is not always possible to relate the different modes and mechanisms of cell death to specific morphological features and triggering events (50). The special properties of muscle fibres as giant syncytial cells with hundreds of nuclei further complicate the classification of any morphological changes as "necrosis" or "apoptosis."

Ligation of Fas (CD95) recruits adaptor molecules (such as procaspase-8 and -10) to the receptor. By being brought into proximity with one another, these procaspases cleave their nearest neighbors and active, mature caspases form (22). The active caspases efficiently cleave procaspase-3 and other executioner caspases, and apoptosis proceeds.

Different groups of investigators found no evidence that apoptosis is a mechanism of muscle fibre injury in human inflammatory myopathies (5, 20, 52) or dystrophies (29). On the other hand, in PM, DM, and IBM, many muscle fibres express Fas (5, 20). What could explain the discrepancy between the expression of the Fas "death receptor" on muscle fibres and the absence of signs of apoptosis? One possibility is that muscle fibres are intrinsically resistant to Fas-mediated classical apoptosis, at least in vivo. Resistance could be related to the peculiar properties of syncytial muscle fibres discussed above, or the expression of specific inhibitory factors such as Bcl-2, or both. Indeed, the majority of Fas+ fibres co-express Bcl-2 (5, 55).

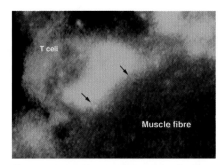

Figure 5. Immunohistochemical analysis of perforin-expressing cells in polymyositis. Co-localization of perforin (red) and CD8 (green) in a T cell by double-fluorescence microscopy. Perforin, which is oriented towards the muscle fibre (arrows), appears yellow due to overlap of the red and green signals.

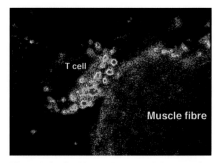

Figure 6. Confocal laser microscopical demonstration of perforin-containing granules (red-yellow) in a T cell contacting a muscle fibre. Note vectorial orientation of perforin towards the contact area. From (21).

Bcl-2 and another anti-apoptotic protein, Bcl-x, have also been localised in atrophic muscle fibres in late-onset spinal muscular atrophy (53). These molecules block apoptosis by preventing the release of mitochondrial proteins like cytochrome C. The release of cytochrome C triggers a series of reactions eventually leading to activation of procaspase-9 (22). Although the Fas-mediated apoptotic pathway does not require the involvement of mitochondria, Bcl-2 can inhibit Fas-triggered apoptosis in some cell types (22).

Bcl-2 is not the only factor protecting muscle fibres from apoptosis. Muscle fibres constitutively express the human IAP (inhibitor of apoptosis)-like protein hILP (human IAP-like protein) (also called XIAP) (36). hILP was found to be expressed in the sarcolemmal region, co-localizing with dystrophin (36). The staining pattern for hILP was essentially identical in normal, PM and IBM muscle. Furthermore, muscle fibres in PM muscle express the anti-apoptotic molecule FLIP (FLICE-inhibitory protein) (45). These authors provided evidence that FLIP indeed protects muscle cells from apoptosis in functional experiments with cultured human myoblasts (45).

Fas expression was observed not only in muscle fibres, but also in inflammatory cells in PM, IBM, DM, and Duchenne muscular dystrophy (5). Immunologically naive peripheral T cells are known to express little or no Fas on their surface, whereas previously activated memory T cells express

relatively high amounts of cell-surface Fas (40). Interestingly, Fas expression in lymphocytes can have different functional consequences (35). In freshly isolated T cells, ligation of Fas with anti-Fas mAb leads to enhanced proliferation, increased expression of activation markers and production of cytokinessuch as interleukin-2, interferon-γ, and TNF-α (40).

By contrast, chronically activated T cells are susceptible to Fas-mediated apoptosis (7, 40). It is therefore thought that Fas is an important factor in the homeostatic regulation of immune responses (35). Fas-mediated costimulation seems to contribute to clonal expansion and effector function of T cells during the early stage of an immune response. Later, Fas-mediated apoptosis helps to eliminate chronically activated T cells (40). It appears that although a proportion of inflammatory cells do express Fas and Fas-L (55), like muscle fibres they are protected from apoptosis by Bcl-x and other anti-apoptotic molecules like cyclin-dependent kinase inhibitors p16 and p57 (55).

In conclusion, the observation that the autoinvasive T cells express and orient perforin towards target muscle fibres is consistent with a secretion- and perforin-dependent cytotoxic mechanism of muscle fibre injury in PM. On the other hand, although many muscle fibres and inflammatory cells express Fas, the nuclear changes typical for apoptosis are essentially absent in the inflammatory myopathies. Resistance to Fas-mediated injury is probably related to the expression of protective (anti-apoptotic) factors in muscle fibres and inflammatory cells.

Future perspectives

Much has been learned in the past two decades about the pathogenesis of the major inflammatory myopathies. Different effector mechanisms have been attributed to PM (mainly T-cell mediated) and DM (mainly antibody-mediated), and a unique γδ-T-cell mediated subtype of PM has been described. Challenges for future research include the identification of the elusive (auto?)antigens and the triggering mechanisms of the immune reactions against muscle fibres. Progress in these areas should lead to advances in therapy.

References

1. Arahata K, Engel AG (1986) Monoclonal antibody analysis of mononuclear cells in myopathies. III: Immunoelectron microscopy aspects of cell-mediated muscle fiber injury. Ann Neurol 19: 112-125

2. Artlett CM, Ramos R, Jiminez SA, Patterson K, Miller FW, Rider LG (2000) Chimeric cells of maternal origin in juvenile idiopathic inflammatory myopathies. Childhood Myositis Heterogeneity Collaborative Group. Lancet 356: 2155-2156

3. Artlett CM, Smith JB, Jimenez SA (1998) Identification of fetal DNA and cells in skin lesions from women with systemic sclerosis. N Engl J Med 338: 1186-1191

4. Bartoccioni E, Gallucci S, Scuderi F, Ricci E, Servidei S, Broccolini A, Tonali P (1994) MHC class I, MHC class II and intercellular adhesion molecule-1 (ICAM- 1) expression in inflammatory myopathies. Clin Exp Immunol 95: 166-172

5. Behrens L, Bender A, Johnson MA, Hohlfeld R (1997) Cytotoxic mechanisms in inflammatory myopathies. Co-expression of Fas and protective Bcl-2 in muscle fibres and inflammatory cells. Brain 120: 929-938

6. Bender A, Ernst N, Iglesias A, Dornmair K, Wekerle H, Hohlfeld R (1995) T cell receptor repertoire in polymyositis: clonal expansion of autoaggressive CD8+ T cells. J Exp Med 181: 1863-1868

7. Brunner T, Mogil RJ, LaFace D, Yoo NJ, Mahboubi A, Echeverri F, Martin SJ, Force WR, Lynch DH, Ware CF, et al. (1995) Cell-autonomous Fas (CD95)/Fas-ligand interaction mediates activation- induced apoptosis in T-cell hybridomas. Nature 373: 441-444

8. Cherin P, Herson S, Crevon MC, Hauw JJ, Cervera P, Galanaud P, Emilie D (1996) Mechanisms of lysis by activated cytotoxic cells expressing perforin and granzyme-B genes and the protein TIA-1 in muscle biopsies of myositis. J Rheumatol 23: 1135-1142

9. Choi YC, Dalakas MC (2000) Expression of matrix metalloproteinases in the muscle of patients with inflammatory myopathies. Neurology 54: 65-71

10. Dalakas MC (1998) Molecular immunology and genetics of inflammatory muscle diseases. Arch Neurol 55: 1509-1512

11. Dalakas MC, Sivakumar K (1996) The immunopathologic and inflammatory differences between dermatomyositis, polymyositis and sporadic inclusion body myositis. Curr Opin Neurol 9: 235-239

12. De Bleecker JL, Engel AG (1994) Expression of cell adhesion molecules in inflammatory myopathies and Duchenne dystrophy. J Neuropathol Exp Neurol 53: 369-376

13. De Bleecker JL, Engel AG (1995) Immunocytochemical study of CD45 T cell isoforms in inflammatory myopathies. Am J Pathol 146: 1178-1187

14. Emslie-Smith AM, Arahata K, Engel AG (1989) Major histocompatibility complex class I antigen expression, immunolocalization of interferon subtypes, and T cell-mediated cytotoxicity in myopathies. Hum Pathol 20: 224-231

15. Emslie-Smith AM, Engel AG (1990) Microvascular changes in early and advanced dermatomyositis: a quantitative study. Ann Neurol 27: 343-356

16. Engel AG, Arahata K (1984) Monoclonal antibody analysis of mononuclear cells in myopathies. II: Phenotypes of autoinvasive cells in polymyositis and inclusion body myositis. Ann Neurol 16: 209-215

17. Engel AG, Hohlfeld R, Banker BQ (1994) The polymyositis and dermatomyositis syndromes. In Myology, AG Engel, C Franzini-Armstrong (eds). McGraw Hill: New York. pp. 1335-1383

18. Furuya T, Hakoda M, Higami K, Ueda H, Tsuchiya N, Tokunaga K, Kamatani N, Kashiwazaki S (1998) Association of HLA class I and class II alleles with myositis in Japanese patients. J Rheumatol 25: 1109-1114

19. Fyhr IM, Moslemi AR, Lindberg C, Oldfors A (1998) T cell receptor beta-chain repertoire in inclusion body myositis. J Neuroimmunol 91: 129-134

20. Fyhr IM, Oldfors A (1998) Upregulation of Fas/Fas ligand in inclusion body myositis. Ann Neurol 43: 127-130

21. Goebels N, Michaelis D, Engelhardt M, Huber S, Bender A, Pongratz D, Johnson MA, Wekerle H, Tschopp J, Jenne D, Hohlfeld R (1996) Differential expression of perforin in muscle-infiltrating T cells in polymyositis and dermatomyositis. J Clin Invest 97: 2905-2910

22. Green DR (2000) Apoptotic pathways: paper wraps stone blunts scissors. Cell 102: 1-4

23. Henkart PA (1994) Lymphocyte-mediated cytotoxicity: two pathways and multiple effector molecules. Immunity 1: 343-346

24. Hohlfeld R, Engel AG (1991) Coculture with autologous myotubes of cytotoxic T cells isolated from muscle in inflammatory myopathies. Ann Neurol 29: 498-507

24a. Hohlfeld R, Engel A, Li K, Harper M (1991) Polymyositis mediated by T Lymphocytes that exp[ress the γ/δ receptor. N Engl J Med 324: 877-881

25. Hohlfeld R, Engel AG (1992) Expression of 65-kd heat shock proteins in the inflammatory myopathies. Ann Neurol 32: 821-823

26. Hohlfeld R, Engel AG (1994) The immunobiology of muscle. Immunol Today 15: 269-274

27. Hohlfeld R, Engel AG, Goebels N, Behrens L (1997) Cellular immune mechanisms in inflammatory myopathies. Curr Opin Rheumatol 9: 520-526

28. Iannone F, Cauli A, Yanni G, Kingsley GH, Isenberg DA, Corrigall V, Panayi GS (1996) T-lymphocyte immunophenotyping in polymyositis and dermatomyositis. Br J Rheumatol 35: 839-845

29. Inukai A, Kobayashi Y, Ito K, Doyu M, Takano A, Honda H, Sobue G (1997) Expression of Fas antigen is not associated with apoptosis in human myopathies. Muscle Nerve 20: 702-709

30. Inukai A, Kuru S, Liang Y, Takano A, Kobayashi Y, Sakai M, Doyu M, Sobue G (2000) Expression of HLA-DR and its enhancing molecules in muscle fibers in polymyositis. Muscle Nerve 23: 385-392

31. Kagi D, Ledermann B, Burki K, Zinkernagel RM, Hengartner H (1996) Molecular mechanisms of lymphocyte-mediated cytotoxicity and their role in immunological protection and pathogenesis in vivo. Annu Rev Immunol 14: 207-232

32. Karpati G, Carpenter S (1993) Pathology of the inflammatory myopathies. In Baillière's Clinical Neurology, M FL (eds). Baillière Tindal: London, U. pp. 527-556

33. Karpati G, Pouliot Y, Carpenter S (1988) Expression of immunoreactive major histocompatibility complex products in human skeletal muscles. Ann Neurol 23: 64-72

34. Kieseier BC, Schneider C, Clements JM, Gearing AJ, Gold R, Toyka KV, Hartung HP (2001) Expression of specific matrix metalloproteinases in inflammatory myopathies. Brain 124: 341-351

35. Krammer PH (2000) CD95's deadly mission in the immune system. Nature 407: 789-795

36. Li M, Dalakas MC (2000) Expression of human IAP-like protein in skeletal muscle: a possible explanation for the rare incidence of muscle fiber apoptosis in T-cell mediated inflammatory myopathies. J Neuroimmunol 106: 1-5

37. Lindberg C, Oldfors A, Tarkowski A (1994) Restricted use of T cell receptor V genes in endomysial infiltrates of patients with inflammatory myopathies. Eur J Immunol 24: 2659-2663

38. Liu CC, Walsh CM, Young JD (1995) Perforin: structure and function. Immunol Today 16: 194-201

39. Liu CC, Young LH, Young JD (1996) Lymphocyte-mediated cytolysis and disease. N Engl J Med 335: 1651-1659

40. Lynch DH, Ramsdell F, Alderson MR (1995) Fas and FasL in the homeostatic regulation of immune responses. Immunol Today 16: 569-574

41. Mantegazza R, Andreetta F, Bernasconi P, Baggi F, Oksenberg JR, Simoncini O, Mora M, Cornelio F, Steinman L (1993) Analysis of T cell receptor repertoire of muscle-infiltrating T lymphocytes in polymyositis. *J Clin Invest* : 2880-2886

42. Mantegazza R, Bernasconi P, Confalonieri P, Cornelio F (1997) Inflammatory myopathies and systemic disorders: a review of immunopathogenetic mechanisms and clinical features. *J Neurol* 244: 277-287

43. Mendell JR, Garcha TS, Kissel JT (1996) The immunopathogenic role of complement in human muscle disease. *Curr Opin Neurol* 9: 226-234

44. Miller FW (1993) Myositis-specific autoantibodies. Touchstones for understanding the inflammatory myopathies. *JAMA* 270: 1846-1849

45. Nagaraju K, Casciola-Rosen L, Rosen A, Thompson C, Loeffler L, Parker T, Danning C, Rochon PJ, Gillespie J, Plotz P (2000) The inhibition of apoptosis in myositis and in normal muscle cells. *J Immunol* 164: 5459-5465

46. O'Hanlon TP, Dalakas MC, Plotz PH, Miller FW (1994a) Predominant TCR-alpha beta variable and joining gene expression by muscle-infiltrating lymphocytes in the idiopathic inflammatory myopathies. *J Immunol* 152: 2569-2576

47. Orimo S, Koga R, Goto K, Nakamura K, Arai M, Tamaki M, Sugita H, Nonaka I, Arahata K (1994) Immunohistochemical analysis of perforin and granzyme A in inflammatory myopathies. *Neuromuscul Disord* 4: 219-226

48. Pluschke G, Ruegg D, Hohlfeld R, Engel AG (1992) Autoaggressive myocytotoxic T lymphocytes expressing an unusual gamma/delta T cell receptor. *J Exp Med* 176: 1785-1789

48a. Reed AM, Picornell YJ, Harwood A, Kredich DW (2000) Chimerism in children with juvenile dermatomyositis. *Lancet* 356: 2156-2157

49. Reed AM, Stirling JD (1995) Association of the HLA-DQA1*0501 allele in multiple racial groups with juvenile dermatomyositis. *Hum Immunol* 44: 131-135

50. Reed JC (2000) Mechanisms of apoptosis. *Am J Pathol* 157: 1415-1430

51. Rider LG, Miller FW (2000) Idiopathic inflammatory muscle disease: clinical aspects. *Baillieres Best Pract Res Clin Rheumatol* 14: 37-54

52. Schneider C, Gold R, Dalakas MC, Schmied M, Lassmann H, Toyka KV, Hartung HP (1996) MHC class I-mediated cytotoxicity does not induce apoptosis in muscle fibers nor in inflammatory T cells: studies in patients with polymyositis, dermatomyositis, and inclusion body myositis. *J Neuropathol Exp Neurol* 55: 1205-1209

53. Tews DS, Goebel HH (1997) Apoptosis-related proteins in skeletal muscle fibers of spinal muscular atrophy. *J Neuropathol Exp Neurol* 56: 150-156

54. Tews DS, Goebel HH (1998) Cell death and oxidative damage in inflammatory myopathies. *Clin Immunol Immunopathol* 87: 240-247

55. Vattemi G, Tonin P, Filosto M, Spagnolo M, Rizzuto N, Tomelleri G (2000) T-cell anti-apoptotic mechanisms in inflammatory myopathies. *J Neuroimmunol* 111: 146-151

56. Wiendl H, Behrens L, Maier S, Johnson MA, Weiss EH, Hohlfeld R (2000) Muscle fibers in inflammatory myopathies and cultured myoblasts express the nonclassical major histocompatibility antigen HLA-G. *Ann Neurol* 48: 679-684

57. Yazici Y, Kagen LJ (2000) The association of malignancy with myositis. *Curr Opin Rheumatol* 12: 498-500

Inclusion body myositis

Reinhard Hohlfeld

DM	dermatomyositis
IBM	inclusion-body myositis
MHC	major histocompatibility complex
PM	polymyositis
s-IBM	sporadic IBM
TCR	T-cell receptor

Definition of entities

Although inclusion body myositis (IBM) is the most frequently occurring inflammatory myopathy in patients older than 50 years, it is often misdiagnosed. The onset of IBM is more insidious than that of dermatomyositis (DM) and polymyositis (PM). Furthermore, IBM patients have a different pattern of weakness, with early weakness and atrophy of the quadriceps, volar forearm muscles (wrist and finger flexors), and ankle dorsiflexors (Table 2, chapter 11.2). Muscle involvement is often asymmetric, in contrast to the symmetric involvement in PM and DM. Note that there are hereditary forms of non-inflammatory inclusion body *myopathy*, which are clinically and structurally different from the more common sporadic inclusion body *myositis* (18). Unlike DM and PM, IBM is not associated with myocarditis or interstitial lung disease, nor is there an increased risk of malignancy. However, up to 15 to 20% of IBM patients have an associated autoimmune disorder.

IBM is strongly associated with the MHC antigens HLA-DR3, DR52, and B8 (2, 16). A candidate region for the susceptibility gene(s) in the HLA region has recently been mapped (21). For further reading about IBM there are several detailed reviews available (3, 4, 7, 8, 10, 17, 18, 24).

Pathophysiology

The aetiology of sporadic IBM remains elusive. A longstanding debate concerns the role of the inflammatory infiltrates in s-IBM. According to one hypothesis, these changes are primary, and in obvious analogy to PM, s-IBM would be considered as an autoimmune disease, apparently mediated by CD8+ cytotoxic T cells. However, immuno-modulatory treatments in most cases do not lead to long-lasting and significant improvement of muscle strength.

According to another hypothesis, the inflammatory changes are secondary. If the latter hypothesis is correct, several possibilities exist for the primary pathogenic trigger: This could be an infectious, metabolic, degenerative, or some other process. The weight of evidence has recently shifted to favor the second hypothesis, but the nature of the triggering event(s) remains unknown (20). A complex pathogenic cascade involving elements of amyloid deposition, oxidative stress, and abnormal signal transduction has been proposed but is speculative (3).

Structural changes

General features. Characteristic light-microscopic features of s-IBM include irregular "rimmed vacuoles" and various degrees of inflammation (Figure 1). Some vacuoles are only slightly rimmed or not rimmed at all. Eosinophilic inclusions are found in the cytoplasm near vacuoles. Intranuclear inclusions are rarely observed. Such nuclei are enlarged, up to 10 μm in diameter, and contain eosinophilic or amphophilic material that displaces the chromatin against the nuclear envelope (9). Biopsy diagnosis of s-IBM is facilitated by fluorescence-enhanced Congo red staining for detection of amyloid deposits and immunocytochemical staining for detection of phosphorylated tau in paired-helical filaments (3). As in PM, the endomysial inflammatory infiltrates are dominated by CD8+ T lymphocytes (Figure 2). In familial IBM inflammatory changes are absent ("familial inclusion body myopathy").

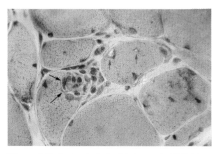

Figure 1. Typical pathological features of s-IBM. Note rimmed vacuoles (red arrows) and invasive inflammatory infiltrate (black arrows). Modified Gomori trichrome stain.

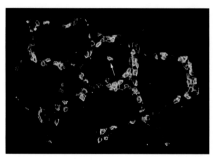

Figure 2. Immunolocalization of CD8 (green) and TCR Vβ5.3 (red) in muscle of a patient with s-IBM. Note that the majority of the infiltrating cells, including two deeply invading T cells, appear yellow (arrow), that is, positive for both markers. From (6).

Ultrastructural studies show abnormal filaments in a proportion of the muscle fibres in all biopsy specimens. The filaments are seen in the nucleus, cytoplasm, or both. The presence of filamentous cytoplasmic inclusions is always associated with fibre damage, whereas fibres with intranuclear filaments may be otherwise structurally normal (24). The paired-helical filaments are 15 to 21 nm in diameter, contain phosphorylated tau protein, and resemble the paired-helical filaments seen in Alzheimer's disease. The cytoplasm of vacuolated muscle fibres also contains thinner Aβ-positive filaments, fine flocculomembranous and amorphous material, myelin-like whorls and other lysosomal debris (3).

Thus, it appears that several "alien" molecules are overexpressed in s-IBM muscle fibres. Some of them are also found in excess in the brain of Alzheimer patients (3), including accumulations of amyloid-β-related protein, phosphorylated tau in the form of paired-helical filaments, and presenilin-1 (3). Additional proteins found in s-IBM include apolipoprotein E, α-synuclein, ubiquitin, α1-antichymotrypsin, basic fibroblast growth factor, and cellular prion protein (PrPc) (3). Because of the overexpression of PrPc, it has even been speculated that IBM might belong to the group of prion diseases. However, this possibility was essentially excluded by the following observations: *i)* both the glycoform profile and size of the normal muscle PrPc are different from those of human brain PrPc, *ii)* increased expression of PrPc is not specific for s-IBM, but also seen in PM, DM, and neurogenic muscle atrophy, and *iii)* only the normal PrPc isoform, but not PrPsc, is detectable in s-IBM (26).

Up to ≈20% of microscopically normal muscle fibres overexpress αB-crystallin, a small heat shock protein (5). The striking frequency of these "X-fibres," which by definition occur independently of inflammatory changes, seems to argue against a primary role of inflammation in the pathogenesis of IBM. Rather, it appears that an unknown "stressor" triggers downstream events including inflammatory reaction (20).

T-cell repertoire studies. The weight of evidence presently indicates that the inflammatory changes seen in s-IBM are secondary to an unknown triggering event. They closely resemble the inflammatory changes seen in PM.

A number of studies have addressed the T cell repertoire expressed in IBM muscle, using immunohistochemistry (23) or PCR (14, 25). Lindberg et al (23) compared the expression of TCR V genes in IBM, PM and DM, using 10 different TCR Vβ-specific monoclonal antibodies. The most abundant TCR Vβ elements detected with these mAbs were Vβ3 and Vβ19. TCR sequences were not reported (23).

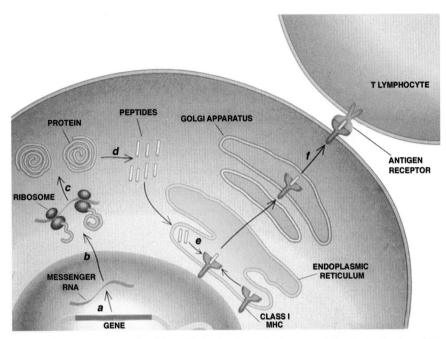

Figure 3. Schematic representation of the MHC class I pathway of antigen presentation. Most antigenic peptides presented in the class I pathway derive from proteins that are synthesized and degraded in the antigen-presenting cell. In principle, these can be foreign (especially viral) or self-proteins. The processed peptides bind to nascent MHC class I molecules. The complex of peptide and MHC molecule is then transported to the cell surface where it is recognized by the antigen-specific T-cell receptor of a CD8+ T cell. In PM and s-IBM, antigenic peptides are recognized on MHC-class I-positive muscle fibres by CD8+ T cells.

Using PCR with TCR V family-specific primers, O'Hanlon et al (25) analysed the TCR repertoire in muscle biopsy specimens from 13 IBM patients. On average, 6 to 7 TCR Vβ families were present per specimen. Vβ3 and Vβ6 were detected more frequently than the other Vβ families. Sequence analysis of the expressed Vβ3 and Vβ6 receptors was done in three patients. In one patient, both the Vβ3 and Vβ6 sequences were heterogeneous. This raised the possibility of a superantigen effect (25). However, in the two other patients, 5 of the 10 sequenced Vβ3 cDNA clones were identical (25). This would be more consistent with clonally dominant T cells recognizing a defined antigen. An additional argument against a superantigen effect is that superantigens typically activate CD4+ T cells by bridging the TCR to HLA class II molecules expressed on other cells (12, 22). However, (11) the autoinvasive cells in muscle are CD8+ rather than CD4+ (19).

Using RT-PCR, Fyhr et al (14) found a limited repertoire of TCRs expressed in muscle of six analysed

patients. TCR Vβ3, 5.2, 8, 12, 14, and 22 were each expressed in at least three cases. No TCR sequences were reported, and PCR was not combined with immunohistochemistry. Finally, using a combination of PCR and immunohistochemistry, we found a high degree of clonal restriction of TCR Vβ families expressed by autoinvasive CD8+ T cell clones in IBM (Figure 2) (6). Using RT-PCR, Fyhr et al found evidence for selective oligoclonal expansion of T cells in muscle as compared to peripheral blood (13, 15). Longitudinal studies revealed that the restricted TCR repertoire persists over time (1). In conclusion, the presently available data indicate that the TCR repertoire expressed in muscle in IBM and PM has strikingly similar features: The autoaggressive T cells are oligoclonal, suggesting that they recognise a limited number of HLA-class-I-associated antigenic peptides (Figure 1, chapter 11.2, Figure 3).

Future perspectives

Identification of the primary pathogenic trigger is clearly the most important goal for future research into the pathogenesis of this puzzling muscle disease. Success in this area will hopefully pave the way for an effective therapy.

References

1. Amemiya K, Granger RP, Dalakas MC (2000) Clonal restriction of T-cell receptor expression by infiltrating lymphocytes in inclusion body myositis persists over time. Studies in repeated muscle biopsies. *Brain* 123: 2030-2039

2. Argov Z, Eisenberg I, Mitrani-Rosenbaum S (1998) Genetics of inclusion body myopathies. *Curr Opin Rheumatol* 10: 543-547

3. Askanas V, Engel WK (2001) Inclusion-body myositis: newest concepts of pathogenesis and relation to aging and Alzheimer disease. *J Neuropathol Exp Neurol* 60: 1-14

4. Askanas V, Engel WK, Mirabella M (1994) Idiopathic inflammatory myopathies: inclusion-body myositis, polymyositis, and dermatomyositis. *Curr Opin Neurol* 7: 448-456

5. Banwell BL, Engel A (2000) AlphaB-crystallin immunolocalization yields new insights into inclusion body myositis. *Neurology* 54: 1020-1021

6. Bender A, Behrens L, Engel AG, Hohlfeld R (1998) T-cell heterogeneity in muscle lesions of inclusion body myositis. *J Neuroimmunol* 84: 86-91

7. Carpenter S (1996) Inclusion body myositis, a review. *J Neuropathol Exp Neurol* 55: 1105-1114

8. Carpenter S, Karpati G (1992) The pathological diagnosis of specific inflammatory myopathies. *Brain Pathol* 2: 13-19

9. Carpenter S, Karpati G, Heller I, Eisen A (1978) Inclusion body myositis: a distinct variety of idiopathic inflammatory myopathy. *Neurology* 28: 8-17

10. Dalakas MC, Sivakumar K (1996) The immunopathologic and inflammatory differences between dermatomyositis, polymyositis and sporadic inclusion body myositis. *Curr Opin Neurol* 9: 235-239

11. Emslie-Smith AM, Arahata K, Engel AG (1989) Major histocompatibility complex class I antigen expression, immunolocalization of interferon subtypes, and T cell-mediated cytotoxicity in myopathies. *Hum Pathol* 20: 224-231

12. Fleischer B (1995) Superantigens. *Acta Pathol Microbiol Immunol Scand* [C] 102: 3-12

13. Fyhr IM, Moslemi AR, Lindberg C, Oldfors A (1998a) T cell receptor beta-chain repertoire in inclusion body myositis. *J Neuroimmunol* 91: 129-134

14. Fyhr IM, Moslemi AR, Tarkowski A, Lindberg C, Oldfors A (1996) Limited T-cell receptor V gene usage in inclusion body myositis. *Scand J Immunol* 43: 109-114

15. Fyhr IM, Oldfors A (1998b) Upregulation of Fas/Fas ligand in inclusion body myositis. *Ann Neurol* 43: 127-130

16. Garlepp MJ, Laing B, Zilko PJ, Ollier W, Mastaglia FL (1994) HLA associations with inclusion body myositis. *Clin Exp Immunol* 98: 40-45

17. Garlepp MJ, Mastaglia FL (1996) Inclusion body myositis. *J Neurol Neurosurg Psychiatry* 60: 251-255

18. Griggs RC, Askanas V, DiMauro S, Engel A, Karpati G, Mendell JR, Rowland LP (1995) Inclusion body myositis and myopathies. *Ann Neurol* 38: 705-713

19. Hohlfeld R, Engel AG (1994) The immunobiology of muscle. *Immunol Today* 15: 269-274

20. Karpati G, Hohlfeld R (2000) Biologically stressed muscle fibers in sporadic IBM: a clue for the enigmatic etiology? *Neurology* 54: 1020-1021

21. Kok CC, Croager EJ, Witt CS, Kiers L, Mastaglia FL, Abraham LJ, Garlepp MJ (1999) Mapping of a candidate region for susceptibility to inclusion body myositis in the human major histocompatibility complex. *Immunogenetics* 49: 508-516

22. Kotzin BL, Leung DYM, Kappler JW, Marrack P (1995) Superantigens and their potential role in human disease. *Adv Immunol* 54: 99-166

23. Lindberg C, Oldfors A, Tarkowski A (1994) Restricted use of T cell receptor V genes in endomysial infiltrates of patients with inflammatory myopathies. *Eur J Immunol* 24: 2659-2663

24. Mikol J, Engel AG (1994) Inclusion body myositis. In *Myology Basic and Clinical*, AG Engel, C Franzini-Armstrong (eds). McGraw-Hill, Inc, New York. pp. 1384-1398

25. O'Hanlon TP, Dalakas MC, Plotz PH, Miller FW (1994b) The alpha beta T-cell receptor repertoire in inclusion body myositis: diverse patterns of gene expression by muscle-infiltrating lymphocytes. *J Autoimmun* 7: 321-333

26. Zanusso G, Vattemi G, Ferrari S, Tabaton M, Pecini E, Cavallaro T, Tomelleri G, Filosto M, Tonin P, Nardelli E, Rizzuto N, Monaco S (2001) Increased expression of the normal cellular isoform of prion protein in inclusion-body myositis, inflammatory myopathies and denervation atrophy. *Brain Pathol* 11: 182-189

Viral myositis

Leila Chimelli
Edson Elias da Silva

car	Coxsackievirus and adenovirus receptor
CK	creatine kinase
EM	electron microscopy
HA	haemagglutinin
HIV	human immunodeficiency virus
HTLV	human T-cell lymphotropic virus
NA	neuroaminidase
RNP	ribonucleoprotein
TSP	tropical spastic paraparesis

Acute myositis may occur in patients with serologic or virologic evidence of recent viral infection. The clinical syndrome, although usually mild, may be severe with rhabdomyolysis (11). Several different viruses can induce myositis; the best known being the influenza and Coxsackie viruses. Myopathies caused by retroviruses such as human immunodeficiency virus (HIV) and human T-cell lymphotropic virus type 1 (HTLV-1) are now well documented (2).

Influenza virus myositis

Definition of entity. This is a distinctive clinical syndrome, usually in adults, which can be seen within the first week after an attack of influenza. It is induced by 2 immunological types of influenza viruses (A, B) known to cause infection of the respiratory tract. In most studies, the incidence of myositis has not been determined; however, in one outbreak of influenza B it seemed to affect 21% of patients (7).

The condition is characterised by severe pain, tenderness, and sometimes swelling, usually of the calf, but sometimes also of the thigh muscles (8). Myalgia, the commonest manifestation, starts about a week after the onset of influenza and persists for another week or two. There may be a moderate rise in serum CK levels. In children it is usually a benign and self-limited disorder, the calf muscles being predomi-

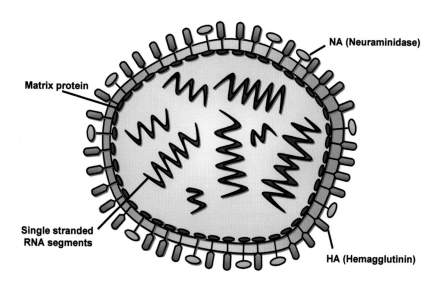

Figure 1. Schematic model for Influenza A virion particles indicating the location of a lipid bilayer in which are inserted glucoprotein peplomers (hemagglutinin and neuraminidase), the matrix protein and the eight segmented single-stranded genomic RNA segments.

nantly affected. In rare cases, the muscle disease is severe with myoglobinuria and a risk of renal failure. The infection can be identified by rising blood antibody titres (15, 18).

Molecular pathogenesis. The family *orthomixoviridae* comprises the three genera of influenza viruses, A, B, and C. Influenza A, the most studied member of the family, contains eight segments of minus-sense single strand RNA molecules in the form of ribonucleoprotein (RNP). Complete nucleotide sequences for many influenza A and B viruses have been obtained. The genome is surrounded by a lipid envelope derived from the host membrane, spikes on the surface consisting of haemagglutinin (HA) and neuraminidase (NA), and the inner side of the envelope is lined by the matrix protein (M) (Figure 1). The capsid influenza A virus haemagglutinin binds to a negatively charged terminal sialic acid (influenza A receptor) present in a number of oligosaccharide chains that are covalently attached to cell surface glycoprotein or glycolipids. The pres-

Benign acute myositis
Influenza A and B
Parainfluenza
Adenovirus 2
Acute rhabdomyolysis
Influenza A and B
Coxsackie B5
Echovirus 9
Adenovirus 21
Herpes simplex
Epidemic pleurodynia (Bornholm disease)
Coxsackie B5 (also B1, B3 and B4)
Subacute/chronic myositis
HIV myopathy
HTLV-1 myopathy
Dermatomyositis-like syndrome
(Echovirus) + agammaglobulinaemia
Epstein-Barr virus

Table 1. Major types of virus-induced muscle changes and their corresponding infectious agent.

ence of sialic acid on most cell surfaces accounts for the ability of influenza virus to attach to many types of cells (17). The myositis is probably not related to viral infection of the muscle itself, as the virus usually remains confined to the respiratory tract and draining lymph nodes. It may be caused by one or more cytokines (pyrogens) produced in the respiratory tract and released into the bloodstream to produce systemic signs of viral infection; however, the susceptibility of human muscle to the virus has been demonstrated in tissue culture. The recovery of influenza viruses from the muscle biopsies of a few patients supports a causal relationship, but clinical timing of the myalgia suggests mediation by an immunogenic mechanism (7).

Structural changes. Muscle biopsies show necrosis of a few muscle fibres without inflammatory reaction during the first 24 hours of muscle symptoms. Five to 10 days later there are signs of regeneration, interstitial mononuclear and polymorphonuclear leukocytes, in addition to some necrotic fibres. Although in some cases electron microscopy (EM) did not demonstrate virus-like particles in muscle, in one adult with severe necrotizing myopathy and myoglobinuria in which influenza B virus was isolated, EM showed viral particles within membrane-bound vacuoles near the sarcolemma (7).

Acute Coxsackie virus myositis

Definition of entity. A clinical syndrome associated with Coxsackievirus infection characterised by widespread acute myositis, which may be severe, coursing with myoglobinuria. It produces epidemics in summer and fall. A few patients develop symptoms of epidemic pleurodynia (Bornholm disease), a self-limiting acute inflammatory myopathy, particularly in children 5 to 15 years of age. Myositis is usually caused by Coxsackievirus group B, and B5 is associated particularly with epidemic pleurodynia.

Non-specific muscle aches, often exacerbated by exercise, are the main complaints. Weakness may not be present, and the symptoms slowly resolve within seven days. Bornholm disease course with acute onset of severe pain and tenderness in the muscles of the chest, back, shoulders, or abdomen.

Molecular pathogenesis. Coxsackieviruses are divided into groups A (23 serotypes) and B (6 serotypes). These viruses belong to the genus *enterovirus* of the *Picornaviridae*, a family of small, non-enveloped, positive-strand RNA viruses (12). Enterovirus virions are 27 nm in diameter, consisting of a capsid with 60 subunits, each with 4 proteins, (VP1 through VP4), and arranged in an icosahedral symmetry around the RNA genome. X-ray diffraction studies have revealed the three-dimensional molecular structure of the poliovirus, the most studied of the enteroviruses. VP1 is the most external and immunodominant of the capsid proteins and a number of major neutralising sites are located in the VP1 proteins of many picornaviruses (9).

Despite much research and the simple nature of the enteroviruses, several steps of the virus growth cycle are not completely understood, including the site and mode of virus entry and its genome release into the cytoplasm. A cell may be susceptible to infection only if a specific and functional viral receptor is present at the plasma membrane. The virus-receptor interaction causes conformational changes in the capsid structure that are necessary to release the genome into the cytoplasm. Group B coxsackieviruses and adenoviruses share the same cell receptor identified as a 46 Kda member of the superfamily immunoglobulin. This receptor is called *car* (Coxsackievirus and adenovirus receptor) (4).

The virus is transmitted by contact with infected individuals and materials such as sewerage. Viraemia occurs early in the infection and the virus is shed in faeces for days or occasionally weeks. The virus is myotropic but immunological mechanisms may play a role in the pathogenesis of the disease (7). Evidence that enteroviruses can be myotoxic is derived from animal experiments in which infection with certain Coxsackievirus and other picornaviruses can cause myositis and myocarditis.

Healthy human muscle in culture can be infected with these viruses providing additional support for their myotoxic potential (3).

Structural changes. Muscle biopsies from some adult cases with myoglobinuria have shown rhabdomyolysis, regenerating fibres, and mononuclear inflammatory cells. Fibre necrosis may selectively involve type 1 fibres; all in the same stage of necrosis or regeneration depending upon the time of the biopsy. Intracytoplasmic crystalline arrays of virus-like particles characteristic of picornavirus virions have been seen by EM in one case, although not confirmed by cytochemical stains (7).

Acute myositis during infection with other viruses

This includes mononucleosis with serological evidence of Epstein-Barr virus infection, parainfluenza virus, cytomegalovirus, HIV, herpes simplex virus, respiratory syncicial virus, echovirus, and adenovirus; the two latter occasionally coursing with rhabdomyolysis and myoglobinuria. Echovirus has also been implicated in a subacute form of dermatomyositis-like syndrome in patients with agammaglobulinaemia. Hepatitis C virus has been associated with inflammatory myopathy, as demonstrated by PCR (16).

In addition, many arboviruses, *e.g.* dengue and yellow fever, can induce acute myositis, producing pain in joints, tendons, and muscles (7). In 12 out of 15 biopsies from patients with dengue (10), a syndrome coursing with severe myalgia, fever, cutaneous rash, and headache, mild to moderate perivascular mononuclear infiltrate was observed. Three of them had rare foci of myonecrosis.

Retroviral-related myopathies

HIV (human immunodeficiency virus) and HTLV (human T-cell lymphotropic virus) belong to *retroviridae* family. The most interesting feature of the retrovirions is the presence of reverse transcriptase, an enzyme that transcribes viral RNA into provirus DNA that is integrated into host-cell genome. HIV is the human prototype of the genus *lentivirus*. The mature HIV virion is a spherically shaped particle with a diameter of ~110 nm. The outer envelope is acquired during virion budding and contains spikes formed by the two major viral-envelope glycoproteins (gp 120 and gp41). The central core contains: four viral proteins—p24 (the major capsid protein), p17 (a matrix protein), p9, and p7; 2 copies of the HIV RNA genome (2 identical copies of single-stranded RNA, about 9-kb long) to which p7 and p9 are bound; and 3 viral enzymes (reverse transcriptase, integrase, and protease) essential for viral replication (Figure 2). The HIV-1 life cycle begins with the binding of the viral attachment protein (SU) with their specific receptor, CD4 present at the T-helper cell surface (1).

Excluding the neurogenic atrophies, muscle involvement in HIV-infected patients usually falls into one of the following categories (5): *i)* HIV-associated myopathy, a myopathy that meets the criteria for polymyositis in the majority of patients, and in some, those for acquired nemaline myopathy, *ii)* zidovudine myopathy, a reversible mitochondrial myopathy (chapter 14), *iii)* the HIV-wasting syndrome and other AIDS-associated cachexia, *iv)* opportunistic infections and tumour infiltration, and *v)* vasculitis and iron deposits.

HIV myopathy. *Definition of entity.*

A myopathy of subacute onset and slow progression characterised by endomysial inflammation (HIV polymyositis), muscle fibre necrosis with minimal primary inflammation, and rarely, nemaline bodies (chapter 4.4). Since these features usually coexist in various degrees, the term HIV myopathy is used to designate the morphological spectrum of a clinically homogeneous myopathy. Muscle involvement may occur at all stages of HIV infection, and represents the first manifestation of the disease in some patients. With improved treatment and survival of

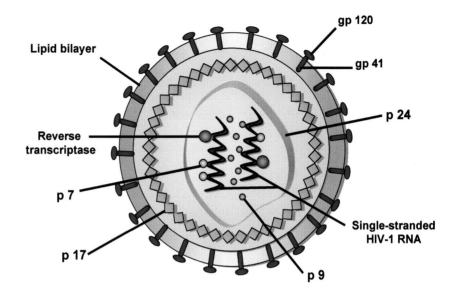

Figure 2. Schematic model for HIV-1 virion particles indicating the names and location of virus proteins, genomic RNA, and envelope.

AIDS patients, the prevalence of HIV myopathy has increased (2).

The clinical and laboratory findings are similar to those in patients with adult polymyositis. Some patients may develop a subacute limb girdle myopathy (2).

Molecular pathogenesis. Immunopathologic studies have shown that HIV antigen is detectable only in interstitial mononuclear cells, not in muscle cells. CD8+ cells and macrophages invade or approach muscle cells expressing MHC-1 antigen in the first stage of muscle cell destruction. The immunological features of HIV polymyositis are similar to those found in idiopathic polymyositis, suggesting that HIV infection can trigger the immune disturbance that leads to the development of the polymyositis syndrome. It has been proposed that this immune response results from molecular mimicry, since retroviral polypeptides coded for the *gag* gene react with certain anti-ribonuclear proteins in the cell. The studies suggest that the HIV proviral genome is not integrated into the muscle fibre DNA (2). Therefore, HIV-polymyositis does not seem to be due to occult persistent viral infection of the muscle fibres as demonstrated by PCR on muscle cultures, suggesting a remote effect of the virus on the muscle tissue, possibly mediated by cytokines

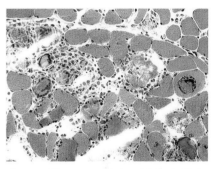

Figure 3. HIV myopathy. Endomysial lympho-histiocytic infiltration around necrotic and regenerating fibres. H& E. ×200.

and interferons. On the other hand, HIV seroconversion may be associated with myalgia and myoglobinuria, suggesting that HIV may directly invade muscle cells early in the infection (2).

Structural changes. There are perivascular, perimysial or endomysial inflammatory cells, mostly lymphocytes and macrophages, surrounding necrotic fibres (Figure 3). CD8+ cells expressing activation antigens such as MHC class II (HLA-DR) antigens, and sarcolemmal expression of MHC class 1 (HLA-ABC) antigens are observed in the fibres. Nemaline bodies (Chapter 4. 4) may occur and occasionally are the predominant finding; more commonly, they are associated with inflammatory infiltrate or the use of AZT. EM shows disorganisation of myofibrillar structures, occasionally rods and osmio-

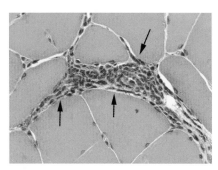

Figure 4. HTLV1-associated myositis showing endomysial lymphocytic infiltration (arrows). H&E. ×400

philic cytoplasmic degradation products. In some cases there are tubuloreticular inclusions in the capillary endothelial cells (2).

The HIV wasting syndrome. This is characterised by extreme fatigue, muscle wasting with normal CK levels, and mild proximal muscle weakness, which is disproportionate to the loss of muscle bulk. Biopsies may show severe type 2 fibre atrophy.

HTLV-1 polymyositis. *Definition of entity.* An inflammatory myopathy with features of polymyositis including muscle weakness and elevated CK in blood, associated with HTLV-1 infection, which is associated with adult T-cell leukaemia/lymphoma. Seroepidemiologic studies revealed a high HTLV-I seropositive rate (>10%) among healthy adults in southwesthern Japan and moderate rates in the Caribbean, West Africa, Colombia, Brazil, Peru, Papua New Guinea, Seychelles, Ivory Cost and Australia. It is occasionally endemic elsewhere (6, 13). The transmission involves several cells but mainly CD4 lymphocytes, occurs in a manner similar to that described for HIV, but is less effective in whole blood transfusion and in needle sharing by injection drug users. Vertical transmission occurs postnatally.

Myositis occurs either alone or as a complication of tropical spastic paraparesis (TSP), the syndrome particularly associated with HTLV-1 infection. It has been frequently observed in TSP patients submitted to muscle biopsy in Caribbean countries (14); 85% of Jamaican patients with polymyositis had circulating HTLV-1 antibodies (15).

Pathogenesis. HTLV1 can be cultured from peripheral blood lymphocytes and can infect CD8+ and T4+ cells, but it does not appear to infect human myotubes in tissue culture. In polymyositis associated with HTLV-1, the primary endomysial cells are CD8+ cytotoxic T cells, which along with macrophages invade or surround necrotic MHC-1 positive muscle fibres. This suggests the occurrence of a T-cell-mediated and MHC-1 restricted cytotoxic process, identical to that described for HIV myopathy (2).

Structural changes. There is perimysial or interstitial inflammatory response, muscle fibre necrosis, and phagocytosis (Figure 4). Immunocytochemical studies occasionally reveal viral antigens only in CD4+ perimysial lymphoid cells but not within the muscle fibres. An in situ hybridisation study showed HTLV1 particles within the muscle fibre of a patient co-infected with HIV and HTLV1. Perinuclear staining with immune HTLV-1 immunoglobulin in muscle fibres has been shown in polymyositis associated with TSP, confirmed by the presence of HTLV1-antigen by the polymerase chain reaction (15).

Future perspectives

The occurrence of infections with influenza virus may decrease as long as vaccination becomes more popular in most parts of the world. Other acute viral infections may still occur, either in sporadic or epidemic forms; the latter, particularly arboviruses, may be prevented by controlling the proliferation of the transmitter insect. As for those transmitted sexually or by blood transfusions, such as HIV and HTLV 1 infections, it is expected that prevention, widespread control of blood donors, massive use of antiretroviral agents, and eventually vaccination, may reduce the number of infected patients.

References

1. Coffin JM (1996) Retroviridae. In *Fields Virology*, BN Fields, DM Knipe, RM Chanock, JL Melnick, TP Monath, B Roizman, SE Straus (eds). Lippincott Raven Publishers: New York. pp. 655-712

2. Dalakas MC (1994) Retrovirus-related muscle diseases. In *Myology*, AJ Engel, C Franzini-Armstrong (eds). Mc Graw-Hill: New York. pp. 1419-1437

3. Dalakas MC (1995) Enterovirus and human neuromuscular diseases. In *Human Enterovirus Infections*, HA Rotbart (eds). ASM Press: Washington DC. pp 387-398

4. Flint SJ, Enquist LW, Krug RM, Racaniello VR, Skalka AM (2000) *Principles of Virology- Molecular Biology, Pathogenesis, and Control* (eds). ASM Press: Washington DC.

5. Gherardi RK (1994) Skeletal muscle involvement in HIV-infected patients. *Neuropathol Appl Neurobiol* 20: 232-237

6. Gotuzzo E, Arango C, Queiroz-Campos A, Isturiz RE (2000) Human T-cell lymphotropic virus-I in Latin America. *Infect Dis Clin North Am* 14: 211-239

7. Hays AP, Gamboa ET (1994) Acute viral myositis. In *Myology*, A Engel, J., C Franzini-Armstrong (eds). Mc Graw-Hill: New York. pp. 1399-1418

8. Heiffener Jr RD (1993) Inflammatory myopathies. A review. *J Neuropathol Exp Neurol* 52: 339-350

9. Hogle JM, Chow M, Filman DJ (1985) The three dimensional structure of poliovirus at 2,9A resolution. *Science* 229: 1358-1365

10. Malheiros SM, Oliveira AS, Schmidt B, Lima JGC, Gabbai AA (1993) Dengue. Muscle biopsy findings in 15 patients. *Arq Neuropsiquiatr* 51: 159-164

11. Mastaglia FL, Walton J (1982) Inflammatory myopathies. In *Skeletal muscle pathology*, F Mastaglia, J Walton (eds). Churchill Livingstone: London. pp. 360-365

12. Melnick JL (1996) Enteroviruses: poliovirus, coxsackievirus, echovirus, and newer enteroviruses. In *Fields Virology*, BN Fields, DM Knipe, RM Chanock, J Melnick, TP Monath, B Roizman, SE Straus (eds). Lippincott-Raven Publishers: New York. pp. 655-712

13. Montgomery RD (1989) HTLV-1 and tropical spastic paraparesis. 1. Clinical features, pathology and epidemiology. *Trans R Soc Trop Med Hyg* 83: 724-728

14. Smadja D, Bellance R, Cabre P, Kerjean J, Lezin A, Vernant JC (1995) Atteintes du système nerveux périphérique et du muscle squelettique au cours des paraplégies associées au virus HTLV-1. Étude de 7 cas observé en Martinique. *Rev Neurol (Paris)* 151: 190-195

15. Swash M, Schwartz MS (1997) *Neuromuscular Diseases. A Practical Approach to Diagnosis and Management.* Springer-Verlag: London.

16. Villanova M, Caudai C, Sabatelli P, Toti P, Malandrini A, Luzi P, Maraldi NM, Valensin PE, Merlini L (2000) Hepatitis C virus infection and myositis: a polymerase chain reaction study. *Acta Neuropathol (Berl)* 99: 271-276.

17. Weis W, Brown JH, Cusak S, Paulson JC, Skehel JJ, Wiley DC (1988) Structure of Influenza virus

hemagglutinin complexed with its receptor, sialic acid. *Nature* 333: 2079-2081

18. Weller RO, Cumming WJK, Mahon M (1998) Diseases of muscle. In *Greenfield´s Neuropathology,* DI Graham, PL Lantos (eds). Arnold: London. pp. 489-581

Bacterial myositis

Leila Chimelli

CK	creatine kinase
SPEA	streptococcal pyrogenic exotoxin A

Skeletal muscles are quite resistant to bacterial invasion. Even in cases of severe bacteraemia, abscesses in muscles are uncommon. However, an increased frequency of bacterial myositis in the last decades is due to the growing number of immunocompromised patients. Pyomyositis and clostridial myositis are the best known bacterial inflammatory myopathies, although others may occasionally be seen.

Pyomyositis

Definition of entity. In tropical areas there is a strange predisposition for suppuration in skeletal muscles with formation of large abscesses called "tropical pyomyositis." When it occurs in the temperate zone, the affected individual has usually been on a recent visit to a tropical area. It may occur without any antecedent illness or other predisposing factors. It may also be associated with trauma, malnutrition, diabetes mellitus, acute viral infection, suppurative arthritis, osteomyelitis, haematogenous spread of a bacterial infection even with negative blood cultures, or be a rare complication of a muscle biopsy or an intramuscular injection (2). Non-tropical pyomyositis are most frequently seen among the following categories: the elderly bedridden who develop abscesses spreading from bedsores, intravenous drug users, burn victims, immunocompromised patients (eg, AIDS and after chemotherapy for cancer), splenectomy patients, and steroid users (1, 4, 6). However, the source of infection is often obscure; there may be only a trivial scratch of the overlying skin. Subclinical myopathy, secondary

to the malignancy or drugs used in treating the malignancy, or both, may predispose to pyomyositis (7).

In the vast majority of cases (85%), *Staphylococcus aureus* can be cultured from the abscesses (12); in 5%, no organisms can be found. Pyomyositis has been reported to be caused also by *Streptococcus pyogenes*, *Salmonella*, and *Pneumococcus* (3).

There is painful swelling of muscle, usually quadriceps or glutei, but biceps and pectoral muscles may also be involved. Bilateral involvement occurs more frequently in patients with AIDS. The swelling is initially hard, but becomes fluctuant within a few days requiring surgical drainage (12). There may be fever, leucocytosis with eosinophilia, and raised CK. Muscle images reveal an enhancing lesion with a fluid density. Haematogenous dissemination and myoglobinuria have been reported. Despite considerable muscle destruction, functional recovery is usually good (2, 8).

Molecular pathogenesis. Since the initial inflammatory infiltrates are mainly lymphocytic and invasion of polymorphonuclear leukocytes comes later, the bacterial invasion may merely be a secondary process that develops in an acute primary inflammatory focus of unknown origin (2). The pathogenesis in AIDS is unknown, but may be due to deficits of neutrophil functioning and the common colonisation of HIV-positive patients by *S. aureus* (1).

Until recently, the study of virulence mechanisms of gram-positive cocci relied primarily on biochemical and immunological analysis because genetic tools were not available. Putative virulence factors can now be tested for their importance in infection by constructing mutant strains that no longer produce them and testing the effect of the mutation in an animal model. As for

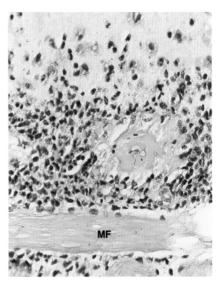

Figure 1. Pyomyositis. Note massive infiltration of inflammatory cells including polymorphonuclear eosinophils surrounding muscle fibres (MF). H & E. ×400.

regulation of *S. pyogenes* virulence genes, it seems that expression of M protein, C5a peptidase, and at least some of the M-like proteins are regulated at the transcriptional level in response to carbon dioxide levels. Increased levels of carbon dioxide are associated with increased production of these proteins. One regulatory gene associated with regulation by carbon dioxide, the *mry*, encodes a transcriptional activator that appears to be one component of the regulatory system (9).

Structural changes. An abscess is visible as a zone of muscle destruction with a core containing polymorphonuclear leucocytes and surrounded by a fibrous capsule. Fibres adjacent to the abscess may be compressed or necrotic. The initial dense inflammatory infiltrates are mainly lymphocytic, and only later is there massive invasion of neutrophils. In tropical cases, eosinophils may be present (Figure 1). The necrotic process may extend beyond the muscle fibres to the vessels and interstitial tissues.

Clostridial myositis

Definition of entity. A rare myositis caused by *Clostridium welchii*, which develops subsequent to contamination of severe deep lacerating puncture wounds of the limbs or after compound comminuted fractures or burns. It is rare in civilian practice although it still occurs. It may develop without trauma, usually in a debilitated patient with a bowel carcinoma (2). There are local symptoms and signs with pain, swelling, serosanguinous exudate, and brownish discoloration of the overlying skin, as well as systemic signs, eg, fever, tachycardia, and prostration.

Pathogenesis. Clostridium welchii produces a toxin and a number of enzymes including collagenases and hyaluronidase. As a result of its action on cell membranes, it may be responsible for initiating necrosis of muscle fibres and interstitial tissues, vascular congestion, fibrin exudation, and haemorrhage (2).

Structural changes. The affected muscle becomes greatly softened, presumably due to the enzyme activity of clostridial organisms. Microscopically, the muscle fibres show extensive necrosis and infiltration with polymorphonuclear leukocytes. If the infection is controlled and necrotic muscle tissue is removed, muscle regeneration will occur but is usually not effective; marked fibrosis and atrophy usually result (2).

Necrotizing fasciitis and myonecrosis "flesh eating infection"

Necrotizing fasciitis and myonecrosis, also known as "flesh eating infection," is a rare and life threatening disease, most often caused by group A *beta-haemolytic streptococcus pyogenes* (5, 10). The condition usually presents itself as a post-operative complication, but only rarely following non-surgical trauma. It may be lethal, due to its severity and because of the difficulty to reach a correct early diagnosis. The absence of immunity against certain streptococcal proteins may increase the severity of infection. In this disease, a bacterial antigen (streptococcal pyrogenic exotoxin A) probably acts as a "superantigen" triggering the destruction of the muscles (11) (Chapter 17).

S. pyogenes has a number of strategies for evading the host's defences: *i)* M protein, an antiphagocytic surface component, *ii)* a protease that cleaves C5a so that it no longer attracts phagocytes, and *iii)* surface proteins related to M protein that bind the Fc portions of antibodies, host proteases inhibitors, or other plasma proteins (9). In a series of 20 cases reported by Haywood et al (5), there was no correlation with the M type or the streptococcal pyrogenic exotoxin genotype and outcome. Treatment requires a combined medical-surgical approach.

Myositis due to other bacterial infections

Myositis due to other bacterial infections such as tuberculosis and syphilis are rare and reports date back many decades (2). The rare involvement of muscle in actinomycosis usually results from direct extension from a neighbouring infective focus in the pleura or skin. This will lead to the formation of abscesses and fistulas which discharge purulent material with the characteristic yellow granules containing colonies of the infective agent (8). In leprosy, in addition to muscle involvement secondary to peripheral neuropathy, Werneck et al (13) reported an interstitial inflammatory myopathy particularly in lepromatous form. Bacilli are seen inside macrophages around vessels in connective tissue septa, between muscle fibres, and also in nerve branches causing signs and symptoms of denervation in the muscles.

Future perspectives

Some of these diseases are closely related to economic and sanitary conditions. However, immunosupression, much more frequent than in the past, contributes to the occurrence of some infections even in developed countries. Prevention and the improvement of sanitary conditions and medical care for immunosuppressed patients and those with chronic debilitating diseases are the most important goals to be achieved in order to reduce the prevalence of the bacterial influences on muscles. In some cases, muscle biopsy is recommended in order to perform an early diagnosis and treatment with appropriate antibiotics.

References

1. Al-Tawfiq JA, Sarosi GA, Cushing HE (2000) Pyomyositis in the acquired immunodeficiency syndrome. *South Med J* 93: 330-334

2. Carpenter S, Karpati G (1984) *Pathology of Skeletal Muscle.* Churchill Livingstone: New York.

3. Collazos J, Mayo J, Martinez E, Blanco MS (1999) Muscle infections caused by Salmonella species: case report and review. *Clin Infect Dis* 29: 673-677

4. Demir M, Cakir B, Vural O, Muammer Karakas H, Kara M, Cicin I (2000) Staphylococcal pyomyositis in a patient with non-Hodgkin's lymphoma. *Ann Hematol* 79: 279-282

5. Haywood CT, McGeer A, Low DE (1999) Clinical experience with 20 cases of group A streptococcus necrotizing fasciitis and myonecrosis: 1995 to 1997. *Plast Reconstr Surg* 103: 1567-1573

6. Hossain A, Reis ED, Soundararajan K, Kerstein MD, Hollier LH (2000) Nontropical pyomyositis: analysis of eight patients in an urban center. *Am Surg* 66: 1064-1066

7. Keith BD, Bramwell VH (2000) Pyomyositis after chemotherapy for breast cancer. *Am J Clin Oncol* 23: 42-44

8. Mastaglia FL, Walton J (1982) *Skeletal muscle pathology.* Churchill Livingstone: London

9. Salyers AA, Whitt DD (1994) *Bacterial pathogenesis. A molecular approach.* ASM Press: Washington

10. Schwartz SN, Roman DL, Grosserode MH, Rowland MD (1995) Stretptococcal necrotizing fasciitis ("flesh-eating strep infection"). *J Okla State Med Assoc* 88: 472-474

11. Sriskandan S, Unnikrishnan M, Krausz T, Cohen J (1999) Molecular analysis of the role of streptococcal pyrogenic exotoxin A (SPEA) in invasive soft-tissue infection resulting from Streptococcus pyogenes. *Mol Microbiol* 33: 778-790

12. Swash M, Schwartz MS (1997) *Neuromuscular Diseases. A Practical Approach to Diagnosis and Management.* Springer Verlag: London

13. Werneck LC, Teive HA, Scola RH (1999) Muscle involvement in leprosy. Study of the anterior tibial muscle in 40 patients. *Arq Neuropsiquiatr* 57: 723-734

Fungal, protozoal, and other parasitic infections

Ana Lia Taratuto
Leila Chimelli

CSF	cerebrospinal fluid
CT	computer tomography
EITH	enzyme-linked immunotransfer blot
EMG	electro myography
RFLP	restriction fragment length polymorphism
RLB	reverse line blot
TGR	toxoplasma gondii gene

Fungal myositis

Fungal infections in the muscle are uncommon (13). However, during recent decades their incidence has increased due to the growing number of immunocompromised patients, the widespread use of immunosuppressive drugs, a larger ageing population with an increased number of malignancies, and the spread of AIDS (3).

Sporotricosis, histoplasmosis, mucormycosis, candidiasis, and cryptococcosis may cause myositis. Muscular involvement is usually restricted to one single muscle or a group of muscles causing an abscess, eg, in sporotrichosis and histoplasmosis. Mucormycosis, in its rhinocerebral form, can spread into the orbit, where it produces ophthalmoplegia, proptosis, oedema of the lids, and occasionally, blindness. The ocular muscles may be involved (Figure 1). Diffuse muscular involvement is almost always associated with disseminated candidiasis, as in patients with systemic malignancy, or in cryptococcosis of immunosuppressed patients (25). The clinical syndrome in candidiasis is manifested by few, papular cutaneous rashes, and widespread muscle weakness with muscle tenderness. Muscle biopsy reveals haemorrhagic necrosis of muscle fibres, acute inflammation and fungi can be identified (13).

Protozoal and other parasitic myositis (Table 1)

The alterations induced by parasites in skeletal muscle are focal, resulting in localised inflammation, or diffuse, resulting in polymyositis; they reflect either a systemic parasitic infection or a specific predilection of the organism for muscle, as in trichinosis. Within the tissue each parasite displays distinctive features that permit its recognition. Protozoa are usually within the fibres, while cestodes and nematodes may be found within or between the fibres, and course with local mass and calcification

Toxoplasmosis

Definition of entity. An infection caused by an intracellular protozoan *Toxoplasma gondii*, encysting most commonly in skeletal muscle, myocardium, and brain. Domestic cats are definitive hosts and the main reservoir, where the entire life cycle is completed. Humans either acquire the infection through intake of poorly cooked meat of infected animals containing cysts, ingesting oocysts from faecal contaminated hands or food, organ transplantation, blood transfusion, or transplacental transmission (10, 27, 30, 34). Serological prevalence data are representative of the worldwide distribution of the acquired infection as disclosed by the third National Health and Nutritional Assessment Survey (24).

Acquired toxoplasmosis in immunocompetent hosts is often asymptomatic, but 10 to 20% of patients with acute infection may develop mild febrile symptoms and lymphadenopathy, which remit spontaneously. Muscle ache and rash may express mild acquired infection, which may course with polymyositis and dermatomyositis syndromes. In immunosuppression, disease dissemination occurs, including uveitis and chorioretinitis, as observed in the congenital form, when myositis may also occur. Anti-*Toxoplasma* antibody titres are higher in polymyositis than in patients with other myopathies

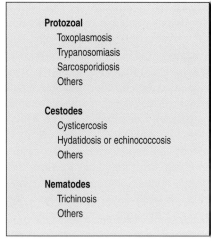

Protozoal
  Toxoplasmosis
  Trypanosomiasis
  Sarcosporidiosis
  Others

Cestodes
  Cysticercosis
  Hydatidosis or echinococcosis
  Others

Nematodes
  Trichinosis
  Others

Table 1. Organisms causing protozoal and other parasitic myositis.

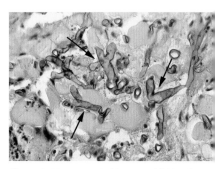

Figure 1. *Mucormycosis (Zygomycosis).* Broad non-septate hyphae (arrows) branching at right angles within necrotic muscle fibres from a bone marrow transplanted host. PAS staining. ×300.

and in the general population (5, 20). Since immunoglobulin (Ig) G titres may be high after primary infection, high or rising IgM level is a more reliable indicator of acute infection.

Pathogenesis. After acquiring the infection from mice, cats complete the entire protozoal cycle, shedding resistant oocysts in their faeces, which survive for several months. In humans, after ingestion of oocysts or raw meat containing cysts, bradyzoites are released into the digestive tract where after binary fission, tachyzoites proliferate intracellularly, disrupt host cells and enter leukocytes, disseminating widely. As host immune response develops, they may persist indefinitely encysted as bradyzoites.

Immunosuppression favours a newly acquired infection or reactivation of a chronic one with dissemination to lymph nodes, muscle, myocardium, liver and especially CNS (1). Given the association between toxoplasmosis and polymyositis, it is still controversial whether the latter is an immunological complication of the former, or whether treatment-induced immunosuppression predisposes to infection.

Toxoplasma gondii (TGR) genes comprise a family of non-coding sequences. By restriction fragment length polymorphism (RFLP) analysis of the PCR amplified TGR sequences, seven groups of isolates have been discerned, including at least 20 new TGR sequences. Genetic distance between isolates may prove useful for tracing routes of infection (14). A new quantitative PCR method (real-time PCR) seems to be as sensitive as conventional nested PCR to detect toxoplasma DNA in human blood, CSF or amniotic fluid (18). In immunocompromised patients, the type of infecting parasitic strain (studied by PCR/RFLP on locus SAG2, which enables to classify strain as type I, II or III) hardly influences the course of disease and supports specific prophylaxis irrespective of strain genotype (15). By using *T. gondii* ITS1-derived primers and a fluorescent probe via real-time PCR, a highly sensitive and specific method has been developed to detect and quantitate *T. gondii* in animal tissue samples, compatible with automation technology for slaughterhouse use (16).

Structural changes. Toxoplasma may be recognised by light microscopy within cysts ranging from 10 to 100 μm, laden with thousands of tightly packed bradyzoites, or in macrophages or other cells, especially muscle, as oval or crescent-shaped trophozoites 2 to 8 μm in length. Immunohistochemistry is useful to demonstrate free trophozoites in necrotic areas. In muscle, there is overt inflammatory reac-

tion with lymphocytes, macrophages, and at times, giant cells. MHC class I and II antigens are present in blood vessels and inflammatory cells, even in the absence of organisms (21).

American trypanosomiasis (Chagas' disease)

Definition of entity. A protozoal infection caused by the *Trypanosoma cruzi* and transmitted by *reduviid* buds (*Triatoma magista*), discovered by Chagas in 1909 in Brazil and later described in other countries of Latin America and Asia. Transmission can also occur through blood transfusion, breast feeding, transplacental, accident in laboratories, and through organ transplants (4). It has multiple clinical presentations with particular involvement of the heart and digestive system causing megavisceras. An inflammatory myopathy and evidence of denervation are the main findings in skeletal muscle (4). In the acute phase, the manifestations are directly related to the parasitism: swollen eyelids and face, toxaemia, and febrile illness. In addition, weakness, myalgia, and erythema, suggesting polymyositis, may be observed in the early phase. In the chronic phase, in addition to the cardiac and digestive symptoms, a peripheral neuropathy leads to muscle denervation. The diagnosis is made by serological tests (4).

Pathogenesis. As the insects bite the victims, parasites are eliminated in the faeces and can enter through the skin wound, around which a firm nodule develops. After the acute phase, when circulating parasites are numerous, their number decrease. In the chronic phase, the host immune response is more important for the development of the lesions. A wide range of autoreactive antibodies and T cells directed to host organs occur. Any cell or organ can be infected, but the protozoan has a particular tropism for muscle tissue, both smooth and striated. In the congenital infection, muscle fibres may also be infected (Figure 2).

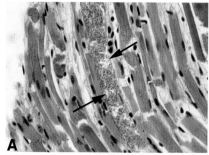
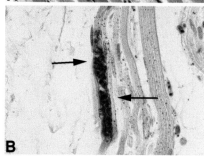

Figure 2. *Myositis in congenital trypanosomyasis. Skeletal muscle from a baby who died just after birth. Note cluster of T. cruzi within a muscle fibre (arrows) stained with H&E* **A.** *confirmed with immunohistochemistry* **B.** ×400. *Illustration kindly provided by Dr Ana Maria Lana, Belo Horizonte, Brazil.*

The alterations in muscle correlate with the presence of circulating antibodies to endocardium, blood vessels of heart, and interstitium of myocardium. These antibodies react with the plasma membrane of skeletal muscle fibres and endothelial cells of intramuscular blood vessels. Immune complexes consisting of IgG and complement are bound to the plasma membrane of skeletal muscle and endothelial cells in the same location as the antibodies (1). However, Zhang and Tarleton (42), using *in situ* polymerase chain reaction analysis for the detection of kinetoplast DNA of *T. cruzi* in murine models of Chagas' disease, demonstrated an absolute correlation between the persistence of parasites and the presence of disease in muscle tissue. In their experience, clearance of parasites from tissues, presumably by immunologic mechanisms, correlates with a decrease in inflammatory responses and the resolution of the disease.

Structural changes. In the acute form the local inflammation around the injection site results in a chagoma. Subsequently, in muscle and other tissues, the parasites multiply within the cells, which rupture, causing inflammation and local damage. The inflammatory infiltrates consist of histiocytes, lymphocytes, and plasma cells in the perimysium, particularly perivascular, but may extend into the endomysium. Parasites are detected in clusters among the inflammatory cells and within histiocytes. Muscle fibres show various stages of degeneration and regeneration apart from signs of vasculitis (4).

Parasitism of autonomic ganglia and nerve fibres of the cardiac plexus and superficial plexus of Meissner and Auerbach may be responsible for the cardiopathy or megavisceras. Neurogenic atrophy due to lesions in anterior horn neurones and motor nerves is noted in the chronic phase (33).

African trypanosomiasis

African trypanosomiasis or sleeping sickness is caused by *Trypanosoma brucei gambiense* and *Trypanosoma brucei rhodesiense*, transmitted by the bite of the TseTse fly. The muscle is affected during the second stage of the disease, 1 to 5 weeks after the bite, and is associated with malaise and fever as a part of the systemic disease. There is myocarditis, polymyositis with perimysial and endomysial infiltration by lymphocytes, plasma cells, and histiocytes (4).

Trypanosomes can be detected in a blood smear only when the concentration is more than 2000 organisms per millilitre. In buffy coat samples, the parasite can be recognised when the concentration is as low as 70 to 100 organisms per millilitre. Other useful methods to detect the organisms are filtration of blood through a small anion exchange column and indirect fluorescence antibody. Serum immunoglobulins are elevated, particularly the IgM. A DNA probe is now available for documenting the genetic sequences unique to this parasite (1).

Sarcosporidiosis

Definition of entity. A protozoal infection caused by *Sarcocystis linde-*

manni, which may encyst in skeletal and cardiac muscle fibres of various domestic and wild animals. Muscle involvement in man is uncommon, usually asymptomatic, and may be an incidental biopsy or autopsy finding. Cases have been described from Southeast Asia, India, Central and South America, Africa, Europe, United States, and China (1). Symptomatic infection courses with fever, weakness, loss of tendon reflexes, preceded by localised swelling, pain and tenderness.

Pathogenesis. Humans, the intermediate host, become infected by ingesting meat, vegetables and water contaminated with sporocysts, which liberate sporozoites in the intestine. These enter endothelial cells, where they develop to schizonts and produce merozoites, which migrate to muscle, becoming encysted as sarcocysts.

Initially, the wall of the vacuole is closely apposed to the cell membrane of the parasite. The cytoplasm of the host cell is separated from the ground substance of the cyst by a dense trilaminar membrane that probably originates as the membrane of the parasitoforous vacuole. Pouches of this membrane insert into the host cytoplasm, whereas the inner surface is relatively smooth. There is no correlation between the thickness of the cyst wall and the size of the mature cyst. As early as 40 days after infection the wall is very well developed, and it changes very little after 325 days (1).

Structural changes. Grossly, the muscle is often normal or contains small, pale intramuscular streaks or bodies, known as Miescher's tubules. Microscopically, they are cylindrical compartmentalised cysts; so-called sarcocysts varying in length and deeply embedded within the muscle fibres. The cysts are filled with many sporozoites, initially found in muscle fibres, and subsequently enlarge to lengths of 1 to 2 mm and 100 to 200 μm in diameter. Subacute or chronic inflammation may be inconspicuous consisting of

signs of myositis, often with eosinophils (1).

Microsporidiosis

Microsporidiosis is caused by *Microsporidia, zoonotic protozoa,* a rare human pathogen prior to 1985, when *Enterocytozoon bieneusi* was described in HIV-infected patients with chronic diarrhoea. Polymyositis occurred in an immunocompromised man with progressive generalised weakness. The parasites present as membrane enclosed clusters of spores, also found in macrophages and stain with PAS (1).

The organism enters the body through the gastrointestinal epithelium as well as through open wounds. In order to infect the host, the parasite emits a tubular filament that penetrates the host cell membrane, allowing the infective sporoplasm to be injected directly into the host cytoplasm. After multiple divisions within the host cell, each resultant organism develops a thick membrane to become a sporant and, through further development, a spore. Accumulation of numerous mature spores results in rupture of the host cell, followed by elimination of the spores in the faeces and their ingestion by another host.

Malaria

Malaria, an infection caused by protozoa of the genum *Plasmodium,* is transmitted by infected anopheline mosquitoes. Only *P. falciparum* can damage skeletal muscle, causing single muscle fibre necrosis in the acute stage (1). The degree of alteration depends on the severity of the disease (6). The pathogenesis of the muscle fibre degeneration in unknown. It may be the same or similar mechanisms as in other acute febrile illnesses, or the result of an active invasion of the muscle fibre by the parasite. The muscle appears to be an important site for *P. falciparum* sequestration, which could contribute to metabolic and renal complications (7).

Cysticercosis

Definition of entity. A worldwide disease caused by *Cysticercus cellulosae*, the larval form of the pork tapeworm cestode *Taenia solium*, which is encysted in subcutaneous tissue, skeletal and heart muscle, eye, and brain. Its true overall incidence has probably been underestimated and there is no reliable data regarding muscle involvement. The disease affects around 50 million people worldwide and is endemic in several countries of Latin America, Africa and Asia, as well as in some Eastern European countries, but not in Australia. It is frequent among Latin American immigrants to the United States. The prevalence of infection may be underestimated since only about half of neurocysticercosis cases diagnosed by CT are seropositive (26, 34, 39, 40). Immunosuppression may increase the frequency of this disease in endemic areas.

Clinical features vary according to the number and location of the cysts. Due to its symptoms and signs, such as mass effect and/or CSF obstruction, neurocysticercosis may overshadow muscle involvement. On occasion it presents itself as one or more small subcutaneous nodules, which lie between muscle fibres. Myalgia, fever, headache and vomiting may occur during the acute phase. More rarely, disseminated cysticercosis may show pseudohypertrophy of muscles without weakness associated with seizures and dementia (39). For antibody detection, there is a specific immunoblot assay, termed the enzyme-linked immunotransfer blot or EITB, which employs parasites glycoproteins. A reaction to one or more 9 to 50 kd band is nearly 100% specific for *T. solium* infection with a high degree of sensitivity (38, 40).

Though unsuitable for serological diagnosis, PCR–based methods readily identify *T. solium* mitochondrial cytochrome oxidase I gene sequences (37). Characteristic restriction patterns for *T. solium* proglottids from human carriers in endemic regions have been disclosed in PCR products containing the ribosomal 5.8S gene plus internal transcribed spacer regions following digestion with Alu I, Dde I, or Mbo I (22).

Pathogenesis. Humans are the only definitive hosts and develop the adult tapeworm after eating poorly cooked pork meat containing encysted larvae. The cyst wall is digested, the scolex is released and attached to the small intestine mucosa where it grows into an adult tapeworm and eliminates gravid egg-laden proglottids into faeces. The life cycle is completed when ova are eaten by the pig, the most common intermediate host. Humans acquire cysticercosis as incidental intermediate hosts by ingesting food contaminated with *T. solium* ova from another human's infected faeces or by auto reinfection (10, 30).

Structural changes. Muscle biopsy disclosing encysted larvae may prove diagnostic, particularly in chronic cases. *C. cellulosae* cysts, ranging from 5 mm to almost 3 to 4 cm in diameter, consist of a thin translucent wall filled by clear fluid, a scolex with a spiral canal, and a rostellum with four suckers and a double row of hooklets (Figure 3). The cyst wall has 3 layers: *i)* the external 3-mm thick folded eosinophilic cuticular layer, beneath which are bundles of muscle fibres, is covered with microtrichia, *ii)* the middle cellular layer and *iii)* the internal reticular layer consisting of a fibrous network with a few calcified bodies. The parasite may remain viable for several years; inflammation mostly occurs after its degeneration due to cyst fluid permeation and includes responses by lymphocytes, plasma cells and eosinophils. Deep cysts may elicit considerable granulation tissue reaction with foreign body giant cells, at times surrounded by a fibrous capsule, which may become calcified (34).

Trichinosis

Definition of entity. A worldwide zoonosis caused by a nematode

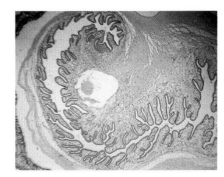

Figure 3. *Cysticercosis.* C. cellulosae with characteristic cyst thin wall and spiral canals. H&E ×100.

Trichinella spp, which lacks a free living stage. Although its incidence has declined over the last half century, it is still endemic worldwide, sparing only Australia and certain Pacific Islands (12). Sporadic outbreaks, some related to horse, boar, puma, and black bear meat ingestion have been reported from North and South America, Europe, and Asia (23, 34, 36).

Clinical symptoms appear some two weeks after intake of contaminated food and include vomiting and diarrhoea (enteric phase), followed by periorbital and facial oedema, fever, myalgia and proximal weakness (acute systemic phase). Erythematous changes may mimic dermatomyositis. Contractures may develop and even affect jaw opening. EMG shows both myopathic changes and fibrillation potential as in idiopathic polymyositis. Several organs may be involved such as lung, heart, and brain. Hypereosinophilia is generally present. Immunodiagnostic test based on IgG antibodies is the most sensitive diagnostic method (23). Positive reaction can be detected in serum samples from 80 to 100% of patients with symptomatic trichinosis 3 to 5 weeks after infection.

Pathogenesis. Human and lower animal infection with predominant muscle involvement is acquired through ingestion of poorly cooked meat, mainly pork, containing infective encysted larvae. Domestic transmission can involve pigs, rats, dogs, cats, and even horses. Wild transmission has been observed in sylvatic mammals. A complete life cycle develops in a single

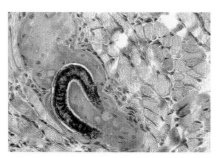

Figure 4. *Trichinosis.* Host nurse cell with faint basophilic cytoplasm and prominent nuclei harbouring a *Trichinella spiralis* larva. PAS ×300.

host harbouring adult worms in the small intestine, from which newborn larvae migrate and encyst in striated muscle. Ingested larvae reach the small intestine, lose their capsule and invade the mucosa. Adult worms develop in duodenum and jejunum. Viviparous female begin to deposit newborn larvae which enter the bloodstream, migrate to skeletal muscle and become encysted, remaining viable for several years (8, 11).

Although PCR is unsuitable for serological diagnosis, as the larva is only found briefly in the bloodstream, it is useful for genotyping larvae from human muscle biopsies, as well as of pigs and wild hosts. A reverse line blot (RLB) assay based on PCR using single larvae identified 24 Trichinella strains of different genotypes, relying on hybridization of the amplified 5S ribosomal DNA intergenic spacer regions to specific membrane-bound oligonucleotide probes (28). Nested multiplex PCR, following first round PCR with primer sets specific for gap regions of the expansion segment V region of ribosomal DNA, has been used to differentiate encapsulated from non-encapsulated Trichinella genotypes from single muscle larvae (41).

Structural changes. Muscles most frequently involved are diaphragm, intercostal, biceps, pectoral, gastrocnemius, back and lumbar region, extraocular, masticatory, and tongue muscles to a widely variable degree. Muscle biopsy is highly diagnostic after the third week in clinically affected muscles and may disclose *T. spiralis* larvae with antigen-producing stichosomes

and a central rudimentary digestive tube together with a thin muscular coat beneath a superficial cuticle, coiled within a muscle fibre host nurse cell surrounded by an eosinopihlic, PAS-positive capsule.

"Nurse cells" containing encysted larvae are multinucleated; their histochemical profile is suggestive of regeneration (Figure 4) (1, 8). Cryostat sections incubated with positive human serum for *T. spiralis* and tested by indirect immunofluorescence may also clearly disclose the larvae (36). Inflammatory cells may even be seen at a distance from encysted larvae and include monocytes, plasma cells, eosinophils, and T lymphocytes, mainly of the suppressor/cytotoxic phenotype (11).

Echinococcosis or Hydatidosis

Definition of entity. A human disease variably affecting lung, liver, brain, striated muscle tissue including periorbital, vertebrae, kidney, and pericardium, caused by the larval stage of cestodes. These are tapeworms of the *Echinococcus* genus, mainly *E. granulosus,* responsible for cystic, and *E. multilocularis*, responsible for the much rarer alveolar echinococcosis. Muscle involvement has been reported in about 5% of humans with extrahepatic lesions (2), which is the third common site (39). Reported figures for the unilocular form due to *E. granulosus* per 100 000 inhabitants may range from 1.2 cases in the Middle East to as many as 75 in South America, mostly acquired in childhood (31). It is more frequent in sheep-raising areas in North Africa, Argentina, Brazil, Australia, and New Zealand. *E. multilocularis* is found in cold areas including Alaska (northwestern United States), central Europe, China, Russia, and Turkey (35).

Both alveolar and cystic forms feature muscle involvement including isolated primary hydatidosis of peripheral muscles. Patients may remain asymptomatic for long periods. As the cyst slowly develops, it appears as a muscle tumour mass affecting paravertebral,

limb girdle, orbital, and more rarely, long limb muscles. Symptoms relate to both cyst location and size-requiring surgery for certain sites. Orbital cysts are usually manifested by proptosis and extraocular muscle paresis (35). Ultrasonography, computed tomography, and magnetic resonance imaging are useful for diagnosis. Immunodiagnostic tests vary according to the form of disease (19).

Pathogenesis. Cestodes parasitize the gut of the dog, wild canides, and other carnivorous definitive hosts, involving as intermediate hosts both domestic and wild animals harbouring the larval form or hydatid cyst (17). Humans and sheep become accidental intermediate hosts by ingesting eggs eliminated in the faeces of definitive hosts. An hexacanth embryo penetrates the intestinal wall and migrates by the portal system to the liver where hydatid cysts are formed and may metastasise to lung, brain, striated muscle, vertebrae, kidney and pericardium. To complete the life cycle, the hydatid cyst must be ingested by the definitive host. The parasite evades host immune attack by diverse mechanisms including a barrier for host cells due to hydatid cyst laminated cuticle (35).

Since the parasite is not found in the bloodstream, PCR is not used for serological human diagnosis. However, PCR followed by sequencing or RFLP is useful for strain identification from fine needle aspiration or surgically removed cysts. Both nuclear (ribosomal ITS1) and mitochondrial (ND1) sequences have been used to characterise human *E. granulosus* isolates (32). Likewise faecal adult parasites, especially from dogs and foxes infested by *E. multilocularis*, whose target sequence is mitochondrial 12S rRNA gene, may be readily identified (9). In Argentina, *E. granulosus* G2 and G6 genotypes in humans have been documented by PCR ribosomal ITS-1 DNA (rDNA) RFLP analysis, and sequencing of the mitochondrial cytochrome C oxidase subunit 1(CO1) and NADH dehydrogenase 1(ND1) genes (29).

Structural changes. The multilocular alveolar cyst has a thin outer membrane and a highly invasive germinal layer. The unilocular hydatid cyst is spherical and contains transparent fluid surrounded by a 2-layer capsule. The outer cuticle is white, elastic, acellular, non-nucleated, and PAS-positive. The inner germinal layer is granular, syncytial and nucleated, generating scolices with suckers and a double row of hooks, as well as small daughter vesicles (Figure 5). Host reaction is minimal, except in the liver where there is a thick adventitial capsule. When cysts degenerate, an epithelioid and giant cell reaction may take place to phagocyte the cuticle. Reabsorption occurs and amorphous necrotic debris are surrounded by reactive tissue and may become calcified (35).

Other parasitic diseases

Coenurosis, sparganosis, visceral larva migrans (*Toxocara canis*), cutaneous larva migrans (*Ancylostoma caninum*) and dracunculosis have all been reported to involve muscles (1).

Future perspectives

In the past, with the exception of those related to immunodeficiency, parasitic myopathies were confined to particular geographic regions. At present, because all countries are easily reached by travellers, some of these diseases are becoming more common in areas where they had not been seen before. Most of these diseases are closely related to economic and sanitary conditions, poverty, cultural and dietary habits, and immigration. Outbreaks, as in trichinosis, may occur due to consumption of pork meat in regions having poor sanitary inspection or inadequate follow up of sanitary laws. However, immunosupression, much more frequent than in the past, also contributes to the occurrence of some infections; in endemic regions, reactivation of Chagas' disease has occurred in haemophilic patients who became immunodeficient because of HIV infection through factor VIII transfusions. Prevention and improvement in

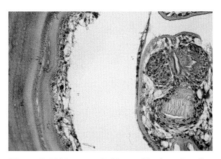

Figure 5. *Echinococcosis.* External laminated acellular PAS positive cuticle, inner nucleated germinal layer and scolex with refringent hooks and suckers (right). PAS ×400.

sanitary conditions are the most important goals to be achieved in order to reduce the prevalence of the parasitic myopathies. Muscle biopsy is highly recommended in order to obtain an early diagnosis.

References

1. Banker BQ (1994) Parasitic Myositis. In *Myology*, AJ Engel, C Franzini-Armstrong (eds). Mc Graw-Hill: New York. pp. 1453-1455

2. Bhabha SK, Bharucha NE, Bharucha EP (1996) Fungal and parasitic infections. In *Neurology in Clinical Practice*, WG Bradley, RB Daroff, GM Fenichel, DC Marden (eds). Butterworth-Heinemann: Boston. pp. 1244-1275

3. Chimelli L, Mahler-Araujo MB (1997) Fungal infections. *Brain Pathol* 7: 613-627.

4. Chimelli L, Scaravilli F (1997) Trypanosomiasis. *Brain Pathol* 7: 599-611.

5. Cuturic M, Hayat GR, Vogler CA, Velasques A (1997) Toxoplasmic polymyositis revisited: case report and review of literature. *Neuromuscul Disord* 7: 390-396.

6. Davis TM, Supanaranond W, Pukrittayakamee S, Holloway P, Chubb P, White NJ (2000) Progression of skeletal muscle damage during treatment of severe falciparum malaria. *Acta Trop* 76: 271-276

7. Davis TME, Pongponratan E, Supanaranond W, Pukrittayakamee S, Helliwell T, Holloway P, White NJ (1999) Skeletal muscle involvement in Falciparum Malaria: biochemical and ultrastructural study. *Clin Infect Dis* 29: 831-835.

8. Despommier D, Symmans WF, Dell R (1991) Changes in nurse cell nuclei during synchronous infection with Trichinella spiralis. *J Parasitol* 77: 290-295.

9. Dinkel A, von Nickisch-Rosenegk M, Bilger B, Merli M, Lucius R, Romig T (1998) Detection of Echinococcus multilocularis in the definitive host: coprodiagnosis by PCR as an alternative to necropsy. *J Clin Microbiol* 36: 1871-1876

10. Ellison D, Love S, Chimelli L, Harding B, Lowe J, Roberts G, Vinters H (1998) *Neuropathology. A reference text of CNS pathology.* Mosby: London.

11. Gherardi R, Baudrimont M, Gaulard P, Gray F, Poirier J (1989) Pathology of muscle in trichinosis: A series of 18 cases. *J Neuropathol Exp Neurol* 48: 373

12. Grove DI (1990) Tissues nematodes (trichinosis). In *Principles and practice of infections diseases*, GL Mandell, RG Douglas, JE Bennet (eds). Churchill Livingstone: New York. pp. 2140-2141

13. Heiffener JRD (1993) Inflammatory myopathies. A review. *J Neuropathol Exp Neurol* 52: 339-350

14. Hogdall E, Vuust, J., Lind P, Petersen E (2000) Characterisation of Toxoplasma gondii isolates using polimerase chain reaction (PCR) and restriction fragment length polymorphism (RFLP) of the non-coding Toxoplasma gondii (TGR)-gene sequences. *Int J Parasitol* 30: 853-858

15. Honore S, Couvelard A, Garín YJ, Bedel C, Henin D, Darde ML, Derouin F (2000) Genotyping of Toxoplasma gondii strains from immunocompromised patients. *Pathol Biol* (Paris) 48: 541-547

16. Jauregui LH, Higgins J, Zarlenga D, Dubey JP, Lunney JK (2001) Development of a real-Time PCR assay for detection of Toxoplasma gondii in pig and mouse tissues. *J Clin Microbiol* 39: 2065-2071

17. Kammerer WS (1993) Echinococcosis affecting the central nervous system. *Semin Neurol* 13: 144-147.

18. Kupferschmidt O, Kruger D, Held TK, Ellerbrok H, Siegert W, Janitschke K (2001) Quantitative detection of Toxoplasma gondii DNA in human body fluids by TaqMan polymerase chain reaction. *Clin Microbiol Infect* 7: 120-124

19. Lightowlers MW, Gottstein B (1995) Echinococcosis/hydatidosis: antigens, immunological and molecular diagnosis. In *Echinococcus and hydatid disease*, RCA Thompson, AJ Lymbery (eds). CAB International: London. pp. 355-410

20. Magid SK, Kagen LJ (1983) Serologic evidence for acute toxoplasmosis in polymyositis- dermatomyositis. Increased frequency of specific anti-toxoplasma IgM antibodies. *Am J Med* 75: 313-320

21. Matsubara S, Takamori M, Adachi H, Kida H (1990) Acute toxoplasma myositis: an immunohistochemical and ultrastructural study. *Acta Neuropathol* 81: 223-227

22. Mayta H, Talley A, Gilman RH, Jimenez J, Verastegui M, Ruiz M, García HH, Gonzalez AE (2000) Differentiating Taenia solium and Taenia saginata infections by simple hematoxylin-eosin staining and PCR-restriction enzyme analysis. *J Clin Microbiol* 38: 133-137

23. Murrell KD, Bruschi F (1994) Clinical trichinellosis. *Prog Clin Parasitol* 4: 117-150

24. National Center for Health Statistics (1994) *Plan and operation of the third National Health and Nutrition Examination Survey.* Monthly vital statistics report: Hyattsville, MD: US Department of Health and Human Services, Public Health Services DC.

25. O'Neill KM, Ormsby AH, Prayson RA (1998) Cryptococcal myositis: a case report and review of the literature. *Pathology* 30: 316-317.

26. Pittella JE (1997) Neurocysticercosis. *Brain Pathol* 7: 681-693.

27. Remington JS, McLeod R, Desmonts G (1995) Toxoplasmosis. In *Infectious diseases of the fetus & newborn infant,* JS Remington, JO Klein (eds). W.B. Saunders Co: Philadelphia. pp. 140-266

28. Rombout YB, Bosch S, Van der Giessen JW (2001) Detection and identification of eight Trichinella genotypes by reverse line blot hybridization. *J Clin Microbiol* 39: 642-646

29. Rozenzvit MC, Zhang LH, Kamenetzky L, Canova SG, Guarnera EA, Mc Manus DP (1999) Genetic variation and epidemiology of Echinococcus granulosus in Argentina. *Parasitology* 118: 523-530

30. Scaravilli F, Cook GC (1997) Parasitic and fungal infections. In *Greenfield´s Neuropathology*, DI Graham, PL Lantos (eds). Arnold: London. pp. 65 -101

31. Schantz PM, Chai J, Craig PS, Eckert J, Jonkins DJ, Macpherson CNL, Thakur A (1995) Epidemiology and control. In *Echinococcus and Hydatid Disease*, RCA Thompson, AJ Lymbery (eds). CAB International: London. pp. 234-231

32. Scott JC, Stefaniek J, Pawlowski ZS, Mc Manus DP (1997) Molecular genetic analysis of human cystic hydatid cases from Poland: identification of a new genotypic group (G9) of Echinococcus granulosus. *Parasitology* 114: 37-43

33. Taratuto A, Pagano MA, Fumo T, Sanz OP, Sica RE (1978) Histological and histochemical changes of the skeletal muscle in human chronic Chagas' disease. *Arq Neuropsiquiatr* 36: 327-331

34. Taratuto AL (1997) Bacterial, Fungal, Protozoal and Parasitic Infections. In *Neuropathology The Diagnostic Approach*, JH Garcia (eds). Mosby: St.Louis. pp. 321-352

35. Taratuto AL, Venturiello SM (1997) Echinococcosis. *Brain Pathol* 7: 673-679

36. Taratuto AL, Venturiello SM (1997) Trichinosis. *Brain Pathol* 7: 663-672

37. Theis JH, Cleary M, Syvanen M, Gilson A, Swift P, Banks J, Johnson E (1996) DNA-confirmed Taenia solium cysticercosis in black bears (Ursus americanus) from California. *Am J Trop Med Hyg* 55: 456-458

38. Tsang VCW, Wilson M (1995) Taenia solium cysticercosis: an under-recognized but serious public health problem. *Parasitol Today* 11: 124-126

39. Wadia NH, Katrak SM (1999) Muscle Infection: Viral, parasitic, bacterial and spirochetal. In *Muscle Diseases*, AH Schapira, RC Griggs (eds). Butterworth-Heinemmann: Woburn MA. pp. 339-362

40. White CA (2000) Neurocysticercosis: Updates and epidemiology, pathogenesis, diagnosis and management. *Ann Rev Med* 51: 187-206

41. Zarlenga DS, Chute MB, Martin A, Kapel CM (1999) A multiplex PCR for unequivocal differentiation of all encapsulated and non-encapsulated genotypes of Trichinella. *Int J Parasitol* 29: 1859-1867

42. Zhang L, Tartelon RL (1999) Parasite persistence correlates with disease severity and localization in chronic Chagas' disease. *J Infect Dis* 180: 480-486

CHAPTER 12

Toxic and iatrogenic disorders

When compared to neurons, even peripheral ones, the vulnerability of skeletal muscle fibres is much lower to exogenous agents, such as medications, environmental pollutants, industrial toxins, etc. However, there are clear examples of myotoxicity brought about by a number of these substances. Their recognition is of great importance since their elimination usually cures the disease.

Furthermore, the mechanism of action of some of these myotoxic agents have been useful in determining molecular functions in muscle cells. For example, the toxicity of Zidovudine in the treatment of AIDS was instrumental in throwing light upon human mitochondrial DNA turnover. Another example of this is myosin depletion syndrome brought about by the use of high dose corticosteroids and muscle paralysis due to depolarizing agents. These points are discussed in detail in this chapter.

Toxic and iatrogenic disorders

Zohar Argov
Waney Squier

Definition of entity

Numerous drugs have myotoxic side effects (Table 1) (2, 10, 16). In some, an adverse reaction is a rare "idiosyncratic" effect, eg, 0.1 to 0.5% of all patients taking one of the cholesterol lowering statins (15), while in others it is an expected complication of accumulated drug dose, eg, prolonged steroid therapy (6). The main clinical diagnostic clue is the appearance of neuromuscular symptoms after exposure to a medication or a toxin. This could be an acute episode, for instance rhabdomyolysis, or a very prolonged process over months. The clinical presentations are *i)* focal myopathy, *ii)* acute painful weakness, *iii)* a painless weakness, *iv)* chronic painful weakness, *v)* chronic painless weakness, *vi)* myalgia only, or *vii)* CK elevation only.

The toxic myopathies with massive necrosis are usually of rapid onset and in many instances painful. Even in the less rapidly progressive cases, muscle pain and tenderness may be a feature. Proximal musculature is mainly affected. The serum CK is always elevated, at times to very high level with myoglobinuria. Inflammatory myopathies are frequently associated with muscle tenderness and myalgia. Vacuolar and mitochondrial abnormalities are usually painless, but CK may still be elevated. Type 2 atrophy is painless and steroid myopathy affects mainly the lower limb girdle musculature without CK elevation. In most toxic myopathies the EMG is abnormal although this may be less conspicuous in steroid and other slowly progressive myopathies.

Drug	Major pathology	Mechanism of toxicity
Alcohol		
acute	Necrosis	Unclear
chronic	Type 2 atrophy	Reduced efficiency of protein synthesis
Aluminum-containing vaccins	Macrophagic myofaciitis	Unclear
Amiodarone	Vacuoles (myeloid bodies) Necrosis	Lysosomal inhibition (drug-induced lipidosis)
Amphotericin B	Vacuoles	Potassium loss, impaired osmotic balance
Chloroquine	Vacuoles (myeloid bodies) Necrosis	Lysosomal inhibition (drug-induced lipidosis)
Cocaine	Necrosis	Vasoconstriction
Colchicine	Autophagic vacuoles (spheromembranous bodies)	Impaired polymerization of microtubules
Corticosteroids	Type 2 atrophy	mRNA inhibition, impaired glycogenolysis
Cyclosporine	Type 2 atrophy	Unknown
D-penicillamine	Inflammation (diffuse) Necrosis	Autoantibody formation, immunomodulation
Emetine (ipecac)	Necrosis	Impaired protein synthesis Mitochondrial inhibition
Epsilon amino caproic acid	Necrosis	Capillary blockade
Fibric acid deriatives (Clofibrate)	Necrosis	Upregulation of lipoprotein lipase
Germanium	Cox negative fibres	Unclear (mitochondrial)
Heroin (other drugs of dependence)	necrosis	Muscle pressure and ischemia
IM injections (chronic)	Fibrosis, nonspecific myopathy	Physical trauma to fibres, Toxic agents
Licorice derivatives (carbenoxolone)	Vacuoles Necrosis	Mineralocorticoid activity
L-tryptophan	Eosinophilic myositis	Allergic reaction
Neuromuscular blockers and steroids (AQM)	Heavy myosin loss Necrosis	Increased proteolysis (chapter 4.8)
Perhexilline	Vacuoles (myeloid bodies) Necrosis	Lysosomal inhibition (drug-induced lipidosis)
Procainamide	Interstitial inflammatory infiltrates	Induction of SLE-like disease
Snake venoms	Necrosis	Activated lipolysis
Statins (HMG CoA reductase inhibitors)	Necrosis	Energy metabolism impairment
Thiazides (other diuretics)	Vacuoles	Potassium loss, impaired osmotic balance
Vincristine	Autophagic vacuoles (spheromembranous bodies)	Impaired polymerization of microtubules
Vitamin E excess	Necrosis, paracrytalline inclusions	Unknown
Zidovudine (other reverse transcriptase inhibitors)	Ragged red fibres Necrosis	Mitochondrial depletion

Table 1. *Toxic and iatrogenic myopathies. Pathology and mechanisms.* "Major pathology" refers both to the most frequent findings and the unique features. "Mechanisms of toxicity" are listed in broad terms and at times represent the best current hypothesis. The text and literature should be consulted for detailed information.

Structural changes and pathophysiology

The pathogenesis of the myotoxicity of many drugs (Table 1) is not well understood. The main mechanism leading to muscular weakness may not be related to the principal pharmacological action. High drug level due to impaired pharmacokinetics, eg, renal failure may be a contributing factor. Combined use of drugs with similar activity enhances the chance for myotoxicity, as is reported for the cholesterol lowering agents of the statins group. Certain combinations of drugs, eg, statins and cyclosporine, may possess increased myotoxicity potential. Gene abnormalities can also play an important role in determining susceptibility to toxic myopathies, eg, anaesthetic induced malignant hyperpyrexia.

Necrotic myopathies. These are frequently observed in several drug-induced myopathies. Necrosis can be seen in the acute phase of rhabdomyolysis as well as in the more subacute forms of the toxic myopathies, which develop over a few weeks (Figures 1, 2). In addition to necrosis, phagocytosis, and regeneration, other nonspecific changes such as central nuclei and fibre size variation are common. The implicated drugs are numerous: the cholesterol lowering agents, especially the HMG CoA reductase inhibitors but also fibric acid derived agents, epsilon aminocaproic acid used in antifibrinolysis, the amoebiasis medication emetine or its derivative ipecac syrup used as an emetic agent, drugs of dependence (mainly heroin and cocaine) and alcohol (acute alcoholic myopathy), hypervitaminosis E, vincristine, cardiac glycosides (scillarin A and B), a variety of drugs injected locally, and many snake venoms. There is a long list of drugs associated with acute rhabdomyolysis (12). General mechanisms leading to necrosis in toxic myopathies have been proposed:

Interference with the normal structure of the muscle membrane. This has been considered to be the cause of the myotoxicity induced by the old generation of cholesterol lowering agents. It was assumed that such drugs led to a defect in the cholesterol-like molecules building the muscle membrane, resulting in increased ionic permeability, especially to calcium, and initiating the cascade of myofibre necrosis.

Lipolytic effects. This is one of the mechanisms by which snake venoms cause muscle cell disruption as part of their overall toxic effect. Increase in lipoprotein lipase activity is thought to be the cause of the myopathy induced by clofibrate and other fibric acid derivatives.

Crush injury. This is the most probable explanation for the rhabdomyolysis caused by many drugs of addiction. It is thought that comatose or motionless patients exert excessive pressure on dependent muscle groups leading to ischaemic necrosis.

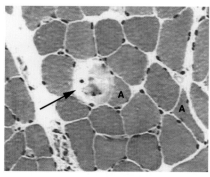

Figure 1. *Pattern of necrosis in toxic disorders.* Very early cell necrosis in a case of drug induced rhabdomyolysis caused by a cholesterol lowering agent. One necrotic fibre is indicated by an arrow. Angular atrophic fibres (A) are also present. H & E.

Impaired oxidative metabolism. This may be due to insufficient blood supply (cocaine-induced vascular constriction) or direct effect on mitochondria.

Vacuolar myopathies. There are 2 types of drug-induced vacuolar myopathy. The first is due to accumulation of autophagic (lysosomal) vacuoles, which contain membranous ("myelin bodies") and other cellular debris. These appear in both fibre types but also in interstitial cells and are typically found in chloroquine-, amiodarone-, perhexilline- and colchicine-related myopathies but also with other drugs (Figure 3). Most are amphiphilic cationic drugs which penetrate the cell and lysosomal membranes in the nonionized state (9). In the lysosomes, they form insoluble complexes with phospholipids and cause alkalinization of the lysosomes. The increase of pH inhibits various enzymes, eg, cathepsins, acid hydrolases resulting in accumulation of phospholipids and neutral lipids (drug-induced lipidosis), glycogen, amyloid and other degradation proteins in the form of membranous or crystal structures. These vacuolar myopathies are often associated with fibre necrosis.

The lysosomal changes associated with vincristine and colchicine show, in addition to the autophagic vacuoles, spheromembranous bodies thought to be derived from the sarcoplasmic reticulum. These drugs inhibit the polymerization of microtubules, possibly by

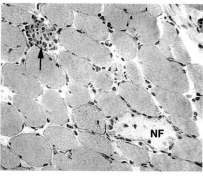

Figure 2. Active necrosis in a case of alcoholic myopathy. Two necrotic fibres are present, one indicated by an arrow is infiltrated with macrophages; another necrotic fibre (NF) is in an early phase of necrosis and appears large and pale.

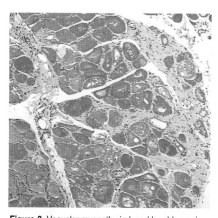

Figure 3. Vacuolar myopathy induced by chloroquine. Paraffine embedded muscle section stained with trichrome showing severe chronic damage with many vacuolated fibres and increased endomysealconnective tissue.

interacting with tubulin, interfering with the conveyance of lysosomes along the microtubular system (13).

The second form of vacuolar myopathy, associated with hypokalaemic agents, is less well defined. The vacuoles are thought to originate from the T tubules (14). Drugs which cause hypokalemic myopathies include the various diuretics especially of the thiazide group, agents used as laxatives (licorice), carbenoxolone, and amphotericin B. Unlike the common muscle picture in periodic paralysis, necrosis is often found in the drug-induced hypokalaemic myopathies. Licorice has mineralocorticoid activity leading to potassium loss in the urine and increased re-uptake of sodium. Similarly, interference with ionic conductance across membranes is probably the main common mechanism of the diuretic

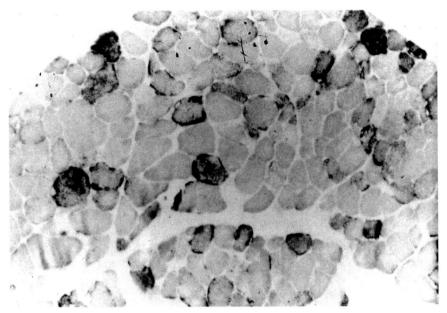

Figure 4. Numerous "ragged blue" muscle fibers, due to massive excess of mitochondria, are present in an HIV seropositive patient with muscle cramps who has been treated preemptively with Zidovudine. Succinic dehydrogenase. ×200. Illustration kindly provided by Dr George Karpati.

side effects on muscle, lowering the potassium and sodium in the interstitial fluid and changing the osmotic balance of the cell. Transient serum potassium levels lower than 2 mM/L are thought to result in swollen and vacuolated fibres.

Mitochondrial defects. The anti-HIV agents that inhibit nucleoside or nucleotide reverse transcriptase deplete mitochondrial DNA. This causes accumulation of abnormal mitochondria and formation of "ragged red fibres" (Figure 4). In most cases of Zidovudine (AZT) myopathy, the mitochondrial abnormalities are associated with other myopathic features and at times by inflammation "the myositis of HIV" (3). Thus, the question whether other toxic mechanisms operate is still unresolved (11). Loss of cytochrome C oxidase activity with mitochondrial abnormalities is also seen in myotoxicity due to the drug germanium.

Type 2 atrophy. Isolated atrophy of type 2 fibres, mainly 2b (chapter 13) is frequently seen in steroid myopathy. The fibres are not angulated and there are no other features of denervation. Impaired protein synthesis and degradation seems to be the main mechanism

by which steroids cause muscle weakness. It is possible that other metabolic effects of steroids such as impaired glycogen metabolism may explain the particular susceptibility of the fast twitch type 2b fibres (6). The fluorinated steroids are more myotoxic than the other steroids.

Chronic alcoholic myopathy and cyclosporin-induced myalgia and weakness are also associated with type 2 atrophy. In alcoholic myopathy, inhibition of translational efficiency of protein synthesis is known to occur. It is not clear whether this is directly due to the effects of ethanol (7).

Inflammatory myopathies. The features of drug induced inflammatory myopathies can be very similar to idiopathic polymyositis with necrosis of fibres and invasion of non-necrotic fibres by lymphocytes (chapter 11.2). The drug most notably associated with inflammatory myopathy is D-penicillamine. It induces several abnormalities in the immune system, especially the enhancement of the production of abnormal autoantibodies including anti-Jo-1 (5). However, D-penicillamine-induced myositis may be cell-mediated via complex autoimmunity mechanisms. Drug-induced inflamma-

tory reaction may be only interstitial (perivascular), as seen in some collagen-vascular disorders. This has been associated with several drugs (phenytoin, procainamide, hydralazine, cimetidine, levodopa and streptokinase). Some of these cases have shown abnormal immune markers, such as positive ANF and high sedimentation rate, indicating a possible generalized autoimmune condition.

An unusual type of inflammatory reaction is eosinophilic myositis and fasciitis, which appeared with the use of L-tryptophan, probably as a result of allergic reaction to a contaminated product. Focal macrophagic myofaciitis has been recently associated with injection of aluminum-containing vaccins (4).

Heavy myosin chain loss. This is a unique disorder associated with acute quadriplegic myopathy (AQM) in intensive care patients. The features of this myosin depletion myopathy are discussed in chapter 4.8. Although the exact mechanism of AQM is not known, the involvement of steroids and nondepolarizing neuromuscular blockers, usually given in combination, is thought to be an important clue to the pathogenesis.

Future perspectives

The rare side effects of drugs on muscles and myopathies due to their infrequent use has not induced many initiatives for further research on their pathogenesis and prevention. Instead, the main therapeutic intervention is stopping the medication. Thus, for many drugs the mechanisms of toxic myopathies are not well studied. However, there are 3 areas in which further research is indicated:

i) Steroid myopathies. Since this group of chemicals will continue to be widely used in the therapy of many disorders, factors which could reduce the frequency of myopathic side effects require controlled studies. It was thought that exercise may reduce the weakness induced by steroids but this has not been confirmed in a well designed experiment. More specific antiinflammatory steroids may be less myotoxic and such agents, eg, deflazacort still require research,

ii) HMG CoA reductase myotoxicity. The wide use of these agents has become a very important part of the prevention of atherosclerotic cardiovascular diseases. It is not clear if patients with high CK before treatment are more susceptible to these agents, especially those with pre-existing myopathies (8). Also, whether mild elevation of CK is an indication for stopping the medication has not been tested (1). Many patients continue to have symptoms and high CK long after the withdrawal of the medication. This phenomenon is not understood.

iii) AQM. Whether other ICU-related factors contribute to the development of this myopathy and how combined use of neuromuscular blockade and steroids should be limited is unclear. The mechanisms of this severe side effect have not been elucidated and a model for this disorder is urgently needed for future therapeutic trials.

References

1. Argov Z (2000) Drug-induced myopathies. *Curr Opin Neurol* 13: 541-545

2. Argov Z, Mastaglia FL (1994) Drug-induced neuromuscular disorders. In *Walton's Disorders of Voluntary Muscle*, J Walton, G Karpati, D Hilton Jones (eds). Churchill-Livingstone: New York. pp. 989-1009

3. Dalakas MC, Illa I, Pezeshkpour GH, Laukaitis JP, Cohen B, Griffin JL (1990) Mitochondrial myopathy caused by long-term zidovudine therapy. *N Engl J Med* 322: 1098-1105

4. Gherardi RKG, Coquet M, Authier F, Moretto P, Cherin P (2000) Macrophagic myofaciitis: a reaction to intramuscular injection of aluminum-containing vaccines. *Arthritis Rheum* 43 (supp 9): S196

5. Jenkins EA, Hull RG, Thomas AL (1993) D-penicillamine and polymyositis: the significance of the anti-Jo-1 antibody. *Br J Rheumatol* 32: 1109-1110

6. Kaminski HJ, Ruff RL (1994) Endocrine myopathies. Hyper- and hypofunction of adrenal, thyroid, pituitary and parathyroid glands and iatrogenic corticosteroid myopathy. In *Myology, Basic and Clinical*, AG Engel, C Frazini-Armstrong (eds). McGraw Hill: New York. pp. 1726-1753

7. Lang CH, Kimball SR, Frost RA, Vary TC (2001) Alcohol myopathy: impairment of protein synthesis and translation initiation. *Int J Biochem Cell Biol* 33: 457-73

8. Leung NM, McQueen MJ (2000) Use of statins and fibrates in hyperlipidemic patients with neuromuscular disorders. *Ann Intern Med* 132: 418-419

9. Lullmann H, Lullmann-Rauch R, Wassermann O (1978) Lipidosis induced by amphiphilic cationic drugs. *Biochem Pharmacol* 27: 1103-1108

10. Mastaglia FL (1992) Toxic myopathies. In *Handbook of Clinical Neurology*, LP Rowland, S DiMauro (eds). Elsevier Publisher: Amsterdam. pp. 595-622

11. Moyle G (2000) Toxicity of anti-retroviral nucloside and nucleotide analogues: is mitochondrial toxicity the only mechanism? *Drug Safety* 23: 467-481

12. Penn AS (1994) Myoglobinuria. In *Myology, Basic and Clinical*, AG Engel, C Frazini-Armstrong (eds). McGraw Hill: New York. pp. 1679-1696

13. Shinde A, Nakano S, Abe M, Kohara N, Akiguchi I, Shibasaki H (2000) Accumulation of microtubule-based motor protein in a patient with colchicine myopathy. *Neurology* 55: 1414-1415

14. Shintani S, Murase H, Tsukagoshi H, Shiigati T (1996) Glycyrrhizin (licorice)-induced kyopkalemic myopathy.Report of two cases and review of the literature. *Eur Neurol* 32: 44-51

15. Tobert JA (1988) Efficacy and long-term adverse effect pattern of lovastatin. *Am J Cardiol* 62: 28J-34J

16. Victor M, Sieb JP (1994) Myopathies due to drugs, toxins, and nutritional deficiency. In *Myology, Basic and Clinical*, AG Engel, C Frazini-Armstrong (eds). McGraw Hill: New York. pp. 1697-1725

CHAPTER 13

Effects of chronic denervation and disuse on muscle

13.1 Effects of denervation on muscle   252
13.2 Effects of disuse on muscle   257

The physical interruption of the motor axon leads to a complex sequence of morphological, molecular and biochemical changes in the denervated muscle fibre. The most conspicuous change is progressive atrophy due to diminishing myofibrillar mass. The expression of some genes is enhanced while others are diminished. These are summarized in a useful table.

Many factors and molecules originating from the motor nerve ("neurotrophic substances" in the old terminology) have been identified and their lack has been correlated with altered gene expression in denervated, or even disused muscle fibres.

Effects of denervation on muscle

Stirling Carpenter

MHC	myosin heavy chain
N-CAM	neural cell adhesion molecule
nNOS	neuronal type nitric oxide synthase
PBEF	pre-B cell enhancing factor
TRAP-1	tumor necrosis factor type-1 receptor associated protein

Definition of entity

Denervation of muscle occurs when the motor axon terminal is lost from the proximity of the muscle endplate. This results in losses of action-current-stimulated acetylcholine release, spontaneous acetylcholine release, and any trophic factors supplied by the nerve to the muscle. The marked alterations that follow may result from lack of acetyl choline produced by the nerve terminal or from the consequent lack of muscle fibre contraction. Lack of trophic factors may also have specific effects. For example, apoptosis can be prevented by exogenous application of neuroregulin to denervated muscle (28).

Effects on gene expression and protein synthesis by the muscle fibre

Denervation has widespread effects on gene transcription and protein synthesis in skeletal muscle. The result of many, though not all, of these changes, is to render the muscle more similar to developing muscle. The full range of these changes has not yet been identified and their causal sequence is still to be determined. Some of the changes are limited in time. Table 1 lists proteins reported to be up-regulated in denervated muscle, and Table 2 lists those down-regulated.

Using RNA fingerprinting with arbitrarily primed PCR (24), four genes were found whose expression was augmented by denervation: glutamine synthetase, tumor necrosis factor type-1 receptor associated protein (TRAP-1), and two novel genes. In addition, four genes were found whose expression was reduced: calpain-3, Pre-B cell

Protein	Reference	Comment
myogenin	Kostrominova (9)	
	Sedehizade (21)	
myoD	Weis (32)	
MRF-4	Weis (31)	transient
glutamine synthase	Tang (24)	
tumor necrosis factor type-1 receptor	Tang (24)	
alpha subunit of the acetyl choline receptor	Sedehizade (21)	
nestin	Vaittinen (29)	
GLUT-4	Jones (6)	
hexokinase	Jones (5)	
guanylate cyclase	Novom (14)	
adenylyl cyclase	Suzuki (14)	decreased activity reported
	Novom (23)	after 2 weeks
embryonic sodium channel (SM2)	Rich (17)	
big Tau	Ng (13)	
beta-tubulin	Ng (13)	
glial cell line derived neurotrophic factor	Lie (11)	
CNTF alpha receptor	Weiss (32)	

Table 1. Proteins (or genes or messages) which are reported to be *up-regulated* in denervated muscle.

Protein	Reference	Comment
calpain-3	Tang (24)	
pre-B cell enhancing factor (PBEF)	Tang (24)	
muscle specific enolase	Tang (24)	
myosin heavy chains	Tang (4)	especially types 1and 2B
	Jakubiec-Puka (24)	
glycogen phosphorylase	Wallis (30)	
GLUT-1	Jones, Fogt (2, 6)	
phosphorylase-b kinase	Wallis (30)	
citrate synthase	Fogt (2)	
proton-linked monocarboxylate transporter	Juel (7)	
muscle-specific enolase	Nozais (15)	
neuronal-type nitric acid synthase (nNOS)	Tews (27)	
parvalbumin	Sedehizade (21)	
cloride channel (CLC-i)	Sedehizade, Rich (17, 21)	

Table 2. Proteins (or their genes or mRNA) which are reported to be *down-regulated* in denervated muscle.

enhancing factor (PBEF), muscle specific enolase, and myosin heavy chain 2B.

The list of genes reported to show increased expression includes those for the myogenic regulatory factors myogenin (9), myoD, and MRF-4 (31). Myogenin and myo-D are virtually absent in normal muscle, while MRF-4 maintains some activity. Its expression returns to normal 14 days after denervation. Immunoblot analysis disclosed a marked overall increase of nestin, an intermediate filament protein, normally limited in mature muscle to the neuromuscular junction (29). After denervation, its immunoreactivity extends widely beyond the NMJ region, as in developing muscle. Reinnervation causes complete reversion.

Messages for several enzymes involved in carbohydrate metabolism are altered. The main muscle glucose transporter, GLUT-4, which mediates insulin stimulated glucose uptake, is downregulated, while GLUT-l, which mediates basal glucose uptake, is upregulated (6). Hexokinase-II protein levels are augmented (5) and phosphorylase-b kinase levels decrease (30), as do those of phosphorylase. The muscle-specific isoform of the glycolytie enzyme, enolase, is normally more highly expressed in fast rat muscle than in slow. After denervation, levels drop significantly in both fast and slow muscle (15). Both muscle isoforms of the proton-linked monocarboxylate transporter, which is responsible for transporting lactic acid across the cell membrane, decrease (7). Guanylate cyclase levels were reported to drop (14). The situation with adenylyl cyclase is complicated: of 4 isoforms, 2 increase and 2 decrease after denervation (23). The response to neurotransmittors was reported increased (23) and, after 2 weeks, decreased (14). Ubiquitin increases along with proteosomal proteolysis (25).

In all experimentally denervated muscles, the total content of myosin heavy chains (MHCs) decreases, more so in the slow than in the fast muscles (3, 4). The proportion of the various MHC isoforms changes in rat muscle. While MHC-1 and MHC-2B decrease, MHC-2A and MHC-2X (which corresponds to human MHC-2B) increase. Embryonic MHC is expressed in some denervated fibres (4).

Denervated muscle displays distinct downregulation of nNOS (neuronal-type nitric acid synthase, or NOS-I) (27) As NO is known to induce growth arrest and collapse of neuronal growth zones, downregulation of NOS may contribute to promotion of axonal regeneration by aiding formation of new endplates. NO is upregulated in reinnervated muscle fibres and thus prevents polyneural hyperinnervation by extrajunctional synapses.

The adult type of sodium channel is unaffected by denervation, but the embryonic type of sodium channel is up-regulated. On the other hand, the muscle chloride channel is down-regulated (17).

Production of glial cell line derived neurotrophic factor is up-regulated in denervation but not in dystrophy of rat muscle (11). This molecule may have a role in reinnervation. Levels of ciliary neurotrophic factor receptor alpha are increased in denervated human muscle but not in dystrophic muscle (32). They are also increased in the urine of patients with amyotrophic lateral sclerosis.

Physiological changes

There is an early reduction of the resting membrane potential by 20 Mv, possibly caused by reduced contribution of Na pumps (17). The reduction in resting membrane potential reduces the proportion of Na channels available for activation. There is also an increase in specific membrane resistance, spread of acetylcholine sensitivity to extrajunctional areas, and reappearance of embryonic tetrodotoxin-resistant Na channels.

Structural changes

Atrophic fibres. The principal change is the presence of atrophic fibres, which are usually angular in cross section and grouped (Figure 1). When large numbers of atrophic fibres occur in conjunction, they may be rounded, suggesting that angular contours result from pressure by nearby normally contracting fibres. In normal muscle, adjacent fibres seldom belong to the same motor unit. Thus, the grouping of atrophic fibres does not conform to the normal pattern and suggests that they may be, to some extent, pushed together. Groups with different degrees of atrophy can often be found, although the degree of atrophy within a group is usually similar. The atrophic fibres in denervation usually are depleted of glycogen (Figure 2) and myophosphorylase. Their membranes

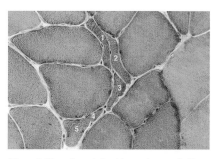

Figure 1. Five adjacent atrophic angular muscle fibres form a sinuous group that indicates denervation. Modified trichrome.

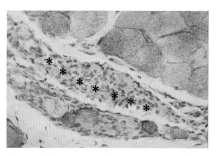

Figure 2. The very atrophic rounded muscle fibres that form a central band indicated by stars * contain almost no PAS-stainable glycogen, in contrast to the large fibres at the bottom and top.

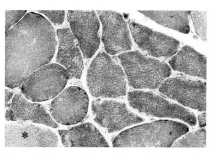

Figure 3. A group of somewhat atrophic, somewhat angular fibres here show strong oxidative enzyme activity in contrast to paler large fibres in the periphery; one indicated by a star *. The pattern of the intermyofibrillar staining in the atrophic fibres is changed from a network to a series of points, reflecting the altered orientation of mitochondria in denervated fibres. NADH-tetrazolium reductase.

are positive for N-CAM (neural cell adhesion molecule). With oxidative enzyme reactions, they usually stain darkly (Figure 3), probably reflecting increased packing density of mitochondria. The loss of calibre occurs at the same time as loss of myofibrils so that cytoplasmic zones devoid of myofibrils are not seen, at least until atrophy is extreme. Lipofuscin granules, visible as yellow pigment or by their acid phosphatase positivity, increase in number.

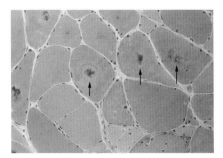

Figure 4. Targets appear on the modified trichrome as dark greenish dots or smudges within muscle fibres. Examples indicated by arrows.

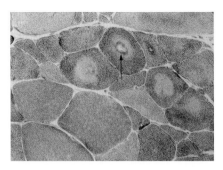

Figure 5. Targets are best displayed on oxidative enzyme reactions. They are pale, usually rounded areas that lack activity. Sometimes, as here in one fibre, an extra zone of increased activity occurs (arrow). NADH-tetrazolium reductase.

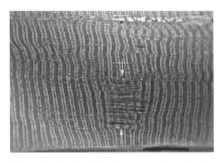

Figure 6. On longitudinal resin sections, Z disc streaming appears as dark streaks that run between Z discs parallel to the fibre axis. Paraphenylene diamine, phase optics.

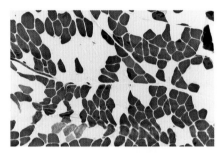

Figure 7. Type grouping consists of blocks of one fibre type interspersed with solid blocks of the other fibre type. The pattern indicates reinnervation, but does not indicate how recently it occurred. ATPase pH9.4

Fibres undergoing severe atrophy may not have sufficient cytoplasm to be identifiable on general tissue stains, although an ATPase may reveal presence of some myosin. Eventually, atrophic fibres may lose all myofibrils. Clumps of nuclei in very atrophic fibres on cross section are often seen in adult denervation although they also occur in myotonic dystrophy and inclusion body myositis.

In chronic denervation with reinnervation in adult patients (such as that seen with a chronic neuropathy), there is usually reactive hyperplasia of the innervated fibres. This may be accompanied by discrete fibre necrosis, probably reflecting excessive stress on the hypertrophied fibres.

Fibrosis may accompany severe denervation atrophy, but it is never composed of dense parallel collagen bundles as in Duchenne dystrophy. It is looser, with randomly oriented collagen fibrils and participation of elastic fibres. These can be identified on the modified trichrome or by their osmiophilia on semithin resin sections.

Nuclear changes. Although denervated muscle under the microscope usually seems to contain an excess of nuclei, there is actually a considerable loss of myonuclei (20). The nuclear/cytoplasmic ratio increases greatly. Most of the loss has been attributed to apoptosis, as shown by the TUNEL technique and ELISA, but not all studies have shown it (12, 18, 26). In one model, neuroregulin, which is normally secreted by the nerve terminal, prevented apoptosis (28). Satellite cells proba-

bly become activated, proliferate, and fuse with muscle fibres during the first few weeks, but their numbers then decrease significantly (1, 16, 20).

Targets. Target fibres are frequently seen in denervating conditions although they may reflect reinnervation rather than denervation. A target on the modified trichrome stain appears as a dark green blotch towards the center of a fibre (Figure 4). Oxidative enzyme reactions show targets as rounded areas without reaction product (Figure 5). Sometimes a ring of increased reactivity surrounds the central area of loss. Targets have a limited longitudinal extent, unlike central cores, with which they can be confused. They are virtually limited to type 1 fibres. On ATPase reactions, they may show a central zone of pallor indicating a loss of myosin. On semithin resin sections (Figure 6) or by electron microscopy, targets are seen to be areas of Z disc streaming occurring within a larger zone of myofibrils that lack mitochondria. Probably related to targets is the phenomenon of motheaten fibres, which show small focal patches of absence of mitochondria without Z disc streaming.

Type grouping. Type grouping indicates reinnervation, but the reinnervation may have taken place at any time in the past. In normal muscle, the 2 fibre types are interspersed rather like a checker board. In many chronic denervating conditions, surviving axons will generate sprouts that reinnervate dener-

vated fibres. This results in solid areas of type 1 fibres interspersed with solid areas of type 2 fibres (Figure 7). As a rough guide more than 13 adjacent fibres of a single fibre type can be considered type grouped. On the other hand, if there is marked predominance of one fibre type in a biopsy, its fibres will be grouped, and without another biopsy it may be impossible to distinguish very large type groups from mere universal predominance, whose significance is usually unclear.

Fibre type specificity. In most denervated adult muscle the atrophic fibres include both fibre types, and no fibre type is specifically spared. However, there is a tendency for type 2 fibres to show the effects of denervation more rapidly than type 1 fibres. This is probably the reason why, in some situations of denervation, more type 2 fibres than type 1s are affected.

Denervation in infants. In infantile spinal muscular atrophy (Werdnig-Hoffman disease or SMAI), there is a

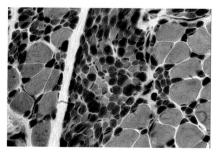

Figure 8. In infantile spinal muscular atrophy biopsy usually shows some greatly hypertrophied fibres. They are almost always of type 1, whereas the normal sized fibres are of type 2, and atrophic fibres are mixed. ATPase pH 9.4.

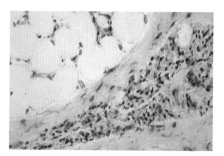

Figure 9. Vimentin (brown) is immunostained in the atrophic fibres of infantile spinal muscular atrophy, while the hypertrophied fibres are negative.

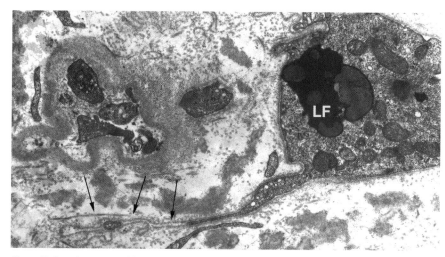

Figure 10. Part of a very atrophic muscle fibre contains a dark mass of lipofuscin (LF). An empty sleeve of basal lamina projects beyond a thin cytoplasmic extension of the cell (arrows). Nearby is the thick basal lamina of a destroyed capillary. Some elastic fibres are present in the background.

particular fibre type pattern. Hypertrophied fibres, which presumably retain innervation, are exclusively of type 1, normal sized fibre are largely of type 2, and atrophic fibres are a mixture of type 1 and type 2, usually with type 1 predominating (Figure 8). It is not clear whether this pattern is merely the typical reaction to denervation at this age or is specific to infantile SMA. Although it was found in some infants with neuropathy, we now know that neuropathy can occur with certain large deletions in the region of the SMA gene (8). In infantile SMA, vimentin-positive fibres are frequent (Figure 9), as well as alkaline phosphatase-positive fibres (19)

Reflecting the fact that immature motor neurons do not develop compensatory sprouting, motor units in SMA1 are not enlarged. In contrast, SMA3 shows a pattern of fascicular denervation with extensive type grouping (19)

Electron microscopy. The most characteristic ultrastructural feature of denervation is the presence of empty sleeves of basal lamina projecting from the surface of the muscle fibre (Figure 10). Usually they are seen at 3 or more sites around its periphery. These redundant basal lamina sleeves remain in continuity with the basal lamina that is apposed to the plasma membrane. This phenomenon appears relatively specific, although no rigorous evaluation of its specificity has been reported. It is not ordinarily seen in disuse. It is possibly related to changes in alpha-dystroglycan in the plasma membrane (10).

A second feature which appears somewhat specific for a denervating process at some stage in its evolution, is the presence of myofibrils oriented in three perpendicular axes. This may well be related to reinnervation.

Various nonspecific ultrastructural changes may be seen within denervated fibres, such as Z-disc streaming, smallness of myofibrils, disoriented isolated thick filaments, and stacking of triads to form pentads. Mitochondria change the orientation of their long axes from largely transverse to longitudinal. This was seen in rats after 6 days of denervation (22).

Future directions

Systematic studies using cDNA and oligonucleotide microarrays should reveal the true extent of alteration of gene expression in denervation.

References

1. Bornemann A, Maier F, Kuschel R (1999) Satellite cells as players and targets in normal and diseased muscle. *Neuropediatrics* 30: 167-175

2. Fogt D, L,, Slentz M, J,, Tischler M, E,, Henrickson E, J. (1997) GLUT-4 protein and citrate synthase activity in distal or proximally denervated rat soleus muscle. *Am J Physiol* 272: R429-R432

3. Huey KA, Bodine SC (1998) Changes in myosin mRNA and protein expression in denervated rat soleus and tibialis anterior. *Eur J Biochem* 256: 45-50.

4. Jakubiec-Puka A, Ciechomska I, Morga J, Matusiak A (1999) Contents of myosin heavy chains in denervated slow and fast rat leg muscles. *Comp Biochem Physiol B Biochem Mol Biol* 122: 355-362.

5. Jones JP, Roberts BR, Tapscott EB, Dohm GL (1997) Transcriptional regulation of hexokinase II in denervated rat skeletal muscle. *Biochem Biophys Res Commun* 238: 53-55.

6. Jones JP, Tapscott EB, Olson AL, Pessin JE, Dohm GL (1998) Regulation of glucose transporters GLUT-4 and GLUT-1 gene transcription in denervated skeletal muscle. *J Appl Physiol* 84: 1661-1666.

7. Juel C, Halestrap AP (1999) Lactate transport in skeletal muscle—role and regulation of the monocarboxylate transporter. *J Physiol Lond* 517: 633-642

8. Korinthenberg R, Sauer M, Ketelson UP, Hanemann CO, Stoll G, Graf M, Baborie A, Volk B, Wirth B, Rudnik-Schoneborn S, Zerres K (1997) Congenital axonal neuropathy caused by deletions in the spinal muscular atrophy region. *Ann Neurol* 42: 364-368

9. Kostrominova TY, Macpherson PC, Carlson BM, Goldman D (2000) Regulation of myogenin protein expression in denervated muscles from young and old rats. *Am J Physiol Regul Integr Comp Physiol* 279: R179-188.

10. Leschziner A, Moukhles H, Lindenbaum M, Gee SH, Butterworth J, Campbell KP, Carbonetto S (2000) Neural regulation of alpha-dystroglycan biosynthesis and glycosylation in skeletal muscle. *J Neurochem* 74: 70-80.

11. Lie DC, Weis J (1998) GDNF expression is increased in denervated human skeletal muscle. *Neurosci Lett* 250: 87-90

12. Migheli A, Mongini T, Doriguzzi C, Chiado-Piat L, Piva R, Ugo I, Palmucci L (1997) Muscle apoptosis in humans occurs in normal and denervated muscle, but not in myotonic dystrophy, dystrophinopathies or inflammatory disease. *Neurogenetics* 1: 81-87.

13. Ng DC, Carlsen RC, Walsh DA (1997) Neural regulation of the formation of skeletal muscle phosphorylase kinase holoenzyme in adult and developing rat muscle. *Biochem J* 325: 793-800.

14. Novom S, Lewinstein C (1977) Adenylate cyclase and guanylate cyclase of normal and denervated skeletal muscle. *Neurology* 27: 869-874

15. Nozais M, Merkulova T, Keller A, Janmot C, Lompre AM, D'Albis A, Lucas M (1999) Denervation of rabbit gastrocnemius and soleus muscles: effect on muscle-specific enolase. *Eur J Biochem* 263: 195-201.

16. Ontell M (1974) Muscle satellite cells: a validated technique for light microscopic identification and a quantitative study of changes in their population following denervation. *Anat Rec* 178: 211-227.

17. Rich MM, Kraner SD, Barchi RL (1999) Altered gene expression in steroid-treated denervated muscle. *Neurobiol Dis* 6: 515-522

18. Rodrigues A, Schmalbruch H (1995) Satellite cells and myonuclei in long-term denervated rat muscles. *Anat Rec* 243: 430-437.

19. Schmalbruch H, Haase G (2001) Spinal muscular atrophy: present state. *Brain Pathol* 11: 231-247

20. Schmalbruch H, Lewis DM (2000) Dynamics of nuclei of muscle fibers and connective tissue cells in normal and denervated rat muscles. *Muscle Nerve* 23: 617-626.

21. Sedehizade F, Klocke R, Jockusch H (1997) Expressin of nerve-regulated genes in muscles of mouse mutants affected by spinal muscular atrophies and muscular dystrophies. *Muscle Nerve* 20: 186-194

22. Stonnington HH, Engel AG (1973) Normal and denervated muscle. A morphometric study of fine structure. *Neurology* 23: 714-724.

23. Suzuki A , Shen T, Ouyard M, Best-Belpomme M, Hanoune J, Def N (1998) Expression of adenyl cyclase mRNAs in the denervated and in the developing mouse skeletal muscle. *Am J Physiol* 274: C1674-C1685

24. Tang H, Cheung WM, Ip FC, Ip NY (2000) Identification and characterization of differentially expressed genes in denervated muscle. *Mol Cell Neurosci* 16: 127-140.

25. Tawa NE, Odessey R, Goldberg AL (1997) Inhibitors of the proteasome reduce the accelerated proteolysis in atrophying rat skeletal muscles. *J Clin Invest* 100: 197-203.

26. Tews DS, Goebel HH (1997) Apoptosis-related proteins in skeletal muscle fibers of spinal muscular atrophy. *J Neuropathol Exp Neurol* 56: 150-156.

27. Tews DS, Goebel HH, Schneider I, Gunkel A, Stennert E, Neiss WF (1997) Expression of different isoforms of nitric oxide synthase in experimentally dener-vated and reinnervated skeletal muscle. *J Neuropathol Exp Neurol* 56: 1283-1289.

28. Trachtenberg JT (1998) Fiber apoptosis in developing rat muscles is regulated by activity neuregulin. *Dev Biol* 196: 193-203.

29. Vaittinen S, Lukka R, Sahlgren C, Rantanen J, Hurme T, Lendahl U, Eriksson JE, Kalimo H (1999) Specific and innervation-regulated expression of the intermediate filament protein nestin at neuromuscular and myotendinous junctions in skeletal muscle. *Am J Pathol* 154: 591-600.

30. Wallis MG, Appleby GJ, Youd JM, Clark MG, Penschow JD (1999) Reduced glycogen phosphorylase activity in denervated hindlimb muscles of rat is related to muscle atrophy and fibre type. *Life Sci* 64: 221-228

31. Weis J, Kaussen M, Calvo S, Buonanno A (2000) Denervation induces a rapid nuclear accumulation of MRF4 in mature myofibers. *Dev Dyn* 218: 438-451.

32. Weis J, Lie DC, Ragoss U, Zuchner SL, Schröder JM, Karpati G, Farruggella T, Stahl N, Yancopulos GD, DiStefano PS (1998) Increased expression of CNTF receptor alpha in denervated human skeletal muscle. *J Neuropathol Exp Neurol* 57: 850-857

Effects of disuse on muscle

Stirling Carpenter

CK	creatine kinase
N-CAM	neural cell adhesion molecule

Definition of entity

Disuse implies that the connection of motor axon to muscle is preserved, but that there is much less stimulation of the muscle than normal action potentials arriving through the nerve. Spontaneous miniature endplate potentials, and theoretically, trophic influences would be preserved. Animal experiments designed to reproduce the effects of disuse have utilized tetrodotoxin block of sodium channels in axons, hindleg suspension, or casting. None of these methods reproduces exactly the chronic disuse encountered in many human patients. The rat muscles mostly used in such experiments have a relatively uniform fibre composition that differs from the mixed state of normal human muscles.

Metabolic studies

Hindlimb suspension resulted in upregulation of message for muscle CK and glyceraldehyde-3-phosphatase dehydrogenase in rat soleus muscle. Type 2X myosin heavy chain (corresponding to human type 2B) was upregulated subsequently (4). Casting in a shortened position resulted in marked loss of carbonic anhydrase III in the soleus but not plantaris, and loss of phosphoglucose-isomerase in plantaris but not soleus (3). Decreased phosphorylation of regulatory myosin light chains was found after tetrodotoxin block in rat gastrocnemius (8). ATP-ubiquitin-dependent proteolysis is increased in simulated weightlessness, as well as in denervation atrophy (1). In tetraplegic patients, upregulation of uncoupling proteins 2 and 3 has been reported (6), as also occurs in denervation. Disuse atrophy is associated with an absolute increase in the number of

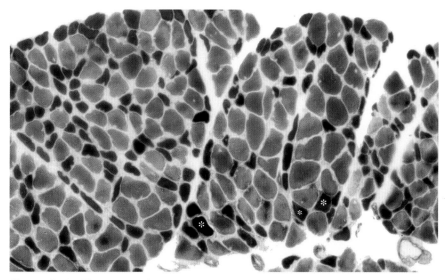

Figure 1. On this ATPase reaction after acid preincubation, most of the type 2 fibres (dark fibres) are atrophic and angular, although they are not grouped. Examples indicated by a star. This is characteristic of disuse atrophy.

glucocorticoid receptors in muscle cells (5).

Structural changes

The majority of studies indicate that the principal finding is atrophy of the type 2 fibres (Figure 1), especially type 2B (2). They usually become angular and may appear to group themselves to a mild extent. Occasionally, they seem to predominate on the periphery of fascicles, mimicking perifascicular atrophy (chapter 11.2). They do not reach the extreme degrees of atrophy that denervated fibres do, nor do they assume such bizarre shapes. N-CAM does not appear on the fibre surfaces. Extrajunctional acetylcholine receptors are much fewer (7) and target fibres do not occur. Electron microscopy does not show the redundant sleeves of basal lamina that are typical of denervated fibres.

Type 2 fibre atrophy is also seen in myasthenia gravis (chapter 9.1), chronic steroid myopathy, cachexia (chapter 15.1), some noncachectic patients with carcinoma, protein malnutrition, and polymyalgia rheumatica.

References

1. Attaix D, Taillandier D, Temparis S, Larbaud D, Aurousseau E, Combaret L, Voisin L (1994) Regulation of ATP-ubiquitin-dependent proteolysis in muscle wasting. *Reprod Nutr Dev* 34: 583-597

2. Bishop DL, Milton RL (1997) The effects of denervation location on fiber type mix in self-reinnervated mouse soleus muscles. *Exp Neurol* 147: 151-158.

3. Brownson C, Loughna P (1996) Alterations in the mRNA levels of two metabolic enzymes in rat skeletal muscle during stretch-induced hypertrophy and disuse atrophy. *Pflugers Arch* 431: 990-992.

4. Cros N, Muller J, Bouju S, Pietu G, Jacquet C, Leger JJ, Marini JF, Dechesne CA (1999) Upregulation of M-creatine kinase and glyceraldehyde3-phosphate dehydrogenase: two markers of muscle disuse. *Am J Physiol* 276: R308-316

5. DuBois DC, Almon RR (1980) Disuse atrophy of skeletal muscle is associated with an increase in number of glucocorticoid receptors. *Endocrinology* 107: 1649-1651.

6. Hjeltnes N, Fernstrom M, Zierath JR, Krook A (1999) Regulation of UCP2 and UCP3 by muscle disuse and physical activity in tetraplegic subjects. *Diabetologia* 42: 826-830.

7. Pestronk A, Drachman DB, Griffin JW (1976) Effect of muscle disuse on acetylcholine receptors. *Nature* 260: 352-353.

8. Takekura H, Kasuga N, Kitada K, Yoshioka T (1996) Morphological changes in the triads and sarcoplasmic reticulum of rat slow and fast muscle fibres following denervation and immobilization. *J Muscle Res Cell Motil* 17: 391-400.

CHAPTER 14

Endocrine disorders and myotrophic molecules

The effect of certain hormones on various aspects of the skeletal muscle fibre biology has been well recognized. The role of thyroid hormones and corticosteroids are particularly well researched and increasingly understood in molecular terms.

More recently, specific myotrophic factors have been identified. These molecules, that may originate from within or from without the muscle fibres, have a net anabolic effect. The best known example is insulin-like growth factor 1 (IGF1), which has therapeutic potential. Other such molecules seem to include beta-adrenergic agonists and creatine monohydrate. This chapter provides and up-to-date account about the molecular and specific pathological aspects of this important topic.

Endocrine disorders and myotrophic molecules

Michael Rose
Robert Griggs

ALS	amyotrophic lateral sclerosis
CK	serum creatinine
MND	motor neurone disease

Definition of entities

Disorders of muscle can arise from a variety of endocrine diseases including those affecting glucocorticoid, thyroid, parathyroid, growth hormone, and insulin levels. Either an excess or deficiency of each of these hormones can present with muscle dysfunction, which shares common themes regardless of the hormone involved. Typically, there is predominant proximal weakness with varying degrees of muscle wasting. In many cases the weakness is disproportionate to the degree of wasting and is associated with minor non-specific myopathic changes in muscle histology. This suggests that functional rather then structural change underlies the weakness.

Thus, in a book entitled *Structural and Molecular Basis of Skeletal Muscle Disease,* this chapter is distinguished by the paucity of any molecular basis for these acquired myopathies, and in most cases, the absence of any specific structural skeletal muscle pathology. Indeed, prominent muscle symptoms without equivalent pathological change should prompt inclusion of endocrine myopathies in the differential diagnosis. The importance of these diseases and the justification for their inclusion in this book lies in the gratifying improvement in muscle symptoms that follows the correction of the abnormal hormone level. Many hormones and hormone regulatory proteins are an important factor in maintaining normal muscle performance and are thus regarded as myotrophic factors. This is particularly evident in considering the changes in muscle function seen with ageing.

Thyroid hormone associated muscle disorders

Clinical features. *Hyperthyroid myopathy.* Although hyperthyroidism is more commonly seen in females than males and has an increasing incidence from the age of 50 years and older, the myopathy associated with it affects males and females equally (48). Usually it is a slowly progressive, painless proximal weakness that is over-shadowed by the systemic symptoms of hyperthyroidism. Although it may be present in up to 80% of cases of hyperthyroidism, it is only a presenting feature in 5% of cases. There may be a predilection for wasting of periscapular muscles with scapular winging. Occasionally there is distal as well as proximal muscle weakness, and very rarely, isolated distal weakness may be seen. Bulbar involvement with dysphagia may occur. In addition to weakness some cases may also have muscle cramps and fasiculations, occasionally of a degree that is mistaken for motor neurone disease/amyotrophic lateral sclerosis (31). Rarely, there may be acute presentation of muscle weakness with myoglobinuria occurring in a thyroid storm. Otherwise acute muscle weakness with hyperthyroidism should prompt a check for a co-existing autoimmune disease namely myasthenia gravis. The creatine kinase (CK) level is usually normal and often low. Electromyography shows myopathic change, and may do so even in those with no muscle involvement on examination. Muscle biopsy shows non-specific myopathic changes with fibre atrophy affecting both fibre types. The symptoms improve within months of the correction of the high thyroid hormone level. Many of the systemic symptoms including those of myopathy improve with β blockers (44).

Hyperthyroid periodic paralysis. Hyperthyroidism is a cause of secondary hypokalaemic periodic paralysis. It was first described in males of Asian origin and remains more common in that ethnic group and gender (33). As with primary hypokalaemic periodic paralysis, attacks of weakness are most often confined to the limbs, and may be precipitated by rest after exercise and carbohydrate load. The weakness is associated with a proportionate degree of hyporeflexia. It may last from hours to days and may recur at a variable frequency up to several per week. The thyroid disorder may be subtle even on biochemical testing and may require persistence and a high level of suspicion to demonstrate (16). An abnormally low circulating TSH level is the most sensitive test; thyroid hormone levels can be normal. The index for suspicion for secondary hyopkalaemic periodic paralysis is heightened if the age of onset is greater than 30-years-old. Correction of the thyroid disorder removes the likelihood of further attacks of periodic paralysis, but attacks do recur if thyroid levels are allowed to rise again (40)

Thyroid eye disease. There are a number of ocular muscle manifestations that can occur in thyroid disease. Hyperthyroid ophthalmopathy is a mild or asymptomatic lid lag or retraction that correlates with the degree of hyperthyroidism and improves with β adrenergic blocking drugs (9). Dysthyroid eye disease is unrelated to the thyroid hormone level and is most often associated with thyroid antibodies as seen in Graves disease and to a lesser extent in Hashimoto's thyroiditis. Features include painful swelling of orbital muscles leading to exophthalmos, sometimes with associated exposure keratitis, a restrictive ophthalmoparesis, and a compressive optic neuropathy (20). The ocular involvement is usually asymmetrical and progresses over a 6 to 18 month period. Corticosteroids and immunosuppressive treatments are used to improve symptoms but occasionally surgical decompression is required to prevent visual loss. Delayed treatment may result in persistent symptoms.

Hypothyroid myopathy. This may occur in up to 40% of those with hypothyroidism. There is a slow onset of mild proximal weakness with muscle swelling, stiffness, cramps, and pain as common additional features. Muscle relaxation maybe impaired causing "pseudomyotonia." In Hoffmann's syndrome, all these features are present together with marked muscle hypertrophy (24). Myoglobinuria can occur. Hypothyroid myopathy has been described as a treatable cause of dropped head syndrome (5). In children, a combination of weakness, slow movements, muscle hypertrophy, and stunted growth was described by Kocher and by Debré and Sémélaigne (2, 39). Hypothyroidism can aggravate coexisting myasthenia gravis (23). Some patients have myoedema which refers to percussion provoked, electrically silent, localised muscle contraction causing mounding. Tendon reflexes are reduced or delayed. The CK is usually high, sometimes with a tenfold rise. The EMG shows myopathic changes and may show spontaneous activity such as fibrillation potentials and sharp waves. A small proportion of patients with hypothyroidism develop myotonia, and in such patients this and other symptoms result from unmasking of an underlying myopathy: myotonic dystrophy type 2, or PROMM (18). The symptoms of hypothyroid myopathy improve in a matter of months following thyroid replacement therapy.

Pathogenesis. With excess thyroid hormone levels there is a multitude of metabolic changes in muscle. Some of these might be thought to be advantageous to muscle function such as the increase in mitochondrial activity and lipid oxidation, the enhanced response of the muscle to catecholamines, and the increased speed of muscle contraction and relaxation. However, these are accompanied by the impairment of muscle glucose uptake, depletion of glycogen, net catabolism of muscle protein, and intracellular potassium loss leading to an overall decline in muscle performance with weakness and fatigue (22).

The aetiology of thyrotoxic periodic paralysis is uncertain. The fact that it has been reported in families suggest an underlying channelopathy. However, the search for both sodium and calcium channel mutations have thus far been unrevealing (26, 27, 34). It is not known whether particular polymorphisms of the same skeletal calcium channel gene, as is implicated in primary hypokalaemic periodic paralysis, predisposes to thyrotoxic induced periodic paralysis. Thyroid hormone given to those with primary hypokalaemic periodic paralysis does not induce attacks of periodic paralysis. Thyroid hormone excess increases Na-K pump numbers, particularly in those with thyrotoxic periodic paralysis, and there is an increased uptake of potassium into muscle during attacks. Calcium pump activity is decreased in thyrotoxic periodic paralysis. How this might relate to muscle membrane depolarisation and inexcitability in thyrotoxic periodic paralysis is unclear (29, 54, 57).

The mild ophthalmopathy seen in thyrotoxicosis is caused by the increased β-adrenergic sensitivity of the ocular muscles induced by the excess thyroid level (52). The more pronounced ophthalmopathy associated with Graves and Hashimoto's diseases is autoimmune in aetiology with thyroid specific antibodies cross reacting with ocular muscle. The specificity of the antibodies for ocular rather than skeletal muscle may be a manifestation of the differing antigenic epitopes present on these two types of muscle; not surprising given their dissimilar physiological characteristics (3, 21). The previously given alternative explanation for the isolated orbital involvement, namely that the ocular contents may be exposed to higher antibody concentrations due interconnecting lymphatic pathways between the thyroid gland and the orbits, seems less plausible (25).

In hypothyroidism there is a general slowing of metabolic processes such as those of glycogenolysis, lipolysis, and mitochondrial respiration which may impair muscle energy production (50). Muscle protein turnover is also impaired. Reduced myosin ATPase activity and calcium uptake by the sarcoplasmic reticulum reduces muscle force generation and slows muscle relaxation. The cause of the marked muscle hypertrophy seen in some cases is obscure since although accumulation of myxoid like material in muscle fibres has been seen in some cases, in most the muscle biopsy is normal (32).

Corticosteroid hormone associated muscle disorders

Clinical features. *Glucocorticosteroid excess; Cushing's syndrome, Iatrogenic corticosteroids*. Glucocorticoid excess leads to a painless symmetrical proximal muscle wasting and weakness affecting the legs more than the arms. It is usually associated with features of systemic glucocorticoid excess. It occurs in up to 80% of cases with Cushing's syndrome. Iatrogenic steroids, especially the 9-α-fluorinated ones like triamcinolone, betamethasone, or dexamethasone can cause dose dependent muscle wasting and weakness within weeks. This can be ameliorated by limitation of the steroid dose, alternate day use, attention to exercise, and a high protein diet. CK in all these cases is normal. EMG may show myopathic features, while muscle biopsy shows type 2 fibre atrophy (1, 36).

Myosin loss myopathy occurs most often when corticosteroids are administered to patients who have concomitant neuromuscular blockade, particularly if there is also sepsis (4, 11). The commonest scenario in which it is seen is in patients with severe asthma requiring ventilation (53). It has also been seen where corticosteroids have been used in those with "physiological," rather than pharmacological neuromuscular blockade, such as is seen in myasthenia (41). There is acute or sub-acute generalised weakness with a proximal emphasis which in severe cases may affect neck, face, and extraocular muscles. There may be associated myoglobinuria. The tendon reflexes are often depressed. The CK may be high, but not necessarily, and in any case will drop to normal levels after a couple of weeks. Nerve conduction studies may show evidence of coexisting "critical care neuropathy." EMG may show a variety of results including being normal, showing myopathic features, spontaneous activity such as fibrillations and positive sharp waves, and being electrically silent. Muscle biopsy may show patchy or complete loss of myosin within muscle fibres best seen on ATPase stain at pH 9.4. Such affected fibres are generally scattered throughout the muscle biopsy.

ACTH excess. ACTH excess, as seen in those with Nelson's syndrome, where the high ACTH results from destruction of the adrenal glands, can be associated with a myopathy similar to that seen in corticosteroid excess even where patients have been treated with corticosteroid replacement therapy (45). However, modern day diagnostic and treatment techniques have probably consigned Nelson's syndrome to the history books.

Corticosteroid deficiency; Addison's disease. Up to half of patients with adrenocorticosteroid deficiency, regardless of the cause, develop a mild proximal symmetrical weakness usually with a normal CK, EMG, and a normal or non-specifically abnormal muscle biopsy. In some cases there is associated myalgia. Rarely, there may be respiratory muscle involvement. A similar picture with prominent muscle pain can be precipitated by abrupt withdrawal of long standing steroid therapy due to suppression of the pituitary adrenal axis by the steroid treatment (35).

Corticosteroid deficiency is a rare cause of secondary hyperkalaemic periodic paralysis (8).

Pathogenesis. Corticosteroids in excess are known to depress glycolysis with relative insulin resistence, and to a lesser extent, mitochondrial oxidative phosphorylation. Since type 2B muscle fibres are more dependant on glycolysis than are type 1 and 2A fibres, this may explain their selective vulnerability to fibre atrophy. The effects of excess corticosteroids on muscle protein turnover are complex. The is a net catabolic effect. Protein synthesis is reduced and this reduction is accelerated where there is concomitant sepsis, dennervation, or lack of exercise. Protein catabolism has been thought to be increased, but lately, evidence suggests that catabolism is actually decreased. Thus, the net muscle protein catabolism results from the fact that protein synthesis is more significantly reduced as compared with the decrease in muscle breakdown (14, 49). Except in the case of acute myosin loss, it is possible that most of the muscle protein loss affects non-contractile proteins since it has proved difficult to demonstrate reduced force generation in muscle exposed to high corticosteroid levels (22).

In Addison's disease mineralocorticoid deficiency results in hyponatraemia and hypovolaemia which contribute to hypotension. The impaired mineralocorticoid activity results in hyperkalaemia with reduced intracellular potassium levels. There is a tendency to fasting hypoglycaemia and depletion of muscle glycogen stores. All of these factors may contribute to weakness and fatigue. The impaired potassium handling may contribute to the periodic paralysis that may occur.

Growth hormone associated muscle disorders

Clinical features. A painful progressive proximal weakness with fatiguability and occasional muscle hypertrophy can occur late in the course of growth hormone excess (acromegaly). In such cases the CK may be only mildly elevated if at all, and the EMG shows myopathic features. The muscle

biopsy may be normal or show a variety of non-specific changes including fibre atrophy or hypertrophy and occasional necrotic fibres. The muscle weakness improves with normalisation of the growth hormone levels (30, 43).

Pathogenesis. Growth hormone increases protein synthesis but despite the resulting increase in muscle mass the muscle force generation is decreased. This may be due to growth hormones action in reducing muscle ATPase activity and reducing sarcolemmal excitability. Insulin resistence and impaired glucose metabolism may contribute to the fatigue and weakness (22, 56).

Insulin associated muscle disorders

Clinical features. Primary generalised muscle weakness is not a feature of diabetes nor of hypoglycaemia. Proximal weakness that does occur is more likely to be due to a neuropathy such as is seen in femoral neuropathy (diabetic amyotrophy) and is painful and most often unilateral. Thus, painless bilateral proximal weakness suggestive of a myopathy occurring in a diabetic patient should prompt a search for causes other than diabetes.

Young patients with poorly controlled diabetes as evidenced by retinopathy, nephropathy, or neuropathy may develop acutely painful, swollen, and tender muscles in either the anterior or posterior thigh, sometimes with a palpable mass. This is often unilateral but sequential bilateral involvement may occur. The pain, tenderness, and swelling usually settle spontaneously, but may recur on the same or opposite side. The CK remains normal. Diagnosis is best made by CT or MRI imaging, which usually shows the focal abnormalities of quadriceps or hamstring muscles. Muscle biopsy is not usually required but shows muscle infarction with areas of necrosis and haemorrhage, and associated inflammatory infiltrates (6, 10).

Flier's syndrome is an ill understood combination of muscle pain, cramps, and fatigue but without weakness. It may be associated with diabetes due to marked insulin resistence. Additional features may include acanthosis nigracans and progressive hand and foot enlargement. The CK may show as much as a fivefold elevation. Muscle biopsy shows no distinctive features. Patients may get symptom relief with phenytoin (12).

Parathyroid associated muscle disorders

Clinical features. Hyperparathyroidism may be primary, due to parathyroid adenoma, or secondary, due to chronic renal disease. Primary hyperparathyroidism may present with muscle stiffness and proximal weakness particularly of the lower limbs. This may be a associated with muscle atrophy, fasiculations, and hyperreflexia. Both the CK and the muscle biopsy may be normal but EMG may show myopathic features. Secondary hyperparathyroidism especially with chronic renal failure may be missed as the calcium level can be normal. However, the alkaline phosphatase is elevated, and phosphate and vitamin D level may be low. The high PTH, low phosphate, and vitamin D may all contribute to the lower limb proximal weakness seen in this situation (13, 42, 58).

In hypoparathyroidism, the effects of peripheral nerve hyperexcitability with tetany and muscle spasm predominate. The muscle spasm can give rise to elevated CK levels (51).

Pathophysiology. Both excess PTH and deficiency of vitamin D cause perturbations in calcium and phosphate levels, but these may not be sufficient to account for the weakness and pain associated with these disease states. Excess PTH reduces the calcium sensivity of the muscle contractile system and deficiency of vitamin D metabolites may exacerbate this effect.

Hormones as trophic factors

Many factors both neuronal and myogenic contribute to the maintenance of normal neuromuscular func-

tion. With ageing, muscle fibre numbers, muscle mass, and muscle strength all show a slow decline, contributing to the muscle atrophy, weakness and fatigue associated with increasing age. Reduced muscle mass may be explained by a decline in anterior horn cell numbers, reduced central activation of muscle, and slowing in muscle synthesis perhaps with accelerated muscle catabolism occurring during intercurrent illness. In part, some of the muscle changes may result from reduced hormone levels such as those of testosterone, growth hormone, insulin-like growth factor 1 (IGF-1), dehydroepiandrosterone (DHEA) oestradiol, and progesterone (19). During exercise training, expression of IGF-1 is up-regulated and contributes to the shift from carbohydrate to fat as the preferred fuel for exercising muscle (15). Increasing IGF-1 expression in rats has been shown to reverse some of the effects of ageing on muscle (7, 37, 38). Administration of exogenous testosterone (55) or growth hormone (59) has improved aspects of muscle structure and function seen in ageing Not surprisingly there has been an interest in using such hormones and trophic factors as potential treatments in wasting neuromuscular disease (17, 28, 46, 47).

References

1. Afifi AK, Bergman RA, Harvey JC (1968) Steroid myopathy. Clinical, histologic and cytologic observations. *Johns Hopkins Med J* 123: 158-173

2. Afifi AK, Najjar SS, Mire-Salman J, Bergman RA (1974) The myopathology of the Kocher-Debre-Semelaigne syndrome. Electromyography, light- and electron-microscopic study. *J Neurol Sci* 22: 445-470

3. Ahmann A, Baker JR, Jr., Weetman AP, Wartofsky L, Nutman TB, Burman KD (1987) Antibodies to porcine eye muscle in patients with Graves' ophthalmopathy: identification of serum immunoglobulins directed against unique determinants by immunoblotting and enzyme-linked immunosorbent assay. *J Clin Endocrinol Metab* 64: 454-460

4. Al-Lozi MT, Pestronk A, Yee WC, Flaris N, Cooper J (1994) Rapidly evolving myopathy with myosin-deficient muscle fibers. *Ann Neurol* 35: 273-279

5. Askmark H, Olsson Y, Rossitti S (2000) Treatable dropped head syndrome in hypothyroidism. *Neurology* 55: 896-897

6. Banker BQ, Chester CS (1973) Infarction of thigh muscle in the diabetic patient. *Neurology* 23: 667-677

7. Barton-Davis ER, Shoturma DI, Musaro A, Rosenthal N, Sweeney HL (1998) Viral mediated expression of insulin-like growth factor I blocks the aging-related loss of skeletal muscle function. *Proc Natl Acad Sci U S A* 95: 15603-15607

8. Bell H, Hayes WL, Vosburgh J (1965) Hyperkalemic paralysis due to adrenal insufficiency. *Arch Intern Med* 115: 418

9. Bouzas AG (1980) The Montgomery Lecture, 1980. Endocrine ophthalmopathy. *Trans Ophthalmol Soc U K* 100: 511-520

10. Chester CS, Banker BQ (1986) Focal infarction of muscle in diabetics. *Diabetes Care* 9: 623-630

11. Danon MJ, Carpenter S (1991) Myopathy with thick filament (myosin) loss following prolonged paralysis with vecuronium during steroid treatment. *Muscle Nerve* 14: 1131-1139

12. Flier JS, Young JB, Landsberg L (1980) Familial insulin resistance with acanthosis nigricans, acral hypertrophy, and muscle cramps. *N Engl J Med* 303: 970-973

13. Frame B, Heinze EG, Jr., Block MA, Manson GA (1968) Myopathy in primary hyperparathyroidism. Observations in three patients. *Ann Intern Med* 68: 1022-1027

14. Goldberg AL, Goldspink DF (1975) Influence of food deprivation and adrenal steroids on DNA synthesis in various mammalian tissues. *Am J Physiol* 228: 310-317

15. Goldspink DF, Cox VM, Smith SK, Eaves LA, Osbaldeston NJ, Lee DM, Mantle D (1995) Muscle growth in response to mechanical stimuli. *Am J Physiol* 268: E288-297

16. Griggs RC, Bender AN, Tawil R (1996) A puzzling case of periodic paralysis. *Muscle Nerve* 19: 362-364

17. Griggs RC, Pandya S, Florence JM, Brooke MH, Kingston W, Miller JP, Chutkow J, Herr BE, Moxley RT, 3rd (1989) Randomized controlled trial of testosterone in myotonic dystrophy. *Neurology* 39: 219-222

18. Griggs RC, Sansone V, Lifton A, Moxley RT (1997) Hypothyroidism unmasking proximal myotonic myopathy. *Neurology* 48: A267 (Abstract)

19. Griggs RC, Welle SL (2001) Aging of the neuromuscular system: hormonal, cellular and molecular factors.

20. Hallin ES, Feldon SE (1988) Graves' ophthalmopathy: II. Correlation of clinical signs with measures derived from computed tomography. *Br J Ophthalmol* 72: 678-682

21. Hiromatsu Y, Fukazawa H, Guinard F, Salvi M, How J, Wall JR (1988) A thyroid cytotoxic antibody that cross-reacts with an eye muscle cell surface antigen may be the cause of thyroid-associated ophthalmopathy. *J Clin Endocrinol Metab* 67: 565-570

22. Kaminski HJ, Ruff RL (1994) Endocrine myopathies. In *Myology*, AG Engel, C Franzini-Armstrong (eds). McGraw-Hill: New York. pp. 1726-1753

23. Kiessling WR, Pflughaupt KW, Ricker K, Haubitz I, Mertens HG (1981) Thyroid function and circulating antithyroid antibodies in myasthenia gravis. *Neurology* 31: 771-774

24. Klein I, Parker M, Shebert R, Ayyar DR, Levey GS (1981) Hypothyroidism presenting as muscle stiffness and pseudohypertrophy: Hoffmann's syndrome. *Am J Med* 70: 891-894

25. Kriss JP, Konishi J, Herman M (1975) Studies on the pathogenesis of Graves' ophthalmopathy (with some related observations regarding therapy). *Recent Prog Horm Res* 31: 533-566

26. Kufs WM, McBiles M, Jurney T (1989) Familial thyrotoxic periodic paralysis. *West J Med* 150: 461-463

27. Leung AK (1989) Familial thyrotoxic periodic paralysis. *West J Med* 151: 209

28. Lynch GS, Cuffe SA, Plant DR, Gregorevic P (2001) IGF-I treatment improves the functional properties of fast- and slow- twitch skeletal muscles from dystrophic mice. *Neuromuscul Disord* 11: 260-268

29. Marx A, Ruppersberg JP, Pietrzyk C, Rudel R (1989) Thyrotoxic periodic paralysis and the sodium/potassium pump. *Muscle Nerve* 12: 810-81

30. Mastaglia FL, Barwich DD, Hall R (1970) Myopathy in acromegaly. *Lancet* 2: 907-909

31. McComas AJ, Sica RE, McNabb AR, Goldberg WM, Upton AR (1974) Evidence for reversible motoneurone dysfunction in thyrotoxicosis. *J Neurol Neurosurg Psychiatry* 37: 548-558

32. McDaniel HG, Pittman CS, Oh SJ, DiMauro S (1977) Carbohydrate metabolism in hypothyroid myopathy. *Metabolism* 26: 867-873

33. McFadzean AJ, Yeung R (1967) Periodic paralysis complicating thyrotoxicosis in Chinese. *Br Med J* 1: 451-455

34. McFadzean AJ, Yeung R (1969) Familial occurrence of thyrotoxic periodic paralysis. *Br Med J* 1: 760

35. Mor F, Green P, Wysenbeek AJ (1987) Myopathy in Addison's disease. *Ann Rheum Dis* 46: 81-83

36. Muller R, Kugelberg E (1959) Myopathy in Cushing's syndrome. *J Neurol Neurosurg Psychiatry* 22: 314-319

37. Musaro A, McCullagh K, Paul A, Houghton L, Dobrowolny G, Molinaro M, Barton ER, Sweeney HL, Rosenthal N (2001) Localized Igf-1 transgene expression sustains hypertrophy and regeneration in senescent skeletal muscle. *Nat Genet* 27: 195-200

38. Musaro A, McCullagh KJ, Naya FJ, Olson EN, Rosenthal N (1999) IGF-1 induces skeletal myocyte hypertrophy through calcineurin in association with GATA-2 and NF-ATc1. *Nature* 400: 581-585

39. Najjar SS (1974) Muscular hypertrophy in hypothyroid children: the Kocher-Debre- Semelaigne syndrome. A review of 23 cases. *J Pediatr* 85: 236-239

40. Okihiro MM, Nordyke RA (1966) Hypokalemic periodic paralysis. Experimental precipitation with sodium liothyronine. *Jama* 198: 949-951

41. Panegyres PK, Squier M, Mills KR, Newsom-Davis J (1993) Acute myopathy associated with large par-enteral dose of corticosteroid in myasthenia gravis. *J Neurol Neurosurg Psychiatry* 56: 702-704

42. Patten BM, Bilezikian JP, Mallette LE, Prince A, Engel WK, Aurbach GD (1974) Neuromuscular disease in primary hyperparathyroidism. *Ann Intern Med* 80: 182-193

43. Pickett JB, Layzer RB, Levin SR, Scheider V, Campbell MJ, Sumner AJ (1975) Neuromuscular complications of acromegaly. *Neurology* 25: 638-645

44. Pimstone N, Marine N, Pimstone B (1968) Beta-adrenergic blockade in thyrotoxic myopathy. *Lancet* 2: 1219-1220

45. Prineas J, Hall R, Barwick DD, Watson AJ (1968) Myopathy associated with pigmentation following adrenalectomy for Cushing's syndrome. *Q J Med* 37: 63-77

46. Rabkin JG, Ferrando SJ, Wagner GJ, Rabkin R (2000) DHEA treatment for HIV+ patients: effects on mood, androgenic and anabolic parameters. *Psychoneuroendocrinology* 25: 53-68

47. Rabkin JG, Wagner GJ, Rabkin R (2000) A double-blind, placebo-controlled trial of testosterone therapy for HIV-positive men with hypogonadal symptoms. *Arch Gen Psychiatry* 57: 141-147; discussion 155-146

48. Ramsay I (1974) *Thyroid disease and muscle dysfunction.* Year Book Medica: Chicago.

49. Rifai Z, Welle S, Moxley RT, 3rd, Lorenson M, Griggs RC (1995) Effect of prednisone on protein metabolism in Duchenne dystrophy. *Am J Physiol* 268: E67-74

50. Schwartz HL, Oppenheimer JH (1978) Physiologic and biochemical actions of thyroid hormone. *Pharmacol Ther [B]* 3: 349-376

51. Shane E, McClane KA, Olarte MR, Bilezikian JP (1980) Hypoparathyroidism and elevated muscle enzymes. *Neurology* 30: 192-195

52. Sharma VK, Banerjee SP (1978) b-adrenergic receptors in rat skeletal muscle. Effects of thyroidectomy. *Biochim Biophys Acta* 539: 538-542

53. Shee CD (1990) Risk factors for hydrocortisone myopathy in acute severe asthma. *Respir Med* 84: 229-233

54. Shizume K, Shishiba Y, Sakuma M, Yamauchi H, Nakao K, Okinaka S (1966) Studies on electrolyte metabolism in idiopathic and thyrotoxic periodic paralysis. I. Arteriovenous differences of electrolytes during induced paralysis. *Metabolism* 15: 138-144

55. Snyder PJ, Peachey H, Hannoush P, Berlin JA, Loh L, Lenrow DA, Holmes JH, Dlewati A, Santanna J, Rosen CJ, Strom BL (1999) Effect of testosterone treatment on body composition and muscle strength in men over 65 years of age. *J Clin Endocrinol Metab* 84: 2647-2653

56. Stern LZ, Payne CM, Hannapel LK (1974) Acromegaly: histochemical and electron microscopic changes in deltoid and intercostal muscle. *Neurology* 24: 589-593

57. Takagi A, Schotland DL, DiMauro S, Rowland LP (1973) Thyrotoxic periodic paralysis. Function of sarcoplasmic reticulum and muscle glycogen. *Neurology* 23: 1008-1016

58. Turken SA, Cafferty M, Silverberg SJ, De La Cruz L, Cimino C, Lange DJ, Lovelace RE, Bilezikian JP (1989) Neuromuscular involvement in mild, asymptomatic primary hyperparathyroidism. *Am J Med* 87: 553-557

59. Welle S, Thornton C, Statt M, McHenry B (1996) Growth hormone increases muscle mass and strength but does not rejuvenate myofibrillar protein synthesis in healthy subjects over 60 years old. *J Clin Endocrinol Metab* 81: 3239-3243

CHAPTER 15

Miscellaneous myopathies

15.1 Cancer-related muscle diseases   266
15.2 Effects of ageing on skeletal muscles and their clinical significance   270
15.3 Hereditary inclusion body myopathies   274
15.4 Marinesco-Sjögren syndrome   277
15.5 Osteomalacia myopathy   279
15.6 Vitamin E deficiency   282
15.7 Amyloid myopathy   284
15.8 Rare myopathies of childhood   287

The existence of this chapter is evidence of the fact that in many muscle diseases we do not yet know the molecular-cellular background, which necessitated their grouping in a special category. We trust that with the passage of time more of these and more diseases will be classifiable in one of the specific chapters based on identified pathogenic mechanism.

Cancer-related muscle disease

Tahseen Mozaffar
Alan Pestronk

CK	serum creatine kinase
EMG	electromyography
IgM	immunglobulin M
Ryr	ryanodine receptors

Definition of entities

Cancer-related muscle diseases are usually paraneoplastic disorders. Paraneoplastic syndromes occur in association with neoplasms, but lying anatomically remote from them (7, 16-18, 21, 22). Paraneoplastic myopathies can be due to one of several underlying etiologies including immune, metabolic, and endocrine. Immune paraneoplastic syndromes are commonly associated with humoral immune mechanisms. Since the spectrum of responses shown by different paraneoplastic myopathies to

treatments is wide (Table 1), and the possible treatments often have prominent side effects or high cost, an accurate, well-documented biopsy diagnosis is important before embarking on therapy.

Type 2 muscle fibre atrophy

Type 2 muscle fibre atrophy is the most common paraneoplastic myopathy (18). The associated clinical syndrome is encountered in about 5% of all patients with cancer. It is especially common (almost 100%) later in the course of neoplasms when weight loss is more than 15% (cachexia), and with neoplasms of the pancreas and stomach. Loss of muscle mass occurs out of proportion to changes in other organ systems. Clinically, muscle wasting is

often more prominent than muscle weakness. Weakness is proximal and symmetric, and mild to moderate in degree. The clinical myopathy syndrome is often associated with a mild sensory-motor neuropathy. This combination of myopathy and neuropathy produces a pattern of weakness that is most prominent in proximal and distal muscles, with sparing of strength in intermediate muscles. Type 2 muscle fibre atrophy may be associated with most neoplasms. It may also be related to medications, such as dexamethasone, that are used in treating neoplasms. Serum creatine kinase (CK) is normal. The weakness is usually reversible when the neoplasm responds to treatment, and with adequate nutrition and exercise.

Myopathy syndrome	Age/ Sex (M:F)	Clinical Features	CK	EMG	Associated malignancies	Muscle pathology	Outcome
Type 2 muscle fibre atrophy	All 1:1	Weakness: Proximal Wasting: Prominent Progression: Slow Weight loss	Normal	Normal	All Late in course	Type 2B fibre atrophy	Prognosis dependent on: Nutrition Malignancy treatment
Paraneoplastic necrotizing myopathy	17-87 4:3	Weakness: Proximal; Symmetric Cranial nerve Dysphagia ± Facial weakness Progression: Rapid (weeks)	Increased 10×-100×	Myopathic Irritable	Adenocarcinoma Lung	Myopathy: Active, little inflammation	Myopathy Corticosteroid responsive Prognosis dependent on: Malignancy treatment
Amyloid	26-80 3:1	Weakness: Proximal ± Distal Muscle enlargement Cardiomyopathy Hepatomegaly Progression: Slow	Normal - Increased 70×	Myopathic Irritable 55%	Multiple myeloma Monoclonal gammopathy	Myopathy: Chronic Amyloid: Perivascular Endomysium	Slowly progressive weakness
Anti-decorin antibody	55	Weakness: Proximal Progression: Slow	Increased 2× to 5×	Myopathic Irritable	Monoclonal gammopathy Waldenström's macroglobulinemia	Myopathy: Chronic Abnormal myonuclei IgM in endomysium	Slowly progressive weakness
Scleromyxedema	29-77 3:2	Weakness: Proximal Progression: Slow Skin: Rash; Raynaud's Lung disease	Normal - Increased 5×	Myopathic Irritable	Acute leukemia Multiple myeloma Monoclonal gammopathy	Myopathy: Active. Perifascicular atrophy Vacuoles	Myopathy? Treatment Prognosis dependent on: Malignancy treatment
Granulomatous myositis	29-63 M>F	Weakness: Proximal Joint contractures Myocarditis Other immune disorders	Increased 3×	Myopathic Irritable	Thymoma	Myopathy: Active Inflammation: Endomysial Granuloma	Myopathy? Corticosteroid responsive Prognosis dependent on: Malignancy treatment

Table 1. Features of cancer-related myopathies.

The mechanisms producing type 2 muscle fibre atrophy are not entirely understood (24). Muscle wasting may be related to cytokines, including tumor necrosis factor-α, interleukins 1 and 6, and interferon-γ. The effects of these cytokines may mimic those of leptin and alter body weight regulation. Lysosome (cathepsin) and proteasome pathways may be involved. A tumor product, proteolysis-inducing factor, initiates muscle protein degradation by activating proteasome pathways.

Pathologically, the small type 2 muscle fibres are angular and scattered through the biopsy (for illustrations, see chapter 13). On routine histochemical stains, type 2 atrophy has many similarities to the changes that occur with acute partial denervation. The process is defined by ATPase stains which show that most of the smallest muscle fibres are type 2, staining darkly at pH 9.4 and lightly at pH 4.3. Most of the largest muscle fibres are type 1. Early in the course of disease, type 2B muscle fibres, with intermediate degrees of staining at ATPase pH 4.6, may be selectively atrophied. In this instance, the largest muscle fibres are composed of both types 1 and 2. Later in the course of disease, even the larger type 1 muscle fibres in the biopsy are somewhat atrophied, but the population of type 2 fibres remains significantly smaller than type 1. These pathological patterns are similar whether the type 2 muscle fibre atrophy occurs in association with neoplasms or other systemic disorders, disuse, malnutrition, and weight loss from other causes. Several features, other than ATPase staining, may distinguish the small angular muscle fibres in type 2 atrophy from denervation atrophy. Typically, the small type 2 fibres are randomly distributed through the biopsy and do not occur in the groups seen with denervation atrophy. In type 2 atrophy, the small muscle fibres are pale on NADH stain and do not stain strongly with non-specific esterase.

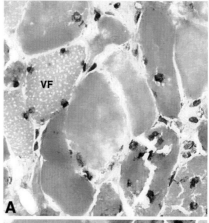

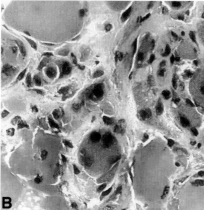

Figure 1. *Paraneoplastic necrotic myopathy.* **A.** In this region of muscle most muscle fibres are undergoing necrosis. Some fibres are pale. Other fibres are somewhat fragmented and invaded by phagocytic cells. Occasional muscle fibres have small vacuoles (VF) through the sarcoplasm that probably reflect dilated sarcoplasmic reticulum. H&E. **B.** Later phases of the necrotic pathology. Small basophilic, regenerating muscle fibres are present. Phagocytosis is more advanced. Some pale, necrotic fibres are present. H&E.

Paraneoplastic necrotizing myopathy

This rare disorder presents most commonly with an acute onset of weakness in patients over 40 years of age (12). Weakness is typically proximal and symmetric. It may progress over a few months to produce severe disability. Myalgias are common. Levels of serum CK are elevated from 8 to 100 times normal. Necrotizing myopathy most commonly occurs in association with adenocarcinoma and non-small cell cancer of the lung, but has been described in the setting of a wide variety of other neoplasms. Weakness often improves with corticosteroid treatment; however, survival is depend-

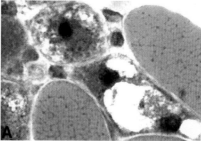

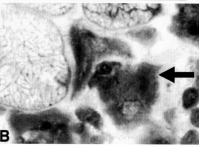

Figure 2. *Scleromyxedema.* **A.** Vacuoles are present in several muscle fibers. H & E. **B.** Large mononuclear cells in perimysium have prominent PAS staining of the cytoplasm (arrow). Original slides courtesy of Dr. A. Verity, UCLA and Drs. T. Medsger and J. Martinez, University of Pittsburgh.

ent on the ability to treat the associated neoplasm.

Pathologically, the hallmark of paraneoplastic necrotizing myopathy is the patchy presence of regions containing numerous necrotic muscle fibres but little inflammation (Figure 1). Muscle fibre necrosis is active, with many fibres having pale staining cytoplasm in H&E stain, with or without phagocytic infiltration into the sarcoplasm. Abundant small basophilic muscle fibres with large nuclei manifest active regeneration. The pattern of patchy regions, or groups of necrotic and regenerating muscle fibres, differs from that seen with acute rhabdomyolysis in which the necrotic fibres are more typically scattered throughout the biopsy. On histochemical staining (NADH-tetrazolium reductase), many muscle fibres have coarse internal architecture. Type 2C fibres, with intermediate staining at ATPase pH 4.3, are often abundant. Alkaline phosphatase staining of endomysial and perimysial connective tissue is often prominent. Inflammation consists mainly of phagocytic cells associated with necrotic muscle fibres. Foci of lymphocytic inflammatory infiltrates are uncommon. The lack of

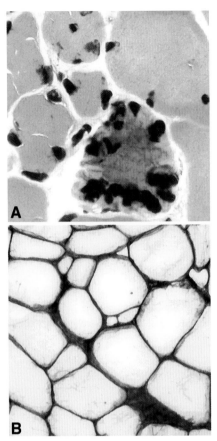

Figure 3. *Anti-decorin antibody associated myopathy.* **A.** Muscle fibres are variably sized. Small fibres are polygonal or rounded. Endomysial connective tissue spaces between muscle fibres are increased. Nuclei have an unusual configuration in some muscle fibres. H& E. **B.** IgM (brown staining) deposited around muscle fibres throughout the endomysial connective tissue.

inflammation suggests that humoral mechanisms, or cytokines, could play an important role in the pathogenesis of this, probably immune, myopathy. Overall, this pattern of muscle pathology has specificity for paraneoplastic necrotizing myopathy and strongly indicates an extensive evaluation for an associated neoplasm.

Scleromyxedema

Scleromyxedema is a multisystem disorder associated with monoclonal gammopathies (M-proteins) involving skin, muscle and other tissues (6, 10, 25). The skin lesions include disseminated papules, plaques, and infiltrative lesions distributed in a symmetric pattern on the face, neck, and arms. Skin pathology involves accumulation of mucopolysaccharides in the upper der-

mis, fibroblast proliferation, and inflammation (6, 25). A slowly progressive proximal, symmetric myopathy occurs in 25% of patients. It is often associated with dysphagia involving the upper esophagus. Other systemic features can include Raynaud's phenomenon, interstitial lung disease, encephalopathy, and weight loss. The disease course varies from spontaneous resolution to progressive disability. Serum CK is elevated in 60% of patients. Electrodiagnostic testing shows an irritative myopathy. The associated M-protein is most commonly IgG λ. Myeloma occurs in 10% of patients. In some cases, weakness associated with the myopathy may improve with immunosuppression. However, long term morbidity is high due to complications of the associated neoplasm.

Muscle pathology can include muscle fibre regeneration, and some necrosis, in perifascicular regions, and scattered through the biopsy. Some muscle fibres have unusual vacuolar changes (Figure 2) that differ from those in storage disorders and inclusion body myopathies. Scattered lymphocytic infiltrates may occur.

Myopathy with anti-Decorin antibodies

This pathologically distinctive, slowly progressive myopathy has onset in the seventh decade, and an association with a monoclonal IgM antibody (2-4). The monoclonal serum IgM binds to decorin, a proteoglycan located in the muscle basal lamina. Weakness is proximal and symmetric. Laboratory testing shows a mildly elevated serum CK and myopathic EMG. Serum IgM binds to endomysial connective tissue in normal muscle. The antigenic epitope on decorin is a chondroitin sulfate moiety.

Muscle pathology shows chronic myopathic changes with variable muscle fibre size and increased endomysial connective tissue (Figure 3). There is little active necrosis or regeneration, and no inflammation. In some muscle fibres, myonuclei are large and have

bizarre shapes. IgM is deposited diffusely in the endomysial connective tissue.

Other cancer associated myopathies

Rippling muscle syndrome. This condition includes cramps induced by exercise or touching muscle (14). Onset is in the fourth to sixth decades. Muscle contractions have a rapid onset, are uncomfortable, and last for a brief period, ie, up to 30 seconds. Acquired rippling muscle syndromes are associated with thymomas and myasthenia gravis. Corticosteroids have been reported to be a useful treatment. Muscle pathology includes inflammation. Myopathic changes are not described.

Amyloid myopathy. This myopathy produces slowly progressive weakness with onset in the sixth to ninth decades (13, 19, 23, 26). Weakness is proximal and symmetric, and respiratory failure may occur. Muscles, including the tongue, may become enlarged. Systemic features of amyloidosis are often present, but the myopathy may be a presenting feature. Serum CK is usually normal. Patients frequently (60%) have a serum M-protein, most often κ or λ light chain disease. Muscle biopsies show myopathic changes with variation in muscle fibre size, some necrosis, and regeneration. Stains for amyloid include Congo red, crystal violet, and thioflavin S. Amyloid may be deposited in the endomysium and around small to moderate sized vessels in the perimysium. In some cases immunostaining of muscle can define the type of immunoglobulin or other protein forming the amyloid deposits. For further reading and illustrations see chapter 15.7.

Inflammatory myopathies including otherwise typical polymyositis or dermatomyositis, are statistically associated with neoplasms (5, 9) (chapter 11.2). The specific association depends, in part, on tumor types, age, and ethnic background. There may be a stronger association between inflammatory myopathies and neoplasm in patients over 40 years of age. There is no clear evidence of an association in children. In white, Northern Europeans there is a stronger association of neoplasm with dermatomyositis than polymyositis. For dermatomyositis, there is a 3-fold increased risk of neoplasms. The strongest associations are with ovarian and lung cancers with squamous or adenomatous cell origin. For poly-myositis, there is a 1.4-fold increased risk of neoplasms. The strongest asso-ciation is with non-Hodgkin lym-phoma. In Asians there is a strong asso-ciation between dermatomyositis and nasopharyngeal carcinoma, especially in patients over 40 years of age (1, 11). Granulomatous myositis occurs with thymoma (and myasthenia gravis or neuromyotonia) (8, 15). The presence of antibodies to ryanodine receptors (RyR) may predict the presence of myositis or myocarditis (15). For typi-cal dermatomyositis or polymyositis, no specific morphologic features have been defined that are predictive of an associated neoplasm.

Endocrine myopathies can be asso-ciated with secretory neoplasms (chap-ter 12). Proximal weakness associated with corticosteroid or ACTH produc-tion is probably the best documented clinical example of this group of disor-ders (20). Corticosteroid-induced weak-ness has been associated with type 2 muscle fibre atrophy, type 2B muscle fibre predominance, or myosin-loss myopathy.

References

1. Abraham SC, DeNofrio D, Loh E, Minda JM, Tomaszewski JE, Pietra GG, Reynolds C (1998) Desmin myopathy involving cardiac, skeletal, and vas-cular smooth muscle: report of a case with immuno-electron microscopy. *Hum Pathol* 29: 876-882

2. Al-Lozi M, Pestronk A (1999) Organ-specific autoan-tibodies with muscle weakness. *Curr Opin Rheumatol* 1: 483-488

. Al-Lozi MT, Pestronk A, Choksi R (1997) A skeletal muscle-specific form of decorin is a target antigen for serum IgM M-protein in a patient with a proximal myopathy. *Neurology* 49: 1650-1654

. Al-Lozi MT, Pestronk A, Yee WC, Flaris N (1995) myopathy and paraproteinemia with serum IgM bind-ing to a high-molecular- weight muscle fiber surface protein. *Ann Neurol* 37: 41-46

5. Callen JP (1994) Myositis and malignancy. *Curr Opin Rheumatol* 6: 590-594

6. Dinneen AM, Dicken CH (1995) Scleromyxedema. *J Am Acad Dermatol* 33: 37-43

7. Giometto B, Taraloto B, Graus F (1999) Autoimmu-nity in paraneoplastic neurological syndromes. *Brain Pathol* 9: 261-273

8. Herrmann DN, Blaivas M, Wald JJ, Feldman EL (2000) Granulomatous myositis, primary biliary cirrho-sis, pancytopenia, and thymoma. *Muscle Nerve* 23: 1133-1136

9. Hill CL, Zhang Y, Sigurgeirsson B, Pukkala E, Mellemkjaer L, Airio A, Evans SR, Felson DT (2001) Frequency of specific cancer types in dermatomyositis and polymyositis: a population-based study. *Lancet* 357: 96-100

10. Launay D, Hatron PY, Delaporte E, Hachulla E, Devulder B, Piette F (2001) Scleromyxedema (lichen myxedematosus) associated with dermatomyositis. *Br J Dermatol* 144: 359-362

11. Leow YH, Goh CL (1997) Malignancy in adult der-matomyositis. *Int J Dermatol* 36: 904-907

12. Levin MI, Mozaffar T, Al-Lozi MT, Pestronk A (1998) Paraneoplastic necrotizing myopathy: clinical and pathological features. *Neurology* 50: 764-767

13. Mandl LA, Folkerth RD, Pick MA, Weinblatt ME, Gravallese EM (2000) Amyloid myopathy masquerad-ing as polymyositis. *J Rheumatol* 27: 949-952

14. Muller-Felber W, Ansevin CF, Ricker K, Muller-Jenssen A, Topfer M, Goebel HH, Pongratz DE (1999) Immunosuppressive treatment of rippling muscles in patients with myasthenia gravis. *Neuromuscul Disord* 9: 604-607

15. Mygland A, Vincent A, Newsom-Davis J, Kaminski H, Zorzato F, Agius M, Gilhus NE, Aarli JA (2000) Autoantibodies in thymoma-associated myasthenia gravis with myositis or neuromyotonia. *Arch Neurol* 57: 527-531

16. Newsom-Davis J (1999) Paraneoplastic neurologi-cal disorders. *J R Coll Physicians Lond* 33: 225-227

17. Pestronk A (2001) Paraneoplastic syndromes. Neu-romuscular Disease Center at Washington University in Saint Louis. *http://wwwneurowustledu/neuromuscu-lar*

18. Posner JB (1995) *Neurologic Complications of Cancer.* FA Davis: Philadelphia

19. Prayson RA (1998) Amyloid myopathy: clinico-pathologic study of 16 cases. *Hum Pathol* 29: 463-468

20. Rebuffe-Scrive M, Krotkiewski M, Elfverson J, Bjorntorp P (1988) Muscle and adipose tissue mor-phology and metabolism in Cushing's syndrome. *J Clin Endocrinol Metab* 67: 1122-1128

21. Rees J (1998) Paraneoplastic syndromes. *Curr Opin Neurol* 11: 633-637

22. Rudnicki SA, Dalmau J (2000) Paraneoplastic syn-dromes of the spinal cord, nerve, and muscle. *Muscle Nerve* 23: 1800-1818

23. Spuler S, Emslie-Smith A, Engel AG (1998) Amy-loid myopathy: an underdiagnosed entity. *Ann Neurol* 43: 719-728

24. Tisdale MJ (2001) Loss of skeletal muscle in can-cer: biochemical mechanisms. *Front Biosci* 6: D164-174

25. Verity MA, Toop J, McAdam LP, Pearson CM (1978) Scleromyxedema myopathy. Histochemical and elec-tron microscopic observations. *Am J Clin Pathol* 69: 446-451

26. Voulgarelis M, Goutas N, Skopouli FN (1999) A 47-year-old woman with persistent watery diarrhea, pro-teinuria, proximal weakness and monoclonal gam-mopathy. *Clin Exp Rheumatol* 17: 351-354

Effects of ageing on skeletal muscles and their clinical significance

George Karpati

mtDNA	mitochondrial DNA
nNOS	nitric oxide synthase
OXPHOS	oxidative phosphorylation

Ageing of skeletal muscle fibres has a 2-fold practical significance. Firstly, in the case of late-onset myopathies, it is presumed that certain ageing changes in skeletal muscles predispose to the development of these types of diseases. The best example is oculopharyngeal dystrophy (4), a genetic disease; however, clinical symptoms do not usually manifest until the fifth-seventh decade. Sporadic inclusion body myositis (16), a non-genetic disease, is another example of such a situation. The second importance of the ageing process of muscle is that it tends to produce a decline in muscle function that is discernible in the activities of daily living, and this decline may be grafted on top of any neuromuscular disease that may develop in old age. This Chapter will briefly summarise the essential current information with respect to these two issues.

Decline of skeletal muscle structure and function in old age

For this communication, old age is defined as being above age 65. This is an arbitrary limit, since the ageing process already starts in early life. However, it is true that the tempo of ageing accelerates over age 60 and it affects many organs. The muscle mass is reduced by as much as 40% between ages 24 to 80 years (14, 18). This appears to be due mainly to shrinkage of the histochemical type 2 fibres (21) and, perhaps, even to apoptosis of muscle fibres (23). Parallel with the muscle atrophy, maximal force generation of limb muscle declines by about 15% between ages 50 to 75 years (9) and approximately by a further 30% between ages 70 to 80 years. The oxidative capacity of muscle cells sig-

nificantly declines particularly for fatty acids (28). Ageing changes of collagen and other elements of the intramuscular connective tissue would predict that the elastic elements would have reduced compliance (5).

There are certain characteristics of skeletal muscle fibres that have appreciable relevance and impact on the ageing process (Table 1). The muscle fibre is a *multinucleated* cell. This implies that apoptotic death of muscle fibres, which would be expected to occur during ageing, cannot take place to any major extent. For details see chapter 1.

Muscle fibres are *post-mitotic cells*, which has relevance to ageing since toxic substances and deleterious molecules must be cleared by a very efficient system normally assigned for this role, ie, ubiquitin-proteosomal system, antioxidants. Otherwise, potentially damaging molecules would remain in the muscle fibre indefinitely and could behave as an old age related negative factor. Lipofuscin appears to be such a substance but deleterious effects have not, thus far, been assigned to this material (38). However, this issue seems to be very relevant to highly reactive oxygen radicals.

The fact that certain muscle fibres are *highly oxidative cells*, particularly histochemical type 1 (slow-twitch) fibres (34), entails the risk of generat-

ing harmful oxygen radicals that may outstrip the neutralising capacity of the counteracting molecules (eg, peroxidases, superoxide dismutase, glutathione) (35) even though there is some evidence that gene expression related to these antioxidant molecules tend to increase with age.

Because the structural and functional integrity of the muscle fibre is greatly dependent on *long-term motor neuronal input*, any old age-related loss or deterioration of motor neurones, or of their function, could exert a significant negative effect on the ageing muscle fibres. Several "trophic" molecules have been identified that are normally transferred from the motor nerve terminal to the muscle fibres (11). Some of these molecules, eg, agrin (11), have presumed transcriptional or translational activities. Thus, a neurogenic element of muscle fibre ageing is quite possible and might contribute to the reduced myofibrillar volume with proportionately or disproportionately reduced force generation.

Since muscle fibres greatly depend on a critical level of *contractile usage* (37) for maintaining their structural and functional integrity, a major reduction of this could also result in significant atrophy. The relatively high prevalence of mental depression or discouragement, joint disease such as osteoarthri-

1. Reduction of motor neuronal trophic input
2. Reduction of androgenic hormone level and/or their tissue receptors
3. Satellite cells' proliferative exhaustion
4. Increased oxidative stresses mediated by free oxygen radicals and NO
5. Impaired proteosomal proteolysis
6. Impaired DNA repair
7. Impaired ATP generation through decline of glycolytic metabolism and mitochondrial OXPHOS
8. Increased and/or mishandled antigenic load
9. Impaired capillarity of muscle causing relative ischemia

Table 1. Major cellular and molecular factors or events that could negatively affect adged skeletal muscle fibers and might predispose them to a heightened response to pathogenic stimuli.

is, osteoporosis, and cardiovascular or pulmonary disease in old age would tend to reduce contractile usage of muscles ("deconditioning"), and thus promote their structural and functional decline.

Adequate quantitative or qualitative *nutrition* (37) is of paramount importance to assure normal structure and function of muscle fibres. Chronically reduced total calorie intake, a real risk in old age, will lead to some degree of cachectic atrophy.

Ageing changes facilitate or trigger late-onset skeletal muscle diseases

There are a number of cellular and molecular events in the ageing skeletal muscle that could create a favourable biological milieu for the appearance of symptomatic muscle disease. Increasing oxidative stress and declining neuronal trophic function have already been cited. In addition, there are 2 major factors that could also play a role: *i)* age-related exhaustion of the proliferative and differentiating capacity of muscle satellite cells (39), and *ii)* age-related alteration of gene expression characteristics of the muscle fibre (19, 20, 29, 32, 33).

Reduced capacity of satellite cells.
Satellite cells are myogenic cells that are normally in a dormant (G_0) state and are situated in the space between the basal lamina and plasma membrane of muscle fibres. In response to only partially understood molecular triggers during normal growth, as well as work hypertrophy or regeneration, they proliferate and fuse with either the parent fibre (growth and hypertrophy) or with each other (regeneration) (39). If an overabundant demand for regeneration arises, eg, in Duchenne muscular dystrophy, the repeated cycles of regeneration may cause satellite cells to reach the limits of the so-called Hayflick constraint.

In other words, a genetically programmed limit to further cell division precludes further regenerative activity of the available satellite cells. In certain situations, this "regenerative exhaus-

tion" may be an important factor in old age. For example, the nearly invariable decline of the strength of the iliopsoas muscle after age of 80 may very well be due to the fact that normally this muscle is subjected to a great deal of lengthening contractions with necrotic consequences requiring constant regeneration. In light of the above, it would not be surprising if a proportion of the satellite cells in such muscle would prematurely exhaust its capacity to contribute to effective regeneration.

Altered gene expression. Alteration of gene expression in old age (19, 20, 29, 32, 33) is probably the most active area of research in the biology of ageing. Several models and techniques have been used to determine the level of changes in gene expression in older *vs.* younger animals and humans. These included the study of transgenic models (25) and premature ageing syndromes, such as Progeria and Werner syndrome (26). The most informative technique was the use of oligonucleotide gene arrays. Membranes containing DNA of several thousand major genes were hybridised with pure mRNA extracted from the test tissues.

The most extensive study of this type was published by Lee et al (19) using an oligonucleotide array corresponding to 6347 genes (5-10% of the mouse genome). Hybridisation profile was established by using mRNA from gastrocnemius muscles of 5 months old (young) and 30 months old (aged) mice. They scored the hybridisation signals as being "significant," if a molecule showed a greater than 2-fold difference between muscles of young and old of either upregulation or downregulation. Approximately 1% of the studied genes showed a significantly increased signal, while about 1% showed significantly reduced level of signal in the muscles of old animals vs. the younger ones. This was interpreted to mean that about 1% of the genes showed a higher or lower level of gene expression (and/or mRNA stability) in the aged animals.

Among the upregulated genes there were 2 noteworthy classes that suggested particular metabolic trends in ageing muscles: *i)* genes pertaining to cellular stress responses, such as those encoding heat-shock proteins, DNA-repair molecules, and molecules combating deleterious oxygen radicals. The largest increase was shown for mitochondrial-sarcomeric creatine kinase, which is designed to boost ATP production, and *ii)* genes pertaining to neuronal regeneration (neurite extension and sprouting). These results imply adaptive mechanisms by the cell to minimise the deleterious effects of general cellular stress, DNA damage, and oxygen radical-induced other cell damage. Additionally, the upregulation of gene expression related to regenerative motor neuronal activity as a response to natural age-related motor neuron fall out is also understandable.

The most important reduced gene expression related to those proteins that regulate glycolysis, cholesterol and fatty acid synthesis, and mitochondrial oxidative phosphorylation as well as those molecules that form proteosomal subunits. Further evidence from other sources also indicates various types of old age-related mitochondrial damage (1, 7, 8, 12, 17). For example, total mitochondrial DNA, as well as molecules responsible for mitochondrial biogenesis, decline.

A very interesting aspect of the experiments by Lee et al (19) is that a 24% calorie restriction starting at 2 months of age has mitigated or eliminated the observed alterations in gene expression profile and significantly increased the longevity of the animals. Calorie restriction caused further alterations in the gene expression profile in muscle (13) by upregulating genes related to protein synthesis and turnover (2), as well as energy metabolism, eg, gluconeogenesis and fatty acid biosynthesis. Genes related to proteins that are instrumental in reducing macromolecular damage have been enhanced by calorie restriction (24). These factors are illustrated in Table 2 (3, 22, 27, 36).

Upregulated gene expression	Downregulated gene expression

1. Genes related to various cellular stresses
 	
  a. Heat-shock
 	
  b. DNA repair molecules
 	
  c. Oxygen radical scavengersor neutralizers
 	
2. Genes related to repairing neuronal injury:
 	
  a. Trophic factors to promote neurite extension and sprouting subserving reinnervation of muscles
	1. Genes related to energy metabolism and reduced ATP generation
	
	  a. Reduced glycolysis with reduced ATP generation
	
	  b. Reduced OXPHOS and mitochondrial ATP generation

Table 2. Significant alterations of gene expression in aged skeletal muscles vs young ones.

While it is not clear if the cited alterations of gene expression are key factors in triggering the appearance of the clinical phenotype of late-onset myopathies, it is conceivable that they play a role. However, the other previously listed factors and circumstances may also contribute. It is important to realise that the study by Lee et al (19) only probed up to 10% of the genome. Indeed, in the rest of the genome, other relevant upregulation or downregulation of genes may well have been present in old age. These might include a change in expression of androgen hormones (6) and/or their receptors which are known to decline in old age. Increased gene expression of pro-apoptotic molecules and an increased IGF1 level may also be uncovered. Furthermore, a reduced capillarity of aged muscles was not reflected by an alteration of gene expression of endotheliotrophic molecules. Additionally, the demonstrated toxicity of nNOS (30, 31) in aged muscles was not reflected in the published gene expression profile.

An additional genomic event that received a great deal of attention is the decline in telomerase activity and the shortening of telomere in cells of aged tissues (10). Skeletal muscle being a post-mitotic cell, this change is probably of limited significance, since telomere shortening is predicated on cell division.

Notwithstanding the above reservations, the cited factors may well have a significant role in facilitating or triggering the phenotypic expression of late-onset myopathies. One such mechanism could be the decline of a compensating molecule that postpones the deleterious effects of a genetic determined deficiency of a protein. This could, perhaps, apply to the late-onset of oculopharyngeal dystrophy although this is only a hypothesis. Another mechanism of old age onset could be an old age-related upregulation of a protein molecule that was generated as a result of a dominant-negative mutation. This could also explain the late-onset of oculopharyngeal dystrophy.

Perhaps the most readily explainable mechanism, by which old age by itself can produce a phenotypically distinct disease, exists in late-onset mitochondrial myopathy (15). In this condition, over many years, the increasing number of naturally occurring multiple mtDNA deletions reach such a high degree in certain muscle fibre segments that OXPHOS and ATP generation is significantly compromised. This occurs by a regional clonal expansion of a deleted (at multiple sites) mtDNA copy arising from still unknown reasons. A role for oxidative stress has been suspected but not proven in this process. It would be of interest to determine if caloric restriction would, at least partially, counteract this change, and thus, would eliminate the suppression of OXPHOS even in the natural ageing process.

Future perspectives

An exhaustively detailed analysis of all gene expression changes in ageing muscle would help in the further understanding of the cellular and molecular mechanisms that operate in old age onset muscle diseases. This research is now largely facilitated by the availability of the findings of the universal genome projects and the various DNA chip technologies that permit the screening quantitatively, simultaneously, and cost-effectively of the expression profile of tens of thousands of genes.

References

1. Barazzoni R, Short KR, Nair KS (2000) Effects aging on mitochondrial DNA copy number and cytochrome c oxidase gene expression in rat skeletal muscle, liver, and heart. *J Biol Chem* 275: 3343-3344

2. Beaufrere B, Boirie Y (1998) Aging and protein metabolism. *Curr Opin Clin Nutr Metab Care* 1: 85-8

3. Bejma J, Ji LL (1999) Aging and acute exercise enhance free radical generation in rat skeletal muscle. *J Appl Physiol* 87: 465-470.

4. Brais B, Bouchard JP, Xie YG, Rochefort DL, Chretien N, Tome FM, Lafreniere RG, Rommens J, Uyama E, Nohira O, Blumen S, Korczyn AD, Heutink Mathieu J, Duranceau A, Codere F, Fardeau Rouleau GA, Korcyn AD (1998) Short GCG expansions in the PABP2 gene cause oculopharyngeal muscular dystrophy. *Nat Genet* 18: 164-167.

5. Brown M, Fisher JS, Salsich G (1999) Stiffness and muscle function with age and reduced muscle use. *Orthop Res* 17: 409-414.

6. Clague JE, Wu FC, Horan MA (1999) Difficulties measuring the effect of testosterone replacement therapy on muscle function in older men. *Int J Androl* 2 261-265.

7. Cormio A, Lezza AM, Vecchiet J, Felzani G, Marangi L, Guglielmi FW, Francavilla A, Cantatore P, Gadaleta

ta MN (2000) MtDNA deletions in aging and in nonmitochondrial pathologies. *Ann N Y Acad Sci* 908: 299-301.

8. Cottrell DA, Blakely EL, Borthwick GM, Johnson MA, Taylor GA, Brierley EJ, Ince PG, Turnbull DM (2000) Role of mitochondrial DNA mutations in disease and aging. *Ann N Y Acad Sci* 908: 199-207.

9. Danneskiold-Samsoe B, Kofod V, Munter J, Grimby G, Schnohr P, Jensen G (1984) Muscle strength and functional capacity in 78-81-year-old men and women. *Eur J Appl Physiol Occup Physiol* 52: 310-314

10. Decary S, Hamida CB, Mouly V, Barbet JP, Hentati F, Butler-Browne GS (2000) Shorter telomeres in dystrophic muscle consistent with extensive regeneration in young children. *Neuromuscul Disord* 10: 113-120.

11. Fuhrer C, Gautam M, Sugiyama JE, Hall ZW (1999) Roles of rapsyn and agrin in interaction of postsynaptic proteins with acetylcholine receptors. *J Neurosci* 19: 6405-6416.

12. Fukagawa NK, Li M, Liang P, Russell JC, Sobel BE, Absher PM (1999) Aging and high concentrations of glucose potentiate injury to mitochondrial DNA. *Free Radic Biol Med* 27: 1437-1443.

13. Hansen BC, Bodkin NL, Ortmeyer HK (1999) Calorie restriction in nonhuman primates: mechanisms of reduced morbidity and mortality. *Toxicol Sci* 52: 56-60.

14. Janssen I, Heymsfield SB, Wang ZM, Ross R (2000) Skeletal muscle mass and distribution in 468 men and women aged 18-88 yr. *J Appl Physiol* 89: 81-88.

15. Johnston W, Karpati G, Carpenter S, Arnold D, Shoubridge EA (1995) Late-onset mitochondrial myopathy. *Ann Neurol* 37: 16-23.

16. Karpati G (1997) Inclusion body myositis. *The Neurologist* 3: 201-208

17. Kovalenko SA, Kopsidas G, Islam MM, Heffernan D, Fitzpatrick J, Caragounis A, Gingold E, Linnane AW (1998) The age-associated decrease in the amount of amplifiable full-length mitochondrial DNA in human skeletal muscle. *Biochem Mol Biol Int* 46: 1233-1241.

18. Larsson L (1978) Morphological and functional characteristics of the ageing skeletal muscle in man. A cross-sectional study. *Acta Physiol Scand Suppl* 457: 1-36

19. Lee CK, Klopp RG, Weindruch R, Prolla TA (1999) Gene expression profile of aging and its retardation by caloric restriction. *Science* 285: 1390-1393.

20. Lee DH, Lockhart DJ, Lerner RA, Schultz P (2000) Mitotic misregulation and human aging. *Science* 287: 2486-2492

21. Lexell J, Taylor CC, Sjostrom M (1988) What is the cause of the ageing atrophy? Total number, size and proportion of different fiber types studied in whole vastus lateralis muscle from 15- to 83-year-old men. *J Neurol Sci* 84: 275-294.

22. Locke M (2000) Heat shock transcription factor activation and hsp72 accumulation in aged skeletal muscle. *Cell Stress Chaperones* 5: 45-51.

23. Malmgren LT, Jones C, Bookman LM (1999) Stereological study of apoptosis in the aging human thy-

roarytenoid muscle. *NIH-NIA Grant Abstract #298*, date 2/15/99 session K2 poster

24. Merry BJ (2000) Calorie restriction and age-related oxidative stress. *Ann N Y Acad Sci* 908: 180-198.

25. Musaro A, Rosenthal N (1999) Transgenic mouse models of muscle aging. *Exp Gerontol* 34: 147-156.

26. Nehlin JO, Skovgaard GL, Bohr VA (2000) The Werner syndrome. A model for the study of human aging. *Ann N Y Acad Sci* 908: 167-179.

27. Pansarasa O, Bertorelli L, Vecchiet J, Felzani G, Marzatico F (1999) Age-dependent changes of antioxidant activities and markers of free radical damage in human skeletal muscle. *Free Radic Biol Med* 27: 617-622.

28. Pastoris O, Boschi F, Verri M, Baiardi P, Felzani G, Vecchiet J, Dossena M, Catapano M (2000) The effects of aging on enzyme activities and metabolite concentrations in skeletal muscle from sedentary male and female subjects. *Exp Gerontol* 35: 95-104.

29. Petropoulou C, Chondrogianni N, Simoes D, Agiostratidou G, Drosopoulos N, Kotsota V, Gonos ES (2000) Aging and longevity. A paradigm of complementation between homeostatic mechanisms and genetic control? *Ann N Y Acad Sci* 908: 133-142.

30. Richmonds CR, Boonyapisit K, Kusner LL, Kaminski HJ (1999) Nitric oxide synthase in aging rat skeletal muscle. *Mech Ageing Dev* 109: 177-189.

31. Richmonds CR, Kaminski HJ (2000) Nitric oxide myotoxicity is age related. *Mech Age Develop* 113: 183-191

32. Schachter F (2000) Genetics of survival. *Ann N Y Acad Sci* 908: 64-70.

33. Slagboom PE, Heijmans BT, Beekman M, Westendorp RG, Meulenbelt I (2000) Genetics of human aging. The search for genes contributing to human longevity and diseases of the old. *Ann N Y Acad Sci* 908: 50-63.

34. Slater CR, Harris JB (1994) The anatomy and physiology of the motor unit. In *Disorders of voluntary muscles*, JN Walton, G Karpati, D Hilton-Jones (eds). Churchill Livingston: Edinburgh. pp. 3-32

35. Spiers S, McArdle F, Jackson MJ (2000) Aging-related muscle dysfunction. Failure of adaptation to oxidative stress? *Ann N Y Acad Sci* 908: 341-343.

36. Squier TC, Bigelow DJ (2000) Protein oxidation and age-dependent alterations in calcium homeostasis. *Front Biosci* 5: D504-526.

37. Starling RD, Ades PA, Poehlman ET (1999) Physical activity, protein intake, and appendicular skeletal muscle mass in older men. *Am J Clin Nutr* 70: 91-96.

38. Terman A, Brunk UT (1998) Lipofuscin: mechanisms of formation and increase with age. *Apmis* 106: 265-276.

39. Webster C, Blau HM (1990) Accelerated age-related decline in replicative life-span of Duchenne muscular dystrophy myoblasts: implications for cell and gene therapy. *Somat Cell Mol Genet* 16: 557-565.

Hereditary inclusion body myopathies

Zohar Argov
Dov Soffer

DMRV	distal myopathy with rimmed vacuoles
HIBM	hereditary inclusion body myopathy
QSM	quadriceps-sparing myopathy

Definition of entities

Hereditary inclusion body myopathies (HIBM) are a heterogeneous group of muscle diseases with the following broad-term diagnostic criteria: *i)* primarily limb muscle weakness (ophthalmoplegia or facial weakness are possible), *ii)* onset in adolescence or early adulthood (earlier onset has been recorded), *iii)* at least 2 affected members in the same family (typical phenotype in a known ethnic cluster suffices), *iv)* presence of rimmed vacuoles and 15 to 21 nm tubular filamentous inclusions in myofibres, and *v)* no inflammation (1, 7).

Molecular genetics and pathophysiology

The proposed classification (Table 1) is similar to those used in other hereditary neuromuscular disorders (1). Dominantly-inherited adult disorders with distal weakness and rimmed vacuoles prevalent in Scandinavia (eg, Welander distal myopathy linked to chromosome 2p13 and Finnish tibial muscular dystrophy linked to chromosome 2q) may be related to HIBM sharing common pathophysiological processes.

Structural changes

Light microscopy. Except for the lack of inflammation, the light microscopic features of HIBM (Figures 1, 2) are almost identical to those of sporadic IBM. Typical biopsy shows vacuolated myofibres associated with variable degrees of neurogenic and myopathic features, and endomysial fibrosis (2, 5, 10, 14).

The number of vacuolated fibres ranges from the very few to up to 70%

of the fibres. On cryostat sections, the vacuoles are typically rimmed by granular eosinophilic material that is also present in their lumen; consequently, they are called "rimmed vacuoles." These granules stain purple-red with the modified Gomori trichrome stain, and are dissolved on paraffin sections making the identification of vacuolated myofibres in such preparations very difficult. The vacuoles may be rounded, cleft-like, or irregularly shaped. They are often subsarcolemmal, but can be located in the centre of the fibre;

HIBM1-autosomal dominant types

Type	Characteristics
HIBM1A	Adult onset (4-5th decade) proximal and distal limb muscle weakness. Linkage to chromosome 8 was detected in one family.
HIBM1B	Fascioscapulohumeral dystrophy-like disorder appearing either distally in hand muscles at early childhood or proximally in the legs. Gene site is unknown.
HIBM1C	Proximal weakness affecting primarily the pectoral and quadriceps muscles, external ophthalmoplegia and joint contractures. Onset can be traced to early childhood with further deterioration during adulthood. Myosin 2A gene on chromosome 17 is mutated (8).
HIBM1D	Variable onset from teenage to early 6th decade with distal weakness in the legs. Progression to the proximal and bulbar musculature. Linkage to chromosome 19p13.
HIBM1E	A distal myopathy of late onset, around age 60 manifesting first in the posterior leg and thigh muscles. Gene site is unknown.

HIBM2-autosomal recessive types

Type	Characteristics
HIBM2A	This unique quadriceps-sparing myopathy (QSM) (2, 13) starts in young adulthood and slowly pro-gresses to affect all limb muscles, except the quadriceps which remains strong even at advanced age. This prototypic disorder was first identified in Iranian Jews (12) but QSM type of HIBM exists in other communities: Afghani Iraqi Jews, Egyptian Jews (with facial involvement), non Jews from India, Caucasian from the USA, Denmark and Italy, Hispanic from Mexico and Arab Bedouins (1, 3). The disease in most of the reported families was linked to chromosome 9p1 (11).
HIBM2B	Japanese adult-onset distal myopathy with rimmed-vacuole (DMRV). The main difference from HIBM2A is the involvement of the quadriceps about a decade later. The gene site is however similar at chromosome 9p1-q1 (7).
HIBM2C	Myopathy associated with white matter abnormalities on brain MRI. The Tunisian form is linked to chromosome 9p1-q1.
HIBM2D	Oculopharyngodistal myopathy. Gene site is unknown.
HIBM2E	Scapuloperoneal syndrome with rimmed vacuoles that may be defined as HIBM. Gene site is un-known.

Table 1. Classification of hereditary inclusion body myopathies.

they are single or multiple, and measure 2 to 25 microns in diameter.

Involved muscle fibres may be normal in size or atrophic, and are either of type 1 or type 2. In many cases small, refractive, eosinophilic inclusions are seen in the cytoplasm, usually near the vacuoles. Less commonly, intranuclear inclusions are present.

Neurogenic changes include the presence of angular atrophic fibres, either randomly scattered or grouped in nuclear clumps. Other common myopathic changes include marked variation in fibre size, presence of hypertrophied fibres, central nuclei, muscle fibre splitting, and scattered myofibre necrosis and regeneration. In addition, there is interstitial fibrosis and adipose replacement. Amyloid deposits are rare in HIBM.

Immunohistochemistry. The SM-31 monoclonal antibody directed against 200 kD phosphorylated neurofilaments (cross reacting with hyperphosphorylated tau) stains "squiggly" inclusions, corresponding to the "paired helical filaments" in sporadic IBM (4). It was suggested that SMI-310 (another monoclonal antibody to phosphorylated neurofilament) can separate between the hereditary and sporadic forms of IBM since strong immunoreactivity is seen only in the latter (3, 11). Accumulation within abnormal muscle fibres of several proteins that are characteristic of Alzheimer's disease brain (eg, beta-amyloid, epitopes of beta-amyloid precursor protein, apolipoprotein E, presenilin 1, cellular prion protein and alpha-synuclein) have been detected (3, 4).

Electron microscopy. A diagnostic hallmark of HIBM (Figures 3, 4) is the collection of 15 to 21 nm cytoplasmic tubolofilaments (5, 10) that may also be present in the nuclei of myofibres. The tubulofilaments are thicker, longer, and less regularly spaced than the adjacent thick myofilaments (5). They are randomly dispersed, but sometimes run parallel to one another. The filamentous inclusions are typically present near the

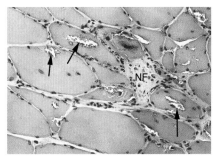

Figure 1. *Rimmed vacuoles.* There are several rimmed vacuoles (arrows), one necrotic fibre (NF), others with central nuclei and splitting. Haematoxylin and eosin.

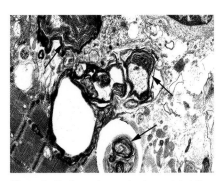

Figure 3. Electron micrograph of vacuolated fibre showing membranous whorls, so-called "myeloid bodies" (arrows) and cytoplasmic debris.

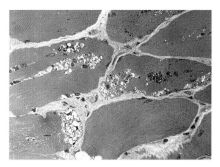

Figure 2. Rimmed vacuoles containing cytoplasmic membranous debris as seen in a semithin epoxy resin section. Toluidine blue.

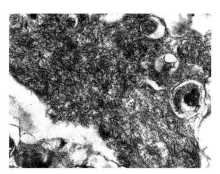

Figure 4. A tubulofilamentous cytoplasmic inclusion adjacent to a vacuole containing membrane fragments and debris.

vacuoles, and a minimum of 3 vacuolated fibres must be scrutinised to detect them with confidence. These inclusions are thought to be made up of paired helical filaments (4). The nonmembrane bound vacuoles are filled with degradation products consisting of membranous whorls, the so-called "myeloid structures"; membrane fragments; and debris. Other ultrastructural findings include the occurrence of cytoplasmic bodies and occasional abnormal mitochondria.

Future perspectives

It is clear that the HIBM heterogeneous group will be divided into different conditions as disease-responsible defective genes are identified. These disorders may share a common pathway of muscle cellular death that is different from the common necrosis seen in other hereditary myopathies. Apoptosis may play a more important role in HIBM, and the similarities between neuronal degeneration and HIBM may become more clear.

Recently, the gene for the QSM type of HIBM was identified (6). It encodes a key enzyme of the sialic acid metabolism. It remains to be determined how this results in the obeserved myopathic changes, but other forms of recessive HIBM may harbor mutations in this gene too

References

1. Argov Z, Eisenberg I, Mitrani-Rosenbaum S (1998) Genetics of inclusion body myopathies. *Curr Opin Rheumatol* 10: 543-547

2. Argov Z, Yarom R (1984) "Rimmed vacuole myopathy" sparing the quadriceps. A unique disorder in Iranian Jews. *J Neurol Sci* 64: 33-43

3. Askanas V, Engel WK (1998) Sporadic inclusion-body myositis and hereditary inclusion-body myopathies: current concepts of diagnosis and pathogenesis. *Curr Opin Rheumatol* 10: 530-542

4. Askanas V, Engel WK (2001) Inclusion-body myositis: newest concepts of pathogenesis and relation to aging and Alzheimer disease. *J Neuropathol Exp Neurol* 60: 1-14

5. Carpenter S (1996) Inclusion body myositis, a review. *J Neuropathol Exp Neurol* 55: 1105-1114

6. Eisenberg I, Avidan N, Potikha T, Hochner H, Chen M, Olender T, Barash M, Shemesh M, Sadeh M, Grabov-Nardini G, Shmilevich I, Friedmann A, Karpati G, Bradley WG, Baumbach L, Lancet D, Ben Asher E,

Beckmann JS, Argov Z, Mitrani-Rosenbaum S (2001) UDP-N-Acetylglucosamine 2-epimerase/N-acetylman-nosamine kinase is mutated in recessive hereditary inclusion body myopathy. *Nat Genet* 29: 83-87

7. Griggs RC, Askanas V, DiMauro S, Engel A, Karpati G, Mendell JR, Rowland LP (1995) Inclusion body myositis and myopathies. *Ann Neurol* 38: 705-713

8. Ikeuchi T, Asaka T, Saito M, Tanaka H, Higuchi S, Tanaka K, Saida K, Uyama E, Mizusawa H, Fukuhara N, Nonaka I, Takamori M, Tsuji S (1997) Gene locus for autosomal recessive distal myopathy with rimmed vacuoles maps to chromosome 9. *Ann Neurol* 41: 432-437

9. Martinsson T, Oldfors A, Darin N, Berg K, Tajsharghi H, Kyllerman M, Wahlstrom J (2000) Autosomal dominant myopathy: missense mutation (Glu-706 → Lys) in the myosin heavy chain IIa gene. *Proc Natl Acad Sci USA* 97: 14614-14619

10. Mikol J, Engel AG (1994) Inclusion body myositis. In *Myology: Basic and Clinical*, AG Engel, C Frazini-Armstrong (eds). McGraw-Hill: New York. pp. 1384-1398

11. Mirabella M, Alvarez RB, Bilak M, Engel WK, Askanas V (1996) Difference in expression of phosphorylated tau epitopes between sporadic inclusion-body myositis and hereditary inclusion-body myopathies. *J Neuropathol Exp Neurol* 55: 774-786

12. Mitrani-Rosenbaum S, Argov Z, Blumenfeld A, Seidman CE, Seidman JG (1996) Hereditary inclusion body myopathy maps to chromosome 9p1-q1. *Hum Mol Genet* 5: 159-163

13. Sadeh M, Argov Z (1997) Hereditary inclusion body myopathy in Jews of Persian origin: Clinical and laboratory data. In *Inclusion Body Myositis and Myopathies*, V Askanas, WK Engel, G Serratrice (eds). Cambridge University Press: Cambridge. pp. 191-199

14. Sadeh M, Gadoth N, Hadar H, Ben-David E (1993) Vacuolar myopathy sparing the quadriceps. *Brain* 116: 217-232

Marinesco-Sjögren syndrome

Caroline A. Sewry

Definition of entity

Marinesco-Sjögren syndrome (OM-IN 248800) is a rare degenerative, spinocerebellar disorder in which the most prominent features are cerebellar ataxia, congenital cataracts and mental retardation (2, 6). Additional features include ptosis, strabismus, microcephaly, short stature, hypergonadotropic hypogonadism, joint laxity, and a variety of skeletal abnormalities, including pigeon chest, contractures and scoliosis. Hypotonia and muscle weakness, affecting several muscle groups, are early features (4, 5). Serum creatine kinase activity (CK) may be elevated, but is not a consistent feature; acute rhabdomyolysis with very elevated CK can also occur (3).

Molecular genetics and pathophysiology

Evidence indicates autosomal recessive inheritance; however, linkage and the gene(s) responsible have not been identified. Linkage to the locus for hypergonadotropic hypogonadism was suggested, but not substantiated, in one study (7).

The precise cause(s) of Marinesco-Sjögren syndrome have not been determined. A lysosomal storage disorder (11) and vitamin E deficiency (1) have been proposed, as well as the suggestion that apoptosis and nuclear changes may have a primary role (8).

Structural changes

Light microscopy. The pathological features of muscle biopsies are myopathic (Figure 1). They include variation in fibre size, an increase in internal nuclei, and mild necrosis and regeneration. Rimmed vacuoles and autophagic vacuoles are common (Figure 1). An increase in connective tissue and fat can also occur and appearances resembling congenital muscular dystrophy have been observed (9). Mitochondrial

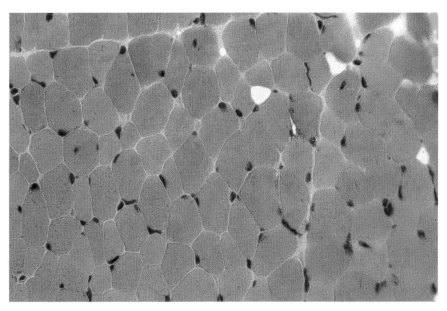

Figure 1. Muscle section stained with haematoxylin and eosin showing variation in fiber size, occasional internal nuclei and a peripheral vacuole. Magnification: ×102.

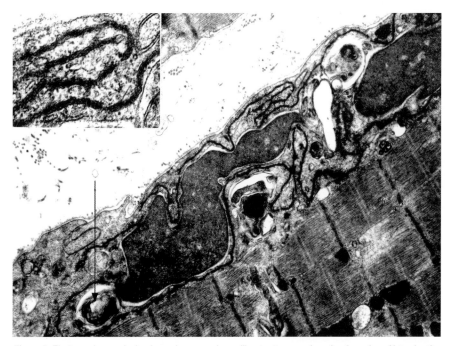

Figure 2. Electron micrograph showing a dense membrane-like structure round a pyknotic nucleus. Note also the myelin whorl (arrow). Insert (upper left) is a higher magnification of the dense membrane-like structure. Magnification: ×15000, insert ×51000.

changes presenting as ragged-red fibres have also been reported (10). Type 1 predominance is a common, but not universal feature; a deficiency of 2B fibres and an increase in 2C fibres can also occur.

Immunocytochemistry. Extensive immunocytochemical studies have not been reported, although dystrophin expression was normal in the cases studied by Tachi et al (9). A small number of fibres expressing foetal myosin may occur, suggesting a little regeneration following muscle damage. Studies of emerin and lamin expression have not revealed any changes to the nuclear membrane.

Electron microscopy. Membranous whorls often occur, particularly in perinuclear regions. Mitochondria may also show abnormalities (5, 10) and some nuclei may be pyknotic and have dense heterochromatin. A unique feature is a dense double membrane structure, of unknown origin (Figure 2), associated with a proportion of nuclei (4, 5). In the author's experience this structure has only been observed in Marinesco-Sjögren syndrome, but it is not clear if it is a consistent feature.

Future perspectives

Identifying the genetic cause of Marinesco-Sjögren syndrome is likely to occur before the origin of the dense membranous structure and the underlying pathogenesis of all the diverse clinical features have been determined. The application of modern pathological tools, such as immunocytochemistry, has not been extensively used, but may be useful in the elucidation of some pathological aspects.

References

1. Aguglia U, Annesi G, Pasquinelli G, Spadafora P, Gambardella A, Annesi F, Pasqua AA, Cavalcanti F, Crescibene L, Bagala A, Bono F, Oliveri RL, Valentino P, Zappia M, Quattrone A (2000) Vitamin E deficiency due to chylomicron retention disease in Marinesco-Sjögren syndrome. *Ann Neurol* 47: 260-264

2. Marinesco G, Draganesco S, Vasiliu D (1931) Nouvelle maladie familiale caracterisee par une cataracte congenitale et une arret du development somato-neuro-psychique. *Encephale* 26: 97-109

3. Muller-Felber W, Zafiriou D, Scheck R, Patzke I, Toepfer M, Pongratz DE, Walther U (1998) Marinesco Sjögren syndrome with rhabdomyolysis. A new subtype of the disease. *Neuropediatrics* 29: 97-101

4. Sasaki K, Suga K, Tsugawa S, Sakuma K, Tachi N, Chiba S, Imamura S (1996) Muscle pathology in Mari-nesco-Sjögren syndrome: a unique ultrastructural feature. *Brain Dev* 18: 64-67

5. Sewry CA, Voit T, Dubowitz V (1988) Myopathy with unique ultrastructural feature in Marinesco-Sjögren syndrome. *Ann Neurol* 24: 576-580

6. Sjögren T (1947) Hereditary congenital spinocerebellar ataxia combined with congenital cataract and oligophrenia. *Acta Psychiat Neurol Scand* 46 (suppl.): 286-289.

7. Skre H, Berg K (1977) Linkage studies on Marinesco-Sjögren syndrome and hypergonadotropic hypogonadism. Clin Genet 11: 57-66

8. Suzuki Y, Murakami N, Goto Y, Orimo S, Komiyama A, Kuroiwa Y, Nonaka I (1997) Apoptotic nuclear degeneration in Marinesco-Sjögren syndrome. *Acta Neuropathol (Berl)* 94: 410-415

9. Tachi N, Nagata N, Wakai S, Chiba S (1991) Congenital muscular dystrophy in Marinesco-Sjögren syndrome. *Pediatr Neurol* 7: 296-298

10. Torbergsen T, Aasly J, Borud O, Lindal S, Mellgren SI (1991) Mitochondrial myopathy in Marinesco-Sjögren syndrome. *J Ment Defic Res* 35: 154-159

11. Walker PD, Blitzer MG, Shapira E (1985) Marinesco-Sjögren syndrome: evidence for a lysosomal storage disorder. *Neurology* 35: 415-419

Osteomalacia myopathy

James M. Gilchrist

DBP	vitamin D-binding protein
PTH	parathyroid hormone
SOC	store-operated calcium
VDR	vitamin D receptor

Definition of entity

Osteomalacia is the abnormal mineralization of bone after closure of epiphyseal plates. Causes of osteomalacia myopathy are listed in Table 1 (6). Bone pain is the most common initial complaint of osteomalacia, but proximal arm and leg weakness from myopathy is very common, occurring in 73 to 97% of cases. Increased deep tendon reflexes are also commonly seen. Short stature and kyphoscoliosis can be seen in longstanding cases. The weakness is by no means specific to osteomalacia, but the combination of pain, hyperactive reflexes and proximal weakness should immediately key the clinician to consider this diagnosis.

Laboratory abnormalities in osteomalacia vary according to the cause. Alkaline phosphatase level is the most sensitive screening test, being elevated in 80 to 90% of patients. In vitamin D deficiency, low serum calcium, phosphorus and 25(OH)D vitamin D levels, increased parathyroid hormone (PTH) levels, decreased urinary calcium levels and increased urinary phosphorus levels are common, but their absence does not exclude the diagnosis. Patients with chronic phosphorus depletion will have low serum phosphorus, normal serum calcium, increased urinary calcium and absent urinary phosphorus. Patients with hypophosphatemia from urinary loss will have normal serum calcium, low serum phosphorus, low urine calcium and high urine phosphorus levels. Creatine phosphokinase levels are usually normal and only infrequently elevated.

On radiological examination, pseudofractures and biconcave vertebral bodies are seen in two thirds of patients, with osteopenia/osteoporosis the most common findings. Bone densitometry is not helpful, but bone biopsy is diagnostic. Major histological findings are increased osteiod surface, increased thickness of the osteoid seam, and an abnormal calcification front. Electromyography reveals small, polyphasic and brief motor unit potentials without fibrillations or positive waves, indicating a non-destructive myopathy, a finding common to all endocrine-related myopathies

Molecular genetics and pathophysiology

The term vitamin D (calciferol) incorporates both vitamin D_2 (ergocalciferol) and vitamin D_3 (cholecalciferol), both of which are produced by a thermal photolysis in the epidermis and neither of which are biologically active. In the liver, vitamin D is converted to 25(OH)D and in the kidney, 25(OH)D is converted to 1,25(OH)$_2$D, the primary active metabolite, and less importantly, 24,25(OH)$_2$D. Vitamin D and its metabolites are bound in the blood by vitamin D-binding protein (DBP), which vastly outnumbers all of the vitamin D metabolites, leaving approximately 0.03 to 0.04% of total 25(OH)D and 1,25(OH)$_2$D concentration as biologically active hormone. Dietary supplementation is important when exposure to ultraviolet light is inadequate.

The primary target organs of vitamin D metabolites are intestine, bone and kidney. The role of vitamin D metabolites in skeletal muscle is a work in progress, however, it appears vitamin D exerts its actions via both a nuclear, gene-based mechanism and by a more rapid, non-genomic mechanism with an obscure physiologic importance.

The effects of 1,25(OH)$_2$D in muscle, as in its main target organs, in large part proceeds through interaction with the vitamin D receptor (VDR), located in the nucleus. The VDR is homologous to many other nuclear hormone receptors and when activated by 1,25(OH)$_2$D, forms a heterodimer with

Vitamin D Deficiency	
Decreased bioavailability	Insufficient sunlight, nutritional deficiency, urinary loss, malabsorption
Abnormal metabolism	Liver disease, chronic renal disease, vitamin D-resistant rickets type 1 (a-1-hydroxylase deficiency), oncogenic hypophosphatemia, chronic acidosis, anticonvulsants
Abnormal target tissue response	Vitamin D-resistant rickets type 2 (mutant VDR), gastrointestinal disorders
Hypophosphatemia	
Decreased intestinal absorption	Malnutrition, malabsorption, aluminum hydroxide antacids
Increased renal loss	Oncogenic hypophosphatemia, Fanconi syndrome
Calcium Deficiency	
Primary Bone Matrix Disorders	Hypophosphatasia (alkaline phosphatase deficiency), fibrogenesis imperfecta ossium, axial osteomalacia
Inhibitors of Mineralization	Aluminum, etidronate, flouride

Table 1. Causes of osteomalacia, and osteomalacia myopathy.

the retinoid X receptor. This complex then binds to regulatory portions of the promoter regions (called vitamin D response elements, or VDREs) of specific genes. Other proteins called co-activators are recruited to bridge the gap to the transcription initiation complex (TATA box proteins) and transcription of RNA begins (6). Vitamin D metabolites increase levels of troponin C and the uptake of calcium by sarcoplasmic reticulum (5), but how this plays out in normal or abnormal muscle physiology is unknown.

The non-genomic vitamin D activities in muscle control intracellular calcium availability, through calcium influx via L-type voltage-gated calcium channels, store-operated calcium (SOC) entry, or release from intracellular calcium storage (9). Activation of a poly-phosphoinositol-phospholipase C complex leads to increased intracellular calcium release, activating a calmodulim-mediated influx via SOC entry, under the possible control of protein kinase C (8). Non-genomic actions of vitamin D metabolites also appear to regulate various signal transduction pathways including a GTP-dependent adenyl cyclase/cAMP/protein kinase A system (7). Experimental evidence supports a role for non-genomic vitamin D activity in myoblast proliferation and differentiation (1).

It is unknown which physiologic action of vitamin D deficiency is responsible for causing osteomalacia myopathy. Certainly the therapeutic improvement obtained by vitamin D supplementation in most cases supports the theory that inadequate vitamin D effect is at the heart of osteomalacia myopathy. Whether the syndrome arises because of inactivation of nuclear genetic transcription, impaired regulation of RNA transcription, altered calcium metabolism, disordered signal transduction via cyclic AMP or GMP, or effects on excitation-contraction coupling is unknown. In patients with hypophosphatemic osteomalacia without vitamin D deficiency, myopathy may be due to inability to phosphory-late proteins or synthesize ATP.

Secondary hyperparathyroidism is frequent in osteomalacia. Parathyroid hormone also does not exert its primary effects upon muscle, but cell surface receptors for PTH stimulate adenyl cyclase leading to increased cAMP production. Elevated PTH may be involved in osteomalacia myopathy by increased calcium activating a neutral cytoplasmic protease, leading to increased protein degradation and disruption of myofibre contractile mechanisms (4).

Structural changes

The pathological changes of muscle in osteomalacia myopathy are non-specific and do not lend themselves to a satisfying correlation with molecular abnormalities. The most common finding is type 2 fibre atrophy, which is of some interest given reports of depressed myofibrillar ATPase activity in vitamin D deficient animal models (4). Scattered myonecrosis and internal nuclei, and disruption of the intermyofibrillar network have been reported on both light and electron microscopy (10).

Tubular aggregates were reported in a single case of osteomalacia myopathy (2). They are felt to derive from sarcoplasmic reticulum and are thought to be equivalent to hypertrophied sarcoplasmic reticulum, serving as a calcium sink. This may be a reactive rather than degenerative change in response to increased calcium influx to prevent calcium accumulation leading to irreversible contraction and myonecrosis, which is somewhat confusing in osteomalacia myopathy given the presumed effect of vitamin D deficiency on decreasing muscle calcium influx.

A single case of osteomalacia myopathy with lobulated fibres has been reported (3), a finding of unknown significance. The lobulated fibres contained mitochondrial aggregates, focal areas of Z-line streaming and disrupted myofibrils, all suggestive of myofibre disruption.

Future perspectives

Our understanding of the ultimate cause of osteomalacia myopathy is dependent upon a further elucidation of the function of vitamin D metabolites in normal and abnormal skeletal muscle, including the role of the VDR and of the putative cell membrane receptor involved in the rapid, non-genomic actions of vitamin D. The lack of specific pathologic findings at the light or ultrastructural levels implies that the dysfunction is physiological or biochemical, as does the often rapid response to treatment. Animal models of vitamin D deficiency, studied with modern molecular and biochemical methods, are slowly revealing clues, but a holistic picture remains elusive. The coexistence of vitamin D deficiency and hyperparathyroidism in many cases of osteomalacia also requires a better understanding of the role of PTH in skeletal muscle.

The relevance and prevalence of relative vitamin D deficiency in certain potentially at-risk populations also needs further explication. Non-pathologic levels of vitamin D deficiency may cause declines in muscle function. Studies in the elderly, the homebound, and the malnourished ill may reveal remediable findings. A particularly at-risk population would seem to be intensive care unit patients with multi-organ failure.

References

1. Capiati DA, Tellez-Inon MT, Boland RL (1999) Participation of protein kinase C alpha in 1,25-dihydroxy-vitamin D3 regulation of chick myoblast proliferation and differentiation. Mol Cell Endocrinol 153: 39-45

2. Doriguzzi C, Mongini T, Jeantet A, Monga G (1984) Tubular aggregates in a case of osteomalacic myopathy due to anticonvulsant drugs. Clin Neuropathol 3: 42-45

3. Guerard MJ, Sewry CA, Dubowitz V (1985) Lobulated fibers in neuromuscular diseases. J Neurol Sci 69: 345-356

4. Kaminski HJ, Ruff RL. Endocrine myopathies, in Myology, Engel AC Franzini-Armstrong C, Editors. 1994, McGraw-Hill: New York. p. 1745-1786

5. Pointon JJ, Francis MJ, Smith R (1979) Effect of vitamin D deficiency on sarcoplasmic reticulum function and troponin C concentration of rabbit skeletal muscle. Clin Sci (Colch) 57: 257-263

6. Shoback D, Marcus R, Bikle D, Strewler G. Mineral metabolism & metabolic bone disease, in *Basic and Clinical Endocrinology*, Greenspan FS Gardner DG, Editors. 2001, Lange Medical Books/McGraw-Hill: New York. p. 273-333

7. Vazquez G, de Boland AR, Boland RL (1997) 1 alpha,25-(OH)2-vitamin D3 stimulates the adenylyl cyclase pathway in muscle cells by a GTP-dependent mechanism which presumably involves phosphorylation of G alphai. *Biochem Biophys Res Commun* 234: 125-128

8. Vazquez G, de Boland AR, Boland RL (1998) 1alpha,25-dihydroxy-vitamin-D3-induced store-operated Ca^{2+} influx in skeletal muscle cells. Modulation by phospholipase C, protein kinase C, and tyrosine kinases. *J Biol Chem* 273: 33954-33960

9. Vazquez G, Selles J, de Boland AR, Boland R (1999) Rapid actions of calcitriol and its side chain analogues CB1093 and GS1500 on intracellular calcium levels in skeletal muscle cells: a comparative study. *Br J Pharmacol* 126: 1815-23

10. Yoshikawa S, Nakamura T, Tanabe H, Imamura T (1979) Osteomalacic myopathy. *Endocrinol Jpn* 26: 65-72

Vitamin E deficiency

P. K. Thomas

AVED	ataxia with isolated vitamin E deficiency
PUFA	polyunsaturated fatty acyl chains
TTPA	alpha tocopherol transfer protein gene

Definition of entities

Vitamin E is the generic term applied to a group of lipid soluble compounds that are derivatives of tocol and tocotrienol, the former possessing saturated and the latter an unsaturated side chain. Alpha-tocopherol has the greatest biological activity and accounts for more than 90% of vitamin E in tissues. Vitamin E deficiency gives rise to a neuromuscular syndrome characterized by ataxia, tendon areflexia, a large fibre sensory neuropathy and muscle weakness (7) and, although less well studied, to a myopathy (4, 5, 12).

Acquired. Prolonged severe lack of vitamin E is necessary for the development of the deficiency syndrome. This is encountered in chronic cholecystasis or cystic fibrosis in children (3, 14) or chronic intestinal malabsorbstion in adults (5). A similar disorder can be induced in primates (11), rats (18) and the quokka (8). Myopathy is more severe in vitamin E deficient rats than in the human disorder (16). Both in the human disorder (17) and the experimental animal disease (2), improvement may take place with vitamin E replacement.

Inherited. Abetalipoproteinaemia (Bassen-Kornzweig disease) gives rise to intestinal malabsorption including defective absorption of vitamin E. A disorder resembling Friedreich's ataxia phenotypically with a nodding head tremor as a particular feature and lacking cardiac involvement was originally considered to be due to a selective deficiency of vitamin E absorption (6, 15). It is now referred to as "ataxia with isolated vitamin E deficiency" (AVED). It

is of autosomal recessive inheritance, has been mapped to chromosome 8q13.1-q13.3 (1), and has been shown to be due to mutations in the alpha tocopherol transfer protein gene (TTPA) (13). TTPA is probably involved in the incorporation of alpha tocopherol into very low density lipoproteins secreted by the liver that are implicated in the recycling of plasma vitamin E that otherwise would be eliminated (19).

Molecular biology and pathogenesis. Vitamin E is concentrated in the hydrophobic interior of membranes where it acts as an antioxidant, quenching lipid peroxidation. Membranes that possess a high proportion of polyunsaturated fatty acyl chains (PUFA) and less sphingomyelin and more susceptible to damage by free radicals. Mitochondria contain large amounts of vitamin E, and mitochondrial membranes

contain a high proportion of PUFAs (10). A necrotizing myopathy develops in vitamin E deficient rats (2, 9). Thomas et al (16) studied this phenomenon and showed that it was associated

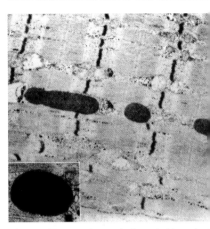

Figure 1. Electron micrograph of muscle biopsy from a patient with vitamin E deficiency showing a row of discrete, dense membrane- limited deposits between myofibrils. The inset shows details of the central inclusion. From H.E. Neville *et al*, *Neurology* 33: 483-488, 1983, with permission.

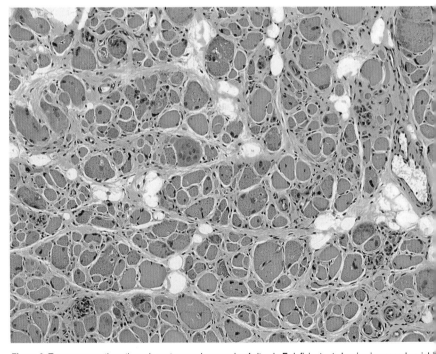

Figure 2. Transverse sections through gastrocnemius muscle of vitamin E deficient rat showing increased variability in muscle fibre size, fibre splitting, increased numbers of internally placed sarcolemmal nuclei, and fibre necrosis with infiltration with inflammatory cells. H&E.

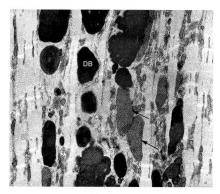

Figure 3. Electron micrograph of longitudinal section through the gastrocnemius muscle of a vitamin E deficient rat showing extensive deposition of electron dense bodies (DB) and accumulations of honeycomb structures (arrows).

with a generalized abnormality of the mitochondrial respiratory chain and a reduction in the fluidity of the mitochondrial membranes, although whether these changes were responsible for the muscle fibre damage and necrosis was not established.

Structural changes

Only a mild degree of neuropathy develops in vitamin E deficiency states in man and usually in conjunction with an ataxic syndrome (4, 12). Neville et al (12) examined muscle biopsies from four patients, in only one of which was there evidence of muscle fibre necrosis. All showed the presence of multiple large dense inclusions with a diameter of 1 to 2 μm and a length of 3 μm (Figure 1). They possessed features both of secondary lysosomes and lipopigment and were thought probably to represent the result of disordered intracellular lipid peroxidation.

In experimental vitamin E deficiency in rabbits and rats (16), a necrotizing myopathy develops within a few months (Figure 2). Dense bodies similar to those observed in the human biopsy specimens are also present (Figure 3). They tend to lie in rows between the myofilaments and are associated with collections of tubules derived from the T system.

Future perspectives

There is strongly suggestive evidence that the myopathy of vitamin E deficiency is related to oxidative damage to mitochondria produced by free radicals. Further studies need to be undertaken to explore this in greater detail and to establish whether the defects of mitochondrial respiratory chain function that have been detected, or possibly damage to mitochondrial DNA, are the cause of the muscle fibre disturbances.

References

1. Ben Hamida C, Doerflinger N, Belal S, Linder C, Reutenauer L, Dib C, Gyapay G, Vignal A, Le Paslier D, Cohen D, et al. (1993) Localization of Friedreich ataxia phenotype with selective vitamin E deficiency to chromosome 8q by homozygosity mapping. *Nat Genet* 5: 195-200

2. Dahlin KJ, Chan AC, Benson ES, Hegarty PV (1978) Rehabilitating effect of vitamin E therapy on the ultrastructural changes in skeletal muscles of vitamin E-deficient rabbits. *Am J Clin Nutr* 31: 94-99

3. Elias E, Muller DP, Scott J (1981) Association of spinocerebellar disorders with cystic fibrosis or chronic childhood cholestasis and very low serum vitamin E. *Lancet* 2: 1319-1321

4. Guggenheim MA, Ringel SP, Silverman A, Grabert BE, Neville HE (1982) Progressive neuromuscular disease in children with chronic cholestasis and vitamin E deficiency: clinical and muscle biopsy findings and treatment with alpha-tocopherol. *Ann N Y Acad Sci* 393: 84-95

5. Harding AE, Muller DP, Thomas PK, Willison HJ (1982) Spinocerebellar degeneration secondary to chronic intestinal malabsorption: a vitamin E deficiency syndrome. *Ann Neurol* 12: 419-424

6. Harding AE, Matthews S, Jones S, Ellis CJ, Booth IW, Muller DP (1985) Spinocerebellar degeneration associated with a selective defect of vitamin E absorption. *N Engl J Med* 313: 32-35

7. Harding AE (1987) Vitamin E and the nervous system. *Crit Rev Neurobiol* 3: 89-103

8. Kakulas BA. Man, Marsupials and Muscle. vol. 1. 1982, Nedlands: University of Western Australia Press.

9. Machlin LJ, Filipski R, Nelson J, Horn LR, Brin M. (1977) Effects of a prolonged vitamin E deficiency in the rat. *J Nutr* 107: 1200-1208

10. Molenaar I, Vos J, Hommes FA (1972) Effect of vitamin E deficiency on cellular membranes. *Vitam Horm* 30: 45-82

11. Nelson JS, Fitch CD, Fischer VW, Broun GO, Chou AC (1981) Progressive neuropathologic lesions in vitamin E-deficient rhesus monkeys. *J Neuropathol Exp Neurol* 40: 166-186

12. Neville HE, Ringel SP, Guggenheim MA, Wehling CA, Starcevich JM (1983) Ultrastructural and histochemical abnormalities of skeletal muscle in patients with chronic vitamin E deficiency. *Neurology* 33: 483-488

13. Ouahchi K, Arita M, Kayden H, Hentati F, Ben Hamida M, Sokol R, Arai H, Inoue K, Mandel JL, Koenig M (1995) Ataxia with isolated vitamin E deficiency is caused by mutations in the alpha-tocopherol transfer protein. *Nat Genet* 9: 141-145

14. Rosenblum JL, Keating JP, Prensky AL, Nelson JS (1981) A progressive neurologic syndrome in children with chronic liver disease. *N Engl J Med* 304: 503-508

15. Stumpf DA, Sokol R, Bettis D, Neville H, Ringel S, Angelini C, Bell R (1987) Friedreich's disease: V. Variant form with vitamin E deficiency and normal fat absorption. *Neurology* 37: 68-74

16. Thomas PK, Cooper JM, King RH, Workman JM, Schapira AH, Goss-Sampson MA, Muller DP (1993) Myopathy in vitamin E deficient rats: muscle fibre necrosis associated with disturbances of mitochondrial function. *J Anat* 183: 451-461

17. Tomasi LG (1979) Reversibility of human myopathy caused by vitamin E deficiency. *Neurology* 29: 1182-1186

18. Towfighi J (1981) Effects of chronic vitamin E deficiency on the nervous system of the rat. *Acta Neuropathol* 54: 261-267

19. Traber MG, Sokol RJ, Burton GW, Ingold KU, Papas AM, Huffaker JE, Kayden HJ (1990) Impaired ability of patients with familial isolated vitamin E deficiency to incorporate alpha-tocopherol into lipoproteins secreted by the liver. *J Clin Invest* 85: 397-407

Amyloid myopathy

P. K. Thomas
Stirling Carpenter

AA	serum amyloid A protein
AL	amyloid derived from immunoglobulin light chains
TTR	transthyretin

Definition of entity

Amyloid material appears amorphous and eosinophilic on light microscopy and stains metachromatically with methyl or crystal violet. It is fluorescent with thioflavin S or T and exhibits red-green dichroism when stained with Congo red and viewed with polarization optics. However, it is more sensitive to fluorescence microscopy on Congo red stained sections using rhodamine optics or a Texas red filter. Ultrastructurally, amyloid is composed of masses of unbranched straight 8 to 15 nm filaments. These must be distinguished from the 10 nm microfilaments (oxytalan fibres) which occur normally in small numbers between muscle fibres. They are formed by type VI collagen and, in contrast to the straight amyloid filaments, are frequently curved.

A considerable number of different proteins can give rise to amyloid. The list includes immunogobulin light chains, transthyretin, gelsolin, apolipoprotein A-l, serum amyloid A protein, beta-microglobulin, beta-amyloid, and prion protein. The relative resistance of amyloid to proteolysis is related to the beta-pleated configuration of the amyloidogenic protein. Whatever the nature of the amyloid, as long as it is extracellular, a number of other molecules are associated with it. These include apolipoprotein E, heparan sulfate proteoglycan, chondroitin sulphate proteoglycan, collagen IV, merosin, and fibronectin (8). Most deposits also contain amyloid protein P, a pentagonal glycoprotein.

While most types of amlyloid are extracellular, some Congo red positivity is seen within muscle fibres in rela-tion to the rimmed vacuoles of inclusion body myositis (10) and oculopharyngeal dystrophy (18). As explained in chapter 15.3, this may be related to beta-amyloid or tau deposition (2). Beta-amyloid is also seen in the vacuoles of experimental chloroquine myopathy along with cathepsin D (17).

Clinical phenotypes. In immunoglobulin-related amyloidosis, asymptomatic involvement of skeletal muscle has been reported. Trotter et al (16) found 10 patients (mostly with plasma cell dyscrasias) that had amyloid in their skeletal muscle. All 10 had evidence of neuropathy, but none of them were considered to have a myopathy. However, there are many reports that identify amyloid myopathy as causing muscular weakness, usually proximally, rarely distally, and sometimes associated with post-exercise myalgia (4, 5, 7, 11, 14). Almost all of these cases are secondary to immunoglobulin abnormality. In addition, rarer patients have diffuse enlargement of muscles, which are firm and ligneous (9) with macroglossia, dysphagia, and dysphonia (19). The tendon reflexes may show slow contraction and relaxation, similar to the changes seen in myxoedema. If peripheral neuropathy is associated with amyloid myopathy, there may be distal sensory loss in the limbs, tendon areflexia, and symptoms of autonomic dysfunction (13).

Acquired amyloidosis

Amyloid derived from immunoglobulin light chains (AL amyloidosis) occurs secondary to multiple myeloma, malignant lymphoma, or Waldenström's macroglobulinaemia; or to a seemingly nonmalignant immunocyte dyscrasia, which sometimes reflects a "smouldering" myeloma. Cases of "primary amyloidosis," in which no cause is obvious, are most likely to have AL amyloidosis. The amyloid is more often derived from lambda than kappa light chains, either from just the variable portion or the complete chain. Peripheral neuropathy occurs in 5 to 10% of patients. Extensive deposition in muscle can lead to amyloid myopathy as described above. AA amyloidosis, which is seen in patients with chronic infections, and in which the amyloid is derived from serum amyloid A protein, does not show muscle involvement (20). For additional information see chapter 15.1.

Inherited amyloidosis

Peripheral neuropathy, initially giving rise to small fibre involvement with pain and temperature sensory loss and autonomic dysfunction, is the dominant presentation in hereditary amyloidosis related to mutations in the gene for transthyretin (TTR) (13). Cardiomyopathy and involvement of other viscera also occurs. Deposition of some amyloid in muscle is not rare, but it would be exaggerated to call this myopathy (20). Neuropathy also occurs with amyloid derived from apolipoprotein A (12), but muscle involvement has not been reported. Mutated gelsolin can also cause amyloid neuropathy (6). One case was reported of myopathy in which the deposits were immunopositive for gelsolin, but the patient had no other manifestation (14).

When the type of amyloidosis is not certain clinically, immunostaining of the deposits can be helpful. Some cases still remain to be classified. Bruni et al (3) described a familial case of chronic proximal myopathy, resembling a limb girdle dystrophy, in which muscle biopsy demonstrated copious amyloid around vessels. The nature of the amyloid was not established. There was no associated cardiomyopathy or peripheral neuropathy and no evidence of plasma cell dyscrasia.

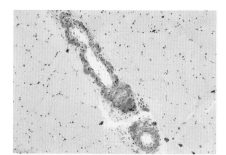

Figure 1. Congo red stain showing amyloid deposition around intramuscular blood vessels.

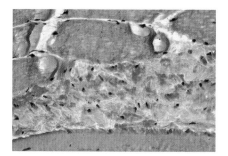

Figure 2. Congo red stain showing endomysial amyloid deposits.

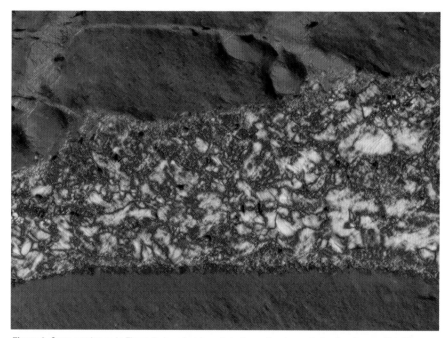

Figure 3. Same section as in Figure 2 viewed under polarization optics demonstrating "apple-green" birefringence of deposits.

Structural changes

Deposits of amyloid in muscle are present around blood vessels (Figure 1), as well as coating one or more sides of varying numbers of muscle fibres (Figures 2, 3). There is a predilection for the external surface of muscle fibres on the periphery of fascicles. Sometimes there is extensive encirclement of virtually all fibres. Patients with this pattern tend to have the hypertrophic clinical picture. As mentioned above, small amounts of amyloid are most easily detected with Congo red and fluorescence microscopy. Certain fibres coated with amyloid are somewhat atrophic and have a characteristic concave shape bordering the deposit. Necrotic or regenerating fibres may be present (14). Neurogenic atrophy related to neuropathy is often seen in the specimen.

On electron microscopy, amyloid deposits are found around vessels (Figures 4, 5), intermingling with reduplications of basal lamina. They may also be seen adjacent to muscle fibres, impinging on their basal lamina, which may be reduplicated, lifted, or partly effaced (Figure 6). At high resolution on longitudinal views, an amyloid fibril

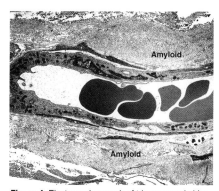

Figure 4. Electron micrograph of triceps muscle biopsy specimen showing amyloid deposits surrounding a blood vessel.

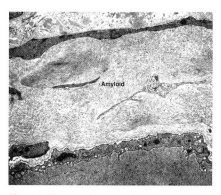

Figure 5. Electron micrograph of triceps muscle biopsy specimen showing amyloid fibrils in vessel wall.

appears as 2 osmiophilic lines separated by a narrow clear space. On transverse sections they appear tubular. Subsarcolemmal zones of muscle fibres

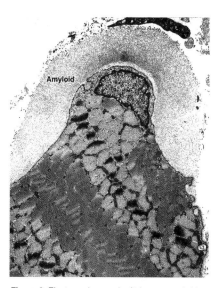

Figure 6. Electron micrograph of triceps muscle biopsy specimen showing amyloid fibrils deposited around a muscle fibre and an adjacent capillary.

coated with amyloid tend to have increased numbers of mitochondria, cisternae of rough endoplasmic reticulum, and myeloid structures (14). Residues of papillary projections from the surface of the fibre were also described.

Future perspectives

There are a number of unsolved questions in amyloidosis. Amyloidogenesis is not well understood. What is the role of the various basal lamina proteins which, in experimental amyloidosis, are co-deposited with the amyloid (8). In some types of amyloid, the formative protein is a mutated version; however, this is probably just related to the likelihood of forming beta-pleated sheets. The tissue localization of various forms of amyloid is puzzling. In some examples of AL amyloidosis, why is skeletal muscle predominantly affected? What causes the muscle weakness in patients with amyloid myopathy when they may have little evidence of fibre loss?

Very little is known about how amyloid damages cells. No evidence for apoptotic nuclei was found in 10 muscle specimens (14), and in only one case of myopathy out of 10 was membrane attack complex found on the surface of muscle fibres (14). A purely physical space-taking effect is sometimes evoked. Vascular obstruction has been suggested. Encasement of muscle fibres by amyloid might impede the passage of nutrients (14). Amyloid deposition has a peculiar affinity for basal laminae. This is seen in relation to muscle fibres, as well as to vessels, and in peripheral nerves, where the Schwann cell basal laminae, mainly those of unmyelinated and small myelinated axons, are invaded by amyloid fibrils (15). In experimental AA amyloidosis where basal lamina components are co-deposited with amyloid, perlecan gene expression is induced even before the appearance of the amyloid (1). Further metabolic interactions between amyloid and adjacent cells remain to be found.

References

1. Ailles L, Kisilevsky R, Young ID (1993) Induction of Perlecan gene expression precedes amyloid formation during experimental murine AA amyoloidogenesis. *Lab Invest* 69: 443-448

2. Askanas V, Engel WK, Alvarez RB (1992) Light and electron microscopic localization of beta-amyloid protein in muscle biopsies of patients with inclusion-body myositis. *Am J Pathol* 141: 31-36

3. Bruni J, Bilbao JM, Pritzker PH (1977) Myopathy associated with amyloid angiopathy. *Can J Neurol Sci* 4: 77-80

4. Fisher R, Thompson RA (1958) Primary amyloidosis. *Can Med Ass J* 78: 264-266

5. Lange RK (1970) Primary amyloidosis of muscle. *South Med J* 63: 321-323

6. Levy E, Haltia M, Fernandez-Madrid I, Koivunen O, Ghiso J, Prelli F, Frangione B (1990) Mutation in gelsolin gene in Finnish hereditary amyloidosis. *J Exp Med* 172: 1865-1867

7. Lubarsch (1929) Zur Kenntnis ungewöhnlicher Amyloidablagerungen. *Virchows Arch (Path Anat)* 271: 867-889

8. Lyon AW, Narindrasorasak S, Young ID, Anastassiades T, Couchman JR, McCarthy KJ, Kisilevsky R (1991) Co-deposition of basement membrane components during the induction of murine splenic AA amyloid. *Lab Invest* 64: 785-790

9. Martin JJ, Van Bogaert L, Van Damme J, Peremans J (1970) Sur une pseudo-myopathie ligneuse generalisee par amyloidose primaire endomysiovasculaire. *J Neurol Sci* 11: 147-166

10. Mendell JR, Sahenk Z, Gales T, Paul L (1991) Amyloid filaments in inclusion body myositis. Novel findings provide insight into nature of filaments. *Arch Neurol* 48: 1229-1234

11. Mollow H, Lebell S (1932) Zur Klinik der systematisierten Amyloidablagerung. *Wien Arch Inn Med* 22: 205-228

12. Nichols WC, Gregg RE, Brewer HB, Benson MD (1990) A mutation in apolipoprotein A-I in the Iowa type of familial amyloidotic polyneuropathy. *Genomics* 8: 318-323

13. Reilly M, Thomas PK (1998) Amyloid neuropathy. In *Autonomic Failure A Textbook of Clinical Disorders of the Autonomic Nervous System*, CJ Mathias, R Bannister (eds). Oxford UP: pp. 410-418

14. Spuler S, Emslie-Smith A, Engel AG (1998) Amyloid myopathy: an underdiagnosed entity. *Ann Neurol* 43: 719-728

15. Thomas PK, King RH (1974) Peripheral nerve changes in amyloid neuropathy. *Brain* 97: 395-406

16. Trotter N, Engel WK, Ignaczak TF (1977) Amyloidosis with plasma cell dyscrasia: an overlooked cause of adult sensorimotor neuropathy. *Arch Neurol* 34 : 209-214

17. Tsuzuki K, Fukatsu R, Takamaru Y, Kimura K, Abe M, Shima K, Fujii N, Takahata N (1999) Immunohistochemical evidence for amyloid beta in rat soleus muscle in chloroquine-induced myopathy. *Neurosci Lett* 182: 151-154

18. Villanova M, Kawai M, Lubke U, Oh SJ, Perry G, Six J, Ceuterick C, Martin JJ, Cras P (1993) Rimmed vacuoles of inclusion body myositis and oculopharyngeal muscular dystrophy contain amyloid precursor protein and lysosomal markers. *Brain Res* 603: 343-347

19. Whitaker JN, Hashimoto K, Quinones M (1977) Skeletal muscle pseudohypertrophy in primary amyloidosis. *Neurology* 27: 47-54

20. Yamada M, Tsukagoshi H, Hatakeyama S (1988) Skeletal muscle amyloid deposition in AL- (primary or myeloma-associated), AA(secondary), and prealbumin-type amyloidosis. *J Neurol Sci* 85: 223-232

Rare myopathies of childhood

Hans H. Goebel

Definition of entity

This chapter concerns certain rare myopathies of childhood marked by distinct structural abnormalities. Some of them have recently been assessed during an ENMC workshop (22). These rare congenital myopathies have been grouped as "probable" because of some familial cases; "possible" because of several sporadic patients; and "doubtful" because of rarity or uniqueness of sporadic cases.

Other, even rarer myopathies are cap disease (17), broad A band disease (33), lamellar body myopathy (22), tubular arrays myopathy (4), sarcotubular myopathy (28), and finger-print body myopathy (15, 16) of which little corroborating data has been provided. A more thorough discussion of problems of classification and definition of these and other congenital myopathies have been presented elsewhere (23).

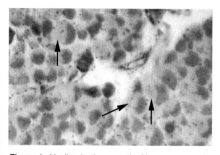

Figure 1. *Hyaline body myopathy.* Numerous muscle fibres contain large non-sarcomeric plaques of light, hyaline bodies. Modified trichrome stain. Examples indicated by arrows.

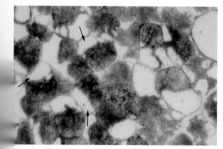

Figure 2. Hyaline bodies do not display oxidative enzyme activity. Examples indicated by arrows. NADH-tetrazolium reductase.

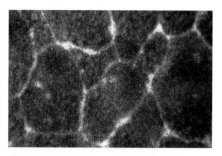

Figure 3. Hyaline bodies show ATPase activity.

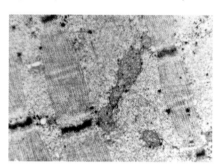

Figure 4. By electron microscopy hyaline bodies can be seen as fine granular material.

Hyaline body myopathy

Hyaline body myopathy was originally termed "familial myopathy with probable lysis of myofibrils in type I fibres" (8). Hyaline bodies (Figures 1-4) consist of plaques of granular non-structured material within muscle fibres. The clinical spectrum is diverse, encompassing sporadically (2, 11), autosomal recessively (siblings) (8, 29), and autosomal dominantly (32) affected patients, but affected genes are unknown. Onset of muscle weakness may be in childhood (8) or adulthood (2, 39).

As hyaline bodies are rich in myofibrillar ATPase—histochemically they lack oxidative enzyme activities—and myosin (2, 11, 32), hyaline body myopathy may represent another, though genetically less well-defined protein surplus myopathy (25, 26).

Cylindrical spirals myopathy

This myopathy, first observed in 2 independent adults (10), is charac-

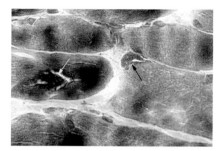

Figure 5. *Cylindrical spirals myopathy.* Subsarcolemmal and central red plaques represent aggregates of cylindrical spirals. Examples indicated by arrows. Modified trichrome stain.

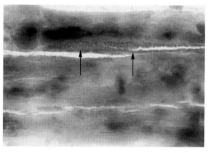

Figure 6. A long subsarcolemmal red-stained structure representing cylindrical spirals within a muscle fibre.

terised by an aggregation of so-called cylindrical spirals representing lamellae of unknown origin, sometimes connected to (41) or resembling tubular aggregates (12).

Although most patients with cylindrical spirals myopathy have been sporadic, autosomal dominant (41) and autosomal recessive (5) familial occurrences have been observed, but genes have not been identified. Cylindrical spirals have been seen in young children (1, 24) and adults (21, 36). Cylindrical spirals have not exclusively been associated with a neuromuscular disorder (36). They may be seen in D-2-hydroxyglutaric aciduria (1) with CNS symptoms such as seizures (1, 24). Muscle symptoms consist of cramps (5, 41) and weakness (21, 41).

Morphologically, aggregates of cylindrical spirals (Figures 5-8) are often located beneath the plasma mem-

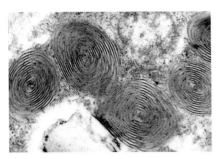

Figure 7. Ultrastructure of cylindrical spirals.

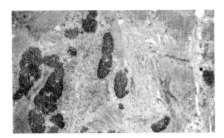

Figure 10. Ultrastructure of several dark reducing bodies.

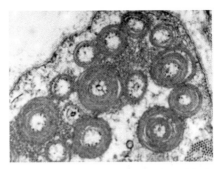

Figure 8. Ultrastructure of concentric laminated bodies.

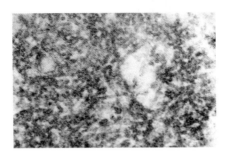

Figure 11. At higher magnification a reducing body consists of electron dense tubules.

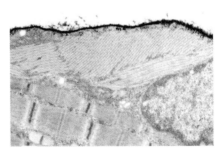

Figure 13. An aggregate of longitudinally cut tubules beneath the dark sarcolemma in a muscle fibre.

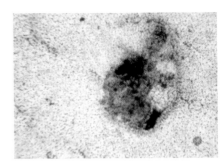

Figure 9. *Reducing body myopathy.* A muscle fibre shows bluish formazan deposits, reducing bodies, MAG reaction without substrate.

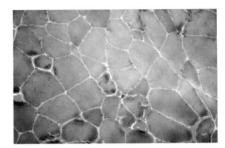

Figure 12. *Tubular aggregate myopathy.* Several muscle fibres contain peripheral bright red aggregates of tubules. Modified trichrome stain. Courtesy of Dr. Sydney Schochet, West Virginia University.

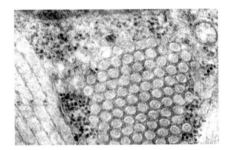

Figure 14. Tubular ultrastructure sectioned transversely and longitudinally.

brane of the muscle fibre. They appear as red plaques in the modified trichrome stain and have defied any immunohistochemical reaction with a wide variety of antibodies: troponin T, vimentin, actin, α-actinin, desmin, β-spectrin, dystrophin, nebulin, vinculin, tropomyosin, and α- and β-tubulin (36). Only their close proximity to tubulovesicular structures, apparently of the sarcotubular system, and their resemblance to tubular aggregates suggest a relationship to the sarcotubular system. Cylindrical spirals may appear similar to concentric laminated bodies, a non-specific feature in muscle fibres of different neuromuscular disorders (20).

Reducing body myopathy

Reducing body myopathy was first described in 2 unrelated young children as a fatal myopathy (6) and has later been seen in a benign form (34) of adult onset (30).

Reducing bodies (Figures 9-11) are circumscribed granular or tubular inclusions, which, in conjunction with menadione, reduce nitroblue tetrazolium to formazan in a non-enzymatic reaction. The origin of reducing bodies is still unknown and they do not show any immunohistochemical signs of desmin, vimentin, ubiquitin, spectrin,

laminin, and α-actinin (31). Reducing bodies reacting with anti-dystrophin antibodies resembling granulofilamentous material (19), and additional desmin storage (3) are further features. Granular and tubular inclusions, often surrounding the muscle fibre nucleus (31), occasionally resemble nuclei without nuclear membranes (6, 9). A similar histochemical "reducing" reaction has been observed in inclusions of childhood acid maltase deficiency (27).

As patients have only been sporadically identified, no genetic data have accrued, thus, leaving documentation of a familial form of reducing body as the first step towards genetic clarification.

Tubular aggregate myopathy

Tubular aggregate myopathy is defined by the accumulation of tubular aggregates within muscle fibres (18). The individual tubules are thought to be derived from the sarcoplasmic reticulum of the muscle fibre (40).

Although tubular aggregates may be a non-specific myopathological feature (eg, in periodic paralyses [38], alcoholic myopathy [14], or congenital myasthenic syndrome) both frequency of tubular aggregates, as well as familial occurrence (eg, autosomal dominant [7, 37] and autosomal recessive [13]), attest to their nosological significance. However, no gene locus/loci and no mutant proteins have been identified

Onset of clinical symptoms, usually muscle weakness, but also myalgia and cramps, may commence early (42) or late in life (37).

Morphologically, tubular aggregates (Figures 12-14) may occur in both fibre types, but rarely in type 2 fibres only (13). They may be seen in virtually all muscles (42), in 50 to 90% (35, 37) of the muscle fibres. These aggregates appear red in the modified trichrome stain, bluish in the haematoxylin eosin stain. Although they react prominently in the NADH preparation, they do not in mitochondrial preparations such as COX and SDH; an important differential diagnostic phenomenon to exclude mitochondrial aggregates.

Future perspectives

Linkage studies, perhaps in conjunction with the exploration of candidate genes, ought to be performed on informative patients and families with these rare neuromuscular disorders.

References

1. Baker NS, Sarnat HB, Jack RM, Patterson K, Shaw DW, Herndon SP (1997) D-2-hydroxyglutaric aciduria: hypotonia, cortical blindness, seizures, cardiomyopathy, and cylindrical spirals in skeletal muscle. *J Child Neurol* 12: 31-36

2. Barohn RJ, Brumback RA, Mendell JR (1994) Hyaline body myopathy. *Neuromuscul Disord* 4: 257-262

3. Bertini E, Salviati G, Apollo F, Ricci E, Servidei S, Broccolini A, Papacci M, Tonali P (1994) Reducing body myopathy and desmin storage in skeletal muscle: morphological and biochemical findings. *Acta Neuropathol* 87: 106-112

4. Bourque PR, Lach B, Carpenter S, Rippstein P (1999) Myopathy with hexagonally cross-linked tubular arrays: a new autosomal dominant or sporadic congenital myopathy. *Ann Neurol* 45: 512-515

5. Bove KE, Iannaccone ST, Hilton PK, Samaha F (1980) Cylindrical spirals in a familial neuromuscular disorder. *Ann Neurol* 7: 550-556

6. Brooke MH, Neville HE (1972) Reducing body myopathy. *Neurology* 22: 829-840

7. Cameron CH, Allen IV, Patterson V, Avaria MA (1992) Dominantly inherited tubular aggregate myopathy. *J Pathol* 168: 397-403

8. Cancilla PA, Kalyanaraman K, Verity MA, Munsat T, Pearson CM (1971) Familial myopathy with probable lysis of myofibrils in type I fibers. *Neurology* 21: 579-585

9. Carpenter S, Karpati G, Holland P (1985) New observations in reducing body myopathy. *Neurology* 35: 818-827

10. Carpenter S, Karpati G, Robitaille Y, Melmed C (1979) Cylindrical spirals in human skeletal muscle. *Muscle Nerve* 2: 282-287

11. Ceuterick C, Martin JJ, Martens C (1993) Hyaline bodies in skeletal muscle of a patient with a mild chronic nonprogressive congenital myopathy. *Clin Neuropathol* 12: 79-83

12. Danon MJ, Carpenter S, Harati Y (1989) Muscle pain associated with tubular aggregates and structures resembling cylindrical spirals. *Muscle Nerve* 12: 265-272

13. de Groot JG, Arts WF (1982) Familial myopathy with tubular aggregates. *J Neurol* 227: 35-41

14. del Villar Negro A, Merino Angulo J, Rivera Pomar JM, Aguirre Errasti C (1982) Tubular aggregates in skeletal muscle of chronic alcoholic patients. *Acta Neuropathol* 56: 250-254

15. Engel AG, Angelini C, Gomez MR (1972) Fingerprint body myopathy, a newly recognized congenital muscle disease. *Mayo Clin Proc* 47: 377-388

16. Fardeau M, Tome FM, Derambure S (1976) Familial fingerprint body myopathy. *Arch Neurol* 33: 724-725

17. Fidzianska A, Badurska B, Ryniewicz B, Dembek I (1981) "Cap disease": new congenital myopathy. *Neurology* 31: 1113-1120

18. Figarella-Branger D, Pellissier JF, Perez-Castillo AM, Desnuelle C, Pouget J, Serratrice G (1991) [Slowly progressive myopathy with accumulation of tubular aggregates]. *Rev Neurol* 147: 586-594

19. Figarella-Branger D, Putzu GA, Bouvier-Labit C, Pouget J, Chateau D, Fardeau M, Pellissier JF (1999) Adult onset reducing body myopathy. *Neuromuscul Disord* 9: 580-586

20. Gambarelli D, Hassoun J, Pellissier JF, Berard M, Toga M (1974) Concentric laminated bodies in muscle pathology. *Pathol Eur* 9: 289-296

21. Gibbels E, Henke U, Schadlich HJ, Haupt WF, Fiehn W (1983) Cylindrical spirals in skeletal muscle: a further observation with clinical, morphological, and biochemical analysis. *Muscle Nerve* 6: 646-655

22. Goebel HH, Anderson JR (1999) Structural congenital myopathies (excluding nemaline myopathy, myotubular myopathy and desminopathies): 56th European Neuromuscular Centre (ENMC) sponsored International Workshop. December 12-14, 1997, Naarden, The Netherlands. *Neuromuscul Disord* 9: 50-57

23. Goebel HH, Fidzianska A (1996) Classification of congenital myopathies. In *Handbook of Muscle Disease*, RJM Lane (eds). Marcel Dekker, Inc: New York. pp. 65-176

24. Goebel HH, Meier W, Rellensmann G (1995) The nosological connotation of cylindrical spiral myopathy. *Electronic Journal of Pathology and Histology* 1. 3: 953-908

25. Goebel HH, Warlo I (2000) Gene-related protein surplus myopathies. *Mol Genet Metab* 71: 267-275

26. Goebel HH, Warlo IA (2001) Surplus protein myopathies. *Neuromuscul Disord* 11: 3-6

27. Jay V, Christodoulou J, Mercer-Connolly A, McInnes RR (1992) "Reducing body"-like inclusions in skeletal muscle in childhood-onset acid maltase deficiency. *Acta Neuropathol* 85: 111-115

28. Jerusalem F, Engel AG, Gomez MR (1973) Sarcotubular myopathy. A newly recognized, benign, congenital, familial muscle disease. *Neurology* 23: 897-906

29. Karasoy H, Yüceyar N (1999) Hyaline body myopathy presenting as scapuloperoneal syndrome with autosomal recessive inheritance. *Neuromuscul Disord* 9: 514 [abstract G.P.515.518]

30. Keith A, Brownell W (1990) Reducing body myopathy in an adult. *J Neurol Sci* 98: 336 [abstract 4.5.5]

31. Kiyomoto BH, Murakami N, Kobayashi Y, Nihei K, Tanaka T, Takeshita K, Nonaka I (1995) Fatal reducing body myopathy. Ultrastructural and immunohistochemical observations. *J Neurol Sci* 128: 58-65

32. Masuzugawa S, Kuzuhara S, Narita Y, Naito Y, Taniguchi A, Ibi T (1997) Autosomal dominant hyaline body myopathy presenting as scapuloperoneal syndrome: clinical features and muscle pathology. *Neurology* 48: 253-257

33. Mrak RE, Griebel M, Brodsky MC (1996) Broad A band disease: a new benign congenital myopathy. *Muscle Nerve* 19: 587-594

34. Oh SJ, Meyers GJ, Wilson ER, Jr., Alexander CB (1983) A benign form of reducing body myopathy. *Muscle Nerve* 6: 278-282

35. Pierobon-Bormioli S, Armani M, Ringel SP, Angelini C, Vergani L, Betto R, Salviati G (1985) Familial neuromuscular disease with tubular aggregates. *Muscle & Nerve* 8: 291-298

36. Rapuzzi S, Prelle A, Moggio M, Rigoletto C, Ciscato P, Comi G, Francesca F, Scarlato G (1995) High serum creatine kinase levels associated with cylindrical spirals at muscle biopsy. *Acta Neuropathol* 90: 660-664

37. Rohkamm R, Boxler K, Ricker K, Jerusalem F (1983) A dominantly inherited myopathy with excessive tubular aggregates. *Neurology* 33: 331-336

38. Rosenberg NL, Neville HE, Ringel SP (1985) Tubular aggregates. Their association with neuromuscular diseases, including the syndrome of myalgias/cramps. *Arch Neurol* 42: 973-976

39. Sahgal V, Sahgal S (1977) A new congenital myopathy. *Acta Neuropathol (Berl)* 37: 225-230

40. Salviati G, Pierobon-Bormioli S, Betto R, Damiani E, Angelini C, Ringel SP, Salvatori S, Margreth A (1985) Tubular aggregates: sarcoplasmic reticulum origin, calcium storage ability, and functional implications. *Muscle & Nerve* 8: 299-306

41. Taratuto AL, Matteucci M, Barreiro C, Saccolitti M, Sevlever G (1991) Autosomal dominant neuromuscular disease with cylindrical spirals. *Neuromuscul Disord* 1: 433-441

42. Tulinius MH, Lundberg A, Oldfors A (1996) Early-onset myopathy with tubular aggregates. *Pediatr Neurol* 15: 68-71

CHAPTER 16

Neuromuscular resources on the Internet

C omputers and the increasingly easy accessibility of special databases on the Internet revolutionized many aspects of practice and research in myology. The avalanche of new information threatens the clinician and researcher with information overload. However, the convenient accessibility to relevant information in these databases is very helpful and even essential for quick and effective diagnosis and important basic biological information necessary for research. The field of myology is fortunate to have large, user-friendly, up-to-date, well-serviced and economical databases that satisfy these requirements. These resources are excellently outlined in this chapter.

Neuromuscular resources on the Internet

Roberta A. Pagon
Thomas D. Bird
Christine Beahler

The Internet offers a range of resources of varying quality for researchers, clinicians, and patients interested in diseases of muscle. The authors reviewed Web sites known to them using a variety of Web-based searching strategies. In evaluating sites, the authors relied on personal experience in the development of Internet-based resources; in their clinical practice and clinically-oriented research in neurology and medical genetics; and on criteria developed by Mitretek for evaluating Internet health information (Table 1).

Sites included are primary information resources; the authors determined the targeted audience for each site based on type of information and its presentation. Sites that marketed products or services, including clinical services or research programs of a single institution, were excluded. Databases and Internet resources dedicated to genomic researchers were not included based on the assumption that these essential tools for basic science researchers are already known to them.

NHGRI	National Human Genome Research Institute
NLM	National Library of Medicine
OMIM	Online Mendelian Inheritance in Man

Top tier sites for clinicians

GeneClinics

http://www.geneclinics.org

Original full text information on inherited disorders for which testing is available; related links. Developed at the University of Washington, Seattle, 1997. Funded by the National Institutes of Health (NLM and NHGRI) and maintained by an editorial board and staff. Entries are either full-text, highly structured, disease profiles with 10 sections or topic reviews (overviews) 10 to 20 pages long. The site contains ~115 entries (as of 08/01); about one new entry added each week. Expert authors are identified; the peer review process is described; bibliographic citations included. Entries are updated at least annually and dated. Entries are accessed with an internal search engine via disease name, author name, gene symbol, or from a list of disease features. Links to GeneTests (laboratory and clinic directories), genomic resources, full text policy statements on testing, Medline (custom searches), PubMed abstracts, and umbrella and disease specific consumer resources are included. Although the designated audience for GeneClinics is healthcare providers, links to support groups provide consumer information as well.

GeneTests

http://www.genetests.org

International genetics laboratory directory with an emphasis on North American laboratories; US genetics clinic directory; educational materials on general genetic counselling and testing concepts; related links. Developed at Children's Hospital and Regional Medical Center, and University of Washington, Seattle, 1993. Funded by National Library of Medicine (NLM) of the NIH and maintained by a project staff and advisory group. The laboratory directory has listings for 500 laboratories testing for 800 inherited diseases; organised by disease name; testing is categorised as clinical or research; searchable by disease name, primary feature, gene, ancillary service, OMIM number, director name. The Clinic Directory has 950 genetics and prenatal diagnosis clinics organised by US state, city, and population served (prenatal, paediatric, adult) searchable by geography, population served, and medical speciality/disease. Both include links to Web sites, contact information, certification, last update. Entries are updated at least annually and dated. Educational materials are expert-authored, peer-reviewed and include a teaching module PowerPoint® slide show, intended for genetics professionals to use in instruction of non-genetics health care practitioners. Links are included from disease entry to specific OMIM entry (ies); from lab/clinic listing to lab/clinic Web Sites; from educational materials to supporting documentation and umbrella consumer resources. Audience is healthcare providers, researchers, policymakers, and consumers.

Neuromuscular Disease Center

http://www.neuro.wustl.edu/neuromuscular

Extensive indexing and classification of neuromuscular disorders in outline form; related links. Developed by Alan Pestronk, MD, Washington University, St. Louis, Mo. Entries are in loosely structured outline format richly illustrated with graphics. Bibliographic citations included. Revisions and updates from 1996 to 2001 are indicated. Indexing is alphabetical as well as by subject heading: molecular, cellular, pathology; internal search engine is provided. Links to OMIM and SWISS-PROT databases and to patient information, clinical and disease sites, other

---

Credibility: source, currency, relevance/utility, and editorial review process for the information

Content: accuracy, completeness; inclusion of appropriate disclaimer

Disclosure: statement of purpose of the site, as well as any profiling or collection of information associated with using the site

Links: selection, architecture, content, and reciprocal linkages

Design: accessibility, organisation, navigability, and internal search capability

Interactivity: feedback mechanisms, means for exchange of information among users

Caveats: marketing products/services or primary information content provider

Table 1. Mitretek criteria for evaluating the quality of Internet health information. Developed by Mitretek (Mitretek Systems Health Summit Working Group 1999).
Web site: *http://hitiweb.mitretek.org/docs/policy.html*

basic science databases, historical references, treatment sites. Audience is neurologists and others interested in neurosciences.

OMIM: Online Mendelian Inheritance in Man
http://www.ncbi.nlm.nih. gov/omim

Full-text information on inherited disorders and allelic variants abstracted from the medical literature; related links. Developed by Victor A. McKusick, MD, Johns Hopkins University, Baltimore, Maryland (USA), mid 1960s. Funded by National Institutes of Health (NHGRI and NLM) and maintained by an Editorial Board and staff. Entries include all genetic disorders and are full-text, loosely structured, excerpts from published literature, chronologically ordered, organised by phenotype and/or genotype; bibliographic citations included. Entries range in length from 1 paragraph to over 50 pages. Over 10 000 entries currently. Entries may include disease synopses (mini-OMIM). New information added regularly, usually in chronological order. Outdated and/or contradictory information often not deleted. Entries can be searched by title, word, OMIM number, references, allelic variants, clinical synopsis, contributors, gene map disorders. Links to Genomic Databases, PubMed. Audience is researchers, healthcare providers.

Orphanet
http://orphanet.infobiogen.fr

Original full-text information on rare diseases; related links; services in France. Funded by 2 French government agencies: Direction Generale de la Santé and INSERM; maintained by an advisory committee, a scientific committee, and a technical committee/staff. Entries include any disease with prevalence lower than one in 2000 in the European population.

Entries are highly structured with a short clinical summary, accompanied by information on support groups, drug treatment, signs of the disease, clinical services (France only). Bibliographic citations and relevant annotated exter-

nal links are included. Includes 950 disease entries. Entries are original full text information written or assigned by scientific editor, with extensive Advisory Board and Science Board input. Entries are updated at least annually. Indexing is by disease, orphan drugs, active substances, support groups, clinical symptoms, and clinics. Entries also accessible alphabetically, or by internal search engine. Audience is healthcare pro-viders, consumers.

Other clinical sites

REHABinfo Network: Neuromuscular Diseases InfoCenter
http://www.rehabinfo.net/Clearing-house/virtual_library/index.html

Links to resources for select neuromuscular diseases. Developed at Rehab Research and Training Center in Neuromuscular Diseases at UC Davis, Calif. Funded by National Institute on Disability and Rehabilitation (Department of Education). 54 disease entries are accessed through 9 categories; links to OMIM, NORD (National Organization for Rare Disorders), MDA USA, and consumer groups. Audience is healthcare providers and consumers.

Research sites

European Neuromuscular Centre
http://enmc.spc.ox.ac.uk/DC/

Diagnostic criteria for 12 disease categories in full text or outline form from workshops sponsored by ENMC and attended by internationally recognised experts; epidemiological data on neuromuscular diseases by country for 10 diseases prepared by the Research Director, Prof Alan Emery, and Dr Dorkins; workshop proceedings of ~30 European workshops from 1996-1999. Maintained by Dr Huw Dorkins, St. Peter's College, University of Oxford (UK). Access is through alphabetical lists of topics. Links to other neuromuscular disease sites have not been activated. Audience is researchers.

MuscleNET
telethon.bio.unipd.it

Information on neuromuscular disorders and cardiomyopathies. Developed by Fabio D'Alessi and staff at the Laboratory of Human Genetics of the Department of Biology of the University of Padua (Italy). Funded by Telethon-Italy, Muscular Dystrophy Association of Italy (UILDM), and the University of Padua. Internal content is under construction. Many links to World Muscle Society, patient organisations, molecular genetics facilities, full-text resources. Updates are at 3-month intervals by Prof G.A. Danieli, MuscleNET Administrator. Links to Human Muscle Gene Map (HMGM), ARVD.net, GET (Genes Expressed in Tissues) Maps, and GET Profiles. Audience is researchers, health care professionals, patients.

Top tier sites for consumers

Muscular Dystrophy Association (USA)
http://www.mdusa.org

The organisation has a scientific/medical advisory board. The site has current information about many neuromuscular diseases, "Ask the Experts" section with an archive of past questions and answers, articles from MDA newsletter written especially for consumers, and searchable database of 230 Muscular Dystrophy Association clinics. Disease entries include a brief definition, a basic reference section, stories about people with the disease, information on clinical trials, FAQs, simply stated articles, research/medical-related articles, and current news. Most entries are also available in Spanish. Links to major medical/research sites, funding and grant information, clinical trials. Audience is consumers, clinicians, researchers.

Muscular Dystrophy Campaign (UK)
http://www.muscular-dystrophy.org

The organisation has a scientific/medical advisory board. The site has an information library divided into key facts (disease entries), research, care, appliances, education, and living. Each of the 25 disease entries is authored by a health care professional and contains definition, prevalence, inheritance, diagnosis, treatment and current research; includes a glossary. Links to Muscular Dystrophy organisations, support groups, publications, disability sites, sites of people with muscular dystrophy, other relevant sites. Audience is consumers, clinicians, researchers.

University of Kansas Medical Center Genetics Education Center
http://www.kumc.edu/gec/

Includes the "Genetic and Rare Conditions" site (*http://www.kumc.edu/gec/support*) and the Neuromuscular Conditions Information site (*http://www.kumc.edu/gec/support/neuromus.html*). Contains over 550 pages with alphabetical listing of diseases, organisations (international), clinical services (national), genetics professionals and links to national and international organisations, directories of genetic professionals, advocacy groups, sites for children and teens. Audience is geneticists, other health care professionals, educators, and families.

NOAH: New York Online Access to Health
http://www.noah-health.org/english/illness/ neuro/neuropg.html

High quality, bilingual (Spanish and English), full-text health information for consumers. Developed by City University of New York, Metropolitan New York Library Council, New York Academy of Medicine, and New York Public Library with an advisory board of healthcare professionals. Funded by Federal Library Services and Technology Act Funds, Queens Borough Public Library, March of Dimes, Aetna U.S. Healthcare, and NYU Medical Center. Librarians and medical information specialists provide peer review of content from other sites and group them by categories such as "The Basics," "Diagnosis and Management," "Information Resources," "Care and Treat-

ment," etc. Updated frequently and dated. Searching by alphabetical categories and internal search engine. Audience is consumers, especially underserved populations.

Family Village
http://www.familyvillage.wisc.edu/index.html

A global community that integrates information, resources, and communication opportunities on the Internet for persons with cognitive and other disabilities, for their families, and for those that provide services and support.

Genetic Alliance
http://www.geneticalliance.org

The Alliance supports individuals with genetic conditions and their families, educates the public, and advocates for consumer-informed public policies. The Web site has a directory of support organisations, which can be searched alphabetically or by search engine, a glossary of medical terms and a newsletter.

CHAPTER 17

The principles of therapies and prevention based on cellular and molecular mechanisms of muscle disease

17 The principles of therapies and prevention based on cellular and molecular mechanisms of muscle disease   296

The increasing practice of molecular medicine in myology has already had a significant impact on diagnosis and prevention. Molecular therapies have so far been lagging behind. However, a large research effort is underway in preclinical models to develop effective molecular therapies for both genetic and non-genetic muscle diseases. Some of these are on the verge of human trials.

Much professional and lay attention is being directed to various forms of cell, gene end genetic therapies. In addition, the application of custom-designed drugs is gaining grounds. The promise of specific immmunotherapies for the dysimmune muscle diseases is also very encouraging. This chapter provides a synopsis of the principles that underlie these therapeutic modalities.

The principles of therapies and prevention based on cellular and molecular mechanisms of muscle disease

George Karpati
Rénald Gilbert
Maria J. Molnar

AV	adenovirus
AAV	adeno-associated virus
BMD	Becker muscular dystrophy
CAR	Coxsackie-adeno virus receptor
DMD	Duchenne muscular dystrophy
GR	gene replacement
GT	gene treatment
NO	nitric oxide
SR	smooth endoplasmic reticulum

Definition of entity

This chapter is not designed to provide a detailed description of therapies of every muscle disease. That information is available in standard textbooks of myology. Here we discuss only principles of treatment and prevention based on known facts concerning the aetiology and pathogenesis of four major muscle disease categories: *i)* Genetic diseases due to mutation of a single gene, *ii)* autoimmune diseases due to perturbed immunoregulation, *iii)* infectious diseases due to a direct effect of pathogenic microorganism, and *iv)* toxic myopathies due to a direct effect of environmental toxins or drugs.

Targeting genetic muscle diseases

As discussed in chapter 1, in genetic diseases there are 4 sequential sets of events pertaining to the aetiology, pathogenesis and the clinical profile:

i) A gene defect and/or the resultant perturbation of some of the downstream genetic mechanisms.

ii) A total or partial deficiency or functional abnormality of the corresponding protein. Such protein may be a structural molecule or an enzyme or a receptor or a transmitter or a cellular signal transducer or an ion channel component, etc. It may be located in any organelle of the muscle fibres or muscle itself (sarcolemma, sarcoplasmic reticulum, mitochondria, cytoskeleton, myofibrils, Golgi system or cytosol). In the muscle it could be in the extracellular matrix or tendons or in blood vessels.

iii) Disturbance of the biology of the cell(s) and tissue(s) where the deficient or abnormal protein is expressed and plays a significant role. Deleterious effects from this may result in cell death (by necrosis or apoptosis) or some sort of nonlethal cellular disturbance, ie, reduced force generation or interference with excitation-contraction coupling or neuromuscular transmission or abnormal ion channel function.

iv) The pathological cellular and tissue alterations will result in clinical signs and symptoms, which may be specific or nonspecific for a particular disease.

Therapeutic and preventative approaches may be directed at any of the four domains cited above. Some therapies may target more than one of these domains. For example, cell replacement therapy may be used as a cell-mediated gene transfer, or as a replacement of destroyed tissue.

Targeting the gene or downstream genetic mechanisms. *Cell therapy.* This therapeutic modality may be used as a cell-mediated therapeutic gene transfer or a replacement of lost muscle fibres. This procedure consists of injection of large numbers of myogenic precursor cells (myoblasts) into diseased muscles where they fuse with each other or with diseased host muscle fibres, into which they introduce normal copies of the culprit gene (cell-mediated gene therapy). Myoblast transfer has the advantage over direct gene therapy in that it can replace destroyed muscle tissue.

During the 1980s, there was considerable enthusiasm engendered for myoblast transfer; a result of promising experiments in the popular animal model of dystrophin deficiency, the mdx mouse (44, 60). Subsequently, this procedure was applied to Duchenne muscular dystrophy (DMD) patients (40, 50, 67). Myoblast transfer in patients consisted of injections into a single muscle of large numbers of cultured myoblasts that were derived from nonisogenic donors, usually from fathers of the patients. However, when the very large numbers of nonisogenic (or even isogenic from an identical twin) myoblasts were injected into the restricted sites of biceps muscles of DMD patients, no significant number of dystrophin-positive fibres were later observed, and no significant change in muscle strength was demonstrable. It appeared that even if proper immunosuppression was instituted, a very large number of myoblasts died shortly after injection. In addition, a large portion of the small number of surviving myoblasts may have been fusion incompetent due to senescence.

Subsequently, many attempts were made to increase the survival rate of the injected myoblasts including institution of anti-inflammatory cytokines, such as IL1, or matching the myosin isoform profile of donors versus recipients (32, 62). These approaches have not yet been assessed in DMD. Another approach to cell therapy is the use of stem cells. Myoblasts derived from satellite cell cultures apparently contain a small percentage of myogenic cells that are difficult to culture but exhibit characteristics of stem cells. These characteristics include a totally undifferentiated state and immortality. Apparently, such cells have a capacity to differentiate into muscle progenitor cells when they reach muscle where they survive. In fact, it has been demonstrated that even haematopoietic cells have a capacity to differentiate into myogenic stem cells without any prior genetic manipulation (25, 33). However, it has been suggested that certain transcription factors are required for the myogenic differentiation of stem cells. It is conceivable that stem cells from any source may have a similar capacity. However, this approach has not been tested in human muscle disease, and one can foresee considerable challenges in making this an effective treatment for human diseases such as DMD. Perhaps the best therapeutic potential is by embryonic stem cells, which do not pose any immunological problem and can be grown in abundance. However, its use raises considerable ethical, moral and legal issues.

Molecular therapies. Various forms of molecular therapies for genetic skeletal muscle diseases have been contemplated and subjected to preclinical experimentation (43). These are autosomal or X-linked disorders where a specific mutation of one specific gene causes an absence or reduction, or functional impairment of an essential molecule which it encodes. In many instances, the deficiency of the culprit molecule brings about secondary deleterious consequences. For example, dystrophin deficiency in DMD reduces the level of dystroglycans and sarcoglycans at the sarcolemma (58). Several forms of molecular therapies have been investigated (Table 1).

1. Gene replacement. This procedure entails the introduction of normal or, at least, functionally adequate alleles, (usually the coding sequence or cDNA) into cells and tissues in which deleterious effects of the gene defect is maximal. This approach is suitable mainly for recessive diseases due to a single defective gene, eg, DMD. GR may be employed directly, ie, the therapeutic gene is introduced directly into the affected cell tissues, or indirectly, ie, when the diseased cells of the hosts are first removed from the body then transfected or transduced with the therapeutic gene, and subsequently, intro-duced into the host. These approaches represent in vivo versus in vitro gene therapies, respectively.

For good results by GR, several items must be optimized or perfected in preclinical experiments. These include: the determination of the most appropriate transferable gene (cDNA), the promoter, the vector, the route of administration, and the availability of appropriate experimental models in which meaningful endpoints could be quantitatively measured. A brief comment will now be made on each of these items.

a. The transferable gene. Usually only the coding sequence of a gene (cDNA) is transferred. However, in some instances, even the therapeutic cDNA is too large for the capacity of the employed gene vector (*vide infra*). In this case, a truncated cDNA may be used which could still generate a functionally adequate, albeit not perfect, protein. Another issue is the possible immunogenicity of the new protein generated by the transferred gene to which the host has not been properly tolerized during development. This may be a significant factor in dystrophin gene replacement therapy in DMD, which raises the advisability of using a non-immunogenic functional homologue of dystrophin (utrophin).

b. The promoter. There are several useful properties of a promoter that controls the expression of a therapeutic gene in an "expression cassette" (the promoter-cDNA-poly A signal). These properties include efficiency and specificity for a given cell and minimal susceptibility for inactivation. Ideally, the natural promoter would satisfy these criteria, but in many instances the natural promoter is not suitable for this role. In preclinical experiments for dystrophin gene transfer, either constitutive promoters, such as CMV, RSV (2, 63, 68) or a hybrid CB (chicken β-actin promoter and human CMV enhancer; unpublished data) promoter have been used, all of which are efficient but not tissue specific. Thus, if and when the vector carrying the therapeutic gene expression cassette is disseminated throughout the body, expression of the therapeutic gene may prove to be deleterious in some tissues outside the target. This could be particularly problematic if germ cell expression occurs. The most useful promoter for muscle gene transfer has been the full-length or abridged muscle creatine kinase (MCK) promoter/enhancer unit (18, 42, 47). However, the risk of late promoter inactivation in the context of episomal vectors appears to be a major problem (*vide infra*).

c. The vector. Large pieces of DNA, the usual expression cassettes used for therapeutic GR, will not readily enter the treatable target cells in which they must reach the nucleus (in nuclear gene defects) for proper expression. Thus, for efficient GT, various vectors have been used for this purpose, including non-viral or viral vectors. The ideal characteristics of a gene vector include: efficiency for a given cell type (which can even vary in different developmental stages of the same cell type), lack of immunogenicity, lack of non-immune-type of toxicity, harmless integration into the host-genome, and relatively easy and cost-effective production of high vector particle number per volume in a GMP mode. It turns out that presently none of the used vectors conform perfectly to these requirements.

Non-viral vectors include circular or supercoiled plasmids, cationic liposomes, protein ligands, and microspheres (7, 69, 72). Efficiency of entry of these vectors to muscle fibres in vitro is relatively low after direct injection, and their applicability for effective GR treatment of muscle is presently doubtful. The only possible exception are plasmids which, unless percutaneous electroporation is used, transfect very few muscle fibres when injected directly into muscle (52). Plasmids also seem to transfect a significant number of muscle fibres if injected intra-arterially (13). The immunogenicity of plasmids also appears to be minimal. The longevity of the plasmid-based therapeutic transgene expression in muscle has not been precisely determined.

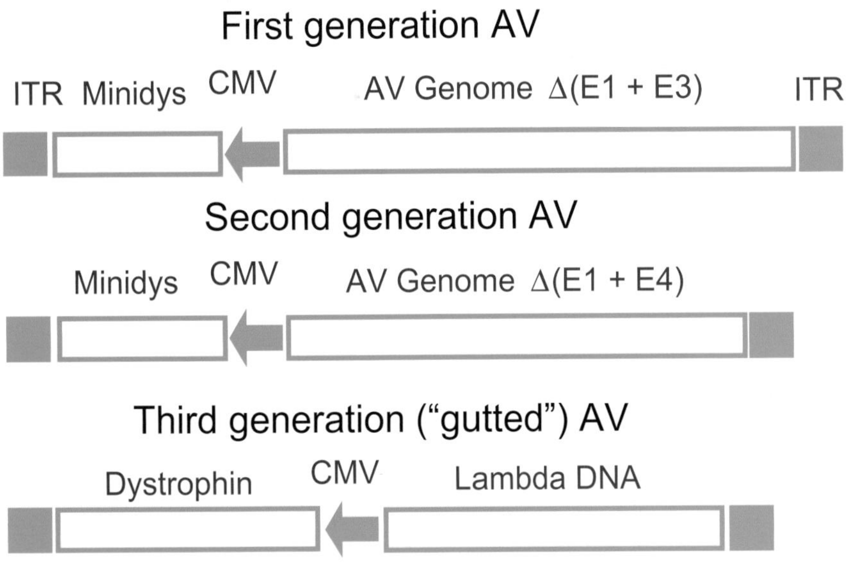

First generation AV

ITR Minidys CMV AV Genome Δ(E1 + E3) ITR

Second generation AV

Minidys CMV AV Genome Δ(E1 + E4)

Third generation ("gutted") AV

Dystrophin CMV Lambda DNA

Figure 1. Different generations of therapeutic adenovirus vectors capable of transferring dystrophin cDNA to skeletal muscle. **A**. First generation AV (E1/E3-deleted). **B**. Second generation AV (E1/E4-deleted). **C**. Third generation AV or "gutted" AV which lacks all viral genes and can carry the full-length dystrophin cDNA (13-kb). The smaller insert capacity of the first and second generation AV is sufficient only for the shortened Becker minidystrophin cDNA (Minidys) of 6.3-kb. A stuffer DNA derived from the bacteriophage lambda (Lambda DNA) has been inserted into the "gutted virus" in order to maintain the size of the viral DNA to the 30-kb required for packaging. The position of left and right inverted terminal repeats (ITR) is indicated. All cDNAs are regulated by the strong cytomegalovirus (CMV) promoter.

The most efficient and widely used vectors for therapeutic gene delivery have been genetically modified viruses. The most commonly used viral vectors for skeletal muscles are adenovirus (AV) (42, 63) and adeno-associated virus (AAV) (53, 65). In addition, a handful of experiments have been reported with herpes simplex and retroviruses as well (3, 22). Two reports of the use of lentiviruses in skeletal muscle has recently been presented(38, 39).

AVs have many attractive features as therapeutic gene vectors including an ability to infect both dividing and post-mitotic cells, easy production of high titer during cultivation, easy purification, potentially large insert capacity, and practically absent oncogenicity. However, the adenoviral proteins are highly immunogenic and the adenovirus does not integrate into the host genome. Furthermore, the density of primary and secondary receptors at the muscle cell surface (CAR and an integrin dimer, respectively) is scarce in mature muscle fibres (1, 55).

The antigenic AV proteins induce both cellular and humoral immune responses in immunocompetent hosts which greatly limits their usefulness (75). We hypothesize that the episomal existence seems to compromise the longevity of the AV vector, possibly as a result of promoter inactivation (by methylation) or by endonuclease-related damage to the expression cassette. The problem of antigenicity has been minimized by the creation of so-called "gutted" AV vectors which do not have viral genes (45, 59). However, the capsid proteins still evoke some humoral response. The "gutted" adenovirus also has a very large (>30 kb) insert capacity that would accommodate all known gene therapeutic expression cassettes for muscle diseases. The disadvantage of the "gutted" AV is the elaborate system required for its cultivation (helper-dependent system), as well as cumbersome purification. Furthermore, for efficient expression of the transgene proteins, certain AV proteins (including E4) appear to be indispensable, which

can even be provided in trans (6, 12). Unfortunately, this might confer some immunogenicity to the otherwise relatively non-immunogenic gutted AV vector. The different generations of therapeutic adenovirus vectors capable of transferring dystrophin cDNA to skeletal muscles are illustrated in Figure 1.

Another problem of AV vector is the poor uptake into mature muscle fibres (1). This is probably related to the paucity of the primary (coxsackie-adeno virus receptor or CAR) and secondary (integrin dimer) on the surface of muscle fibres (1, 55). An additional hindrance may be the major barrier function of the basal lamina (24). Substantial increase of AV uptake into mature muscle fibres may be achieved by prior upregulation of CAR (transgenically or by CAR gene transfer) (55).

AAV is presently the most ideal therapeutic gene vector for skeletal muscles. Unlike AV, it transduces mature muscle fibres well and integrates into the host genome (17, 73). The major disadvantage of AAV is its relatively small insert capacity (maximum 5 kb) and difficult cultivation. However, it is the ideal therapeutic gene transfer vector for smaller than 4 kb cDNAs, eg, those of the sarcoglycans (31, 48).

d. Route of administration. It is a critically important issue for skeletal muscle, which is widely, distributed tissue representing a large body mass. Multiple intramuscular injections employed in preclinical experiments have little practical usefulness, since the spread of the vector from the injection site is very limited (42, 57). Additionally, some muscles are not easily accessible, eg, diaphragm and intercostals. The ideal route of administration into skeletal muscle is vascular (13). Intravenous administration is not suitable since most vectors through this route end up in the liver (37). Systemic intra-arterial injection (via left cardiac ventricle), which requires a preparation in which a very high particle number per unit per blood volume, is probably not safe as it may evoke a fatal cytokine reaction. This leaves the regional intra-arterial route as the choice of administration. In fact, in rats it has been shown that an efficient transduction of leg muscles could be achieved after injection of AV vectors expressing β-galactosidase into the femoral artery (16). So far, the disadvantage of this approach is the requirement for a usually high volume of the injectate, which can create oedema and ischaemic damage to the muscle. This disadvantage could hopefully be mitigated by the intramuscular use of a vascular permeabilization agent.

e. Experimental models and endpoint determinations. There are 2 kinds of animal models that have been used for preclinical gene therapy trials (4). Natural mutation models include the mdx mouse and the Golden Retriever dogs for dystrophin deficiency, the dy/dy mouse model for merosin deficiency, and the dystrophic hamster for δ-sarcoglycan deficiency. In addition, engineered mouse models, such as transgenics, or gene inactivation models have been useful. For instance, the mdx mouse, in which overexpression of a transgene utrophin was engineered, shows the usefulness of utrophin for gene complementation in dystrophin deficiency (*vide infra*) (66). In addition, α-sarcoglycan mouse knockout models have been used to show the efficiency of α-sarcoglycan gene transfer as a therapeutic agent for both skeletal and cardiac myopathies (4).

In these models, it is of paramount importance that the appropriate endpoints be determined quantitatively to demonstrate the usefulness and safety of the gene transfer. These endpoints include the demonstration of the presence of the transferred gene, as well as its messenger RNA and the corresponding protein product plus the functional improvement that the replacement of the missing protein produced, ie, force generation in the case of skeletal muscle. In terms of safety, attention should be paid not only to possible damage that the vector produces in the target

1.	Gene replacement
2.	Gene or genetic repair
	a. Transcript repair by oligonucleotides
	b. Transsplicing
	c. Direct repair of mutation in DNA by RNA-DNA chimeric oligonucleotides
	d. Triplex forming oligonucelotides and "bifunctional" oligonucleotides
3.	Modification of translation of mutant mRNA ("read-through")
4.	Antisense oligonucleotides for mutant mRNA in dominant diseases
5.	Upregulation of a functional homologue, *i.e.* utrophin for dystrophin deficiency

Table 1. Various forms of gene and genetic therapies with potential application for skeletl muscle diseases.

tissues, but also general toxicity and possible modification of the germ cells.

2. Gene repair. These methods (Table 1) include *transcript repair*, which was stimulated by the discovery of the molecular mechanisms operating in the so-called revertant (dystrophin-positive) fibres in mdx muscles (36). In these fibres, a muscle progenitor cell in early embryogenesis appears to have suffered a second mutation in the dystrophin gene leading to a splicing aberration resulting in skipping exon 23 that contains the pathogenetic translational stop codon. Since the junctions of exons 22 and 24 are in-frame, a nearly full-length (minus exon 23 related sequences) dystrophin is produced. The same strategy can be used in vivo by delivery of an antisense oligonucleotide that targets splice sites flanking genomically deleted or duplicated segments, or exons harboring point mutations in the primary transcript (pre-mRNA) (49). As a result, the processed mRNA would be altered to produce a functional, albeit truncated dystrophin molecule. Additional techniques include, *transsplicing by special ribozymes* of the primary transcripts (61), which can be used to shorten the deleterious trinucleotide repeats that occur, for example, in myotonic dystrophy.

Direct repair of the genomic DNA mutation has been attempted in vitro cell lines (30) (Table 2), but it has not been found to be very effective in vivo experiments in mdx mice. *RNA-DNA chimeric oligonucleotides* used for the same purpose have been somewhat

1.	Auto-antigens, exogenous antigens
2.	Antigen presenting cells (APC)
3.	Class I and class II major histocompat ibilty (MHC) products
4.	T helper lymphocytes
5.	T suppressor lymphocytes
6.	T cytotoxic lymphocytes
7.	Natural killer cells
8.	T cell receptors and intracellular signals
9.	Co-stimulatory factors on APC and lymphocytes
10.	B lymphocytes and plasma cells
11.	Circulating antibodies
12.	Immune cytokines
	a) leucotreins
	b) Interleukins ("good" and "bad")
	c) Interferons ("good")

Table 2. Suspected or proven key molecules in the immunopathology of neuromuscular dysimmune diseases.

more promising in vivo in mdx mice and GRMD dogs (8, 64).

3. Modification of translation of mutant mRNA. In situations when a primary stop codon leads to a truncated and unstable protein, corrupting the ability of the ribosomes to recognize stop codons could be beneficial (71). Aminoglycosides have such an affect on ribosomes as evidenced by the fact that systemic administration of gentamicin to mdx mice produced full-length dystrophin in muscle fibres, presumably by the "read-through" phenomenon (9). However, it appears that in humans, the dose of gentamicin required for such an effect and the generation of large amounts of nontruncated dystrophin would probably require a prohibitively toxic dose of gentamicin and prolonged administration.

4. Upregulation of a functional analogue. The best example of this approach would be the upregulation of extrajunctional utrophin in dystrophin-deficient muscle fibres in mdx or DMD. Utrophin is a close structural and functional homologue of dystrophin encoded by a gene on chromosome 6 in humans (11). There appears to be at least 2 promoters corresponding to 2 utrophin isoforms (A and B) (14). In normal skeletal muscle fibres, utrophin is only expressed at the postjunctional sarcolemma of the neuromuscular junction (probably utrophin A). In the extrajunctional myonuclei, the utrophin transcript is minimal (probably utrophin B), and no histochemically detectable utrophin is present in the extrajunctional sarcolemma by immunocyochemistry (41, 56).

In DMD, there is a certain amount of spontaneous upregulation of the extrajunctional sarcolemmal utrophin, but ultimately, it is probably not sufficient in quantity to stop muscle fibre necrosis. Nevertheless, it might somewhat delay muscle fibre loss in DMD. On the other hand, substantial upregulation of extrajunctional utrophin is capable of markedly mitigating or negating the deleterious effects of dystrophin deficiency. This was demonstrated in transgenic mdx mice in which dystrophin overexpression of the transgene utrophin negated the dystrophin phenotype microscopically and physiologically (21, 66). A similar result was obtained after adenovirus-mediated utrophin gene transfer where overexpression of an abundant extrajunctional utrophin caused substantial mitigation of the dystrophic pathological and physiological phenotype in injected muscles (23, 29). In these experiments, comparison of the relative beneficial effects of utrophin and dystrophin gene replacement indicated that utrophin has some advantage (23). This is probably related to the fact that in dystrophin-deficient hosts, neodystrophin is immunogenic but utrophin is not recognized as such.

The most convenient prospect of treating dystrophin deficiency by extrajunctional utrophin upregulation is to find a nontoxic molecule which could regularly administered to DMD patients, and would sufficiently upregulate extrajunctional utrophin by stimulating transcription (probably utrophin B) or post-transcriptional mechanisms of utrophin production. Certain molecules associated with inflammation (eg, cytokines, stress proteins, NO) are good candidates for this role as muscle inflammation induced in mdx muscle markedly upregulated extrajunctional utrophin with impressive mitigation of the dystrophic features in the involved muscles (74). Presently, no other potentially surrogate molecules of dystrophin have been identified.

Targeting the protein deficiency or abnormality. In this domain we can envisage several strategies including replenishment of the deficient protein, replacement of an abnormal protein, custom designed drug therapy to normalize or near-normalize an abnormal protein, or neutralizing a toxic protein, which is exerting a negative dominant effect.

For replenishment of a deficient protein or replacement of an abnormal protein, certain essential requirements must be met that include the following: *i)* protein must be producable in large quantities in chemically pure form in a GMP mode, *ii)* it must be nontoxic, *iii)* it should not be degraded before entering the target tissue, *iv)* it must have a sufficiently long half-life, and *v)* it should be taken up by the target cells in sufficient quantities.

The applicability of this strategy is presently limited to selective situations in skeletal muscle. The best example is α-glucosidase (acid maltase) replacement intravenously in Pompe's disease where there is a genetic deficiency of this lysosomal enzyme (Chapter 10. 1) (10). Since α-glucosidase is a lysosomal enzyme, the cell has the proper apparatus for the cellular uptake and the lysosomal delivery of the administered protein. The drawback is the

inevitable antibody formation that could reduce the efficiency of the protein upon readministration. Another drawback concerns structural proteins whose deficiency cannot be corrected by protein replacement. This is the situation in many of the muscular dystrophies including DMD/BMD, the limb-girdle dystrophies, or the congenital muscular dystrophies.

Another approach is custom designed drug therapy (43). Certain molecules that could be administered orally or parenterally may alter the abnormal protein in a way that its function is improved or normalized. For example, the effect of quinidine sulphate on the voltage regulated sodium channel is such that it markedly improves the appropriate channel function in the so-called slow channel syndrome (34). The effect is an improvement of abnormal channel dynamics which is the basis of the pathogenesis of this congenital myasthenic syndrome.

In the case of autosomal dominant diseases, if the deleterious protein (which is the product of a mutant allele) is eliminated or neutralized, a therapeutic effect is expected. This could be achieved by the generation of specific intracellular antibodies or by custom designed drugs.

Targeting the abnormal biology of the cell. The genetic deficiency of abnormality of proteins can bring about very many abnormal processes in certain cells. In extreme cases, it leads to cell death by necrosis or apoptosis. There are methods by which the cell is made relatively resistant to these deleterious effects. These methods may be extremely varied and usually include nonspecific measures. Examples of this approach include the administration of myotrophic substances (eg, IGF1) (54), other nonspecific "muscle boosters" (eg, creatine-monohydrate) (70), β adrenergic agonists (eg, clenbuterol, antioxidants, antiapoptotic agents, stress proteins, agents that cause p modification of the cell, calcium scavengers, calcium channel blocking

Afferent arm	1.	Elimination or inactivation of offending antigens
	2.	Disabling antigen presentation
	3.	Disabling sensitization of immune cells
	4.	Inhibiting expansion of immune cell population
Efferent arm	5.	Inhibiting the egress of immune-competent cell from blood to target tissues
	6.	Lysis of immune-competent cells
	7.	Inhibiting the cytotoxic effect on target cells by sensitized lymphocytes
	8.	Removal or neutralization of deleterious antibodies

Table 3. Principal therapeutic strategies for dysimmune muscle diseases.

1.	Blockade of Fc receptors on immune competent cells
2.	Antiidiotypic Ab's in IgG preparations
3.	Neutralize complement
4.	Inhibit deleterious cytokine production/action
5.	Mask MHC class II recognition by immune competent cells

Table 4. How does IgG work?

1.	Targeting a subpopulation of immune cells using lymphocytes, cyclosporin, tacrolimus, ALS, antiCD2, antiCD3, antiCD6, antiCDW52, antiHLADR, and antibodies to T cell receptors.
2.	Anti-idiotypic Aβ's
3.	Interference with co-stimulatory interactions using CTLA4-Iγ, antiVLA4, antiLFA1, antiCAM1, antiHLA Aβ's
4.	Interference with cytokines:
	a. Deleterious cytokines: IFN-γ, IL-2, TNF-α, IL1α, and IL-6
	b. Beneficial cytokines: IFN-α and β, IL-10, TGF-β2
	c. Blockade of deleterious cytokines or receptors (IL-2 toxin, cyclosporin A)

Table 5. Specific immunotherapies targeting a particular immune process or immune "player."

agents (eg, Verapamil), or blockers of SR Ca^{2+} release channel (eg, Dantrium) (27), or corticosteroids that mitigate cellular damage in dystrophin deficiency by unknown mechanisms. Surface membrane "stabilization" or curtailing regeneration failure may play a role (43).

Another potentially useful approach is the avoidance of certain dietary factors and pharmaceutical agents that could make the cell more susceptible to a particular damage. For example, the avoidance of the use of halogenated anesthetics, which appear to augment the functional inadequacy of the calcium release channel of SR in malignant hyperthermia syndrome and may trigger a crisis.

Another way of minimizing the cell's susceptibility to a protein deficiency is altering its physiology or physiological use. For example, the avoidance or reduction of lengthening (eccentric) contractions of muscle in DMD markedly lessens the susceptibility of dystrophinless muscle fibres to necrosis.

Targeting the clinical phenotype. In many instances, the cited therapeutic approaches are still not available, and nonspecific treatment of individual symptoms and signs of the muscle disease is the only resort. This category includes: physiotherapy, occupational therapy, orthotics, surgical procedures, respiratory support, dietary measures, psychological support, and tackling gastrointestinal and genito-urinary complications (51). The importance of these measures must not be underesti-

mated on account of being in the so-called "low-tech" category.

Autoimmune diseases

In this group, the most important diseases include inflammatory myopathy (chapter 11), myasthenia gravis (chapter 9.1) and the Lambert-Eaton myasthenic syndrome (chapter 9.2) (20). In each of these, many features of a characteristic immunopathology have been identified. This was made possible by remarkable advances in the understanding of general cellular and molecular immune regulation and immunopathology. This includes the characterization of key molecules that may be culpable in the dysimmune processes (Table 2). The various types of dysimmune mechanisms (the afferent and efferent arms) that operate in myopathies have also been elucidated. Increasing knowledge in the area permitted, at least conceptually, the development of therapeutic strategies for these diseases, which are outlined in Table 3. In practical terms, therapeutic interventions in dysimmune states can be categorized in three groups: *i)* glob-

al immunosuppression, *ii)* selective immunotherapy and *iii)* specific immunotherapy.

In global immunosuppression, so-called "shot-gun" methods are used to disable many parts of the immune system, irrespective of the specific site of the immunological malfunction. This approach is often linked to the cliche, "to squash a mosquito with a sledge hammer." Nevertheless, this is the most predominant approach in clinical practice with the use of corticosteroids, immunosuppression, plasma exchange, high-dose intravenous immunoglobulin (Table 4), and occasionally, global irradiation of the immune system.

In selective immunotherapy, a particular immunomechanism pertinent to the given disease is disabled. Unfortunately, the availability of this approach is still relatively rare, and it is used sparingly in routine clinical practice. In specific immunotherapy, the treatment targets a specific pathogenic process without any untoward effect on the immune system. Most of these strate-

Infectious myopathies

There are four practically important diseases in this category (chapter 11): human immuno-deficiency-virus (HIV)-induced, acquired immuno-deficiency syndrome (AIDS) (19), influenza-A-related acute inflammatory myopathy (35), trichinella myositis (46), and the so-called "flesh eating disease," due to a virulent strain of β-hemolytic streptococcus (26).

Although the human retrovirus does not enter skeletal muscle fibres but does, in fact, enter interstitial cells, and macrophages in muscle and likely exerts its deleterious effect on muscle fibres indirectly. The pathological picture may still be an inflammatory myopathy, indistinguishable from polymyositis or various noninflammatory myopathies. HIV also activates nonspecific cachectic pathways that cause a massive shift of the anabolic/catabolic steady state in favor of the catabolic side. Direct antiviral therapy targeting HIV is effective in treating muscular complications. However, some of the key drugs, such as zidovudine, may be myotoxic by itself, causing a mitochondrial myopathy—probably on account of inhibiting γ-DNA polymerase (76).

Acute influenza A inflammatory myopathy is poorly responsive to antiDNA viral agents. In the so-called "flesh-eating disease," caused by a very virulent form of β-hemolytic streptococcus, massive necrosis of muscle occurs on a rapid time scale. It appears as if the bacterium becomes a super antigen, perhaps in combination with an endogenous molecule. Unless vigorous treatment is instituted with antibiotics, immunoglobulins, and perhaps limb amputation, the disease can be fatal.

Toxic myopathies

In chapter 14 and in another recently published book chapter (5), this group of diseases is discussed in detail. Relatively few environmental or industrial toxins are myotoxic. By contrast, quite a few classes of drugs have myotoxic side-effects, including cholesterol lowering agents zidovudine (28) and high-dose glucocorticoids, particularly the fluorinated ones, given in high doses over a long period of time to elderly people who suffer malnutrition. A peculiar form of an acute myopathy caused by glucocorticoid excess in muscles, which are mechanically paralyzed, is called the "myosin depletion syndrome" because the thick filaments disintegrate and the myosin monomers are dispersed in the muscle fibre (chapter 4.8). Of course, this functionally disables the sarcomeres and compromises contractile activity. Reassembly of the thick myofilaments from the dispersed myosin monomers appears possible if the offending agent and factors are rapidly removed or corrected. The use of cocaine can produce an acute painful ischaemic myopathy.

Prevention of muscle disease

Genetic muscle diseases. Several methods (15) are at our disposal for the prevention of muscle diseases. For exhaustive discussion of this topic the reader is referred to dedicated texts.

1. Carrier detection by standard techniques and prevention all procreation is presented in carriers of dominant or X-linked recessive diseases.

2. Prenatal diagnosis of a particular disease by mutational analysis of DNA derived from chorionic villus biopsy or cells cultured from amniotic fluid, obtained through amniocentesis. These approaches require the knowledge of the identity of the mutation of a particular gene in the proband and also the acceptance of selective termination of certain pregnancies with positive results on moral/ethical grounds.

3. Preimplantation diagnosis. This is just becoming a practical method of preventing muscle disease and its use is most widespread for myotonic dystrophy. In this approach, ova (obtained by superovulation) are impregnated in vitro and the resultant pre-embryos (8 cell stage) are tested *in* vitro. One or 2 blastomeres of an 8 cell-stage preembryo are isolated and tested by PCR for the pathogenic mutation in question. Because the allele profile in question is the same in all of the 8 blastomeres and a 6 to 7 cell pre-embryo is still viable, this method provides a very reliable identification of a potentially affected embryo, even before implantation. This technique can also be adapted to predict the severity of mitochondrial disease by defining the heteroplasmy ratio in one or two individual isolated blastomeres. This would reflect the heteroplasmy of the remaining blastomeres, and eventually of the individual.

Autoimmune diseases. No preventative measure has been devised thus far.

Infectious and toxic myopathies. Preventative measures follow standard public health procedures whose detailed description is beyond the scope of this chapter.

References

1. Acsadi G, Jani A, Massie B, Simoneau M, Holland P, Blaschuk K, Karpati G (1994) A differential efficiency of adenovirus-mediated *in vivo* gene transfer into skeletal muscle cells of different maturity. *Hum Mol Genet* 3: 579-584

2. Acsadi G, Lochmuller H, Jani A, Huard J, Massie B, Prescott S, Simoneau M, Petrof BJ, Karpati G (1996) Dystrophin expression in muscles of mdx mice after adenovirus-mediated *in vivo* gene transfer. *Hum Gene Ther* 7: 129-140

3. Akkaraju GR, Huard J, Hoffman EP, Goins WF, Pruchnic R, Watkins SC, Cohen JB, Glorioso JC (1999) Herpes simplex virus vector-mediated dystrophin gene transfer and expression in MDX mouse skeletal muscle. *J Gene Med* 1: 280-289

4. Allamand V, Campbell KP (2000) Animal models for muscular dystrophy: valuable tools for the development of therapies. *Hum Mol Genet* 9: 2459-2467

5. Argov Z, Kaminski HJ, Mudallal AA, Ruff RL (2001) Toxic and iatrogenic myopathies and neuromuscular disorders. In *Disorders of Voluntary Muscle*, G Karpati, D Hilton-Jones, RC Griggs (eds). Oxford Unviersity Press: New York. pp. 676-688

6. Armentano D, Zabner J, Sacks C, Sookdeo CC, Smith MP, St George JA, Wadsworth SC, Smith AE, Gregory RJ (1997) Effect of the E4 region on the persistence of transgene expression from adenovirus vectors. *J Virol* 71: 2408-2416

7. Baranov A, Glazkov P, Kiselev A, Ostapenko O, Mikhailov V, Ivaschenko T, Sabetsky V, Baranov V

(1999) Local and distant transfection of mdx muscle fibers with dystrophin and LacZ genes delivered *in vivo* by synthetic microspheres. *Gene Ther* 6: 1406-1414

8. Bartlett RJ, Stockinger S, Denis MM, Bartlett WT, Inverardi L, Le TT, thi Man N, Morris GE, Bogan DJ, Metcalf-Bogan J, Kornegay JN (2000) *In vivo* targeted repair of a point mutation in the canine dystrophin gene by a chimeric RNA/DNA oligonucleotide. *Nat Biotechnol* 18: 615-622

9. Barton-Davis ER, Cordier L, Shoturma DI, Leland SE, Sweeney HL (1999) Aminoglycoside antibiotics restore dystrophin function to skeletal muscles of mdx mice. *J Clin Invest* 104: 375-381

10. Bijvoet AG, Van Hirtum H, Kroos MA, Van de Kamp EH, Schoneveld O, Visser P, Brakenhoff JP, Weggeman M, van Corven EJ, Van der Ploeg AT, Reuser AJ (1999) Human acid alpha-glucosidase from rabbit milk has therapeutic effect in mice with glycogen storage disease type II. *Hum Mol Genet* 8: 2145-2153

11. Blake DJ, Tinsley JM, Davies KE (1996) Utrophin: a structural and functional comparison to dystrophin. *Brain Pathol* 6: 37-47

12. Brough DE, Hsu C, Kulesa VA, Lee GM, Cantolupo LJ, Lizonova A, Kovesdi I (1997) Activation of transgene expression by early region 4 is responsible for a high level of persistent transgene expression from adenovirus vectors *in vivo*. *J Virol* 71: 9206-9213

13. Budker V, Zhang G, Danko I, Williams P, Wolff J (1998) The efficient expression of intravascularly delivered DNA in rat muscle. *Gene Ther* 5: 272-276

14. Burton EA, Tinsley JM, Holzfeind PJ, Rodrigues NR, Davies KE (1999) A second promoter provides an alternative target for therapeutic up-regulation of utrophin in Duchenne muscular dystrophy. Proc Natl Acad Sci USA 96: 14025-14030

15. Bushby K (2001) Genetic counselling in muscle disease. In Disorders of Voluntary Muscle, G Karpati, D Hilton-Jones, RC Griggs (eds). Oxford Unviersity Press: New York. pp. 705-739

16. Cho WK, Ebihara S, Nalbantoglu J, Gilbert R, Massie B, Holland P, Karpati G, Petrof BJ (2000) Modulation of Starling forces and muscle fiber maturity permits adenovirus-mediated gene transfer to adult dystrophic (mdx) mice by the intravascular route. *Hum Gene Ther* 11: 701-714

17. Clark KR, Sferra TJ, Johnson PR (1997) Recombinant adeno-associated viral vectors mediate long-term transgene expression in muscle. *Hum Gene Ther* 8: 659-669

18. Clemens PR, Kochanek S, Sunada Y, Chan S, Chen HH, Campbell KP, Caskey CT (1996) *In vivo* muscle gene transfer of full-length dystrophin with an adenoviral vector that lacks all viral genes. *Gene Ther* 3: 965-972

19. Dalakas MC (1994) Retroviral myopathies. In *Myology*, AG Engel, C Franzini-Armstrong (eds). McGraw-Hill: New York. pp. 1419-1437

20. Dalakas MC (1995) Basic aspects of neuroimmunology as they relate to immunotherapeutic targets: present and future prospects. *Ann Neurol* 37 Suppl 1: S2-13

21. Deconinck N, Tinsley J, De Backer F, Fisher R, Kahn D, Phelps S, Davies K, Gillis JM (1997) Expression of truncated utrophin leads to major functional improvements in dystrophin-deficient muscles of mice. *Nat Med* 3: 1216-1221

22. Dunckley MG, Wells DJ, Walsh FS, Dickson G (1993) Direct retroviral-mediated transfer of a dystrophin minigene into mdx mouse muscle *in vivo*. *Hum Mol Genet* 2: 717-723

23. Ebihara S, Guibinga GH, Gilbert R, Nalbantoglu J, Massie B, Karpati G, Petrof BJ (2000) Differential effects of dystrophin and utrophin gene transfer in immunocompetent muscular dystrophy (mdx) mice. *Physiol Genomics* 3: 133-144

24. Feero WG, Rosenblatt JD, Huard J, Watkins SC, Epperly M, Clemens PR, Kochanek S, Glorioso JC, Partridge TA, Hoffman EP (1997) Viral gene delivery to skeletal muscle: insights on maturation- dependent loss of fiber infectivity for adenovirus and herpes simplex type 1 viral vectors. *Hum Gene Ther* 8: 371-380

25. Ferrari G, Cusella-De Angelis G, Coletta M, Paolucci E, Stornaiuolo A, Cossu G, Mavilio F (1998) Muscle regeneration by bone marrow-derived myogenic progenitors. *Science* 279: 1528-1530

26. File TM, Jr., Tan JS (2000) Group A streptococcus necrotizing fasciitis. *Compr Ther* 26: 73-81

27. Fruen BR, Mickelson JR, Louis CF (1997) Dantrolene inhibition of sarcoplasmic reticulum Ca2+ release by direct and specific action at skeletal muscle ryanodine receptors. *J Biol Chem* 272: 26965-26971

28. Gertner E, Thurn JR, Williams DN, Simpson M, Balfour HH, Jr., Rhame F, Henry K (1989) Zidovudine-associated myopathy. *Am J Med* 86: 814-818

29. Gilbert R, Nalbantoglu J, Petrof BJ, Ebihara S, Guibinga GH, Tinsley JM, Kamen A, Massie B, Davies KE, Karpati G (1999) Adenovirus-mediated utrophin gene transfer mitigates the dystrophic phenotype of mdx mouse muscles. *Hum Gene Ther* 10: 1299-1310

30. Goncz KK, Gruenert DC (2000) Site-directed alteration of genomic DNA by small-fragment homologous replacement. *Methods Mol Biol* 133: 85-99

31. Greelish JP, Su LT, Lankford EB, Burkman JM, Chen H, Konig SK, Mercier IM, Desjardins PR, Mitchell MA, Zheng XG, Leferovich J, Gao GP, Balice-Gordon RJ, Wilson JM, Stedman HH (1999) Stable restoration of the sarcoglycan complex in dystrophic muscle perfused with histamine and a recombinant adeno-associated viral vector. *Nat Med* 5: 439-443

32. Guerette B, Asselin I, Skuk D, Entman M, Tremblay JP (1997) Control of inflammatory damage by anti-LFA-1: increase success of myoblast transplantation. *Cell Transplant* 6: 101-107

33. Gussoni E, Soneoka Y, Strickland CD, Buzney EA, Khan MK, Flint AF, Kunkel LM, Mulligan RC (1999) Dystrophin expression in the mdx mouse restored by stem cell transplantation. *Nature* 401: 390-394

34. Harper CM, Engel AG (1998) Quinidine sulfate therapy for the slow-channel congenital myasthenic syndrome. *Ann Neurol* 43: 480-484

35. Hays AP, Gamboa ET (1994) Acute viral myositis. In *Myology*, AG Engel, C Franzini-Armstrong (eds). McGraw-Hill: New York. pp. 1399-1418

36. Hoffman EP, Morgan JE, Watkins SC, Partridge TA (1990) Somatic reversion/suppression of the mouse mdx phenotype *in vivo*. *J Neurol Sci* 99: 9-25

37. Huard J, Lochmuller H, Acsadi G, Jani A, Massie B, Karpati G (1995) The route of administration is a major determinant of the transduction efficiency of rat tissues by adenoviral recombinants. *Gene Ther* 2: 107-115

38. Johnston JC, Gasmi M, Lim LE, Elder JH, Yee JK, Jolly DJ, Campbell KP, Davidson BL, Sauter SL (1999) Minimum requirements for efficient transduction of dividing and nondividing cells by feline immunodeficiency virus vectors. *J Virol* 73: 4991-5000

39. Kafri T, Blomer U, Peterson DA, Gage FH, Verma IM (1997) Sustained expression of genes delivered directly into liver and muscle by lentiviral vectors. *Nat Genet* 17: 314-317

40. Karpati G, Ajdukovic D, Arnold D, Gledhill RB, Guttmann R, Holland P, Koch PA, Shoubridge E, Spence D, Vanasse M, et al. (1993a) Myoblast transfer in Duchenne muscular dystrophy. *Ann Neurol* 34: 8-17

41. Karpati G, Carpenter S, Morris GE, Davies KE, Guerin C, Holland P (1993b) Localization and quantitation of the chromosome 6-encoded dystrophin- related protein in normal and pathological human muscle. *J Neuropathol Exp Neurol* 52: 119-128

42. Karpati G, Gilbert R, Petrof BJ, Nalbantoglu J (1997) Gene therapy research for Duchenne and Becker muscular dystrophies. *Curr Opin Neurol* 10: 430-435

43. Karpati G, Pari G, Molnar MJ (1999) Molecular therapy for genetic muscle diseases--status 1999. *Clin Genet* 55: 1-8

44. Karpati G, Pouliot Y, Zubrzycka-Gaarn E, Carpenter S, Ray PN, Worton RG, Holland P (1989) Dystrophin is expressed in mdx skeletal muscle fibers after normal myoblast implantation. *Am J Pathol* 135: 27-32

45. Kochanek S, Clemens PR, Mitani K, Chen HH, Chan S, Caskey CT (1996) A new adenoviral vector: Replacement of all viral coding sequences with 28 kb of DNA independently expressing both full-length dystrophin and beta-galactosidase. *Proc Natl Acad Sci USA* 93: 5731-5736

46. Kociecka W (2000) Trichinellosis: human disease, diagnosis and treatment. *Vet Parasitol* 93: 365-383

47. Larochelle N, Lochmuller H, Zhao J, Jani A, Hallauer P, Hastings KE, Massie B, Prescott S, Petrof BJ, Karpati G, Nalbantoglu J (1997) Efficient muscle-specific transgene expression after adenovirus- mediated gene transfer in mice using a 1.35 kb muscle creatine kinase promoter/enhancer. *Gene Ther* 4: 465-472

48. Li J, Dressman D, Tsao YP, Sakamoto A, Hoffman EP, Xiao X (1999) rAAV vector-mediated sarcogylcan gene transfer in a hamster model for limb girdle muscular dystrophy. *Gene Ther* 6: 74-82

49. Mann CJ, Honeyman K, Cheng AJ, Ly T, Lloyd F, Fletcher S, Morgan JE, Partridge TA, Wilton SD (2001) Antisense-induced exon skipping and synthesis of dystrophin in the mdx mouse. *Proc Natl Acad Sci USA* 98: 42-47

50. Mendell JR, Kissel JT, Amato AA, King W, Signore L, Prior TW, Sahenk Z, Benson S, McAndrew PE, Rice R, et al. (1995) Myoblast transfer in the treatment of

Duchenne's muscular dystrophy. *N Engl J Med* 333: 832-838

51. Meola G, Karpati G, Griggs RC (2001) The principles of treatment, prevention and rehabilitation: perspectives on future therapies. In *Disorders of Voluntary Muscle*, G Karpati, D Hilton-Jones, RC Griggs (eds). Oxford Unviersity Press: New York. pp. 739-754

52. Mir LM, Bureau MF, Gehl J, Rangara R, Rouy D, Caillaud JM, Delaere P, Branellec D, Schwartz B, Scherman D (1999) High-efficiency gene transfer into skeletal muscle mediated by electric pulses. *Proc Natl Acad Sci USA* 96: 4262-4267

53. Monahan PE, Samulski RJ (2000) Adeno-associated virus vectors for gene therapy: more pros than cons? *Mol Med Today* 6: 433-440

54. Moxley RT, 3rd (1994) Potential for growth factor treatment of muscle disease. *Curr Opin Neurol* 7: 427-434

55. Nalbantoglu J, Pari G, Karpati G, Holland PC (1999) Expression of the primary coxsackie and adenovirus receptor is downregulated during skeletal muscle maturation and limits the efficacy of adenovirus-mediated gene delivery to muscle cells. *Hum Gene Ther* 10: 1009-1019

56. Nguyen TM, Ellis JM, Love DR, Davies KE, Gatter KC, Dickson G, Morris GE (1991) Localization of the DMDL gene-encoded dystrophin-related protein using a panel of nineteen monoclonal antibodies: presence at neuromuscular junctions, in the sarcolemma of dystrophic skeletal muscle, in vascular and other smooth muscles, and in proliferating brain cell lines. *J Cell Biol* 115: 1695-1700

57. O'Hara AJ, Howell JM, Taplin RH, Fletcher S, Lloyd F, Kakulas B, Lochmuller H, Karpati G (2001) The spread of transgene expression at the site of gene construct injection. *Muscle Nerve* 24: 488-495

58. Ohlendieck K, Matsumura K, Ionasescu VV, Towbin JA, Bosch EP, Weinstein SL, Sernett SW, Campbell KP (1993) Duchenne muscular dystrophy: deficiency of dystrophin-associated proteins in the sarcolemma. *Neurology* 43: 795-800

59. Parks RJ, Chen L, Anton M, Sankar U, Rudnicki MA, Graham FL (1996) A helper-dependent adenovirus vector system: removal of helper virus by Cre-mediated excision of the viral packaging signal. *Proc Natl Acad Sci USA* 93: 13565-13570

60. Partridge TA, Morgan JE, Coulton GR, Hoffman EP, Kunkel LM (1989) Conversion of mdx myofibres from dystrophin-negative to -positive by injection of normal myoblasts. *Nature* 337: 176-179

61. Phylactou LA, Darrah C, Wood MJ (1998) Ribozyme-mediated trans-splicing of a trinucleotide repeat. *Nat Genet* 18: 378-381

62. Qu Z, Huard J (2000) Matching host muscle and donor myoblasts for myosin heavy chain improves myoblast transfer therapy. *Gene Ther* 7: 428-437

63. Ragot T, Opolon P, Perricaudet M (1997) Adenoviral gene delivery. *Methods Cell Biol* 52: 229-260

64. Rando TA, Disatnik MH, Zhou LZ (2000) Rescue of dystrophin expression in mdx mouse muscle by RNA/DNA oligonucleotides. *Proc Natl Acad Sci USA* 97: 5363-5368

65. Snyder RO (1999) Adeno-associated virus-mediated gene delivery. *J Gene Med* 1: 166-175

66. Tinsley JM, Potter AC, Phelps SR, Fisher R, Trickett JI, Davies KE (1996) Amelioration of the dystrophic phenotype of mdx mice using a truncated utrophin transgene. *Nature* 384: 349-353

67. Tremblay JP, Malouin F, Roy R, Huard J, Bouchard JP, Satoh A, Richards CL (1993) Results of a triple blind clinical study of myoblast transplantations without immunosuppressive treatment in young boys with Duchenne muscular dystrophy. *Cell Transplant* 2: 99-112

68. Vincent N, Ragot T, Gilgenkrantz H, Couton D, Chafey P, Gregoire A, Briand P, Kaplan JC, Kahn A, Perricaudet M (1993) Long-term correction of mouse dystrophic degeneration by adenovirus- mediated transfer of a minidystrophin gene. *Nat Genet* 5: 130-134

69. Vitiello L, Chonn A, Wasserman JD, Duff C, Worton RG (1996) Condensation of plasmid DNA with polylysine improves liposome-mediated gene transfer into established and primary muscle cells. *Gene Ther* 3: 396-404

70. Walter MC, Lochmuller H, Reilich P, Klopstock T, Huber R, Hartard M, Hennig M, Pongratz D, Muller-Felber W (2000) Creatine monohydrate in muscular dystrophies: A double-blind, placebo- controlled clinical study. *Neurology* 54: 1848-1850

71. Wilschanski M, Famini C, Blau H, Rivlin J, Augarten A, Avital A, Kerem B, Kerem E (2000) A pilot study of the effect of gentamicin on nasal potential difference measurements in cystic fibrosis patients carrying stop mutations. *Am J Respir Crit Care Med* 161: 860-865.

72. Wolff JA, Malone RW, Williams P, Chong W, Acsadi G, Jani A, Felgner PL (1990) Direct gene transfer into mouse muscle *in vivo*. *Science* 247: 1465-1468.

73. Xiao X, Li J, Samulski RJ (1996) Efficient long-term gene transfer into muscle tissue of immunocompetent mice by adeno-associated virus vector. *J Virol* 70: 8098-8108

74. Yamamoto K, Yuasa K, Miyagoe Y, Hosaka Y, Tsukita K, Yamamoto H, Nabeshima YI, Takeda S (2000) Immune response to adenovirus-delivered antigens upregulates utrophin and results in mitigation of muscle pathology in mdx mice. *Hum Gene Ther* 11: 669-680

75. Yang Y, Nunes FA, Berencsi K, Furth EE, Gonczol E, Wilson JM (1994) Cellular immunity to viral antigens limits E1-deleted adenoviruses for gene therapy. *Proc Natl Acad Sci USA* 91: 4407-4411

76. Yerroum M, Pham-Dang C, Authier FJ, Monnet I, Gherardi R, Chariot P (2000) Cytochrome c oxidase deficiency in the muscle of patients with zidovudine myopathy is segmental and affects both mitochondrial DNA- and nuclear DNA-encoded subunits. *Acta Neuropathol (Berl)* 100: 82-86

Contributors

Dr Anthony Amato
Director of Neuromuscular Service
Brigham and Women's Hospital
75 Francis Street
Boston MA 02115
UNITED STATES
Phone: +1 617 735 5436
Fax: +1 617 730 2885
aamato@partners.org

Dr Louise V. B. Anderson
Neurobiology Department
University Medical School
Framlington Place
Newcastle upon Tyne NE2 4HH
UNITED KINGDOM
Phone: +44 191 222 5728
Fax: +44 191 222 5227
L.V.B.Anderson@newcastle.ac.uk

Dr Kiichi Arahata
Department of Neuromuscular Research
National Institute of Neuroscience
4-1-1 Ogawa-Higashi, Kodaira
Tokyo JP-187-8502
JAPAN
Phone: +81 42 341 2711
Fax: +81 42 346 1742
arahata@ncnaxp.ncnp.go.jp

Dr Zohar Argov
Department of Neurology
Hadassah University Hospital
Jerusalem IL-91120
ISRAEL
Phone: +972 2 6776 938
Fax: +972 2 6437 782
zargov@md.huji.ac.il

Ms Christine Beahler
Health Science and Information Center
University of Washington School of Medicine
Seattle WA 98115
UNITED STATES
Phone: +1 206 221 4674
Fax: +1 206 21 4679

Dr Jacques S. Beckmann
Department of Molecular Genetics
Weizmann Institute of Science
P.O. Box 26
IL-76100 Rehovot
ISRAEL
Phone: +972 8 934 3717
Fax: +972 8 934 4108
beckmann@weizmann.ac.il

Dr Robert J. Beynon
Department of Veterinary Preclinical Sciences
University of Liverpool
Liverpool L69 7ZJ
UNITED KINGDOM
Phone: +44 151 794 4312
Fax: +44 151 794 4243
r.beynon@liv.ac.uk

Dr Thomas D. Bird
Geriatrics Research Service (S182)
VA Medical Center
1660 South Columbian Way
Seattle WA 98108
UNITED STATES
Phone: +1 206 764 2308
Fax: +1 206 764 2569
tomnroz@u.washington.edu

Dr Gisèle Bonne
Hôpital Pitié-Salpêtrière
Institut de Myologie
47 Boulevard de l'Hôpital
FR-75651 Paris Cedex 13
FRANCE
Phone: +33 1 42 16 57 23
Fax: +33 1 42 16 57 00
g.bonne@myologie.chups.jussieu.fr

Dr Bernard Brais
Centre de Resreche du CHUM
Hôpital Notre-Dame-CHUM
1560 rue Shrebrooke est
Montreal Quebec H2L 4MI
CANADA
Phone: + 514 890 8000 ext 25560
Fax: +1 514 412 7525
bernard.bras@umontreal.ca

Dr Robert H. Brown Jr
Cecil B. Day Laboratory for Neuromuscular Diseases
Massachusetts General Hospital
13th Street, Navy Yard
Charleston MA 02129
UNITED STATES
Phone: +1 617 726 5750
Fax: +1 617 726 5677
rhbrown@partners.org

Dr Anna Buj-Bello
Institut de Génétique et de Biologie Moléculaire et Cellulaire
CNRS/INSERM/ULP. BP 163
FR-67404 Illkirch Cedex
FRANCE
Phone: +33 3 88 65 415
Fax: +33 3 88 65 32 46
mtm@igbmc.u-strasbg.fr

Dr Stirling Carpenter
Rua Diogo Afonso 19, IF
PT-4100 Porto
PORTUGAL
Phone: +351 22 616 0862
Fax: +351 22 557 0799
scarp@mail.telepac.pt

Dr Leila Chimelli
Serviço de Anatomia Patológica
Hospital Universitário
Universidade Federal do Rio de Janeiro
Ilha do Fundão
RJ-21941-590 Rio de Janeiro
BRAZIL
Phone: +55 21 5622 450
Fax: +55 215 622 450
chimelli@hucff.ufrj.br

Dr Elias da Silva
Enterovirus Laboratory
Oswaldo Cruz Institute
Avenida Brasil 43656
RJ-21045-900 Rio de Janeiro
BRAZIL
Phone: +55 21 2564 7638
Fax: +55 21 2564 7638
eesilva@gene.dbbm.fiocruz.br

Dr Niklas Darin
Inserm U393, Tour Lavoisier (2e étage)
Hopital Necker Enfants-Malades
149 Rue de Sèvres
F -7573 PARIS CEDEX 15
FRANCE
Phone: +33 1 4438 1584
Fax: +33 1 47348 514
darin@necker.fr

Dr Stefano DiDonato
Istituto Nazionale Neurologico Carlo Besta
Via Celoria 11
IT-20133 Milano
ITALY
Phone: +39 2 2 706 3941
Fax: +39 2 706 38217
didonato@istituto-besta.it

Dr Margaritka Dikova-Sorge
ISN Neuropath Press
Am Steinberg 45
DE 82237 Woerthsee
GERMANY
Phone. +49 8153 984 955
Fax: +49 8153 984956
dikovasorge@aol.com

Dr Salvatore DiMauro
Department of Neurology, Room 420A
630 West 168th Street
Columbia University College of Physicians and Surgeons
New York NY 10032
UNITED STATES
Phone: +1 212 305 162
Fax: +1 212 305 3986
sd12@columbia.edu

Dr Alan E. H. Emery
Department of Neurology
Royal Devon and Exeter Hospital (Wonford)
Barrack Road
Exeter EX2 5DW
UNITED KINGDOM
Phone: +44 1395 445847
Fax: +44 1395 443855
emery@budleigh.demon.co.uk

Dr Andrew G. Engel
Department of Neurology
Neuromuscular Research Laboratory
Guggenheim Building G 801
Mayo Clinic
Rochester MN 55905
UNITED STATES
Phone: +1 507 284 5102
+1 507 284 5831
age@mayo.edu

Dr Renald Gilbert
Montreal Neurological Institute
3801 University Street, Room 628
Montreal QC H3A 2B4
CANADA
Phone: +1 514-398-8528
Fax: +1 514 398 8310
renald.gilbert@mcgill.ca

Dr James M. Gilchrist
Department of Neurology
Brown University School of Medicine
Rhode Island Hospital
Providence RI 02903
UNITED STATES
Phone: +1 401 444 8761
Fax: +1 401 444 5929
james_gilchrist@brown.edu

Dr Hans H. Goebel
Department of Neuropathology
Johannes Gutenberg University
Medical Center
Langenbeckstrasse 1
D-55131 Mainz
GERMANY
Phone: +49 6131 17 7308
Fax: +49 613 117 6606
goebel@neuropatho.klinik.uni-mainz.de

Dr Lev Goldfarb
National Institutes of Health
Bldg 10, Room 4B37
10 Center Drive, MSC 1361
Bethesda MD 20892-1361
UNITED STATES
Phone: +1 301 4021 480
Fax: +1-301 4966 341
goldfarb@codon.nih.gov

Dr Robert Griggs
Department of Neurology
University of Rochester Medical Center
601 Elmwood Avenue, Box 673
Rochester NY 14642
UNITED STATES
Phone: +1 716 275 2541
Fax: +1 716 244 2529
robert_griggs@urmc.rochester.edu

Dr Michio Hirano
Department of Neurology
Columbia-Presbyterian Medical Center
P&S 4-443
630 West 168th Street
New York NY 10032
UNITED STATES
Phone: +1 212 305 1048
Fax: +1 212 305 3986
mh29@columbia.edu

Dr Meng F. Ho
Cecil B. Day Laboratory for Neuromuscular Diseases
Massachusetts General Hospital
Building 114, 16th Street, Navy Yard
Charleston MA 02129
UNITED STATES
Phone: +1 617 726 5750
Fax: +1 617 726 8543
mfho@helix.mgh.harvard.edu

Dr Eric P. Hoffman
Research Center for Genetic Medicine
Children's National Medical Center
111 Michigan Avenue NW
Washington DC 20010
UNITED STATES
Phone: +1 202 884 6011
Fax: +1 202 884 6014
ehoffman@cnmc.org

Dr Reinhard Hohlfeld
Institute for Clinical Neuroimmunology
Ludwig-Maximilians University
Marchionistrasse 15
DE-81366 München
GERMANY
Phone: +49 89 7095 4780
Fax: +49 89 7095 4782
rhohlfel@nro.med.uni-muenchen.de

Dr Karin Jurkat-Rott
Department of Applied Physiology
Current Genetics Group
University of Ulm
Albert-Einsten-Allee 11
DE-89081 Ulm
GERMANY
Phone: +49 50 22065
Fax: +49 50 232 60
karin.jurkat-rott@medizin.uni-ulm.de

Dr Hannu Kalimo
Department of Pathology
University Hospital
Kinakvarnsgatan 10
FIN-205 20 Turku
FINLAND
Phone: +358 2 2611 685
Fax: +358 21 6337 459
hkalimo@utu.fi

Dr George Karpati
Montreal Neurological Institute
Neuromuscular Research Group
3801 University Street
Montreal (Quebec) H3A 2B4
CANADA
Phone: +1 514 398 8528
Fax: +1 514 398 8310
mcgk@musica.mcgill.ca

Dr Nigel G. Laing
Australian Neuromuscular Research Institute
4th Floor "A" Block
Queen Elizabeth II Medical Center
Nedlands Western Australia 6009
AUSTRALIA
Phone: +61 8 9346 2658
Fax: +61 8 9346 3487
nlaing@cyllene.uwa.edu.au

Dr Bethan Lang
Department of Clinical Neurology
Institute of Molecular Medicine
John Radcliffe Hospital
Oxford OX3 9DU
UNITED KINGDOM
Phone: +44 1865 222321
Fax: +44 1865 222402
blang@molbiol.ox.ac.uk

Dr Jocelyn Laporte
Institut de Génétique et de Biologie Moléculaire et Cellulaire
CNRS/INSERM/ULP. BP 163
1 rue Laurent Fries
FR-67404 Illkirch Cedex
FRANCE
Phone: +33 3 88 65 415
Fax: +33 3 88 65 32 46
mtm@igbmc.u-strasbg.fr

Dr Frank Lehmann-Horn
Department of Applied Physiology
University of Ulm
Albert-Einsten-Allee 11
Ulm DE-89081
GERMANY
Phone: +49 50 232 50
+49 731 50 232 60
frank.lehmann-horn@medizin.uni-ulm.de

Dr Nicolas Levy
Inserm U491 "Genetique Medicale et Developpement"
Faculté de Médecine de la Timone
FR-13385 Marseille Cedex 05
FRANCE
Phone: + 33 4 91 25 71 59
Fax: + 33 4 91 80 43 19
Nicolas.Levy@medecine.univ-mrs.fr

Dr Jon Lindstrom
Department of Neuroscience
Medical School of the University of Pennsylvania
217 Stemmler Hall
Philadelphia PA-19104-6074
UNITED STATES
Phone: +1 15 573 2859
Fax: +1 215 573 2015
jslkk@mail.med.upenn.edu

Dr Hanns Lochmüller
Gene Centre and Friedrich-Baur-Institute Munic
Ludwig-Maximilians-Universität
Feodor-Lynen-Strasse 25
DE-81377 München
GERMANY
Phone: +49 89 2180 6887
Fax: +49 89 2180 6999
hanns@lmb.uni-muenchen.de

Dr Julian C. P. Loke
Malignant Hyperthermia Investigation Unit
CCRW 2-830
Toronto General Hospital
200 Elizabeth Street
Toronto, Ontario M5G 2C4
CANADA
Phone: +1-416 340 3128
Fax: +1 416 340 4960
j.loke@utoronto.ca.

Dr David H. MacLennan
Banting and Best Department of Medical Research
University of Toronto
112 College Street
Toronto OntarioM5G 1L6
CANADA
Phone: +1 416 978 6180
Fax: +1 416 978 8528
david.maclennan@utoronto.ca

Mr Duncan A. MacRae
UCLA Medical Center
Neuropathology CHS 18-126
Los Angeles, CA 90095
UNITED STATES
Phone: +1 310 267 0543
Fax: +1 310 267 0545
d_macrae@alumni.utexas.net

Dr Jean-Louis Mandel
Institut de Génétique et de Biologie Moléculaire et Cel-
lulaire
CNRS/INSERM/ULP. BP 163
1 rue Laurent Fries
Illkirch Cedex FR-67404
FRANCE
Phone: +33 3 88 65 32 44
Fax: +33 3 88 65 32 46
mandeljl@igbmc.u-strasbg.fr

Dr Frank T. Martiniuk
Department of Medicine
New York University School of Medicine
550 First Avenue
New York NY 10016
UNITED STATES
Phone: +1 212 562 3616
Fax: +1 212 263 8442
martif02@popmail.med.nyu.edu

Dr Tommy Martinsson
Department of Clinical Genetics
Sahlgrenska University Hospital-East
SE-41685 Gothenburg
SWEDEN
Phone: +46 31 3434803
Fax: +46 31 7504317
Tommy.Martinsson@clingen.gu.se

Dr Berge A. Minassian
Division of Neurology
Department of Paediatrics, Room 6541A
The Hospital for Sick Children
555 University Avenue
Toronto Ontario M5G 1X8
CANADA
Phone: +1 416 813 6291
Fax: +1 416 813 6334
bminass@sickkids.on.ca

Dr Maria Molnar
National Institute of Psychiatry and Neurology
Huvosvolgyi ut 116
Budapest HU-1021
HUNGARY
Phone: +36 20 9363 150
Fax: +36 1 391 5440
molnarm@jaguar.dote.hu

Dr Tahseen Mozaffar
University of California, Irvine
UCIMC Neurodiagnostic Lab
101 The City Drive S, Building 22 C, Rt. 13
Orange CA 92868
UNITED STATES
Phone: +1 714 456 5124
Fax: +1714 4566 908
mozaffar@uci.edu

Dr Josef Müller-Höcker
Pathologisches Institut der LMU
Thalkirchner Straße 36
DE-80337 München
GERMANY
Phone: +49 89 5160 4011
Fax: +49 89 5160 4043
josef.mueller-hoecker@web.de

Dr Ichizo Nishino
Department of Ultrastructural Research
National Institute of Neuroscience
National Center of Neurology and Psychiatry
4-1-1 Ogawahigashi-cho, Kodaira,
Tokyo JP-187-8502
JAPAN
Phone: +81 42 346 1719
Fax: +81 42 346 1749
nishino@ncnp.go.jp

Dr Kinji Ohno
Department of Neurology
Neuromuscular Research Laboratory
Guggenheim Building G 801
Mayo Clinic
Rochester MN 55905
UNITED STATES
Phone: +1 507 284 5102
Fax: +1 507 284 5831
ohnok@mayo.edu

Dr Anders Oldfors
Department of Pathology
Sahlgrenska University Hospital
SE 413 45 Gothenburg
SWEDEN
Phone: +46 31 342 2084
Fax: +46 31 417283
anders.oldfors@path.gu.se

Dr Yngve Olsson
Rudbeck Laboratory, C5
University Hospital
SE-751 85 Uppsala
SWEDEN
Phone: +46 070 342 8117
Fax: +46 18 502 172
Yngve.Olsson@genpat.uu.se

Dr George W. Padberg
Department of Neurology
University Hospital
NL-6500 HB Nijmegen
THE NETHERLANDS
Phone: +31 24 361 8860
Fax: +31 24 354 1122
g.padberg@czzoneu.azn.nl

Dr Roberta A. Pagon
Gene Clinics
Box 358735
9725 3rd Avenue N.E., Suite 610
Seattle WA 98115-2024
UNITED STATES
Phone: +1 206 528 2630
Fax: +1 206 526 2217
bpagon@u.washington.edu

Dr Elena Pegoraro
Department of Neurol and Psychiatr Sciences
Via Giustiani 5
IT - 35128 Padova
ITALY
Phone: +49 8213601
Fax: +49 8751770
elenap@ux1.unipd.it

Dr Alan Pestronk
Department of Neurology
Washington University School of Medicine
660 South Euclid Avenue
MO 63110 St Louis
UNITED STATES
Phone: +1 314 362 6981
Fax: +1 708 810 3157
pestronk@kids.wustl.edu

Dr Dieter E. Pongratz
Friedrich-Baur-Institut bei der Medizinischen Klinik
Klinikum Innenstadt
Universität München
Ziemssenstrasse 1a
DE-80336 München
GERMANY
Phone: +49 89 5437 0962
Fax: +49 895 1604750
dieter.pongratz@fbs.med.uni-muenchen.de

Dr Rosalind C. M Quinlivan
Muscle Clinic
Robert Jones & Agnes Hunt Orthopaedic Hospital
NHS Trust
Oswestry, Shropshire
UNITED KINDDOM
Phone: +441691 404376
Fax: +441691 404376
rcmq37@aol.com

Dr Michael Rose
King's Neurosciences Centre
Department of Neurology
Denmark Hill
London SE5 9RS
UNITED KINGDOM
Phone: +44 20 7346 5355
Fax: +44 20 7346 5353
m.r.rose@kcl.ac.uk

Dr Richard L. Sabina
Department of Biochemistry
Medical College of Wisconsin
8701 Watertown Plank Road
Milwaukee WI 53226
UNITED STATES
Phone: +1 414 456 4697
Fax: +1 414 456 6510
sabinar@post.its.mcw.edu

Dr Rolf Schröder
Department of Neurology
University Hospital
Sigmund-Freud-Strasse
DE-53127 Bonn
GERMANY
Phone: +49 228 287 6391
Fax: +49 228 287 4760
myologie@mailer.meb.uni-bonn.de

Dr Duygu Selcen
Department of Neurology
Neuromuscular Research Laboratory
Guggenheim Building G 801
Mayo Clinic
Rochester MN 55905
UNITED STATES
Phone: +1 507 284 5102
Fax: +1 507 284 5831
duygu.selcen@mao.edu

Dr Caroline A. Sewry
Department of Paediatrics and Neonatal Medicine
Imperial College School of Medicine
Hammersmith Hospital
London W12 ONN
UNITED KINGDOM
Phone: +44 208 383 3148
Fax: +44 208 746 2187
c.sewry@ic.ac.uk

Dr Eric A. Shoubridge
Montreal Neurological Institute
Neuromuscular Research Group
3801 University Street
Montreal (Quebec) H3A 2B4
CANADA
Phone: +1 514 398 1997
Fax: +1 514 398 1509
eric@ericpc.mni.mcgill.ca

Dr Dov Soffer
Pathology Department (Neuropathology)
Hadassah Medical Center
P.O. Box 12000
IL-91120 Jerusalem
ISRAEL
Phone: +972 2 675 8206
+972 2 642 6268
soffer@huji.ac.il

Dr Hiroyuki Sorimachi
Department of Applied Biological Chemistry
Grad. Sch. of Agricultural and Life Sciences
The University of Tokyo
Yayoi, Bunkyo-ku
Tokyo JP-113-0032
JAPAN
Phone: +81 3 5841 8218
Fax: +81 3 5841 8118
ahsori@mail.ecc.u-tokyo.ac.jp

Dr Wayney Squier
Department of Neuropathology
Radcliffe Infirmary
Woodstock Road
Oxford OX2 6HE
UNITED KINGDOM
Phone: +44 1865224508
waney.squier@clneuro.ox.ac.uk

Dr Ana Lia Taratuto
Department of Neuropathology
Inst. de Invest. Neurol. "R. Carrea"
Montañeses 2325 p. 3°ree
AR-1428 Buenos Aires
ARGENTINA
Phone: +5411 4788 3444
Fax: +5411 4784 7620
ataratuto@fleni.org.ar

Dr Franco Taroni
Istituto Nazionale Neurologico Carlo Besta
Via Celoria 11
IT- 20133 Milano
ITALY
Phone: +39 02 2394.284
Fax: +39 2 95441044 2
taroni@tin.it

Dr Peter K. Thomas
The National Hospital for Neurology and Neurosurgery
Queen Square
London WCIN 3BG
UNITED KINGDOM
Phone: +44 20 834 3365
Fax: +44 20 833 2823
pkt.hotline@virgin.net

Dr Charles Thornton
Department of Neurology
University of Rochester Medical Center
601 Elmwood Avenue, Box 673
Rochester NY14642
UNITED STATES
Phone: +1 716 275 2559
Fax: +1 716 244 2529
Charles_Thornton@urmc.Rochester.edu

Ms Angelica Tibbling
Department of Genetics and Pathology
University Hospital
SE-751 85 Uppsala
SWEDEN
Phone: +46 18 611 38 38
Fax. +46 18 50 21 72
angelica.tibbling@genpat.uu.se

Dr Carina Wallgren-Pettersson
The Folkhälsan Institute of Genetics
P.O. Box 211
Topeliuskatu 20
FIN-00251 Helsinki
FINLAND
Phone: +358 434 9354
Fax: +358 9 434 9400
carina.wallgren@helsinki.fi

Dr Maggie C. Walter
Friedrich-Baur-Institute and Gene Center
Munich
GERMANY
Phone: +49 89 5160 7476
Fax: +49 89 5160 7402
Maggie.Walter@lrz.uni-muenchen.de

Dr Angela Vincent
Neurosciences Group
Institute of Molecular Medicine
John Radcliffe Hospital
Oxford OX3 9DU
UNITED KINGDOM
Phone: +44 1865 222321
Fax: +44 1865 222402
avincent@hammer.imm.ox.ac.uk

Acknowledgments

The International Society of Neuropathology provided seed corn money and its Executive Committee headed by Professor Samuel K. Ludwin, Canada supported the idea to produce this muscle book in collaboration with WFN and its Research Group on Neuromuscular Diseases. Professor P. K. Thomas, Head of the Research Group was an invaluable speaking partner particularly at the start of the project.

Professor Paul Kleihues, France, who initiated the ISN book series gave us invaluable advice. Without his help this book would not have been produced in its present form. The Department of Genetics & Pathology, Uppsala University, Sweden gave substantial financial contributions.

An outstanding Volume Editor, George Karpati, Canada, all the distinguished Authors and Advisory Board Members as well as highly professional persons like Duncan MacRae, Margaritka Dikova-Sorge and Angelica Tibbing made the completion of this book possible.

For all this support I am very grateful.

Yngve Olsson
ISN Production Editor

Acknowledgements by the authors of the following chapters:

Chapter 2.3, 2.4. Dysferlinopathies and caveolinopathies. We are very grateful to Drs Keith Ligon and Jennifer A. Chan for assistance with electron microscopy. This work was supported in part by the Muscular Dystrophy Association (USA) and the Cecil B. Day Investment Company.

Chapter 4. Myofibrillar and internal cytoskeletal protein lesions. The editorial assistance by Mrs A. Wöber, photographic work by Mrs I. Warlo, Mrs M. Bousfia and Mr W. Meffert are gratefully acknowledged. The "Deutsche Gesellschaft für Muskelkranke, e.V." Freiburg/Germany, the "European Neuromuscular Centre (ENMC)," Baarn/The Netherlands and the "MAIFOR programme" of the Johannes Gutenberg University, Mainz/Germany supported these studies.

Chapter 5.1.1. Myotonia and paramyotonia and chapter 5.1.2. Dyskalemic episodic weakness. We thank U. Richter for designing the figures. This work was supported by the Interdisciplinary Clinical Research Center of Ulm University funded by the Federal Ministry of Research and the TMR Programme on Excitation-contraction coupling funded by the European Community.

Chapter 5.2. Malignant hyperthermia and central core disease associated with defects in Ca^{2+} channels of the sarcotubular system and Chapter 5.3. Brody disease associated with defects in a Ca^{2+} pump. Parts of the work described in these chapters were supported by grants from the Canadian Institutes of Health Research, the Heart and Stroke Foundation of Ontario, the Canadian Genetic Diseases Network of Centers of Excellence, the Muscular Dystrophy Association of Canada and the Muscular Dystrophy Association (USA).

Chapter 6.1.1. The myotonic dystrophies. Supported by the Muscular Dystrophy Association and the National Institutes of Health (AR46806).

Chapter 6.1.2. PABPN1 dysfunction in oculopharyngeal muscular dystrophy. Thanks to Hugo Lavoie for his help with illustrations and Maria Carmo-Fonseca and Human Molecular Genetics for agreeing to reproduce certain figures.

Chapter 7.1. X-linked myotubular myopathy. We wish to thank all members of the International Consortium on Myotubular Myopathy, for sharing information and for helpful discussions, the ENMC (European Neuromuscular Centre) for organisational support, and Dr V. Biancalana (Strasbourg) for communicating unpublished mutations. The group from France was supported by funds from the Institut National de la Santé et de la Recherche Médicale, the Centre National de la Recherche Scientifique, the Hôpital Universitaire de Strasbourg (HUS), and the Association Française contre les Myopathies (AFM). The group from Finland was supported by the AF1VI and the University of Helsinki.

Chapter 8.2.1. Calpainopathy. The authors sincerely thank Dr Michael Fardeau for illustrations 3 through 6.

Chapter 9.3. Congenital myasthenic syndromes. This work was supported by NIH Grant NS6277 and by research grant from the Muscular Dystrophy Association.

Chapter 10.2. Defects of fatty acid metabolism. We thank Dr. Marina Mora for providing some of the skeletal muscle micrographs. Part of the original work was made possible by the valuable contribution by Drs Silvia Baratta, Patrizia Cavadini, Barbara Garavaglia, Cinzia Gellera, Federica Invernizzi, Eleonora Lamantea and Elisabetta Verderio and the generous support by Telethon-Italia.

Chapter 11. Dysimmune myopathies. The Institute for Clinical Neuroimmunology is supported by the Hermann- and Lilly Schilling Foundation.

Index

A

α7 integrin deficiency: 45
Acetylcholine: 156, 170
Acetylcholine receptors (AchR): 156, 166, 170
    Lambert-Eaton myasthenic syndrome: 166
Acetylcholinesterase (AchE): 156
    deficiency of: 171
Acid α-glucosidase: 134
Acid maltase deficiency: 134
Acromegaly: 262
ACTA 1 gene: 62
Actin: 62
Actinopathy: 62
Acute quadriplegic myopathy: 83
Addison's disease: 262
Adenovirus: 298
Ageing: 270
Alpha-tocopherol transfer protein gene: 282
Amyloid myopathy: 268, 284
    cancer-related muscle disease: 268
Anti-Decorin antibodies: 268
ARCO: 209
Atrophy: 252, 257
    denervation: 253
    disuse atrophy: 257
    neurogenic atrophy: 253
Autophagic vacuole: 143, 145, 277
    Danon disease with: 143
    LAMP-2 deficiency with: 142
    Marinesco-Sjögren syndrome with: 277
    X-linked myopathy with excessive autophagy: 145
Autosomal dominant myosin heavy chain IIa myopathy: 85
Autosomal recessive cardiomyopathy, ophthalmoplegia: 209

B

Bacterial myositis: 236
Bassen-Kornzweig disease: 282
Becker muscular dystrophy (BMD): 6
Bethlem myopathy: 41
Brody disease: 103
Brody syndrome: 103

C

CACNA1S gene: 99
Calcium: 279
    osteomalacia myopathy: 279
Calpain3-deficiency: 148
Cancer-related muscle disease: 266
Cap disease: 287
Carbohydrate metabolism: 182
Carcinoma: 269
    cancer-related muscle disease: 269
Carnitine: 189
Carnitine palmitoyltransferas: 189
Carnitine/acylcarnitine translocase: 189
Catecholaminergic polymorphic ventricular tachycardia: 99
Caveolin: 33
Caveolinopathies: 33
Central core disease: 65, 100
    malignant hyperthermia: 65

RYR 1 gene: 65
Centronuclear myopathy: 57
Chagas' disease: 239
Channelopathies: 90, 95, 99, 156
    calcium channels: 99
    chloride channels: 90, 95
    myasthenia gravis: 156
    sodium channels: 90, 95
Chronic external ophthalmoplegia syndromes: 204
Clostridial myositis: 236
Collagen VI gene mutations
Congenital muscular dystrophy: 45
    α7 integrin deficiency: 45
Congenital myasthenic syndrome: 170
Congenital myopathies: 37, 72
    desmin-related myopathies: 70
    laminin α2 (merosin) gene mutations: 29
    plectin deficiency: 78
Cori-Forbes disease: 186
Corticosteroid hormones: 261
COX: 206
CPEO: 204
Critical illness myopathy: 83
CRYAB mutation: 70
Cryptococcosis: 238
Cylindrical spirals myopathy: 287
Cysticercosis: 240

D

Danon disease: 142
    genetic changes: 142
    LAMP-2 deficiency: 142
    secondary LAMP-2 deficiency: 142
    X-linked vacuolar cardiomyopathy and myopathy: 142
Danon's disease: 146
    X-linked myopathy with excessive autophagy: 146
Debrancher deficiency: 186
Debranching enzyme deficiency: 186
Denervation: 252
Dermatomyositis: 221, 268
    cancer-related muscle disease: 268
Desminopathy: 72
Dilated cardiomyopathy with conduction defects: 49
Disuse atrophy: 257
DMPK: 108
Docosahexaenoic acid: 195
Duchenne muscular dystrophy (DMD): 6
Dunnigan-type familial partial lipodystrophy: 49
Dysferlin: 29
Dyskalemic episodic weakness: 95
Dyssegmental dysplasia: 43
Dystroglycan: 8, 24, 38
Dystrophia myotonica: 108
Dystrophin: 6, 24
    Duchenne muscular dystrophy: 6
    sarcoglycanopathies: 24
Dystrophin-associated glycoproteins: 24, 38
Dystrophinopathies: 7
Dystrophy
    Becker muscular dystrophy: 6
    Duchenne muscular dystrophy: 6
    dystrophia myotonica: 108

limb girdle muscular dystrophy type 2B:
limb-girdle muscular dystrophy type 1C:
Miyoshi myopathy: 29
oculopharyngeal muscular dystrophy: 11

E

Echinococcosis: 242
Emerin: 48, 49
Emery-Dreifuss muscular-dystrophy: 49
Endocrine myopathies: 260, 269
    cancer-related muscle disease: 269
European Neuromuscular Centre: 293
Experimental models: 299

F

Facioscapulohumeral dystrophy: 119
Fast-channel syndromes: 174
Fatty-acid metabolism: 189
Fibre type disproportion: 130
Finger-print body myopathy: 287
Flesh eating infection: 237
Friedreich ataxia: 209
FSHD: 119
Fungal myositis: 238

G

Gene replacement: 297
Gene therapy: 297
GeneClinics: 292
GeneTests: 292
Glycogen: 182
    McArdle's disease: 182
Glycogen phosphorylase: 182
Glycogen storage disease: 134, 182
Glycoproteins: 8

H

Heparin sulfate proteoglycan: 43
Hereditary inclusion body myopathy: 85
Hereditary spastic paraplegia: 209
Hyaline body myopathy: 287
Hydatidosis: 242
Hyperkalemic periodic paralysis: 90, 95
Hyperthyroid myopathy: 260
Hyperthyroid periodic paralysis: 260
Hypokalemic periodic paralysis: 90, 95

Hypophosphatemia: 279
    osteomalacia myopathy: 279
Hypothyroid myopathy: 261

I

Immunotherapy: 301
Infantile hypertrophic cardiomyopathy with e▮pathy: 209
Inflammation: 221, 228
Inflammatory myopathies: 218, 221, 268
    cancer-related muscle disease: 268
    experimental models: 218
    fungal myositis: 238
    parasitic myositis: 238
Insulin associated muscle disorders: 262
Internet: 292

K

Kearns-Sayre Syndrome: 204

L

Lambert-Eaton myasthenic syndrome: 166
    Congenital myasthenic syndrome: 170
Lamellar body myopathy: 287
Lamin A/C gene: 49
Laminin: 8, 25, 37
    laminin a2 (merosin) gene mutations: 37
LAMP 2 deficiency: 142
    Danon diseas: 142
    X-linked vacuolar cardiomyopathy and myopathy: 142
LAMP-2 gene: 142
LAP: 48
Large telomeric deletion disease: 119
Leber hereditary optic neuropathy: 206
Leigh syndrome: 206
Limb girdle muscular dystrophy: 41, 49, 82, 148
    Bethlem myopathy: 41
    collagen VI gene mutations: 42
    myotilinopathy: 82
Limb girdle myopathies
    limb girdle muscular dystrophy type 2B: 29
    limb-girdle muscular dystrophy type 1C: 33
    Miyoshi myopathy: 29
    sarcoglycanopathies: 24
Long-chain acyl-CoA dehydrogenase: 192
Lysosomal storage diseases
    Danon's disease: 142
    lysosomal glycogen storage disease with normal acid maltas: 142
    X-linked vacuolar cardiomyopathy and myopathy: 142
Lysosome integral membrane protein-I: 142
Lysosome-associated membrane-2: 142
Lysosomes: 145

M

Major histocompatibility complex (MHC): 221
Malaria: 240
Malignant hyperthermia: 65, 99
    central core disease: 65
MAN1: 48
Marinesco-Sjögren syndrome: 277
McArdle's disease: 182
MELAS: 206
Merosin: 8, 25, 37
MERRF: 207
MHCDS: 83
Minicore disease: 68
Mitochondria: 202
Mitochondrial diseases: 202
Mitochondrial encephalomyopathies: 202
Mitretek criteria: 292
Miyoshi myopathy: 29
MNGIE: 208
Molecular therapy: 297
MtDNA depletion syndrome: 208
Multicore disease: 68
    malignant hyperthermia and: 68
MuscleNET: 293
Muscular dystrophies: 24, 37
    Becker muscular dystrophy: 6
    Bethlem myopathy: 41
    collagen VI gene mutations: 41
    Duchenne muscular dystrophy (DMD): 6

Emery-Dreifuss muscular dystrophy: 49
    laminin a2 (merosin) gene mutations: 37
    limb girdle muscular dystrophy type 2B: 29
    limb-girdle muscular dystrophy type 1C: 33
    Miyoshi myopathy: 29
    myotilinopathy: 82
    plectin deficiency: 78
    sarcoglycanopathies: 24
Myasthenia: 156, 166, 170
    Lambert-Eaton myasthenic syndrome: 166
    myasthenia gravis: 156
Myasthenia gravis: 156, 170
Myoadenylate deaminase deficiency: 182, 214
Myofibrillar myopathy: 70
Myoneurogastrointestinal encephalopathy: 208
Myopathies:
    actinopathy: 62
    Bethlem myopathy: 41
    central core disease: 65
    centronuclear myopathy: 57
    collagen VI gene mutations: 41
    desmin-related myopathies: 70
    dystrophia myotonica
    Emery-Dreifuss muscular dystrophy: 49
    hereditary inclusion body myopathy: 274
    inflammatory myopathy: 218, 221
    laminin α2 (merosin) gene mutations: 37
    limb girdle muscular dystrophy type 2B: 29
    limb-girdle muscular dystrophy type 1C: 33
    minicore disease: 68
    Miyoshi myopathy: 29
    multicore disease: 68
    myotilinopathy: 82
    myotubular myopathy: 124
    oculopharyngeal muscular dystrophy: 115
    plectin defeciency: 78
    sarcoglycanopathies: 24
    SCARMD: 24
Myophosphorylase deficiency: 182
Myosin heavy chain: 85
Myosin heavy chain depletion syndrome: 83
Myositis: 218, 221, 228
    bacterial myositis: 236
    experimental models: 218
    flesh eating infection: 237
    hereditary inclusion body myopathys: 274
    inclusion bosy myositis: 274
Myotilinopathy: 82
Myotonia: 108
Myotonia congenita Becker: 91
Myotonia congenita Thomsen: 91
Myotonic dystrophy: 108
Myotoxicity: 246
Myotubular myopathy: 57, 124

N

NARP: 206
Necrotic myopathies: 247
Necrotizing fasciitis: 237
Nemaline bodies: 62
    actinopathy with: 62
Neurogenic atrophy: 253
Nuclear protein: 48
Nurim: 48

O

Oculopharyngeal muscular dystrophy: 115
OMIM: 293

OPMD (oculopharyngeal muscular dystrophy): 115
Osteomalacia myopathy: 279

P

PABPN1: 115
Paramyotonia congenita: 91
Paraneoplastic disorder: 266
Paraneoplastic necrotizing myopathy: 267
Parasitic myositis: 238
Parathyroid associated muscle disorders: 263
Pearson's syndrome: 205
Perlecan: 43
Phosphofructokinase deficiency: 185
Plectin deficiency: 78
Polymyositis: 221, 268
    cancer-related muscle disease: 268
Pompe's disease: 134
Prevention: 296
Primary carnitine deficiency: 192
Progressive external ophthalmoplegia: 208
Purine metabolism: 214

R

Ragged-red fibres: 203
Reducing body myopathy: 288
Respiratory chain defects: 202
Rimmed vacuoles: 86, 277
    Marinesco-Sjögren syndrome with: 277
Rippling muscle disease: 33
Rippling muscle syndrome: 268
Ryanoide receptor: 99
RYR 1 gene: 65
    central core disease: 65
RYR gene: 99

S

Sarcoglycan: 8, 24, 37
Sarcosporidiosis: 240
Sarcotubular myopathy: 287
Sarcotubular system: 90, 96, 99
SCARMD: 24
Schwartz-Jampel syndrome: 43
Scleromyxedema: 268
SCN4A gene: 100
SERCA1 gene: 103
Silverman-Handmaker: 43
Slow-channel syndromes: 174
Spheroid bodies: 70, 71
Steroid myopathy: 246
Subacute necrotizing encephalomyelopathy: 206

T

Tarui's disease: 185
Therapy: 296
Thyroid eye disease: 260
Tibial muscular dystrophy: 151, 274
Toxic myopathies: 246
Toxoplasmosis: 238
Treatment: 296
Trichinosis: 241
Tropical pyomyositis: 236
Tubular aggregate myopathy: 288
Tubular arrays myopathy: 287
Type 2 muscle fibre atrophy: 266
    cancer-related muscle disease: 266

V

Vacuolar myopathy: 247
Vitamin D: 279

    osteomalacia myopathy: 279
Vitamin E deficiency: 282

W

Web sites: 292
Welander distal myopathy: 274
Wolf-Parkinson-White syndrome: 208
Wolfram syndrome: 208

X

X-Linked dilated cardiomyopathy: 7
X-linked myopathies: 142
    Danon disease: 142
    myotubular myopathy: 124
    X-linked dilated cardiomyopathy: 7
    X-linked myopathy with excessive autophagy: 145
    X-linked vacuolar cardiomyopathy and myopathy: 142, 145
X-linked myopathy with excessive autophagy: 145
X-linked myotubular myopathy: 124
X-linked vacuolar cardiomyopathy and myopathy: 142
    Danon disease: 142
    genetic changes: 142
    primary LAMP-2 deficiency.: 142
    secondary LAMP-2 deficiency: 142
    structural changes: 143

Z

Zidovudine myopathy: 248